Pulmonary infection in the immunocompromised patient

D1418616

PULMONARY INFECTION IN THE IMMUNOCOMPROMISED PATIENT

STRATEGIES FOR MANAGEMENT

Editors

Carlos Agustí and Antoni Torres

Cap de Servei de Pneumologia i Allèrgia Respiratòria Hospital Clínic de Barcelona, Barcelona, Spain

WILEY-BLACKWELL

A John Wiley & Sons, Ltd., Publication

This edition first published 2009
© 2009 John Wiley & Sons, Ltd

Wiley-Blackwell is an imprint of John Wiley & Sons, formed by the merger of Wiley's global Scientific, Technical and Medical business with Blackwell Publishing.

Registered office: John Wiley & Sons Ltd, The Atrium, Southern Gate, Chichester, West Sussex, PO19 8SQ, UK

Other Editorial Offices:
9600 Garsington Road, Oxford, OX4 2DQ, UK
111 River Street, Hoboken, NJ 07030-5774, USA

For details of our global editorial offices, for customer services and for information about how to apply for permission to reuse the copyright material in this book please see our website at www.wiley.com/wiley-blackwell

Library of Congress Cataloguing-in-Publication Data

Pulmonary infection in the immuno-compromised patient: strategies for management/edited by Carlos Agusti and Antoni Torres.
    p. ; cm.
Includes bibliographical references and index.
ISBN 978-0-470-31957-4 (cloth)
1. Respiratory infections. 2. Lungs–Infections. 3. Immunosuppression–Complications. I. Agusti, Carlos.
II. Torres Marti, A. (Antoni)
    [DNLM: 1. Lung Diseases–complications. 2. Opportunistic Infections–complications. 3. Immunocompromised Host.
4. Lung Diseases–therapy. 5. Opportunistic Infections–therapy. WF 600 P983495 2009]
    RC740.P83 2009
    616.2′4–dc22   2008036179

ISBN 978-0-470-31957-4

A catalogue record for this book is available from the British Library.

Set in 10.5/12.5pt Times by Thomson Digital, Noida, India
Printed in Singapore by Markono Print Media Pte. Ltd.
First printing – 2009

Contents

Preface

The number of immunocompromised patients has increased over the last decade. Improvements in solid-organ and haematopoietic stem cell transplantation techniques, the expanded use of chemotherapic treatments and glucocorticoids use, and the appearance of new immunomodulatory therapies are some of the reasons that justify this increase. The success of the different transplant techniques has generated a great deal of interest in the management of immunocompromised patients among clinicians and basic scientists. The recognition and management of pulmonary complications that result from immunosuppression is a challenging task. The lungs may be injured directly through an infectious or toxic insult. Conversely, lung disease may result as a secondary event. Pulmonary complications in these patients require a multidisciplinary approach that often involves different specialists. This includes an appreciation of the epidemiology of post-transplant pulmonary complications, the differential diagnoses for these processes, the appropriate diagnostic explorations, and the specific treatments and potential interactions.

Our goals in this book are to provide an integrated discussion of progress in a comprehensive fashion. The general aspects of the lung immune defences are reviewed by Drs Patel and Koziel. Microbiological diagnosis and respiratory sampling in this population are a very important issues, related to the adequacy of treatment and mortality. Dr Ieven and Dr Baughman have reviewed both chapters in depth. The radiological approach to the diagnosis of respiratory complications is of particular importance and Dr Franquet presents the different tools that we currently have in our hands.

The remaining chapters of the book are dedicated to the review of respiratory infections regarding different types of immunosuppression: HIV infected patients, neutropenia, haematopoietic stem cell transplantation and chronic steroid treatment. Finally, intensive care management, antibacterial, antifungal and antiviral treatments are updated by experts in these subjects.

As in any multi-author book, the success of the endeavour relates to the commitment and creativity of the collaborating authors; we are extremely thankful for the hard and careful work of each of our contributors. We would also like to thank our colleagues at John Wiley & Sons, Ltd who provided outstanding support for this project.

Carlos Agustí
Antoni Torres

Contributors

Bekele Afessa
Division of Pulmonary and Critical Care
Medicine, Mayo Clinic College of Medicine,
200 First ST, Rochester,
MN 55905, USA
Email: afessa.bekele@mayo.edu

José M. Aguado
Unit of Infectious Diseases, University
Hospital 12 de Octubre, Av. de Andalucía
Km. 5,400. 28041 Madrid, Spain
Email: jaguadog@medynet.com

Carlos Agustí
Institut Clinic de Pneumologia ICPCT,
Hospital Clinic, C/Villarroel, 170, 08036
Barcelona, Spain
Email: CAGUSTI@clinic.ub.es

Robert P. Baughman
University of Cincinnati Medical Center,
1001 Holmes, Eden Avenue, Cincinnati,
OH 45267-0565, USA
Email: baughmrp@ucmail.uc.edu

Natividad Benito
Infectious Diseases Unit, Sant Pau Hospital,
Sant Antoni Maria Claret 167, 08025
Barcelona. Spain
Email: nbenito@santpau.es

Oliver A. Cornely
Uniklinik Köln, Klinik I für Innere Medizin,
Klinisches Studienzentrum, Schwerpunkt
Infektiologie II, Bachemer Strasse 86,
50931 Köln, Germany
Email: Oliver.Cornely@ctuc.de

Santiago Ewig
Thoraxzentrum Ruhrgebiet, Kliniken für
Pneumologie und Infektiologie,
Evangelisches Krankenhaus Herne und
Augusta-Kranken-Anstalt, Bergstrasse 26,
44791 Bochum, Germany
Email: ewig@augusta-bochum.de

Tomás Franquet
Chief of Thoracic Imaging Section,
Department of Radiology, Hospital de Sant
Pau, St. Antoni Maria Claret, 167, 08025,
Barcelona, Spain; and Department of
Radiology, Universitat Autónoma of
Barcelona, Barcelona, Spain
Email: tfranquet@santpau.es

Mitchell Goldman
Division of Infectious Diseases, Indiana
University School of Medicine, Wishard
Memorial Hospital (Room OPW 430),
1001 W. 10th Street, IN 46202, USA
Email: mgoldman@iupui.edu

Didier Gruson
Division of Medical Intensive Care,
University Hospital Bordeaux, Hôpital
Pellegrin, Place Amelie Raba-Léon,
F-33076 Bordeaux Cedex, France

Gilles Hilbert
Division of Medical Intensive Care,
University Hospital Bordeaux, Hôpital
Pellegrin, Place Amelie Raba-Léon, F 33076
Bordeaux Cedex, France
Email: Gilles.hilbert@chu-bordeaux.fr

Andy I.M. Hoepelman
University Medical Center Utrecht,
Division of Medicine, Department
of Internal Medicine and Infectious
Diseases, PO Box 85500,
3508 GA Utrecht, The Netherlands
Email: i.m.hoepelman@umcutrecht.nl

Margareta Ieven
Department of Medical Microbiology,
Faculty of Medicine, University of Antwerp,
Universiteitsplein 1 S3,
B-2610, Wilrijk, Belgium
Email: greet.ieven@uza.be

Michael G. Ison
Northwestern University Feinberg School
of Medicine, Divisions of Infectious Diseases
& Organ Transplantation, Transplant
& Immunocompromised Host Infectious
Diseases Service, 676 N. Street Clair
Street Suite 200, Chicago, IL 60611, USA
Email: mgison@northwestern.edu

Henry Koziel
Division of Pulmonary, Critical Care and
Sleep Medicine, Kirstein Hall, Room E/KSB-
23, Beth Israel Deaconess Medical Center
and Harvard Medical School, 330 Brookline
Avenue, Boston,
MA 02215, USA
Email: hkoziel@bidmc.harvard.edu

Elyse E. Lower
University of Cincinnati Medical Center,
1001 Holmes, Eden Avenue, Cincinnati, OH
45267-0565, USA

Asunción Moreno-Camacho
Infectious Diseases Service,
Hospital Clinic, Villarroel 170,
08036-Barcelona, Spain
Email: amoreno@clinic.ub.es

Jan Jelrik Oosterheert
University Medical Center Utrecht,
Division of Medicine, Department
of Internal Medicine and Infectious
Diseases, PO Box 85500, 3508
GA Utrecht, The Netherlands
Email: j.j.oosterheert@umcutrecht.nl

Naimish Patel
Division of Pulmonary, Critical Care
and Sleep Medicine, Kirstein Hall, Room
E/KSB-23, Beth Israel Deaconess Medical
Center and Harvard Medical
School, 330 Brookline Avenue,
Boston, MA 02215, USA

Steve G. Peters
Division of Pulmonary and Critical Care
Medicine, Mayo Clinic College of Medicine,
200 First St, Rochester,
MN 55905, USA
Email: peters.steve@mayo.edu

Julio C. Medina Presentado
Cátedra de Enfermedades Infecciosas,
Universidad de la República,
Uruguay

Ana Rañó
Institut Clinic de Pneumologia ICPCT,
Hospital Clinic, C/ Villarroel, 170,
08036 Barcelona, Spain

Maria J. Rüping
Uniklinik Köln, Klinik I für Innere Medizin,
Klinisches Studienzentrum, Schwerpunkt
Infektiologie II, Bachemer Strasse 86,
50931 Köln, Germany
Email: Maria.Rueping@ctuc.de

George A. Sarosi
Department of Medicine, Indiana University School of Medicine, Indianapolis VAMC, Room C-7-018, 1461 West 10th Street, IN 46202, USA
Email: george.sarosi@med.va.gov

Andrew F. Shorr
Pulmonary and Critical Care Medicine, Washington Hospital Center, Room 2D-38, 110 Irving Street, NW, Washington, DC 20010, USA
Email: afshorr@dnamail.com

Ayman O. Soubani
Division of Pulmonary, Allergy, Critical Care and Sleep, Wayne State University School of Medicine, Harper University Hospital, 3990 John R- 3 Hudson, Detroit, MI 48201, USA
Email: asoubani@med.wayne.edu

Antoni Torres
Institut Clinic de Pneumologia ICPCT, Hospital Clinic, C/Villarroel, 170, 08036 Barcelona, Spain
Email: ATORRES@clinic.ub.es

Frederic Vargas
Division of Medical Intensive Care, University Hospital Bordeaux, Hôpital Pellegrin, Place Amelie Raba-Léon, F 33076 Bordeaux, Cedex, France

Jörg J. Vehreschild
Uniklinik Köln, Klinik I für Innere Medizin, Klinisches Studienzentrum, Schwerpunkt Infektiologie II, Bachemer Strasse 86, 50931 Köln, Germany
Email: Janne.Vehreschild@ctuc.de

1

Lung immune defences in the immunosuppressed patient

Naimish Patel and Henry Koziel

Division of Pulmonary, Critical Care and Sleep Medicine, Department of Medicine, Beth Israel Deaconess Medical Center and Harvard Medical School, Boston, MA

1.1   Introduction

The respiratory tract is constantly exposed to environmental elements and potential pathogens on a daily basis during the obligatory process of breathing or through subclinical aspiration. To avoid infectious disease pathogenesis in the respiratory tract, a number of elegant, complex and interdependent systems of host defence mechanisms are in place to prevent microorganism colonization of the respiratory epithelium, promote efficient microbe elimination, and maintain sterility of the lower respiratory tract in the healthy host. The layers of host defence mechanisms include physical barriers and secreted chemical factors (operant immediately), innate immune system (operant within minutes to hours), and the adaptive immune system (operant within days). Disruption of any of these components of lung host defence may lower critical threshold for microbial invasion and promote disease pathogenesis. Several acquired immunodeficiency states are associated with frequent and severe respiratory tract infections, and lung infections with opportunistic pathogens. This chapter will review the components of lung host defences in health with particular focus on human data, and discuss perturbations of host defences associated with select specific immunodeficiency states that may promote susceptibility and contribute to pathogensis of respiratory tract infections.

1.2   Host defence function in health

In health, host defence function is provided by three critical integrated components, including (1) physical (or mechanical) and chemical mechanisms; (2) innate immunity; and (3) adaptive immunity. Physical and chemical mechanisms are present and operate continuously and serve as an immediate protective function to microbial challenge. For microbes that circumvent or bypass physical and chemical mechanisms, the innate

Pulmonary Infection in the Immunocompromised Patient, Edited by Carlos Agustí and Antoni Torres
© 2009 John Wiley & Sons, Ltd.

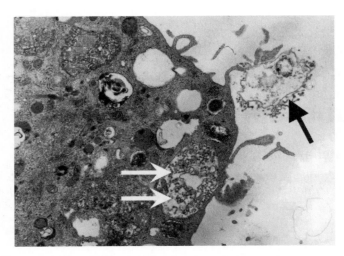

Figure 1.1   Electron micrograph of human alveolar macrophage engaging pneumocystis organisms. Alveolar macrophages represent the predominant immune cells in the alveolar airspace, and critical effector cells in pathogen recognition and elimination. Pneumocystis trophic forms are seen in the process of engagement by macrophage pseudopodia (arrow) and ingested in the macrophage (arrows). *Pneumocystis* is a major opportunistic pathogen responsible for severe pneumonia in the immuno-compromised host. (Electronphoromicrograph courtesy of Angeline Warner, Harvard School of Public Health, Boston, MA).

immune system represents another layer of the host defence response. Cellular and soluble components of innate immunity are constantly present, and are capable of recognizing, engaging and eliminating a broad array of microbes (through molecular recognition of conserved molecular patterns expressed by pathogens but not host cells) within minutes to hours of microbial challenge (Figure 1.1). Through a relatively limited number of secreted and host-cell associated recognition molecules, innate immunity can detect and generate an appropriate antimicrobial response to a broad range of bacteria, fungi and viruses. In health, the majority of daily microbial challenges are likely effectively cleared by these first two layers of host defences, as the majority of living creatures have only mechanical and chemical defences, and innate immunity. If clearance of microbes is not achieved despite activation of innate immune mechanisms, the adaptive immune system can be activated within days to provide an amplified and specific immune response. The adaptive immune response is composed predominantly of B-lymphocytes and T-lymphocytes that recognize specific antigen determinants on pathogens, and ultimately provide lifelong memory against repeated challenges with the same pathogen.

Physical (mechanical) and chemical mechanisms of host defence

Physical barrier and mechanical host defence mechanisms, and chemical host defence mechanisms are constantly available for immediate action in the healthy host. Particle size in part determines fate, as particles and microbes generally exceeding 5 μm can be entrapped as air flows through the tortuous channels of the nasopharynx and by nasal hairs, and through inertial forces are impacted along the tonsilar pillars, glottis, trachea and branching bronchi and bronchioles. Entrapped particles and microbes may be expelled through coughing and sneezing mechanisms. The complex glycoprotein mucins lining the airway epithelial surfaces facilitate particle entrapment, and promote elimination by the cephalad respiratory epithelial cell ciliary movement that allows expectoration or swallowing of mucin-entrapped pathogens. In general, particles and potential pathogens smaller than 5 μm can bypass these mechanical obstacles and gain access to the terminal bronchioles and alveoli. In addition, the respiratory epithelium serves as a critical barrier function. Similar to the function of the skin, the integrity of the mucosal surfaces including the respiratory epithelial cells and associated tight functions remains critical to protective host defence function. The importance of these mechanisms, which operate constantly, is underscored by conditions that interfer with proper function such as mucociliary disease (dynein arm dyskinesia), bronchiectasis (anatomical distortion and scarring of epithelium), and neurological disorders or pharmacological agents that prevent effective cough reflexes.

A number of secreted airway products also contribute to antimicrobial functions by several mechanisms including direct antimicrobial activity, opsonization and agglutinization (Table 1.1). Microbes that pass the physical and mechanical barriers may be eliminated by a range of chemical mediators that are constantly expressed and may be further induced. These mediators include molecules capable of direct antimicrobial effect (ex. lysozyme, lactoferrin, SLPI, complement, α-, β- and θ-defensins and cathelicidins), agents that inhibit microbial growth (ex. transferrin), and molecules that serve as opsonins that facilitate host cell recognition (ex. complement, fibronectin, collectins, SP-A, SP-D, IgA and IgG) or modulate host cell response to pathogens (ex. LPS-binding protein) (Crouch, 1998; Shepherd, 2002; Zhang and Koziel, 2002; McCormack and Whitsett, 2002). Lung collectins, such as surfactant components

Table 1.1 Secreted antimicrobial factors in the airways.

Cathelicidin
Collectins
  SP-A
  SP-D
  mannose binding protein (MBP), or mannose binding lectin (MBL)
Complement
Defensins (α and β)
Fibronectin, vitronectin
Ficolins
Immunoglobulins
  IgA (predominant in upper airways)
  IgG (predominant in lower airways)
Lactoferrin
LPS binding protein (LBP)
Lysozyme
Transferrin

SP-A and SP-D can serve as opsonins and enhanced phagocytosis, agglutination of microbes, and increased bacterial membrane permeability promoting pathogen elimination (Shepherd, 2002). Classical pathway complement proteins C3, C4, C1q and alternative complement pathway component factor B are expressed in the lung alveolar fluid (Watford, Ghio and Wright, 2000), and can provide opsonization of microbes in the respiratory tract.

Innate immunity in the lungs

Innate immunity is an evolutionarily conserved ancient defence mechanism that comprised components that are constantly expressed and available, can be activated within minutes to hours, and can engage potential pathogens upon initial encounter (Martin and Frevert, 2005; Zaas and Schwartz, 2005). The principal cellular components of lung innate immunity include alveolar macrophages, neutrophils, NK cells, dendritic cells and eosinophils. Alveolar macrophages represent the predominant immune cell in the alveolar airspace, accounting for >85% of mobile cells in the alveoli. Neutrophils and eosinophils are generally not present in the alveoli but are recruited in response to chemotactic signals. Natural killer (NK) cells participate in early innate defence through cytotoxic activity against pathogen-infected cells and secretion of cytokines and chemokines that modulate subsequent steps in the adaptive immune response (Biron et al., 1999). Recognition of microbial products by dendritic cells triggers functional dendritic cell maturation and leads to initiation of antigen-specific adaptive immune responses.

The innate immune response is mediated through interactions of microbes or microbial products with the germline-encoded host cell receptors. Innate immune cells such as alveolar macrophages recognize potential pathogens through surface recognition receptors such as mannose receptors, β-glucan receptors, scavenger receptors and Toll-like receptors (TLRs). The family of mammalian TLRs serves a critical role in the early host defence response through recognition of conserved molecules derived from microbial pathogens (Imler and Hossmann, 2001), leading to activation of NF-κB (Beutler, 2000) and MAP kinases (Barton and Medzhitov, 2003), and subsequent transcription and translation of host defence genes (Medzhitov, 2001; Aggarwal, 2003). Expressed on cells near mucosal portals of entry including macrophages (Jones et al., 2001) dendritic cells (Muzio et al., 2000) and lung epithelial cells (Armstrong et al., 2004), mammalian TLR1 through TLR9 represent critical molecules in the first line of host defence to microbes in the lungs. Functional deficiency or genetic deletion of TLR4 increase susceptibility to H. Influenza, S. pneumoniae, and K. pneumoniae respiratory tract infection in murine models (Wang et al., 2002; Branger et al., 2004). Humans with TLR4 mutations are hyporesponsive to inhaled LPS (Arbour et al., 2000). Alveolar macrophage and alveolar epithelial cells exhibit limited responsiveness to TLR4 stimulation due to relatively low membrane expression of the adaptor molecule MD-2 (Jia et al., 2004; Kajikawa et al., 2005). TLR5 polymorphism (TLR5[392stop]) in the ligand binding domain increases susceptibility of humans to Legionella pneumonia (Hawn et al., 2003).

Regulation of activating pattern recognition receptors

Control of inflammatory responses to infectious challenge is of particular importance for the continued normal gas exchange function of the lungs. In general innate receptor activation promotes proinflammatory responses, and cellular innate immune responses (such as macrophages) to antigenic challenge can result in enhanced innate immune response upon future rechallenge by the same antigen (Bowdish *et al.*, 2007). However, concurrent with innate surface membrane and intracellular receptor activation to promote proinflammatory responses, a number of counter regulatory molecules are also activated that likely limit the proinflammatory response to maintain homeostasis and limit collateral damage. Examples of these regulatory molecules for TLRs include: TOLLIP, IRAK-M, sMyD88, ST2, SIGGR, SOCS-1, NOD2, MIF, PR105 and TAM receptor family (TYRO3, AXL and MER) (Rothlin *et al.*, 2007; Liew *et al.*, 2005). Whether these molecules are modulated by immunosuppressive agents or medical conditions associated with immune suppression is not completely understood.

Regulation of innate immunity by secreted products

In addition to serving antimicrobial functions, soluble products can also serve to modulate cellular innate immune response in the lungs. For example, lung collectins such as SP-A can modulate the innate immune response, such as regulating macrophage pattern recognition receptor expression (Beharka *et al.*, 2002) and regulating the generation of macrophage reactive oxygen species (Crowther *et al.*, 2004). SP-A and SP-D bind LPS and prevent interaction with LBP and TLR4-CD14 complex on alveolar macrophages (Borron *et al.*, 2000; Sano *et al.*, 2000) and thus limit activating responses. In addition to hepatic production as an acute phase reactant, LBP is expressed by pulmonary artery smooth muscle cells (Wong *et al.*, 1995) and type-II alveolar epithelial cells (Wong *et al.*, 1995; Dentener *et al.*, 2000). Alveolar lining fluids contain high concentrations of sCD14 and LBP (Martin *et al.*, 1992; Martin *et al.*, 1997b) and thus can modulate TLR4-mediated signaling.

Epithelial cells

Alveolar epithelial cells, in addition to providing a physical barrier function, also contribute to the innate immune response in the lungs. Epithelial cells express defensins HBD-1 and HBD-2 (McCray and Bentley, 1997; Hiratsuka and Al, 1998), and defensins also stimulate IL-8 production by epithelial cells (van Wetering *et al.*, 1997). Epithelial cells express TLRs and CD14, and can thus respond to microbial products analogous to TLR signaling in leukocytes, with release of IL-1β, IL-6, TNF-α, IL-8 and RANTES, GM-CSF, and TGF-β (Diamond, Legarda and Ryan, 2000). Microbes and microbial components (such as lipopolysaccharide, peptidoglycan and flagella) can interact with innate receptors (such as TLR2) expressed on the apical surface of epithelial cells (often in the context of lipid rafts) (Soong *et al.*, 2004), which in turn can promote Ca^{2+} release (Chun, Soong and Prince, 2006) and activate epithelial cell transcription factors such as

NF-kB, AP-1, C/EBP and CREB to promote host defence gene activation. In a murine model, targeted disruption of respiratory epithelial cell NF-κB results in blunted neutrophil recruitment in response to LPS inhalational challenge (Skerrett *et al.*, 2004), suggesting a significant contribution of chemotactic signals by respiratory epithelial cells in the context of TLR stimulation.

Adaptive immunity in the lungs

Generation of adaptive immunity requires the somatic rearrangement of lymphocyte receptors (including B-lymphocyte and T-lymphocyte receptors) that confers antigen specificity directed against specific epitopes expressed by pathogens, amplifying the immune response against pathogens expressing the specific antigen or epitope, and promotes immune memory that allows enhanced immune response upon future rechallenge with the pathogen expressing the same antigen or epitope. Therefore, in contrast to innate immunity, which represents preprogrammed expression of molecules and receptors present at birth, the adaptive immune system is acquired throughout life as a consequence of cumulative challenges with infectious agents.

For persistent infectious challenge, antigens are presented to lymphocytes by lung dendritic cells in regional lymph nodes. As alveolar macrophages are poor antigen-presenting cells, alveolar macrophages may transport antigen to interstitium and/or regional lymph nodes where antigen can be processed by dendritic cells, or perhaps antigen may be processed by alveolar dendritic cells that then may be transported to the regional lymph nodes. Once in the regional lymph nodes, dendritic cells present antigen to responsive T- and B-lymphocytes in the context of MCH molecules to activate the adaptive immune response. B-lymphocytes are activated to produce antibodies directed against specific epitopes, and CD8+ T-lymphocytes target infected cells expressing specific epitopes on the cell surface. Whereas T-lymphocyte receptors can interact with processed or cleaved foreign antigens, B-lymphocyte receptors can interact directly with intact foreign antigens.

Innate immunity regulated by adaptive immunity

Traditionally, innate immunity provided the initial response to contain newly encountered infectious challenge, and with continued activation or overwhelming infection the adaptive immune response is triggered (instructed in part by specific receptors and particular signals generated by the innate immune response). Consequently, the adaptive immune response provided critical regulatory signals that amplified the innate immune effector cells. In this model, the innate immune system provides the initial first line of host defence within minutes and hours of infectious challenge, whereas the regulatory influence of the adaptive immune response occurred within days of the initial infectious challenge (and thought that the adaptive response was able to modulate or regulate the innate response following antigen processing and development of antigen-specific T-lymphocytes and B-lymphocytes). However, recent data suggest that components of the adaptive immune system may regulate the initial innate immune response. In a MHV model of infection, regulation of the host cytokine response to MHV infection was modulated by T-lymphocytes, which required cell–cell contact and was in part MHC-II dependent (Kim *et al.*, 2007). Importantly, this T-lymphocyte-regulated influence of innate immune cell proinflammatory cytokine release (to avoid a 'cytokine storm'-mediated lethality) occurred within 24 hours of new infectious challenge, well in advance of traditional adaptive immune responses.

1.3   Host defence function in select immunocompromised patients

Immunocompromised patients represent a heterogeneous population with genetic or acquired conditions that predispose to infectious complications, including pneumonia. Although immunecompromised patients may share common deficiencies in some components of immunity, certain medical conditions or the use of specific immune modulatory agents target specific components of innate or adaptive immunity, and result in relatively specific functional or quantitative defects in immunity. Recognizing that elimination of certain pathogens or opportunistic microbes may rely predominantly on specific components of innate or adaptive immunity, unique immunodeficiencies associated with certain conditions predispose individuals to certain types of infectious complications (Figure 1.2). The remainder of the chapter will review current under-standing of the mechanisms underlying immunocompromised states in select patient groups, and serves as the basis for discussions in subsequent chapters that focus on specific conditions in greater detail.

HIV infection

HIV is the causative agent of AIDS. As of 2006 more than 30 million people worldwide were living with AIDS, with 4.3 million newly infected with HIV and 2.9 million deaths due to AIDS (Prevention, 2006). Opportunistic infections including tuberculosis remain the major cause of mortality in HIV+ patients worldwide, with more than 60% of deaths in HIV caused by secondary infections (Organization, 2007). The dramatic loss of CD4+ T-lymphocytes accounts for many of the manifestations of AIDS (Douek, Picker and Koup, 2003). Even in the presence of antiretroviral therapy, peripheral CD4+ T-lymphocyte count remains the best factor for predicting the risk of opportunistic infection, although peripheral viral load remains an inde-pendent risk factor (Ledergerber *et al.*, 1999). However, in addition to T-lymphocytes, evidence suggests HIV infection is associated with dysfunction of several other types of immune cells.

CD4+ T-lymphocyte dysfunction

HIV infection is associated with a number of specific quantitative and qualitative abnormalities of CD4+ T-lymphocytes. Progressive depletion of peripheral CD4+

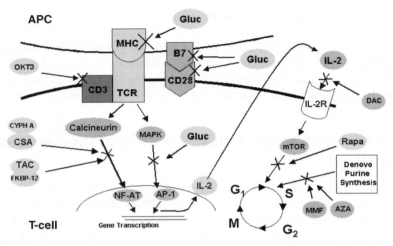

Figure 1.2 Pathways influenced by immune modulating agents: Transplant graft rejection occurs when recipient antigen presenting cells (APC) present alloantigens from the graft to recipient T-cells via MHC Class II. T-cells recognize these antigens via the CD3-T-cell receptor (TCR) complex. This interaction when coupled with co-stimulatory signals such as B7-CD28 results in the activation of calcineurin and mitogen activated protein kinases (MAPK) eventually resulting in T-cell activation. Calcineurin accomplishes this by dephosphorylating, thus activating, the transcriptions factor nuclear factor of activated T-cells (NF-AT), while MAPK activated the transcription factor AP-1. These transcriptions factors stimulate the production of a variety of immune activating cytokines including IL-2. Released IL-2 binds to IL-2 receptor on helper T-cells activating the protein mTOR which results in T-cell expansion by stimulating T-cells to enter the S phase of the cell cycle. Glucocorticoids (Gluc) inhibit expression of MHC and co-stimulatory molecules on APCs and T-cells. Gluc also inhibit MAPK activation. Cyclosporine (CSA) forms a complex with cyclophilin A (CYPH A) and tacrolimus (TAC) after binding to FK-binding protein 12 (FKBP12), and each inactivate calcineurin. Daclizumab (DAC) blocks the IL-2 receptor, while rapamycin (RAPA) inhibits mTOR. Azathioprine (AZA) and mycophenolate mofetil (MMF), both inhibit denova purine synthesis which inhibits DNA synthesis during the S phase in lymphocytes.

T-lymphocytes remains the hallmark of HIV infection, especially advanced AIDS. Current concepts suggest that the CD4+ T-lymphocyte depletion is a consequence of chronic immune activation and not by direct virus-mediated cell death (Brenchley, Price and Douek, 2006). Massive mucosal CD4+ memory T-lymphocyte depletion from the gut lamina propria may lead to increased bacterial translocation, chronically activating innate and adaptive immunity (Brenchley, Price and Douek, 2006; Centlivre et al., 2007; Veazey et al., 1998; Guadalupe et al., 2003; Brenchley et al., 2004). Chronic T-lymphocyte activation generates a continuous supply of HIV targets which eventually surpasses the ability to produce new T-lymphocytes and leads to systemic T-lymphocyte depletion (Brenchley, Price and Douek, 2006). This early preferential loss of CD4+ T-lymphocytes at mucosal sites may also play a role in increasing incidence of infections at these mucosal sites independent of changes in peripheral CD4+ T-cell count (Veazey and Lackner, 2003), as peripheral CD4+ T-lymphocyte counts do not predict local T-lymphocyte responses to microbes such as Hepatitis C virus (Koziel, 2006) or *Mycobacterium tuberculosis* (Breen *et al.*, 2006).

CD4+ T-lymphocyte depletion is also associated with abnormal lymphocyte prolife-rative responses to CMV and HSV in AIDS patients with serologic evidence of prior exposure to these viruses (Sheridan *et al.*, 1984), and decreased proliferative response and IFN-γ secretion to *M. tuberculosis* despite clinical response to highly-active antiretroviral therapy (HAART) (Schluger, Perez and Liu, 2002; Sutherland *et al.*, 2006). Although the ability of T-lymphocytes to produce IFN-γ in response to mitogens or antigens correlates with HIV clinical status, peripheral CD4+ T-lymphocyte count, and predict progression to AIDS (Murray *et al.*, 1985), the above data suggest the abnormalities of T-lymphocyte function may occur early in HIV disease and may not reverse with HAART.

CD8+ T-lymphocyte dysfunction

The absolute numbers of peripheral blood CD8+ T-cells increases rapidly with acute HIV infection and continue to increase with disease progression (Lang *et al.*, 1989; Margolick *et al.*, 1993), a pattern similar to that observed in lungs (Twigg *et al.*, 1999). The intensity of CD8+ T-lymphocyte infiltration of lungs depends on HIV viral load and may portend a poor prognosis (Twigg *et al.*, 1999). CD8+ T-lymphocytes can be infected with HIV, especially in late-stage HIV infection (Livingstone *et al.*, 1996). Similar to CD4+ T-lymphocytes, HIV infects predominantly activated CD8+ T-lymphocytes, which express high levels of CD4 (Kitchen *et al.*, 1998), although the frequency of CD8+ T-lymphocyte infection is low (Brenchley *et al.*, 2004) and the significance is unclear. Evidence, however, suggests functional impairment of CD8+ T-lymphocytes in HIV infection, as CD8+ T-lymphocyte-mediated cytotoxicity in response to influenza virus is reduced in HIV (Shearer *et al.*, 1985), and progressive HIV infection is associated with a loss of IFN-γ producing CD8+ T-lymphocytes specific to CMV(Bronke *et al.*, 2005). CD8+ T-lymphocytes may control HIV repli-cation (Benito, Lopez and Soriano, 2004) and functional impairment in cytokine production, perforin expression, phenotypic maturation, and low proliferation may contribute both to disease pathogenesis and susceptibility to opportunistic infections (Benito, Lopez and Soriano, 2004).

B-lymphocyte dysfunction

HIV infection is characterized by elevated numbers of polyclonal B-cells that sponta-neously secrete immunoglobulins (De Milito, 2004), and patients with AIDS have increases in serum IgA, IgG and IgM (Shirai *et al.*, 1992). Evidence for B-cell dysfunction includes abnormal proliferation (Lane *et al.*, 1983), abnormal differentia-tion (Conge *et al.*, 1998), increased apoptosis (Muro-Cacho, Pantaleo and Fauci, 1995), and reduced capacity to co-stimulate CD4+ T-lymphocytes (Malaspina *et al.*, 2003). HIV infected persons demonstrate abnormal antibody response to pneumococcal vaccine (Ballet *et al.*, 1987) especially in subjects with CD4+ T-lymphocyte count

<500 cells/mm^3 (Rodriguez-Barradas *et al.*, 1992). These abnormalities are associated with specific loss of memory B cell subsets (D'Orsogna *et al.*, 2007) similar to that seen in other immunodeficiencies such as common variable immunodeficiency (Hart *et al.*, 2007). Many B-lymphocyte abnormalities are related to plasma viremia and can be rescued by HAART (Morris *et al.*, 1998; Notermans *et al.*, 2001; Malaspina *et al.*, 2003). The lungs of HIV infected individuals demonstrate elevated B-lymphocytes and immunoglobulin levels (Young *et al.*, 1985; Fahy *et al.*, 2001), although opsonic activity of lung immunoglobulins, specifically to *Pneumococcus*, may be impaired in HIV (Eagan *et al.*, 2007).

Macrophage dysfunction

HIV can infect macrophages by interaction of the HIV gp120 envelope glycoprotein V3 hypervariable loop and macrophage CCR5 [Zhang, 1996 #19] *in vitro* and *in vivo* [Koziel, 1999:23]. Unlike CD4+ T-lymphocytes, HIV infection of macrophages leads to persistent infection with low-level viral replication [Fauci, 1988:20]. The role of macrophages as a reservoir for HIV persistence and the role in HIV pathogenesis remains controversial [Stebbing, 2004:#21] although macrophages may be a major source of HIV replication during opportunistic infections [Orenstein, 1997:22].

Although only 1–10% of alveolar macrophages are infected with HIV [Koziel, 1999:23], these cells demonstrate impaired phagocytosis (Koziel *et al.*, 1998), NF-κB nuclear translocation (Zhang *et al.*, 2004), and respiratory burst response (Koziel *et al.*, 2000) to *Pneumocystis*. Alveolar macrophage functional abnormalities may be specific as phagocytosis of Ig-opsonized erythrocytes (Koziel *et al.*, 1998), opsonized *S. pneumonia* (Gordon *et al.*, 2001), and unopsonized *E. coli* (Elssner *et al.*, 2004) remain intact, whereas phagocytosis of the intracellular pathogen, *M. tuberculosis*, is enhanced (Day *et al.*, 2004; Patel *et al.*, 2007). Alveolar macrophages from asymptomatic HIV+ individuals demonstrate impaired TLR4 signaling (Tachado *et al.*, 2005), and impaired apoptotic response (Patel *et al.*, 2007), β-chemokine and TNFα secretion in response to *M. tuberculosis* (Patel *et al.*, 2007; Saukkonen *et al.*, 2002). Taken together, these studies suggest that HIV is associated with targeted and pathogen-specific alterations in macrophage responses.

Dendritic cell dysfunction

Both myeloid and plasmacytoid dendritic cells (DC) are susceptible to HIV infection, with 1–3% of DCs infected *in vivo* (Wu and KewalRamani, 2006). Both infected DC and uninfected DC that can bind HIV through C-type lectin receptors such as DC-SIGN and mannose receptor (Turville *et al.*, 2002) and are capable of transmitting HIV to T-lymphocytes, a mechanism by which initial infection may be established and by which HIV infection may be maintained and spread in tissues and lymph organs (Wu and KewalRamani, 2006). HIV-mediated modulation of antigen-presenting function of DC may be a key aspect of viral pathogenesis and contributes to viral immune evasion (Wu and KewalRamani, 2006). DC infected *in vitro* or taken from the peripheral blood of HIV+ subjects less efficiently stimulate T-lymphocytes (Macatonia *et al.*, 1990; Knight, Patterson and Macatonia, 1991), and total DCs are decreased in chronic HIV infection (Macatonia *et al.*, 1990). Although total DCs are increased in acute HIV infection, costimulatory receptor expression is decreased (Lore *et al.*, 2002). HIV selectively infects immature DCs, although, unlike with DC infection from other viruses, HIV-infected DC fail to mature in culture and instead stimulate T-lymphocytes to produce an immunosuppressive response with increased levels of IL-10 (Granelli-Piperno *et al.*, 1998; Granelli-Piperno *et al.*, 2004; Granelli-Piperno *et al.*, 2006).

Neutrophil dysfunction

A number of abnormalities of neutrophil function have been observed in HIV infected individuals. Neutrophils are vital for the host defence of both bacterial and fungal organisms (Kuritzkes, 2000). Neutropenia may occur in up to one-third of HIV infected individuals (Kuritzkes, 2000). The expression of CD88, the ligand for complement 5a (C5a), is reduced in neutrophils from HIV+ individuals with corresponding decreases in C5a-mediated neutrophil chemotactic responses (Monari *et al.*, 1999; Meddows-Taylor, Pendle and Tiemessen, 2001). A reduction in neutrophil IL-8 receptor expression and IL-8 mediated chemotaxis has been described in HIV+ individuals (Meddows-Taylor, Martin and Tiemessen, 1998). Additional neutrophil defects include reduced IL-8 production in response to *Cryptococcus* in late stage AIDS (Monari *et al.*, 1999), impaired bacterial killing (Ellis *et al.*, 1988), impaired phagocytosis of *Candida* (Ellis *et al.*, 1988), impaired adhesion molecule expression (Ellis *et al.*, 1988) and impaired respiratory burst activity (Ellis *et al.*, 1988; Elbim *et al.*, 1994).

Organ transplant recipients

Pulmonary complications, especially infectious complications are among the most common in transplant recipients (Kotloff, Ahya and Crawford, 2004). Infections in the transplant patient may increase risk of graft rejection (Hartmann, Sagedal and Hjelmesaeth, 2006; Potena and Valantine, 2007) and conversely graft rejection may increase risk of infection (Hamadani *et al.*, 2007). Allograft rejection is mediated predominantly by CD4+ T-lymphocytes which are activated by either recipient or donor antigen presenting cells(APC) which present both alloantigens and costimulatory molecules (Lindenfeld *et al.*, 2004). This, in turn, leads to T-lymphocyte activation and proliferation, with subsequent activation of immune cells such as B-lymphocytes, CD8+ cytotoxic T-lymphocytes, macrophages and NK cells (Lindenfeld *et al.*, 2004). Immunosuppressive agents administered to organ transplant recipients aim to prevent allograft rejection by inhibiting specific steps in this process. Novel immunotherapy agents have contributed to improved survival in organ transplant patients, although the mechanism of immune suppression can increase susceptibility to infectious complications. Select agents used in organ transplant recipients are discussed below and the modes of action are summarized in Figure 1.2.

Glucocorticoids

Glucocorticoids are potent immunosuppressive agents that inhibit a broad array of cellular processes involved in both allograft rejection and host defence. Glucocorticoids cross the cell membrane, bind to the cytoplasmic glucocorticoid receptor and translocate to the nucleus where the receptor-steroid complex increases expression of specific responsive genes while inhibiting others (Morand, 2007). In T- and B-lymphocytes, major effects are mediated by inhibition of the transcription factors activator protein-1 (AP-1) (Jonat et al., 1990), in part through the induction of MAP kinase phosphatase 1 (MKP-1) (Clark, 2003), and inhibition of nuclear factor kappa-B (NF-κB) (Auphan et al., 1995). These factors modulate the expression of costimulatory molecules, growth factors and cytokines such as IL-2 which inhibit T- and B-lymphocyte proliferation (Morand, 2007). In monocytes, glucocorticoids target cytokine production through a similar mechanism (Lindenfeld et al., 2004), and reduce MHC class II expression (Duncan and Wilkes, 2005). In addition, glucocorticoids retard inflammatory responses by decreasing the production of vasoactive and chemoattractive factors, and decrease neutrophil adherence and migration by inhibiting endothelial expression of adhesion molecules in part by inhibiting phospholipase A_2 (an early enzyme required for the production of leukotrienes and prostaglandins) (Lindenfeld et al., 2004; Duncan and Wilkes, 2005).

Calcineurin inhibitors

Tacrolimus and cyclosporine represent mainstays of transplant immunosuppression therapy allowing the sparing of the more toxic corticosteroids (Haberal et al., 2004). Both agents inhibit the calcium-activated/calmodulin dependent serine threonine phophatase calcineurin which is found predominantly in T-lymphocytes (Kahan, 1989; Ho et al., 1996). Cyclosporine binds an immunophilin called cylcophilin A, while tacrolimus (FK506) binds FK-binding protein 12. In each case the drug-immunophilin complex binds and inactivates calcineurin. Active calcineurin dephosphorylates (thus activates) the transcription factor family nuclear factor of T-lymphocytes (NFAT) (Kapturczak, Meier-Kriesche and Kaplan, 2004), which results in IL-2, IL-4, and CD40 ligand expression (cytokines and surface proteins vital for T-lymphocyte proliferation and activation). In addition, calcineurin inhibition also interferes with NF-κB activation, Na-K-ATPase, IL-3, GM-CSF and nitric oxide synthase while upregulating the immunosuppressive cytokine transforming growth factor-β production (TGF-β) (Kapturczak, Meier-Kriesche and Kaplan, 2004). Upregulation of TGF-β may also be responsible for the fibrosis that occurs in chronic organ rejection (Kapturczak, Meier-Kriesche and Kaplan, 2004). In addition, both drugs inhibit MAP kinase/AP-1 activation (Matsuda et al., 2000) and antigen presentation by dendritic cells (Lee et al., 2005) in a calcineurin-independent manner.

mTOR inhibitors

Rapamycin (sirolimus) is structurally related to FK506 and binds to FK-binding proteins, but does not inhibit calcineurin, and instead binds the kinase mammalian target of rapamycin (mTOR) (Easton and Houghton, 2006). mTOR phosphorylates a variety of proteins important for regulating the cell cycle, and thus mediates the signaling for a variety of growth factor receptors that stimulate the growth and proliferation of T- and B-lymphocytes (Heitman, Movva and Hall, 1991; Ingle, Sievers and Holt, 2000). Rapamycin effetively inhibits lymphocyte proliferation by preventing IL-2 receptor mediated activation of cell cycle progression from G1 to S phase via inhibition of mTOR. In addition, rapamycin inhibits proliferation of smooth muscle, fibroblasts, endothelial cells and a variety of other cell types which gives it potential in both cancer therapy (Easton and Houghton, 2006) and drug eluting stents (Wessely, Schomig and Kastrati, 2006), but may increase the likelihood of complications such as anastomotic dehiscence post-lung transplantation (King-Biggs *et al.*, 2003).

Antimetabolites

Azathioprine (AZA) is a pro-drug of 6-mercaptopurine (6-MP) developed in the 1950s (Duncan and Wilkes, 2005), while Mycophenolate mofetil (MMF) was developed as a more potent and selective replacement for AZA (Duncan and Wilkes, 2005). Both drugs inhibit *de novo* purine synthesis, inhibiting DNA and RNA production, and are considered antimetabolites. Unlike other cell types, lymphocytes depend on both the *de novo* and salvage pathways for purine biosynthesis making these drugs relatively specific for inhibiting T- and B-lymphocyte proliferation (Gummert, Ikonen and Morris, 1999). AZA is metabolized to 6-MP by glutathione (Taylor, Watson and Bradley, 2005), then metabolized to purine anaologs 6-thiouric acid, 6-methyl-MP, and 6-thioguanine triphosphate (6-thio-GTP) which upon incorporation into DNA halts DNA synthesis. This mode of action activity is not specific for lymphocytes which accounts, in part, for decreased specificity of AZA for lymphocytes compared to MMF (Gummert, Ikonen and Morris, 1999). 6-MP is also converted into thioinosinic mercaptopurine, which inhibits *de novo* pathway enzymes phosphoribosyl pyrophosphatase synthase and inosinate monphosphate dehydrongenase (IMPDH), inhibiting synthesis of adenosine monophosphate (AMP), and guanosine monophosphate (GMP). In addition, 6-thio-GTP can inhibit the rhoGTPase rac1 in place of GTP, blocking CD28 costimulation pathways and preferentially causing apoptosis of activated lymphocytes (Tiede *et al.*, 2003).

MMF, a pro-drug of mycophenolic acid (MPA), is a more potent and selective inhibitor of *de novo* purine synthesis with less effect on hematopoietic cells and neutrophils (Duncan, 2005:76). MPA is not a purine analog, but instead inhibits IMPDH by reversibly binding the cofactor site (NAD/H_2O), preventing a critical enzyme in GMP production (Sintchak, 1996:92), and leads to the accumulation of AMP over GMP which feedbacks negatively on proximal enzymes within the *de novo* pathway, and potently inhibits T- and B-lymphocyte proliferation, antibody production, NK cell generation and delayed-type hypersensitivity response (Gummert, Ikonen and Morris, 1999). As guanosine nucleotides are also required for glycosylation of proteins (Laurent *et al.*, 1996), MPA inhibits glycosylation of adhesion molecules, decreasing recruitment of leukocytes to areas of inflammation (Gummert, Ikonen and Morris, 1999).

Antilymphocyte antibodies

Polyclonal antithymocyte globulin (ATG) are purified monomeric anti-human gamma globulins created by immunizing rabbits, horses, or goats with human thymocytes or T cell lines (Haidinger *et al.*, 2007). These agents are typically used for induction or to treat acute rejection (Beiras-Fernandez, Thein and Hammer, 2003). They bind to cell surface receptors, thereby opsonizing lymphocytes for complement-mediated lysis or reticuloendothelial cell-dependant phagocytosis (Beiras-Fernandez, Thein and Hammer, 2003). ATG recognize most molecules involved in the T-lymphocyte activation cascade such as CD2, CD3, CD4, CD8, CD11a, CD18, CD25, HLA DR and HLA class I (Beiras-Fernandez, Thein and Hammer, 2003). Although T cell depletion is the major mechanism of action, additional effects include modulating key cell surface molecules that mediate leukocyte-endothelium interactions, induce B-lymphocyte apoptosis, interfere with DC functional properties and induce regulatory T- and natural killer T-lymphocytes (Mohty, 2007).

Monoclonal antibodies

The first monoclonal antibody used in organ transplantation was OKT3 or Muromonab-CD3, a murine IgG2a monoclonal antibody directed against the human T-lymphocyte surface protein CD3 (Renders and Valerius, 2003). CD3, when complexed with the T cell receptor (TcR), is critical to CD4+ T-lymphocyte activation and to CD8+ T-lymphocyte to binding and lysis of target cells (Chatenoud and Bluestone, 2007). T-lymphocytes exposed to OKT3 subsequently internalize the TcR-CD3 complex, which induce immunosuppressive mechanisms, including: 1) Cell coating preventing T-lymphocyte-cell interactions; 2) T-lymphocyte depletion via destruction of Ab-coated T-lymphocytes; 3) T-lymphocyte anergy via internalization of TcR-CD3 complex (thus low expression of TCR); and 4) upregulation of immune modulating T-regulatory cells (Chatenoud, 2003). The mechanism of T-lymphocyte depletion includes complement mediated cell lysis, antibody dependent cell killing by NK cells or macrophages, and apoptosis via ligation of CD95 (Fas) which occurs in activated T-lymphocytes (Chatenoud, 2003). The latter effect on T regulatory cells may in part account for prolonged OKT3 effects following antibody clearance (Chatenoud and Bluestone, 2007).

Antireceptor antibodies

Daclizumab is a humanized monoclonal antibody directed against the CD25 molecule, a key component of the IL-2 receptor (IL-2R) (Waldmann, 2007), central in promoting T-lymphocyte activation, differentiation and proliferation (Duncan and Wilkes, 2005). The main mechanism of action of daclizumab is to inhibit IL-2 induced T-lymphocyte proliferation. Importantly, daclizumab does not deplete non-CD25+ T-lymphocytes, and thus affords higher specificity than OKT3 or ATG (Duncan and Wilkes, 2005). Other effects include inhibition of CD8+ T-lymphocyte production, immunoglobulin production, and suppression of IL-15 dependant T-lymphocyte proliferation (Waldmann, 2007).

IL-2 is also important in immune regulatory functions such as IL-2 activation-induced cell death and the maintenance and fitness of T-regulatory cells, although the clinical significance in patients treated with Daclizumab is uncertain (Waldmann, 2007). Alemtuzumab (anti-CD52 monoclonal antibody, or Campath) was initially used for the treatment of chronic lymphocytic leukemia, now with increasing off-label use for transplantation induction (Magliocca and Knechtle, 2006). CD52 is a glycoprotein expressed on approximately 95% of peripheral blood lymphocytes, natural killer cells, monocytes, macrophages and thymocytes (almost all mononuclear cells) (Hale, 1990:103). The biological effects may be prolonged, with reduction of T- and B-lymphocytes observed for greater than one year after a single dose (Magliocca and Knechtle, 2006).

Immunodeficiency associated with cancer patients

In patients with malignancy, infections (including pneumonia) are a significant cause of morbidity and mortality (Joos and Tamm, 2005). Neutropenia associated with chemotherapy or hematologic malignancies is the strongest factor for infection risk (Joos and Tamm, 2005). The duration of neutropenia (absolute granulocyte count of $\leq$500 cells/mm^3), is strongly linked to incidence of infections including bacterial and fungal pneumonias (Viscoli, Varnier and Machetti, 2005). Neutrophils are important in the control of *Aspergillus*, in particular killing of hyphael forms (Feldmesser, 2006). Platelets, which are also typically low in neutropenic patients, may also have animicrobial properties against *Staphylococcus*, *Candida* and *Aspergillus* (Yeaman *et al.*, 1992; Yeaman *et al.*, 1996; Christin *et al.*, 1998). Monoclonal antibody therapies, such as Alemtuzumab (used to treat T-lymphocyte lymphomas or leukemias) cause profound cytopenias. Rituximab, a monoclonal antibody to CD20, specficially targets B-lymphocytes (used to treat B-cell lymphomas) but does not induce as profound immunosuppression as alemtuzumab or other chemotherapy agents (Plosker and Figgitt, 2003).

Numerous immune defects have been described in patients with solid and hematologic cancers. Hematologic malignancies, specifically acute leukemias, are associated with neutropenia, impaired neutrophil function (Hubel *et al.*, 1999), and impaired T-lymphocyte activation (Scrivener *et al.*, 2003). Defects in T-lymphocytes function in solid organ malignancies including abnormalites in interferon signaling in T-lymphocytes from melanoma patients (Critchley-Thorne *et al.*, 2007), increased expression of immunosuppressive TGF-β-secreting T-regulatory cells in patients with non-small cell lung cancer and ovarian cancer, and defects in NK cells, cytotoxic T cells, and macrophages in select solid tumours (Elgert, Alleva and Mullins, 1998; Kiessling *et al.*, 1999). In addition to increasing infection risk, tumour-induced immune dysfunction may also contribute to tumour progression (Elgert, Alleva and Mullins, 1998; Kiessling *et al.*, 1999).

Chemotherapy-induced defects in immune function are the major factors in the susceptibility of cancer patients to infection (Joos and Tamm, 2005). Cancer therapy may contribute to structural defects in the lungs, independent of impaired immune cells.

Direct pulmonary toxicity from bleomycin (Sleijfer, 2001), busulfan (Oliner *et al.*, 1961), cyclophosphamide (Malik *et al.*, 1996), methotrexate (Cannon, 1997) and radiotherapy (Abratt *et al.*, 2004) are clinically appreciated. Although the mechanism of drug-induced and radiation-induced lung injury is not well understood, epithelial injury is believed to play a central role (Higenbottam *et al.*, 2004). Lung epithelial injury may increase risk of pulmonary infection due to breakdown of mucosal barriers and impairing lung clearance mechanisms (Blijlevens, Donnelly and de Pauw, 2005), such as impaired respiratory ciliary function described in bone marrow transplant recipients (Au *et al.*, 2001). In addition, breakdown of gastrointestinal mucosal barriers with chemotherapy is believed to be responsible for increased incidence of gram-negative infections (including pneumonia) through hematogenous spread (Viscoli, Varnier and Machetti, 2005).

Immunodeficiency associated with collagen vascular disease

Infections associated with collagen vascular disease are common and can result in high morbidity and mortality (Noel *et al.*, 2001). Immunodeficiency in subjects with collagen vascular disease are attributed to agents used in treatment (Hamilton, 2005) although some immune defects have been attributed directly to collagen vascular diseases. For example, systemic lupus erythematosis (SLE) is associated with a relative T- and B-cell lymphopenia (Banchereau and Pascual, 2006), reduced T-lymphocyte activation (Kyttaris and Tsokos, 2004), and SLE acute exacerbations ('flares') are independent risk factors for infection (Noel *et al.*, 2001).

Various pharmacological agents are used to treat this group of diseases. In addition to immunosuppressive agents such as corticosteroids, AZA, MMF and cyclosporine (described above), other agents include cyclosphosphamide and methotrexate (Ponticelli, 2006). Cyclophosphamide is an alkylating agent that inhibits DNA replication (Martin *et al.*, 1997a), and can induce neutropenia (Martin *et al.*, 1997a), generalized lympho-penia (Cupps and Fauci, 1982), and can impair B-lymphocyte activation, proliferation and differentiation (Zhu *et al.*, 1987). Methotrexate interferes with folate metabolism, and consequently purine and puridine synthesis (Genestier *et al.*, 2000), and results in decreased T- and B-lymphocyte replication, activation and differentiation (Quemeneur *et al.*, 2004). Methotrexate also interferes with neutrophil migration and may decrease leukocyte phagocytic function (Genestier *et al.*, 2000).

A number of monoclonal antibody or soluble receptor antagonists are used to treat Crohn's disease, rheumatoid arthritis and sarcoidosis including rituximab, TNF-α inhibitors, and IL-1 receptor antagonist (Hamilton, 2005; Ponticelli, 2006). These agents are used to neutalize the effects of TNF-α, a critical protein in mediating inflammation (Clark, 2007). The TNF-α inhibitors include infliximab, a chimeric monoclonal antibody, and adalimumab, a fully human monoclonal body, that bind and neutralize both soluble and surface bound TNF-α. Etanercept is a soluble receptor fusion protein that binds to soluble TNF-α less avidly than infliximab (Hamilton, 2005), but also binds lymphotoxin which infliximab does not. TNF-α is particularly important in mediating host-defence against specific organisms such as *M. tuberculosis*

(Patel *et al.*, 2007). In particular, TNF-α is vital to the formation and maintenance of granulomas to destroy pathogens, limit generalized inflammation, and prevent dissemination of pathogens (Algood, Lin and Flynn, 2005). The use of TNF-α inhibitors can be associated with the development of life-threatening disseminated infections that are typically controlled by granulomas, including tuberculosis, histoplasmosis, aspergillosis, Cryptococcus infection, and listeriosis (Hamilton, 2005).

The immunocompromised critically ill patient

Burns, trauma, sepsis and other critical illness place patients at increased risk of nosocomial pneumonias with attendant high mortality (Wunderink, 2005; Church *et al.*, 2006). A number of factors contribute to infection susceptibility, especially mechanical factors including reduced cough and decreased airway protection from delerium, sedatives, analgesics, or pain, supine positioning that may impair mucociliary clearance or increases aspiration risk, direct thoracic wall or pulmonary injury due to chest wall trauma, pulmonary contusion, or smoke inhalation, all of which may also impair cough or mucociliary clearance. The presence of an endotracheal tube bypasses critical upper respiratory tract mechanisms, and provides a direct conduit for microbes into the lower respiratory tract. Furthermore, the normal host bacterial flora is altered due to colonization with ICU-associated microbes and the use of multiple antibiotics (Wunderink, 2005).

Other factors that contribute to infection risk include immunoparalysis associated with critical illness (Wunderink, 2005). Burn trauma patients have decreased expression of HLA-DR in peripheral blood monocytes and elevated expression of IL-10 suggesting decreased immune activation and relative immunosuppression (Sachse *et al.*, 1999), with similar findings noted in patients with other forms of trauma, major surgery, and sepsis (Monneret *et al.*, 2003). These findings correlate with reduced LPS responsiveness (Wolk *et al.*, 1999), increased levels of regulatory T-lymphocytes (Monneret *et al.*, 2003), and increased risk of nosocomial infection (Sachse *et al.*, 1999). There is also evidence for decreased opsonic activity (Saba *et al.*, 1986) and decreased respiratory burst activity in critically ill patients (Zapata-Sirvent and Hansbrough, 1993). Lymphopenia and increased lymphocyte apoptosis also correlates with mortality in sepsis (Hotchkiss *et al.*, 2001) and inhibitors of apoptosis may improve outcomes in sepsis (Hotchkiss *et al.*, 2001). Agents targeted to counteract immunoparalysis in the critically ill may improve outcomes by reducing risks for serious infections.

1.4 Summary and future directions for this field

As our understanding of the barrier and pharmacological defences, the innate immune and adaptive immune systems (and the instructive bidirectional interaction of these systems) in health improves through continued scientific research, an improved understanding of the factors that predispose immunocompromised patients to various infections may be identified as targeted or specific deficiencies in innate or adaptive

Table 1.2 Summary of immunocompromised host populations.

Immunocompromised host	Mechanism(s) of immunocompromise	Predominant area(s) of immune dysfunction	Common infectious organisms
HIV+ Individuals	(1) Direct HIV-mediated effects causing cytotoxicity and dysfunction. (2) Indirect effects through alterations of mucosal immunity	(1) T-cell depletion and dysfunction (2) B-cell dysfunction (3) Marcrophage dysfunction (4) Neutrophil depletions and dysfunction	Community-Acquired Bacterial organisms, *Pneumocystis*, *Mycobacterium tuberculosis*
Transplant Patient	(1) Medication-related immunosuppression	(1) T-cell dysfunction (2) B-cell dysfunction	Community-acquired bacterial organisms, CMV, *Pneumocystis*
Cancer Patient	(1) Chemotherapy related immunosuppression. (2) Direct cancer-induced immunosuppression	(1) Neutropenia (2) barrier dysfunction from chemotherapeutic/radiation injury	Gram-negative bacteria, *Candida* infection, *Aspergillus* infection
Collagen Vascular Disease	(1) Steroids and pharmacologic immunosuppressives (2) Anti-cytokine therapy	(1) T-cells/B-cells dysfunction (2) Granuloma Formation (anti-TNF)	Bacterial Infections Mycobacterium tuberculosis, Histoplasma
Critically Ill Patient	(1) Impaired mucosal barrier function (2) immunoparalysis due to critical illness	(1) impaired ciliary function due to direct lung injury (2) impaired clearance due to intubation, sedation and positioning. (3) impaired T-cell/B-cell function	Bacterial infections, *Candida* infections

immune systems. Understanding the underlying basic mechanisms that contribute to the pathogenesis of infectious diseases will allow development of targeted and novel therapeutic agents for use in immunocompromised hosts for the purpose of augmenting or rescuing immune function and controlling infectious disease in vulnerable patients (Table 1.2).

References

Abratt, R.P., Morgan, G.W., Silvestri, G. and Willcox, P. (2004) Pulmonary complications of radiation therapy. *Clinics in Chest Medicine*, **25**, 167–177.

Aggarwal, B.B. (2003) Signaling pathways of the TNF superfamily: A double-edged sword. *Nature Reviews Immunology*, **3**, 745–756.

Algood, H.M., Lin, P.L. and Flynn, J.L. (2005) Tumor necrosis factor and chemokine interactions in the formation and maintenance of granulomas in tuberculosis. *Clinical Infectious Diseases*, **41** (Suppl 3), S189–S193.

Arbour, N.C., Lorenz, E., Schutte, B.C. *et al.* (2000) TLR4 mutations are associated with endotoxin hyporesponsiveness in humans. *Nature Genetics*, **25**, 187–191.

Armstrong, L., Medford, A.R.L., Uppington, K.M. *et al.* (2004) Expression of functional Toll-like receptor (TLR-)2 and TLR-4 on alveolar epithelial cells. *American Journal of Respiratory Cell and Molecular Biology*, (E-published March 25, 2004).

Au, W.Y., Ho, J.C., Lie, A.K. *et al.* (2001) Respiratory ciliary function in bone marrow recipients. *Bone Marrow Transplantation*, **27**, 1147–1151.

Auphan, N., Didonato, J.A., Rosette, C. *et al.* (1995) Immunosuppression by glucocorticoids: inhibition of NF-kappa B activity through induction of I kappa B synthesis. *Science*, **270**, 286–290.

Ballet, J.J., Sulcebe, G., Couderc, L.J. *et al.* (1987) Impaired anti-pneumococcal antibody response in patients with AIDS-related persistent generalized lymphadenopathy. *Clinical and Experimental Immunology*, **68**, 479–487.

Banchereau, J. and Pascual, V. (2006) Type I interferon in systemic lupus erythematosus and other autoimmune diseases. *Immunity*, **25**, 383–392.

Barton, G.M. and Medzhitov, R. (2003) Toll-like receptor signaling pathways. *Science*, **300**, 1524–1525.

Beharka, A.A., Gaynor, C.D., Kang, B.K. *et al.* (2002) Pulmonary surfactant A up-regulates activity of the mannose receptor, a pattern recognition receptor expressed on human macrophages. *Journal of Immunology*, **169**, 3565–3573.

Beiras-Fernandez, A., Thein, E. and Hammer, C. (2003) Induction of immunosuppression with polyclonal antithymocyte globulins: an overview. *Experimental and Clinical Transplantation*, **1**, 79–84.

Benito, J.M., Lopez, M. and Soriano, V. (2004) The role of CD8+ T-cell response in HIV infection. *AIDS Reviews*, **6**, 79–88.

Beutler, B. (2000) Tlr4: central component of the sole mammalian LPS sensor. *Current Opinion in Immunology*, **12**, 20–26.

Biron, C.A., Nguyen, K.B., Pien, G.C. *et al.* (1999) Natural killer cells in antiviral defense: function and regulation by innate cytokines. *Annual Review of Immunology*, **17**, 189–220.

Blijlevens, N.M., Donnelly, J.P. and De Pauw, B.E. (2005) Microbiologic consequences of new approaches to managing hematologic malignancies. *Reviews in Clinical & Experimental Hematology*, **9**, E2.

Borron, P., Mcintosh, J.C., Korfhagen, T.R. *et al.* (2000) Surfactant-associated protein A inhibits LPS-induced cytokines and nitric oxide production in vivo. *American Journal of Physiology. Lung Cellular and Molecular Physiology*, **278**, 840–847.

Bowdish, D.M.E., Loffredo, M.S., Mukhopadhyay, S. *et al.* (2007) Macrophage receptors implicated in the 'adaptive' form of immunity. *Microbes and Infection/Institut Pasteur*, **9**, 1680–1687.

Branger, J., Knapp, S., Weijer, S. *et al.* (2004) Role of toll-like receptor 4 in gram-positive and gram-negative pneumonia in mice. *Infection and Immunity*, **72**, 788–794.

Breen, R.A., Janossy, G., Barry, S.M. *et al.* (2006) Detection of mycobacterial antigen responses in lung but not blood in HIV-tuberculosis co-infected subjects. *AIDS*, **20**, 1330–1332.

Brenchley, J.M., Hill, B.J., Ambrozak, D.R. *et al.* (2004) T-cell subsets that harbor human immunodeficiency virus (HIV) in vivo: implications for HIV pathogenesis. *Journal of Virology*, **78**, 1160–1168.

Brenchley, J.M., Price, D.A. and Douek, D.C. (2006) HIV disease: fallout from a mucosal catastrophe? *Nature Immunology*, **7**, 235–239.

Bronke, C., Palmer, N.M., Jansen, C.A. *et al.* (2005) Dynamics of cytomegalovirus (CMV)-specific T cells in HIV-1-infected individuals progressing to AIDS with CMV end-organ disease. *The Journal of Infectious Diseases*, **191**, 873–880.

Cannon, G.W. (1997) Methotrexate pulmonary toxicity. *Rheumatic Disease Clinics of North America*, **23**, 917–937.

Centlivre, M., Sala, M., Wain-Hobson, S. and Berkhout, B. (2007) In HIV-1 pathogenesis the die is cast during primary infection. *AIDS*, **21**, 1–11.

Chatenoud, L. (2003) CD3-specific antibody-induced active tolerance: from bench to bedside. *Nature Reviews Immunology*, **3**, 123–132.

Chatenoud, L. and Bluestone, J.A. (2007) CD3-specific antibodies: a portal to the treatment of autoimmunity. *Nature Reviews Immunology*, **7**, 622–632.

Christin, L., Wysong, D.R., Meshulam, T. *et al.* (1998) Human platelets damage Aspergillus fumigatus hyphae and may supplement killing by neutrophils. *Infection and Immunity*, **66**, 1181–1189.

Chun, J., Soong, G. and Prince, A. (2006) Activation of Ca2+ -dependent signaling by TLR2. *Journal of Immunology*, **177**, 1330–1337.

Church, D., Elsayed, S., Reid, O. *et al.* (2006) Burn wound infections. *Clinical Microbiology Reviews*, **19**, 403–434.

Clark, A.R. (2003) MAP kinase phosphatase 1: a novel mediator of biological effects of glucocorticoids? *The Journal of Endocrinology*, **178**, 5–12.

Clark, I.A. (2007) How TNF was recognized as a key mechanism of disease. *Cytokine & Growth Factor Reviews*, **18**, 335–343.

Conge, A.M., Tarte, K., Reynes, J. *et al.* (1998) Impairment of B-lymphocyte differentiation induced by dual triggering of the B-cell antigen receptor and CD40 in advanced HIV-1-disease. *AIDS*, **12**, 1437–1449.

Critchley-Thorne, R.J., Yan, N., Nacu, S. *et al.* (2007) Down-regulation of the interferon signaling pathway in T lymphocytes from patients with metastatic melanoma. *PLoS Medicine*, **4**, e176.

Crouch, E.C. (1998) Collectins and pulmonary host defense. *American Journal of Respiratory Cell and Molecular Biology*, **19**, 177–201.

Crowther, J.E., Kutala, V.K., Kuppusamy, P.K. *et al.* (2004) Pulmonary surfactant protein A inhibits macrophage reactive oxygen intermediate production in response to stimuli reducing MADPH oxidase activity. *Journal of Immunology*, **172**, 6866–6874.

Cupps, T. and Fauci, A. (1982) Corticosteroid-mediated immunoregulation in man. *Immunological Reviews*, **65**, 133–155.

D'Orsogna, L.J., Krueger, R.G., Mckinnon, E.J. and French, M.A. (2007) Circulating memory B-cell subpopulations are affected differently by HIV infection and antiretroviral therapy. *AIDS*, **21**, 1747–1752.

Day, R.B., Wang, Y., Knox, K.S. *et al.* (2004) Alveolar macrophages from HIV-infected subjects are resistant to Mycobacterium tuberculosis *in vitro*. *American Journal of Respiratory Cell and Molecular Biology*, **30**, 403–410.

De Milito, A. (2004) B lymphocyte dysfunctions in HIV infection. *Current HIV Research*, **2**, 11–21.

Dentener, M.A., Vreugdenhil, A.C., Hoet, P.H. *et al.* (2000) Production of acute-phase protein lipopolysaccharide-binding protein by respiratory type II epithelial cells: implications for local defense to bacterial endotoxins. *American Journal of Respiratory Cell and Molecular Biology*, **23**, 146–153.

Diamond, G., Legarda, D. and Ryan, L.K. (2000) The innate immune response of the respiratory epithelium. *Immunological Reviews*, **173**, 27–38.

Douek, D.C., Picker, L.J. and Koup, R.A. (2003) T cell dynamics in HIV-1 infection. *Annual Review of Immunology*, **21**, 265–304.

Duncan, M.D. and Wilkes, D.S. (2005) Transplant-related immunosuppression: a review of immuno-suppression and pulmonary infections. *Proceedings of the American Thoracic Society*, **2**, 449–455.

Eagan, R., Twigg, H.L., 3rd, French, N. *et al.* (2007) Lung fluid immunoglobulin from HIV-infected subjects has impaired opsonic function against pneumococci. *Clinical Infectious Diseases*, **44**, 1632–1638.

Easton, J.B. and Houghton, P.J. (2006) mTOR and cancer therapy. *Oncogene*, **25**, 6436–6446.

Elbim, C., Prevot, M.H., Bouscarat, F. *et al.* (1994) Polymorphonuclear neutrophils from human immunodeficiency virus-infected patients show enhanced activation, diminished fMLP-induced L-selectin shedding, and an impaired oxidative burst after cytokine priming. *Blood*, **84**, 2759–2766.

Elgert, K.D., Alleva, D.G. and Mullins, D.W. (1998) Tumor-induced immune dysfunction: the macrophage connection. *Journal of Leukocyte Biology*, **64**, 275–290.

Ellis, M., Gupta, S., Galant, S. *et al.* (1988) Impaired neutrophil function in patients with AIDS or AIDS-related complex: a comprehensive evaluation. *The Journal of Infectious Diseases*, **158**, 1268–1276.

Elssner, A., Carter, J.E., Yunger, T.M. and Wewers, M.D. (2004) HIV-1 infection does not impair human alveolar macrophage phagocytic function unless combined with cigarette smoking. *Chest*, **125**, 1071–1076.

Fahy, R.J., Diaz, P.T., Hart, J. and Wewers, M.D. (2001) BAL and serum IgG levels in healthy asymptomatic HIV-infected patients. *Chest*, **119**, 196–203.

Fauci, A.S. (1988) The human immunodeficiency virus: infectivity and mechanisms of pathogenesis. *Science*, **239**(4840), 617–622.

Feldmesser, M. (2006) Role of neutrophils in invasive aspergillosis. *Infection and Immunity*, **74**, 6514–6516.

Genestier, L., Paillot, R., Quemeneur, L. *et al.* (2000) Mechanisms of action of methotrexate. *Immunopharmacology*, **47**, 247–257.

Gordon, S.B., Molyneux, M.E., Boeree, M.J. *et al.* (2001) Opsonic phagocytosis of Streptococcus pneumoniae by alveolar macrophages is not impaired in human immunodeficiency virus-infected Malawian adults. *The Journal of Infectious Diseases*, **184**, 1345–1349.

Granelli-Piperno, A., Delgado, E., Finkel, V. *et al.* (1998) Immature dendritic cells selectively replicate macrophagetropic (M-tropic) human immunodeficiency virus type 1, while mature cells efficiently transmit both M- and T-tropic virus to T cells. *Journal of Virology*, **72**, 2733–2737.

Granelli-Piperno, A., Golebiowska, A., Trumpfheller, C. *et al.* (2004) HIV-1-infected monocyte-derived dendritic cells do not undergo maturation but can elicit IL-10 production and T cell regulation. *Proceedings of the National Academy of Sciences of the United States of America*, **101**, 7669–7674.

Granelli-Piperno, A., Shimeliovich, I., Pack, M. *et al.* (2006) HIV-1 selectively infects a subset of nonmaturing BDCA1-positive dendritic cells in human blood. *Journal of Immunology*, **176**, 991–998.

Guadalupe, M., Reay, E., Sankaran, S. *et al.* (2003) Severe CD4+ T-cell depletion in gut lymphoid tissue during primary human immunodeficiency virus type 1 infection and substantial delay in restoration following highly active antiretroviral therapy. *Journal of Virology*, **77**, 11708–11717.

Gummert, J.F., Ikonen, T. and Morris, R.E. (1999) Newer immunosuppressive drugs: a review. *Journal of the American Society of Nephrology*, **10**, 1366–1380.

Haberal, M., Emiroglu, R., Dalgic, A. *et al.* (2004) The impact of cyclosporine on the development of immunosuppressive therapy. *Transplantation Proceedings*, **36**, 143S–147.

Haidinger, M., Geyeregger, R., Poglitsch, M. *et al.* (2007) Antithymocyte globulin impairs T-cell/antigen-presenting cell interaction: disruption of immunological synapse and conjugate formation. *Transplantation*, **84**, 117–121.

Hale, G., Xia, M.Q., Tighe, H.P., Dyer, M.J. and Waldmann, H. (1990) The CAMPATH-1 antigen (CDw52). *Tissue Antigens*, **35**(3), 118–127.

Hamadani, M., Benson, D.M., Jr, Blum, W. *et al.* (2007) Pulmonary Nocardia and Aspergillus co-infection in a patient with chronic graft-versus-host disease. *Transplant Infectious Disease*.

Hamilton, C.D. (2005) Immunosuppression related to collagen-vascular disease or its treatment. *Proceedings of the American Thoracic Society*, **2**, 456–460.

Hart, M., Steel, A., Clark, S.A. *et al.* (2007) Loss of discrete memory B cell subsets is associated with impaired immunization responses in HIV-1 infection and may be a risk factor for invasive pneumococcal disease. *Journal of Immunology*, **178**, 8212–8220.

Hartmann, A., Sagedal, S. and Hjelmesaeth, J. (2006) The natural course of cytomegalovirus infection and disease in renal transplant recipients. *Transplantation*, **82**, S15–S17.

Hawn, T.R., Verbon, A., Lettinga, K.D. *et al.* (2003) A common dominant TLR5 stop codon polymorphism abolishes flagellin signaling and is associated with susceptibility to legionnaires' disease. *The Journal of Experimental Medicine*, **198**, 1563–1572.

Heitman, J., Movva, N.R. and Hall, M.N. (1991) Targets for cell cycle arrest by the immunosuppressant rapamycin in yeast. *Science*, **253**, 905–909.

Higenbottam, T., Kuwano, K., Nemery, B. and Fujita, Y. (2004) Understanding the mechanisms of drug-associated interstitial lung disease. *British Journal of Cancer*, **91** (Suppl 2), S31–S37.

Hiratsuka, T. and Al, E. (1998) Identification of human b-defensin-2 in respiratory tract and plasma and its increase in bacterial pneumonia. *Biochemical and Biophysical Research Communications*, **249**, 943–947.

Ho, S., Clipstone, N., Timmermann, L. *et al.* (1996) The mechanism of action of cyclosporin A and FK506. *Clinical Immunology and Immunopathology*, **80**, S40–S45.

Hotchkiss, R.S., Tinsley, K.W. Swanson, P.E. *et al.* (2001) Sepsis-induced apoptosis causes progressive profound depletion of B and CD4+ T lymphocytes in humans. *Journal of Immunology*, **166**, 6952–6963.

Hubel, K., Hegener, K., Schnell, R. *et al.* (1999) Suppressed neutrophil function as a risk factor for severe infection after cytotoxic chemotherapy in patients with acute nonlymphocytic leukemia. *Annals of Hematology*, **78**, 73–77.

Imler, J.L. and Hossmann, J.A. (2001) Toll receptors in innate immunity. *Trends in Cell Biology*, **11**, 304–311.

Ingle, G.R., Sievers, T.M. and Holt, C.D. (2000) Sirolimus: continuing the evolution of transplant immunosuppression. *Annals of Pharmacotherapy*, **34**, 1044–1055.

Jia, H.P., Kline, J.N., Penisten, A. *et al.* (2004) Endotoxin responsiveness of human airway epithelia is limited by low expression of MD-2. *American Journal of Physiology. Lung Cellular and Molecular Physiology*, **287**, 428–437.

Jonat, C., Rahmsdorf, H.J., Park, K.K. *et al.* (1990) Antitumor promotion and antiinflammation: down-modulation of AP-1 (Fos/Jun) activity by glucocorticoid hormone. *Cell*, **62**, 1189–1204.

Jones, B.W., Heldwein, K.A., Means, T.K. *et al.* (2001) Differential roles of toll-like receptors in the elicitation of proinflammatory responses by macrophages. *Annals of the Rheumatic Diseases*, **60** (supplement), 6–12.

Joos, L. and Tamm, M. (2005) Breakdown of pulmonary host defense in the immunocompromised host: cancer chemotherapy. *Proceedings of the American Thoracic Society*, **2**, 445–448.

Kahan, B.D. (1989) Cyclosporine. *The New England Journal of Medicine*, **321**, 1725–1738.

Kajikawa, O., Frevert, C.W., Lin, S.M. *et al.* (2005) Gene expression of Toll-like receptor 2. Toll-like receptor 4 and MD2 is differentially regulated in, rabbits with Escherichia coli pneumonia. *Gene*, **344**, 193–202.

Kapturczak, M.H., Meier-Kriesche, H.U. and Kaplan, B. (2004) Pharmacology of calcineurin antagonists. *Transplantation Proceedings*, **36**, 25S–32.

Kiessling, R., Wasserman, K., Horiguchi, S. *et al.* (1999) Tumor-induced immune dysfunction. *Cancer Immunology, Immunotherapy*, **48**, 353–362.

Kim, K.D., Zhao, J., Auh, S. *et al.* (2007) Adaptive immune cells temper initial innate responses. *Nature Medicine*, **13**, 1248–1252.

King-Biggs, M.B., Dunitz, J.M., Park, S.J. *et al.* (2003) Airway anastomotic dehiscence associated with use of sirolimus immediately after lung transplantation. *Transplantation*, **75**, 1437–1443.

Kitchen, S.G., Korin, Y.D., Roth, M.D. *et al.* (1998) Costimulation of naive CD8(+) lymphocytes induces CD4 expression and allows human immunodeficiency virus type 1 infection. *Journal of Virology*, **72**, 9054–9060.

Knight, S.C., Patterson, S. and Macatonia, S.E. (1991) Stimulatory and suppressive effects of infection of dendritic cells with HIV-1. *Immunology Letters*, **30**, 213–218.

Kotloff, R.M., Ahya, V.N. and Crawford, S.W. (2004) Pulmonary complications of solid organ and hematopoietic stem cell transplantation. *American Journal of Respiratory and Critical Care Medicine*, **170**, 22–48.

Koziel, M.J. (2006) Influence of HIV co-infection on hepatitis C immunopathogenesis. *Journal of Hepatology*, **44**, S14–S18.

Koziel, H., Kim, S., Reardon, C., Li, X., Garland, R., Pinkston, P. *et al.* (1999) Enhanced *in vivo* human immunodeficiency virus-1 replication in the lungs of human immunodeficiency virus-infected persons with Pneumocystis carinii pneumonia. *American Journal of Respiratory and Critical Care Medicine*, **160**(6), 2048–2055.

Koziel, H., Eichbaum, Q., Kruskal, B.A. *et al.* (1998) Reduced binding and phagocytosis of Pneumocystis carinii by alveolar macrophages from persons infected with HIV-1 correlates with mannose receptor downregulation. *The Journal of Clinical Investigation*, **102**, 1332–1344.

Koziel, H., Li, X., Armstrong, M.Y. *et al.* (2000) Alveolar macrophages from human immunodeficiency virus-infected persons demonstrate impaired oxidative burst response to Pneumocystis carinii in vitro. *American Journal of Respiratory Cell and Molecular Biology*, **23**, 452–459.

Kuritzkes, D.R. (2000) Neutropenia, neutrophil dysfunction, and bacterial infection in patients with human immunodeficiency virus disease: the role of granulocyte colony-stimulating factor. *Clinical Infectious Diseases*, **30**, 256–260.

Kyttaris, V.C. and Tsokos, G.C. (2004) T lymphocytes in systemic lupus erythematosus: an update. *Current Opinion in Rheumatology*, **16**, 548–552.

Lane, H.C., Masur, H., Edgar, L.C. *et al.* (1983) Abnormalities of B-cell activation and immunoregulation in patients with the acquired immunodeficiency syndrome. *The New England Journal of Medicine*, **309**, 453–458.

Lang, W., Perkins, H., Anderson, R.E. *et al.* (1989) Patterns of T lymphocyte changes with human immunodeficiency virus infection: from seroconversion to the development of AIDS. *Journal of Acquired Immune Deficiency Syndromes*, **2**, 63–69.

Laurent, A.F., Dumont, S., Poindron, P. and Muller, C.D. (1996) Mycophenolic acid suppresses protein N-linked glycosylation in human monocytes and their adhesion to endothelial cells and to some substrates. *Experimental Hematology*, **24**, 59–67.

Ledergerber, B., Egger, M., Erard, V. *et al.* (1999) AIDS-related opportunistic illnesses occurring after initiation of potent antiretroviral therapy: the Swiss HIV Cohort Study. *Journal of the American Medical Association*, **282**, 2220–2226.

Lee, Y.R., Yang, I.H., Lee, Y.H. *et al.* (2005) Cyclosporin A and tacrolimus, but not rapamycin, inhibit MHC-restricted antigen presentation pathways in dendritic cells. *Blood*, **105**, 3951–3955.

Liew, F.Y., Xu, D., Brint, E.K. and O'Neill, L.A.J. (2005) Negative regulation of Toll-like receptor-mediated immune responses. *Nature Reviews Immunology*, **5**, 446–458.

Lindenfeld, J., Miller, G.G., Shakar, S.F. *et al.* (2004) Drug therapy in the heart transplant recipient: part I: cardiac rejection and immunosuppressive drugs. *Circulation*, **110**, 3734–3740.

Livingstone, W.J., Moore, M., Innes, D. *et al.* (1996) Frequent infection of peripheral blood CD8-positive T-lymphocytes with HIV-1. Edinburgh Heterosexual Transmission Study Group. *Lancet*, **348**, 649–654.

Lore, K., Sonnerborg, A., Brostrom, C. *et al.* (2002) Accumulation of DC-SIGN+ CD40+ dendritic cells with reduced CD80 and CD86 expression in lymphoid tissue during acute HIV-1 infection. *AIDS*, **16**, 683–692.

Macatonia, S.E., Lau, R., Patterson, S. *et al.* (1990) Dendritic cell infection, depletion and dysfunction in HIV-infected individuals. *Immunology*, **71**, 38–45.

Magliocca, J.F. and Knechtle, S.J. (2006) The evolving role of alemtuzumab (Campath-1H) for immunosuppressive therapy in organ transplantation. *Transplant International*, **19**, 705–714.

Malaspina, A., Moir, S., Kottilil, S. *et al.* (2003) Deleterious effect of HIV-1 plasma viremia on B cell costimulatory function. *Journal of Immunology*, **170**, 5965–5972.

Malik, S.W., Myers, J.L., Deremee, R.A. and Specks, U. (1996) Lung toxicity associated with cyclophosphamide use. Two distinct patterns. *American Journal of Respiratory and Critical Care Medicine*, **154**, 1851–1856.

Margolick, J.B., Donnenberg, A.D., Munoz, A. *et al.* (1993) Changes in T and non-T lymphocyte subsets following seroconversion to HIV-1: stable CD3+ and declining CD3- populations suggest regulatory responses linked to loss of CD4 lymphocytes. The multicenter AIDS cohort study. *Journal of Acquired Immune Deficiency Syndromes*, **6**, 153–161.

Martin, T.R. and Frevert, C.W. (2005) Innate immunity in the lungs. *Proceedings of the American Thoracic Society*, **2**, 403–411.

Martin, T.R., Mathison, J.C., Tobias, P.S. *et al.* (1992) Lipopolysaccharide binding protein enhances the responsiveness of alveolar macrophages to bacterial lipopolysaccharide: implications for cytokine production in normal and injured lungs. *The Journal of Clinical Investigation*, **90**, 2209–2219.

Martin, F., Lauwerys, B., Lefebvre, C. *et al.* (1997a) Side-effects of intravenous cyclophosphamide pulse therapy. *Lupus*, **6**, 254–257.

Martin, T.R., Rubenfeld, G.D., Ruzinski, J.T. *et al.* (1997b) Relationship between soluble CD14, lipopolysaccharide binding protein, and the alveolar inflammatory response in patients with acute respiratory distress syndrome. *American Journal of Respiratory and Critical Care Medicine*, **155**, 937–944.

Matsuda, S., Shibasaki, F., Takehana, K. *et al.* (2000) Two distinct action mechanisms of immunophilin-ligand complexes for the blockade of T-cell activation. *EMBO Reports*, **1**, 428–434.

Mccormack, F.X. and Whitsett, J.A. (2002) The pulmonary collectins, SP-A and SP-D, orchestrate innate immunity in the lung. *The Journal of Clinical Investigation*, **109**, 707–712.

McCray, P.B. and Bentley, L. (1997) Human airway epithelia express a defensin. *American Journal of Respiratory Cell and Molecular Biology*, **16**, 343–349.

Meddows-Taylor, S., Martin, D.J. and Tiemessen, C.T. (1998) Reduced expression of interleukin-8 receptors A and B on polymorphonuclear neutrophils from persons with human immunodeficiency virus type 1 disease and pulmonary tuberculosis. *The Journal of Infectious Diseases*, **177**, 921–930.

Meddows-Taylor, S., Pendle, S. and Tiemessen, C.T. (2001) Altered expression of CD88 and associated impairment of complement 5a-induced neutrophil responses in human immunodeficiency virus type 1-infected patients with and without pulmonary tuberculosis. *The Journal of Infectious Diseases*, **183**, 662–665.

Medzhitov, R. (2001) Toll-like receptors and innate immunity. *Nature Reviews Immunology*, **1**, 135–145.

Mohty, M. (2007) Mechanisms of action of antithymocyte globul: T-cell depletion and beyond. *Leukemia*, **21**, 1387–1394.

Monari, C., Casadevall, A., Pietrella, D. *et al.* (1999) Neutrophils from patients with advanced human immunodeficiency virus infection have impaired complement receptor function and preserved Fcgamma receptor function. *The Journal of Infectious Diseases*, **180**, 1542–1549.

Monneret, G., Debard, A.L., Venet, F. *et al.* (2003) Marked elevation of human circulating CD4+ CD25+ regulatory T cells in sepsis-induced immunoparalysis. *Critical Care Medicine*, **31**, 2068–2071.

Morand, E.F. (2007) Effects of glucocorticoids on inflammation and arthritis. *Current Opinion in Rheumatology*, **19**, 302–307.

Morris, L., Binley, J.M., Clas, B.A. *et al.* (1998) HIV-1 antigen-specific and -nonspecific B cell responses are sensitive to combination antiretroviral therapy. *The Journal of Experimental Medicine*, **188**, 233–245.

Muro-Cacho, C.A., Pantaleo, G. and Fauci, A.S. (1995) Analysis of apoptosis in lymph nodes of HIV-infected persons. Intensity of apoptosis correlates with the general state of, activation of the lymphoid tissue and not with stage of disease or viral burden. *Journal of Immunology*, **154**, 5555–5566.

Murray, H.W., Hillman, J.K., Rubin, B.Y. *et al.* (1985) Patients at risk for AIDS-related opportunistic infections. Clinical manifestations and impaired gamma interferon, production. *The New England Journal of Medicine*, **313**, 1504–1510.

Muzio, M., Bosisio, D., Polentarutti, N. *et al.* (2000) Differential expression and regulation of toll-like receptors (TLR) in human leukocytes: selective expression of TLR3 in dendritic cells. *Journal of Immunology*, **164**, 5998–6004.

Noel, V., Lortholary, O., Casassus, P. *et al.* (2001) Risk factors and prognostic influence of infection in a single cohort of 87 adults with systemic lupus erythematosus. *Annals of the Rheumatic Diseases*, **60**, 1141–1144.

Notermans, D.W., De Jong, J.J., Goudsmit, J. *et al.* (2001) Potent antiretroviral therapy initiates normalization of hypergammaglobulinemia and a decline in HIV type 1-specific antibody responses. *AIDS Research and Human Retroviruses*, **17**, 1003–1008.

Oliner, H., Schwartz, R., Rubio, F. and Dameshek, W. (1961) Interstitial pulmonary fibrosis following busulfan therapy. *The American Journal of Medicine*, **31**, 134–139.

Orenstein, J.M., Fox, C. and Wahl, S.M. (1997) Macrophages as a source of HIV during opportunistic infections. *Science*, **276**(5320), 1857–1861.

Organization, W.H. (2007) TB and HIV/AIDS. 2007 Tuberculosis Facts Sheet, 1–2.

Patel, N.R., Zhu, J., Tachado, S.D. *et al.* (2007) HIV impairs TNF-alpha mediated macrophage apoptotic response to Mycobacterium tuberculosis. *Journal of Immunology*, **179**, 6973–6980.

Plosker, G.L. and Figgitt, D.P. (2003) Rituximab: a review of its use in non-Hodgkin's lymphoma and chronic lymphocytic leukaemia. *Drugs*, **63**, 803–843.

Ponticelli, C. (2006) New therapies for lupus nephritis. *Clinical Journal of the American Society of Nephrology*, **1**, 863–868.

Potena, L. and Valantine, H.A. (2007) Cytomegalovirus-associated allograft rejection in heart transplant patients. *Current Opinion in Infectious Diseases*, **20**, 425–431.

Prevention, CFDCA, (2006) HIV/AIDS Surveillance Report, 2006. HIV/AIDS Surveillance Report, **18**, 1–55.

Quemeneur, L., Beloeil, L., Michallet, M.C. *et al.* (2004) Restriction of de novo nucleotide biosynthesis interferes with clonal expansion and differentiation into effector and memory CD8 T cells. *Journal of Immunology*, **173**, 4945–4952.

Renders, L. and Valerius, T. (2003) Engineered CD3 antibodies for immunosuppression. *Clinical and Experimental Immunology*, **133**, 307–309.

Rodriguez-Barradas, M.C., Musher, D.M., Lahart, C. *et al.* (1992) Antibody to capsular polysaccharides of Streptococcus pneumoniae after vaccination of human immunodeficiency virus-infected subjects with 23-valent pneumococcal vaccine. *The Journal of Infectious Diseases*, **165**, 553–556.

Rothlin, C.V., Ghosh, S., Zuniga, E.I. *et al.* (2007) TAM receptors are pleotropic inhibitors of the innate immune response. *Cell*, **131**, 1124–1136.

Saba, T.M., Blumenstock, F.A., Shah, D.M. *et al.* (1986) Reversal of opsonic deficiency in surgical, trauma, and burn patients by infusion of purified human plasma fibronectin. Correlation with experimental observations. *The American Journal of Medicine*, **80**, 229–240.

Sachse, C., Prigge, M., Cramer, G. *et al.* (1999) Association between reduced human leukocyte antigen (HLA)-DR expression on blood monocytes and increased plasma level of interleukin-10 in patients with severe burns. *Clinical Chemistry and Laboratory Medicine*, **37**, 193–198.

Sano, H., Chiba, H., Iwaki, D. *et al.* (2000) Surfactant proteins A and D bind CD14 by different mechanisms. *The Journal of Biological Chemistry*, **275**, 22442–22451.

Saukkonen, J.J., Bazydlo, B., Thomas, M. *et al.* (2002) Beta chemokines are induced by Mycobacterium tuberculosis and inhibit its growth. *Infection and Immunity*, **70**, 1684–1693.

Schluger, N.W., Perez, D. and Liu, Y.M. (2002) Reconstitution of immune responses to tuberculosis in patients with HIV infection who receive antiretroviral therapy. *Chest*, **122**, 597–602.

Scrivener, S., Goddard, R.V., Kaminski, E.R. and Prentice, A.G. (2003) Abnormal T-cell function in B-cell chronic lymphocytic leukaemia. *Leukemia & Lymphoma*, **44**, 383–389.

Shearer, G.M., Salahuddin, S.Z., Markham, P.D. *et al.* (1985) Prospective study of cytotoxic T lymphocyte responses to influenza and antibodies to human T lymphotropic virus-III in homosexual men. Selective loss of an influenza-specific, human leukocyte antigen-restricted cytotoxic T lymphocyte response in human T lymphotropic virus-III positive individuals with symptoms of acquired immunodeficiency syndrome and in a patient with acquired immunodeficiency syndrome. *The Journal of Clinical Investigation*, **76**, 1699–1704.

Shepherd, V.L. (2002) Distinct roles for lung collectins in pulmonary host defense. *American Journal of Respiratory Cell and Molecular Biology*, **26**, 257–260.

Sheridan, J.F., Aurelian, L., Donnenberg, A.D. and Quinn, T.C. (1984) Cell-mediated immunity to cytomegalovirus (CMV) and herpes simplex virus (HSV) antigens in the acquired immune deficiency syndrome: interleukin-1 and interleukin-2 modify in vitro responses. *Journal of Clinical Immunology*, **4**, 304–311.

Shirai, A., Cosentino, M., Leitman-Klinman, S.F. and Klinman, D.M. (1992) Human immunodeficiency virus infection induces both polyclonal and virus-specific B cell activation. *The Journal of Clinical Investigation*, **89**, 561–566.

Sintchak, M.D., Fleming, M.A., Futer, O., Raybuck, S.A, Chambers, S.P., Caron, P.R. *et al.* (1996) Structure and mechanism of inosine monophosphate dehydrogenase in complex with the immunosuppressant mycophenolic acid. *Cell*, **85**(6), 921–930.

Skerrett, S.J., Liggitt, H.D., Hajjar, A.M. *et al.* (2004) Respiratory epithelial cells regulate lung inflammation in response to inhaled endotoxin. *American Journal of Physiology. Lung Cellular and Molecular Physiology*, **287**, 143–152.

Sleijfer, S. (2001) Bleomycin-induced pneumonitis. *Chest*, **120**, 617–624.

Soong, G., Reddy, B., Sokol, S. *et al.* (2004) TLR2 is mobilized into an apical lipid raft receptor complex to signal infection in airway epithelial cells. *The Journal of Clinical Investigation*, **113**, 1482–1489.

Stebbing, J., Gazzard, B. and Douek, D.C. (2004) Where does HIV live? *The New England Journal of Medicine*, **350**(18), 1872–1880.

Sutherland, R., Yang, H., Scriba, T.J. *et al.* (2006) Impaired IFN-gamma-secreting capacity in mycobacterial antigen-specific CD4 T cells during chronic HIV-1 infection despite long-term HAART. *AIDS*, **20**, 821–829.

Tachado, S.D., Zhang, J., Zhu, J. *et al.* (2005) HIV impairs TNF-alpha release in response to TLR4 stimulation in human alveolar macrophages in vitro. *American Journal of Respiratory Cell and Molecular Biology*, **33**, 610–621.

Taylor, A.L., Watson, C.J. and Bradley, J.A. (2005) Immunosuppressive agents in solid organ transplantation: Mechanisms of action and therapeutic efficacy. *Critical Reviews in Oncology/ Hematology*, **56**, 23–46.

Tiede, I., Fritz, G., Strand, S. *et al.* (2003) CD28-dependent Rac1 activation is the molecular target of azathioprine in primary human CD4+ T lymphocytes. *The Journal of Clinical Investigation*, **111**, 1133–1145.

Turville, S.G., Cameron, P.U., Handley, A. *et al.* (2002) Diversity of receptors binding HIV on dendritic cell subsets. *Nature Immunology*, **3**, 975–983.

Twigg, H.L., Soliman, D.M., Day, R.B. *et al.* (1999) Lymphocytic alveolitis, bronchoalveolar lavage viral load, and outcome in human immunodeficiency virus infection. *American Journal of Respiratory and Critical Care Medicine*, **159**, 1439–1444.

van Wetering, S., Mannesse-Lazeroms, S.P., Van Sterkenberg, M.A. *et al.* (1997) Effect of defensins on interleukin-8 synthesis in airway epithelial cells. *The American Journal of Physiology*, **272**, L888–L896.

Veazey, R. and Lackner, A. (2003) The mucosal immune system and HIV-1 infection. *AIDS Reviews*, **5**, 245–252.

Veazey, R.S., Demaria, M., Chalifoux, L.V. *et al.* (1998) Gastrointestinal tract as a major site of CD4+ T cell depletion and viral replication in SIV infection. *Science*, **280**, 427–431.

Viscoli, C., Varnier, O. and Machetti, M. (2005) Infections in patients with febrile neutropenia: epidemiology, microbiology, and risk stratification. *Clinical Infectious Diseases*, **40** (Suppl 4), S240–S245.

Waldmann, T.A. (2007) Anti-Tac (daclizumab, Zenapax) in the treatment of leukemia, autoimmune diseases, and in the prevention of allograft rejection: A 25-year personal odyssey. *Journal of Clinical Immunology*, **27**, 1–18.

Wang, X., Moser, C., Louboutin, J.P. *et al.* (2002) Toll-like receptor 4 mediates innate immune responses to Haemophilus influenzae infection in mouse lung. *Journal of Immunology*, **168**, 810–815.

Watford, W.T., Ghio, A.J. and Wright, J.R. (2000) Complement-mediated host defense in the lung. *American Journal of Physiology. Lung Cellular and Molecular Physiology*, **279**, 790–798.

Wessely, R., Schomig, A. and Kastrati, A. (2006) Sirolimus and Paclitaxel on polymer-based drug-eluting stents: similar but different. *Journal of the American College of Cardiology*, **47**, 708–714.

Wolk, K., Docke, W., von Baehr, V. *et al.* (1999) Comparison of monocyte functions after LPS- or IL-10-induced reorientation: importance in clinical immunoparalysis. *Pathobiology*, **67**, 253–256.

Wong, H.R., Pitt, B.R., Su, G.L. *et al.* (1995) Induction of lipopolysaccharide-binding protein gene expression in cultured rat pulmonary artery smooth muscle cells by interleukin 1 beta. *American Journal of Respiratory Cell and Molecular Biology*, **12**, 449–454.

Wu, L. and KewalRamani, V.N. (2006) Dendritic-cell interactions with HIV: infection and viral dissemination. *Nature Reviews Immunology*, **6**, 859–868.

Wunderink, R.G. (2005) Nosocomial pneumonia, including ventilator-associated pneumonia. *Proceedings of the American Thoracic Society*, **2**, 440–444.

Yeaman, M.R., Puentes, S.M., Norman, D.C. and Bayer, A.S. (1992) Partial characterization and staphylocidal activity of thrombin-induced platelet microbicidal protein. *Infection and Immunity*, **60**, 1202–1209.

Yeaman, M.R., Soldan, S.S., Ghannoum, M.A. *et al.* (1996) Resistance to platelet microbicidal protein results in increased severity of experimental Candida albicans endocarditis. *Infection and Immunity*, **64**, 1379–1384.

Young, K.R., Jr, Rankin, J.A., Naegel, G.P. *et al.* (1985) Bronchoalveolar lavage cells and proteins in patients with the acquired immunodeficiency syndrome. An immunologic analysis. *Annals of Internal Medicine*, **103**, 522–533.

Zaas, A.K. and Schwartz, D.A. (2005) Innate immunity and the lung: defense at the interface between host and environment. *Trends in Cardiovascular Medicine*, **15**, 195–202.

Zapata-Sirvent, R.L. and Hansbrough, J.F. (1993) Temporal analysis of human leucocyte surface antigen expression and neutrophil respiratory burst activity after thermal injury. *Burns*, **19**, 5–11.

Zhang, L., Huang, Y., He, T., Cao, Y. and Ho, D.D. (1996) HIV-1 subtype and second-receptor use. *Nature*. **383**(6603), 768.

Zhang, J. and Koziel, H. (2002) Alveolar macrophages, in Cellular Aspects of HIV Infection (eds A. Cossarizza and D. Kaplan), Wiley-Liss, Inc, New York.

Zhang, J.M., Zhu, J., Imrich, A. *et al.* (2004) Pneumocystis activates human alveolar macrophage NF-kB signaling through mannose receptors. *Infection and Immunity*, **72**, 3147–3160.

Zhu, L.P., Cupps, T.R., Whalen, G. and Fauci, A.S. (1987) Selective effects of cyclophosphamide therapy on activation, proliferation, and differentiation of human B cells. *The Journal of Clinical Investigation*, **79**, 1082–1090.

2

Microbiological diagnosis of respiratory infections in the immunocompromised

Margareta Ieven

Department of Medical Microbiology, Faculty of Medicine, University of Antwerp, Belgium

2.1 Introduction

Immunodeficient individuals are highly susceptible to exogenous infections and to reactivation of endogenous latent infections that are prevented in immunocompetent persons by normally functioning immune defense mechanisms.

Conditions likely to impair immune defenses are human immunodeficiency virus (HIV) infection, diabetes mellitus, rheumatoid arthritis, corticosteroid therapy, leukemia, lymphoma, cancer and chemotherapy accompanying transplantation of bone marrow as well as solid organ transplantation. With medical progress the number of immunocompromised patients is steadily climbing. The growing use of potent immunosuppressive drugs in the management of lymphoproleferative malignancies results in the number of patients at risk that almost reaches levels encountered in recipients of allogeneic stem cell grafts.

The upper respiratory tractus is permanently exposed to the environmental opportunistic flora and is the preferred initial site of colonization that may result in a local or a generalized infection.

Laboratory procedures for the diagnosis of opportunistic infections are not different from those for non-opportunistic infections, but the main concern is the differentiation between colonization and infection that are in many situations frequently divided by only a thin line. The most reliable procedure remains the identification of the infecting organism in normally sterile specimens. For respiratory infections these are peripheral blood, pleural exudates or deep respiratory specimens obtained either by protected brush (PB) or broncho-alveolar lavage (BAL). Frequently however the seriousness of the disease status of the patient precludes invasive PB and BAL procedures and the only specimen available is sputum. As a last resort transthoracic needle aspiration or open

Pulmonary Infection in the Immunocompromised Patient, Edited by Carlos Agustí and Antoni Torres
© 2009 John Wiley & Sons, Ltd.

lung biopsy can be performed (Nosari *et al.*, 2003). Traditional diagnostic methods however often lack sensitivity, are not available in many contexts and focus on only a few of the large number of aetiological agents. Therefore alternative diagnostic procedures were developed: antigen detection by latex agglutination or immuno-fluorescence (DIF), Elisa, immunochromatography and nucleic acid amplification techniques (NAATs), particularly PCR and NASBA (nucleic acid sequence based amplification).

Over the past two decades, NAATs are revolutionizing the diagnostic procedures for the management of patients with RTI, resulting from a combination of improved sensitivity and specificity, a potential for automatization and the production of very rapid results. NAATs have already become the gold-standard in some diagnostic fields but only a few assays have been approved by the US Food and Drug Administration and fewer still have entered the daily routine diagnosis and management of patients. This can be ascribed to the rapid evolution of the technology, the cost of this technology and the large number of etiological agents, bacterial as well as viral, responsible for community-acquired LRTI.

The list of infections in immunodeficient patients is almost unlimited. Common causes of respiratory infections in the immunocompetent are also found in the immunocompromised patient. The diagnosis of these infections has been described previously and is therefore not the subject of this chapter (Ieven, 2007).

Nevertheless some infections are more prevalent in particular situations of immunodeficiency and merit special discussion. These respiratory infections in immunodeficient patients will be discussed under the following headings:

- HIV infection and *Mycobacterium tuberculosis*.

- HIV infection and non tuberculous Mycobacteria.

- Infections in transplant patients or other immunodeficiencies.

    Cytomegalovirus (CMV);

    Epstein Barr virus;

    Herpes simplex virus (HSV);

    Respiratory viruses;

    Bacterial infections;

    Fungal infections.

2.2   HIV infection and *Mycobacterium tuberculosis*

In 2001–2002 before the era of highly active treatment of HIV infections, respiratory infections accounted in Florida for 49% of hospital admissions of HIV positive patients. Community acquired pneumonia was the cause in 52% of the cases, *Pneumocystis jirovecii* in 24%, non tuberculous mycobacteria (NTM) in 11% and *Mycobacterium tuberculosis* (Mtb) in 9% (Harries, Maher and Nunn, 1998). In Africa, south of the

Sahara, where two thirds of the people are living with HIV, tuberculosis (TB) is by far the most prevalent opportunistic infection and in some countries, causes one third of all AIDS related deaths (Murray, 2005).

HIV infection by impairing cell-mediated immunity appears to be the highest known risk factor for the reactivation of latent tuberculosis. There is also evidence that HIV infected people are more susceptible to a new tuberculous infection and may more rapidly develop overt disease (Daley *et al.*, 1992; Di Perri *et al.*, 1989).

After the introduction of highly active antiretroviral therapy (HAART) the epidemiology and impact of pulmonary infection on HIV patients changed, restoring the tuberculosis situation to the pre-HIV era. Patients receiving HAART are now at increased risk for the development of bacterial pneumonia and non-Hodgkin's lymphoma.

Diagnosis of tuberculosis based on sputum smear microscopy, culture and nucleic acid amplification.

In up to 98% of immunocompetent tuberculosis patients with cavitations, sputum smears are positive for acid-fast bacilli. In HIV positive patients the clinical pattern of pulmonary tuberculosis and the results of sputum smear tests correlate with the host immune status. As HIV induced immunosuppression worsens the clinical and radiographic manifestations of TB become increasingly atypical, with less cavitation and haemophysis, while the sputum smears tend to be acid -fast bacilli negative. (Getahun *et al.*, 2007) Tubercle bacilli do not appear in sputum because of the paucity of pulmonary inflammation and decreased cavitation. In a retrospective study Karstaedt *et al.* 1998 found 68% HIV patients to have smear positive sputum compared with 79% in HIV negative patients. There was also a correlation of smear positivity with the CD4 counts. In a prospective study of 109 sputum culture positive pulmonary tuberculosis cases, 43% of the 72 HIV positive patients had a negative sputum smear compared with 24% of the 37 HIV negative patients (Elliott *et al.*, 1993).

As a result of the lower bacillary load in sputum of HIV infected patients, sputum culture needs more incubation time compared with that of patients without HIV. The use of liquid media can shorten the recovery time of mycobacteria by 15 days compared with standard Loewenstein-Jensen medium (Crump *et al.*, 2003; Hanna *et al.*, 1995).

Mycobacteraemia is detected in many patients with HIV and active tuberculosis.

Although culture remains the gold standard for the detection of *Mycobacterium tuberculosis*, the Food and Drug Administration approved in 1999 a reformulated Amplified Mycobacterium tuberculosis Direct Test (MTD) (Gen-Probe, San Diego, California) for the detection of *Mycobacterium tuberculosis* in acid-fast bacilli (AFB) smear-positive and smear-negative respiratory specimens from patients suspected of having tuberculosis (TB). MTD and the Amplicor Mycobacterium tuberculosis Test (Amplicor) (Roche Diagnostic Systems), previously had been approved for the direct detection of *M. tuberculosis* in respiratory specimens that have positive AFB smears.

For nucleic acids amplification (NAA) tests the CDC updated original guidelines published in 1996 and proposes the following algorithm for using and interpreting NAA test results for managing patients suspected of having TB (CDC, 2000).

The appropriate number of specimens to test with NAA will vary depending on the clinical situation, the prevalence of TB, the prevalence of nontuberculous mycobacteria

(NTM), and the laboratory proficiency. Based on available information, the following algorithm is a reasonable approach for NAA testing of respiratory specimens from patients with signs or symptoms of active pulmonary TB for whom a presumed diagnosis has not been established:

1. Collect sputum specimens on three different days for AFB smear and mycobacterial culture.

2. Perform nucleic acid amplification (NAA) test on the first sputum specimen collected, the first smear-positive sputum specimen, and additional sputum specimens as indicated below.

    (a) If the first sputum specimen is smear-positive and NAA-positive, the patient can be presumed to have TB without additional NAA testing. However, unless concern exists about the presence of non tuberculous mycobacteria (NTM), the NAA test adds little to the diagnostic work-up.

    (b) If the first sputum is smear-positive and NAA-negative, a test for inhibitors should be done. The inhibitor test can be done as an option with Amplicor. To test for inhibitors of MTD, spike an aliquot of the lysated sputum sample with lysed *M. tuberculosis* (approximately 10 organisms per reaction, or an equivalent amount of *M. tuberculosis* rRNA) and repeat the test starting with amplification.

        • If inhibitors are not detected, additional specimens (not to exceed a total of three) should be tested. The patient can be presumed to have NTM if a second sputum specimen is smear-positive, NAA-negative and has no inhibitors detected.

        • If inhibitors are detected, the NAA test is of no diagnostic help. Additional specimens (not to exceed a total of three) can be tested with NAA.

    (c) If sputum is smear-negative and MTD-positive, additional specimens (not to exceed three) should be tested with MTD. The patient can be presumed to have TB if a subsequent specimen is MTD-positive.

    (d) If sputum is smear-negative and MTD-negative, an additional specimen should be tested with MTD. The patient can be presumed not to be infectious if all smear and MTD results are negative. The clinician must rely on clinical judgment in decisions regarding the need for antituberculous therapy and further diagnostic work-up because negative NAA results do not exclude the possibility of active pulmonary TB.

3. If the indicated repeat NAA testing fails to verify initial NAA test results, the clinician must rely on clinical judgment in decisions regarding the need for antituberculous therapy, further diagnostic work-up, and isolation.

4. Ultimately, the patient's response to therapy and culture results is used to confirm or refute a diagnosis of TB.

Cautions

NAA tests can enhance diagnostic certainty, but they do not replace AFB smear or mycobacterial culture, and they do not replace clinical judgment. Clinicians should interpret these tests based on the clinical situation, and laboratories should perform NAA testing only at the request of the physician and only on selected specimens. Laboratorians should not reserve material from clinical specimen for NAA testing if this compromises the ability to perform the other established tests that have better-defined diagnostic utility and implications. Specificity of NAA tests varies between laboratories as a result of unrecognized procedural differences and differences in cross-contamination rates. Multiple specimens from the same patient should not be tested together to reduce risks of methodologic errors. Laboratory directors should provide clinicians with information on the performance of NAA tests in the local setting, including sensitivity and specificity compared with culture for both smear-positive and smear-negative respiratory specimens. Substantial discrepancies can indicate problems with either culture or NAA technique. The number of NAA tests repeated because of failure of negative and positive controls should also be reported. Clinicians should understand the impact that changes in sensitivity, specificity of a test and the prevalence of TB, and of other mycobacterial diseases can have on the predictive value of the NAA test. Information is limited regarding NAA test performance for nonrespiratory specimens, or specimens from treated patients. NAA tests often remain positive after cultures become negative during therapy and can remain positive even after completion of therapy.

2.3 HIV infection and non tuberculous mycobacteria (NTM)

Many different species of NTM produce disease in HIV infected persons and the relative importance of the different species may differ between geographic areas, it is now generally accepted that natural waters and sometimes soil can be a reservoir for most human NTM infections. *Mycobacterium avium* complex (MAC) is always the more prevalent. As an example in one study disease producing NTM in HIV infected persons were in decreasing order: *Mycobacterium avium* complex (MAC) *M. fortuitum*, *M. kansasii*, *M. xenopi*, *M. abscessus* (Miguez-Burbano *et al.*, 2006). *M. malmoense* is a major NTM pathogen in northern Europe. (Tortoli *et al.*, 1997; Enzensberger *et al.*, 1999).

Because NTM are ubiquitous in the environment some specific diagnostic criteria have been proposed to differentiate clinical infection by NTM and colonization of secretions in the absence of clinical disease.

Diagnosis

Diagnostic criteria have been proposed by the American Thoracic Society and by the British Thoracic Society, both are presented since they are slightly different (American Thoracic Society, 2007. In symptomatic patients with infiltrate, nodular or cavitary disease, or a high resolution computed tomography scan which shows multifocal bronchiectasis and/or multiple small nodules, the following apply:

(a)   if three positive sputum/bronchial wash cultures with negative acid-fast bacillus (AFB) smear or two positive cultures and one positive AFB smear in the last 12 months;

(b)   if only one bronchial wash available then a positive culture with a 2+ to 4+ AFB smear or 2+ to 4+ growth on solid media;

(c)   if sputum or bronchial wash are nondiagnostic then a transbronchial or lung biopsy yielding nontuberculous mycobacteria or biopsy showing mycobacterial histo-pathologic features and one or more sputums or bronchial washings are positive for nontuberculous mycobacteria, even if in low numbers.

British Thoracic Society (Henry *et al.*, 2004). Pulmonary disease: *M. kansasii*, *M. avium* intracellulare complex infections, *M. malmoense*, *M. xenopi*. Pulmonary disease is diagnosed when positive cultures develop from specimens of sputum obtained at least seven days apart in a patient whose chest radiograph suggests mycobacterial infection and who may or may not present with symptoms and signs.

In immunocompromised persons, blood cultures are frequently positive for *M. tuberculosis* as well as for NTM (Eng *et al.*, 1989). The difference between the two can easily be made by a microscopic examination of positive cultures, particularly in liquid media: *M. tuberculosis* producing typical cords that are absent in NTM.

2.4   HIV and *Pneumocystis jirovecii*

Pneumocystis jirovecii (formerly known as *P. carinii*) is one of the most frequent and severe opportunistic pathogens in immunocompromised individuals causing severe pneumonia (PCP) in individuals with immune systems impaired by HIV, transplantation or malignancy. Its incidence *increased* significantly after the emergence of HIV. However, after widespread use of antimicrobial prophylaxis and the introduction of HAART there has been a steady decline in the incidence of pneumocystosis in these patients. (Hughes, 1989).

Diagnosis of *Pneumocystis jiroveci*

Detection of *Pneumocystis* by growth in artificial medium or tissue culture is not possible; serologic assays for the detection of antibodies are useful for epidemiologic studies but not for the diagnosis of PCP as most humans become seropositive for *Pneumocystis* antibodies early in life.

Diagnosis is mostly made by Giemsa stain, methenamine silver staining immuno-fluorsence or PCR on sputum or preferentially on BAL fluid (Wakefeld *et al.*, 1990; Brancart *et al.*, 2005).

In contrast to the cyst wall stains, Giemsa stains the nuclei of all the various life cycle stages a reddish purple and the cytoplasm a light blue. Since there are approximately 10-fold more trophic forms than cysts, the sensitivity is likely to be increased. This stain also permits assessment of BAL fluid quality by demonstration of host alveolar macrophages, which should be present in a productive sample.

Increasingly sensitive techniques such as PCR have been developed for detecting *Pneumocystis* DNA in human respiratory samples (broncho alveolar lavage fluid, induced sputum and oropharyngeal washes). The high sensitivity has enabled detection of very low levels of *Pneumocystis,* not detectable by conventional staining techniques (Wakefeld *et al.*, 1990). However, although more sensitive than conventional methods relying on organism detection by microscopic methods, the presence of a specific *Pneumocystis* PCR product has not been strictly correlated with underlying disease: molecular detection techniques have shown that *Pneumocystis* is carried in the lungs of asymptomatic individuals with mild immunosuppression induced by HIV or malignancy (Miller and Huang, 2004; Morris *et al.*, 2004).

2.5   Infections in transplant patients or other immunodeficiencies

The success of transplantation depends on the administration of immunosuppressive drugs to prevent and treat rejection of the graft and graft versus host disease (GvHD) and the administration of anti-infectives either as preemptive therapy of a subclinical infection or as aggressive therapy of a clinical infection. Initially bacterial infections were most problematic. Strategies to control bacterial infections improved, but it was obvious that enhanced use of antibacterials inevitably would be accompanied by selection of resistant organisms. Next to bacteria, viruses demanded more attention, the associated morbidity declined due to advances in rapid diagnostics and the introduction of effective antivirals. Resistant bacteria, particularly gram positive organisms like enterococci and methicillin resistant staphylococci urged vigilance. Today, opportunistic fungi have become the most frequent and most dangerous pathogens with Candida and Aspergillus being the more prominent.

It is useful to divide the timetable after transplantation into three periods. (Afessa and Peters, 2006; Matulis and High, 2002; Marty and Rubin, 2006).

Phase 1, one month post-transplant. There is profound granulocytopenia and mucositis. Infections are typically caused by skin flora and gastro-intestinal organisms.

The responsible organisms are gram positives, streptococci and staphylococci, gram negatives (Enterobacteriaceae, Acinetobacter spp. and *Pseudomonas aeruginosa*) as well as Candida spp. Bacterial infections are thus the primary concern among patients with febrile neutropenia in the early phase, particularly after hematopoietic stem cell transplantation (HSCT). With time the incidence of angioinvasive mould infection (invasive aspergillosis and others) rises. Fever with an unidentified focus that continues after three to five days of broad spectrum antibiotic therapy is frequently related to fungal infections.

Phase 2, days 31–100 post transplant. This is the peak time for reactivation of herpes group viruses especially CMV but also HSV, EBV and Varicella-zostervirus. During this period patients are at risk for community acquired bacterial and viral infections as well as for *Pneumocystis jiroveci*, and Aspergillus infections (Razonable and Paya, 2003).

Phase 3, more than 100 days post transplant and extends until the patients no longer require treatment for chronic GvHD. This period is dominated by whether or not GvHD is occurring with its requirement for prolonged immunosuppression. Recipients are at risk for opportunistic and conventional infections, pneumococcal and viral pneumonia (Rubin, 1996). Treatment for GvHD results in a significant risk of infection with CMV, *Pneumocystis jiroveci* and invasive fungi.

Cytomegalovirus infection

Following primary exposure CMV has the ability to establish lifelong persistent and latent infection. CMV evades the host immune function by several mechanisms and in the immunocompetent individual, the infection is held in check by the host's immune response. Under certain conditions CMV can reactivate resulting in asymptomatic viral shedding or development of disease. In Western Europe 47% of the population is CMV seropositive. CMV is the single most important infectious complication after HSCT and solid organ transplantation with incidences of 15–60% and 20–35% respectively of CMV reactivation and disease (Sandherr *et al.*, 2006). Consensus definitions were established to distinguish between active CMV infection (evidence of CMV replication) CMV syndrome (CMV replication plus fever, weakness, leucopenia, thrombocytopenia) and CMV disease (CMV replication and histopathological evidence of invasive disease of liver, gastrointestinal tract, lung or others.) (Ljungman *et al.*, 2002) CMV seropositive patients are at the highest risk–approximately 70% develop reactivation and 35–40% develop CMV disease–followed by seronegative recipients with a seropositive donor. Twenty per cent of these patients develop a primary infection and 10% CMV disease. (Nichols, 2003). Week 4 from transplantation is the earliest time point to note a significant difference between those patients who eventually develop CMV disease and those who remain asymptomatic (Ghisetti *et al.*, 2004).

After HSCT CMV primarily causes pneumonitis and gastrointestinal disease. Pulmonary localization is the most life threatening. CMV is also associated, though not causally linked to, the development of acute and chronic graft rejection, it predisposes patients to bacterial and fungal superinfections (Zamora, 2004). CMV with or without exogenous factors has been proposed to have a contributory role in the development of bronchiolitis obliterans, but bronchiolitis obliterans occurs exclusively in allogeneic HSCT recipients with graft versus host disease.

Seronegative recipients of CMV-positive donors are at the highest risk of developing severe disease (Zamora, 2004).

Four strategies to prevent CMV infection have been utilized: matching the donor-recipient pair by CMV serologic status, use of CMV negative blood products, antiviral agents to suppress viral replication and immunoglobulin preparations to provide passive immunization.

Antiviral drugs may be used in a prophylactic or in a preemptive manner. In prophylaxis antivirals are administered indiscriminately. The preemptive approach consists of the application of antiviral therapy only when CMV reactivation is documented on serial sampling of blood using highly sensitive assays, thus avoiding overtreatment. Costs of prophylaxis are less than the routine monitoring and preemptive therapy (Fishman *et al.*, 2007). However, prophylaxis is associated with mylotoxicity, increased incidence of invasive fungal infection and late CMV disease due to delayed CMV-specific T-cell recovery (Li *et al.*, 1994) after HSCT. CMV replicates rapidly *in vivo* and the time from the first detection to overt disease may be less than seven days (Emery *et al.*, 2000). Thus rapid detection and monitoring of CMV reactivation is essential for the identification of subjects at high risk of developing CMV disease. Preemptive therapy reduced the incidence of CMV disease to less than 5% in high risk patients during the first 100 days after transplantation, but as a result of delayed CMV-specific immune reconstitution CMV disease now occurs late after transplantation, more than 100 days (Nichols, 2003).

The antigenemia assay is currently used by many centres as a guiding tool for preemptive therapy.

Diagnosis of CMV infection

The methods available for the diagnosis of active CMV infection are: cell culture, an antigenemia assay and the detection of CMV nucleic acids either by hybridization in the clinical sample or after amplification (Mazzulli *et al.*, 1999).

Conventional cell culture and cell vial assays lack sensitivity and do not allow quantitation of the viral load.

The CMV antigenemia assay has been a major advance in the diagnosis of CMV infection in organ transplantation (Razonable and Emery, 2004).

The presence of CMV in blood leucocytes provides an early marker of active CMV infection and is a rapid test for the detection of CMV viremia. The test consists of a number of steps including isolation of blood leukocytes, preparation of microscopic slides, fixation, immunostaining and quantitative scoring. Monoclonal antibodies detect the viral pp65 antigen, a structural late protein, expressed in the nuclei of blood leucocytes during the early phase of the CMV replication cycle. The test is quantitative. It can also be applied on cells obtained by broncho-alveolar lavage (Sia and Patel, 2000). The results may be reported as the number of cells used to prepare the slides or as the result per 50 000 cells. Antigenemia requires the presence of $=+0.5 \times 10^9$/L leucocytes.

In the pp65 antigenemia assay the number of positive cells in the peripheral blood reflects the viral load and high numbers of pp65 positive cells correlate with CMV disease. A small number of antigen positive cells following solid organ transplantation generally indicates asymptomatic infection, whereas large numbers imply an increased likelihood of CMV disease.

Antigenemia has several disadvantages: a low sensitivity for detecting early active CMV infection or disease that may appear before engraftment in HSCT, the lack of leucocytes during the period of aplasia and low positive predictive value for the occurrence of CMV gastroenteritis. CMV antigenemia assay requires processing of the blood samples within a few hours, is labour intensive and cannot be automated. Variations in the methods applied make it difficult to compare results from different laboratories. False negative results may occur in neutropenic patients.

Currently once-weekly blood sampling is often undertaken to determine viral load. In D^+/R^- CMV patients more frequent sampling may prove to be more effective. Monitoring should continue for at least 100 days after HSCT (Razonable et $al.$, 2005).

No universal cut-off point for initiating pre-emptive therapy exists today. Clinically relevant threshold of the number of interpreted peripheral blood leucocytes (PBL) differs among different populations of patients. Thresholds of more than 10 or even >1 or >2 or +3 positive cells per 200 000 PBL cells in samples containing >0.5 × 10^9/L cells has been suggested to guide preemptive therapy (Gentile et $al.$, 2006). Weekly monitoring should continue for at least 100 days after HSCT (Razonable et $al.$, 2005).

Hybrid capture assay (HCA; Digene Diagnostics Inc) uses a RNA probe targeting 17% of the CMV genome. The resulting hybrids are captured by a monoclonal antibody specific for DNA-RNA hybrids, the resulting signal being measured in a luminometer. Qualitative and quantitative results can be obtained (Bhorade et $al.$, 2001).

Nucleic acid amplification tests are extremely sensitive and specific for the detection of viral nucleic acids. The amplification technology made significant progress during recent times as a result of the development of automatic nucleic acid extraction procedures and real time formats providing the possibility for highly reproducible, quantitative results that are largely operator independent, within a short time (4–5 hours). Comparison between previously laboratory-developed PCR assays is impossible due to differences in the origin of samples–whole blood, plasma, serum, PBL, PBMC–primers, probes, cycling programmes and quantitation standards. Several commercial tests are presently available: the Amplicor CMV Monitor assay (Roche), the NucliSens CMV pp67 assay (Biomerieux) and analyte-specific reagents (ASR) (Abbott and Qiagen) to compose CMV DNA assays (Caliendo et $al.$, 2007). Viral loads obtained from plasma specimens tested by the Amplicor, the ARS and the HCA are in very close agreement, the greatest variability being observed near the limit of detection. The performance characteristics and the reproducibility of the tests is similar to those observed for other real-time PCR tests. (Caliendo et $al.$, 2007; Razonable et $al.$, 2005) performed a head to head comparison of CMV detection by PCR on whole blood, plasma, peripheral blood leucocytes and peripheral monocytes. CMV PCR on whole blood was the most sensitive. Plasma does not require lengthy cell preparation procedures and offers much better opportunity to detect CMV viremia during periods of severe cytopenia (Boeckh et $al.$, 2004; Razonable and Emery, 2004).

It was hoped that quantitation of viral load would be useful in preemptive treatment strategies in that certain threshold or increasing levels of viral load could be used to start therapy. Recent evaluations of RT-PCR revealed that PCR and the antigenemia assay could be falsely negative when virus levels are quite low (Thorne et $al.$, 2007), that a negative result does not exclude CMV end-organ disease (Ruell et $al.$, 2007) and that real-time PCR cannot completely replace the antigenemia assay. In general, PCR tends to turn positive earlier than does the antigenemia assay (Sia and Patel, 2000) but the reverse situation has also been observed (Gentile *et al.*, 2006; Boeckh *et al.*, 2004; Ruell *et al.*, 2007).

There is need for a prospective, multicentre study comparing the antigenemia assay with these recently developed standardized quantitative NAATs to evaluate the optimal procedure for the implementation of post transplantation preemptive therapy.

Epstein-Barr virus infection

Epstein-Barr virus (EBV) is a ubiquitous human herpes virus with worldwide distribution.

Severe infections due to primary EBV infection or EBV reactivation, are reported particularly in immunocompromised patients. Discrete pneumonitis develops in 5–10% of all patients with primary EBV infections, but a few cases of severe pneumonitis have also been reported (Haller *et al.*, 1995).

The main manifestation of EBV reactivation is the development of post-transplant lymphoproliferative disease (Sandherr *et al.*, 2006). Although the incidence is low, 0.5–2%, it may be as high as 20% in the presence of three or more risk factors. Risk factors for developing EBV disease are:

- *ex vivo* T-cell depletion;
- treatment with anti-thymocyte globulin for preventing or treating graft versus host disease (GvHD);
- anti-CD3 antibodies for GvHD therapy;
- unrelated or HLA-mismatched transplants.

(Cohen *et al.*, 2007; van Esser *et al.*, 2001; van Esser *et al.*, 2002).

Although respiratory symptoms are not the main manifestation of EBV disease, monitoring of EBV in transplant patients is often recommended and diagnosis is therefore also discussed in this chapter.

Diagnosis of EBV infection

Cultures are usually not helpful in making a diagnosis. Although EBV can be isolated from the nasopharynx, culture techniques are cumbersome and time consuming. EBV DNA detection by PCR techniques may be useful for monitoring progression. Biweekly EBV monitoring is recommended in patients with three or more risk factors for developing EBV reactivation (Sandherr *et al.*, 2006).

A cut off of >500 EBN genome equivalents (GE)/10^5 lymphocytes was indicated as being associated with PTLD in pediatric SOT recipients while asymptomatic SOT recipients were mostly EBV DNA negative or showed very low (<200 GE) EBV DNA levels (Rowe *et al.*, 1997). Not all BMT patients with elevated levels of EBV DNA developed PTLD but all PTLD patients had high DNA levels (Lucas *et al.*, 1998). As with CMV there might be differences in threshold values related to each detection method but the emerging pattern indicates that PTLD is associated with high EBV DNA load in peripheral blood. At present no definitive cut-off values predictive for development of PTLD have been established (Baldanti *et al.*, 2000).

Immunodeficiency and herpes simplex virus infection

Immunocompromised people, especially organ transplant recipients, are at increased risk of widespread and devastating infection of the gastrointestinal or respiratory tract. In adults, HSV infection of the lower respiratory tract is very rare, and has been recorded almost exclusively in combination with severe immunosuppression. HSV has been visualized by immunohistochemistry in lung tissue from burn patients dying with acute lung injury, and occasionally in lower respiratory tract samples from surgical patients in intensive care units (ICUs) (Bruynseels *et al.*, 2003).

Reactivation of herpes simplex virus (HSV) predominantly results in muco-cutaneous infections in less than 1% of transplant patients (Sandherr *et al.*, 2006).

The rate of HSV in the respiratory tract of intensive care patients is found to be high. Most frequently HSV pneumonia may be acquired by endogenous reactivation or it may be introduced from colonized oropharyngeal secretions into the lower respiratory tract (Bruynseels *et al.*, 2003; Cunha *et al.*, 2007).

Diagnosis of HSV can be made by innoculation of clinical specimens (sputum, tracheal specimens, BAL) on to susceptible cell cultures followed by immunofluorecent detection after 24 hours (Bruynseels *et al.*, 2003).

Nucleic acid amplification tests are also extremely sensitive and specific for the detection of HSV nucleic acids. However, as also described for PCR detection of *Pneumocystis*, it is so far not known whether HSV PCR positivity is strictly correlated with underlying disease: molecular detection techniques may also be too sensitive and detect HSV in the lungs of asymptomatic individuals. A quantitative approach to HSV detection in lower respiratory tract samples has been suggested but has not been implemented routinely yet. Clinically relevant thresholds of DNA levels in BAL specimens have not been determined. Quantitation of HSV in BAL specimens could potentially distinguish a lower respiratory tract infection from asymptomatic colonization.

There is a need for a prospective, multicentre study comparing the conventional culture techniques with these recently developed standardized quantitative NAATs to evaluate the optimal procedure for diagnosis and treatment of these infections.

Respiratory virus infections

A multitude of reports have appeared on the epidemiology of ARI but most are restricted to a few viruses (influenza, sometimes together with RSV, to rhino-, metapneumo- or coronaviruses) and/or to some population groups for example; children, adults or old age people. Great variations occur in function of time, place and the age groups studied.

As time progresses the importance of the more recently discovered human bocavirus (Kesebir *et al.*, 2006; Kupfer *et al.*, 2006; McIntosh, 2006; Kleines *et al.*, 2007; Allander *et al.*, 2005) human metapneumovirus infections (Ordas *et al.*, 2006; Dare *et al.*, 2007; van den Hoogen *et al.*, 2001; Boivin *et al.*, 2007) and coronaviruses (Vabret *et al.*, 2006;

Koetz *et al.*, 2006) are becoming more evident. Although the role of these new viruses becomes clearer in specific patient populations, more studies are needed to identify the clinical relevance of some others such as bocavirus.

Up to now, respiratory viruses have not often been considered as possible aetiologic pathogen of pneumonia because they are mostly not routinely investigated. Respiratory viruses have, however, been increasingly recognized as causes of severe lower respiratory tract infections in immunocompromised hosts (Whimbey, Englund and Couch, 1997; Ljungman, 2007; van Elden *et al.*, 2003). Respiratory infections are more common in solid organ recipients, particularly in lung transplant recipients (Kotloff *et al.*, 2004; Dare *et al.*, 2007). Infections are especially dangerous prior to engraftment and during three months after transplantation, in the setting of graft versus host disease. The origin of the infections is community-acquired as well as nosocomial (Barron and Weinberg, 2005).

Respiratory syncytial virus, influenza- and adenovirus infections may be associated with severe infections in transplant patients (Boyton, 2005; Khushalani *et al.*, 2001; Whimbey and Bodey, 1992; La Rosa *et al.*, 2001; Ison *et al.*, 2003; Martino *et al.*, 2005; Chemaly *et al.*, 2006; Feuchtinger, Lang and Handgretinger, 2007). Parainfluenza virus type 3 is the most frequent serotype in lung transplant patients, with a rate of 10–66% of cases (Dignan *et al.*, 2006).

Disseminated adenovirus infections following stem cell transplantation are increasingly recognized particularly in children with an incidence of up to 21% (Chakrabarti *et al.*, 2002). Adenoviremia is detected during an initial asymptomatic stage and can evolve to disseminated disease. The virus probably reactivates from latency to a stage of viremia before it causes symptomatic organ disease. Increasing viral load not simple viremia leads to organ involvement (Chakrabarti, 2007).

Community respiratory viruses are relatively common causes of upper and lower respiratory infections in transplant recipients particularly after HSCT (Dykewicz, 2001). The epidemiology of respiratory viruses closely parallels the occurrence of these infections in the community such that RSV and influenza infections most commonly occur during the well defined winter and early spring 'flu season'. Parainfluenza infections however occur the year round. Adenoviruses consisting of more than 50 different serotypes may manifest as upper respiratory tract infections, gastroenteritis, haemorhagic cystitis, fatal hepatitis, menongoencephalitis or pneumonia (Nichols, 2003; Chakrabarti *et al.*, 2002).

Rhinoviruses until recently were not often detected but several studies in immunocompromised patients with CAP suggest that rhinoviruses may be one of the most frequent viruses identified (Malcolm *et al.*, 2001; Ison *et al.*, 2003).

Among bone marrow recipients Wang *et al.* (2004) found diffuse pulmonary infiltrates in 68 out of 341 (20%) bone marrow recipients. The leading diagnoses were idiopathic interstitial pneumonitis in 40% and CMV pneumonitis in 20% of the cases.

Diagnosis of respiratory virus infections

Antigens of the most common respiratory viruses such as influenza, respiratory syncytial virus (RSV), adenovirus, and parainfluenzaviruses can be detected by direct immunofluorescence or by commercially available enzyme immunoassays. The sensitivities of these tests vary from 50 to >90%. (Covalciuc, Webb and Carlson, 1999; Henrickson, 2004; Landry, Cohen and Ferguson, 2000). Several common respiratory viruses can be detected simultaneously by the use of pooled monoclonal antibodies. For the detection of influenza virus infections, the sensitivity of the immunofluorescence can be increased by innoculation of the clinical sample on appropriate cells followed by immunofluorescence applied after 48 hours. The sensitivity of the direct immuno-fluorecence (DIF) test is lower in adults and older persons than in children (Steininger *et al.*, 2002). Real time multiplex NAATs offer the solution. To cover the wide spectrum of etiologic respiratory agents a number of uni-and/or multiplex reactions are to be performed simultaneously (Lee, Robinson and Khurana, 2006). Templeton developed a two tube real-time multiplex PCR for the diagnosis of influenza A and B and RSV in a first tube and the four parainfluenzaviruses in a second tube (Templeton *et al.*, 2004). The sensitivity was higher than culture or DIF test but no comparisons were made between multiplex reactions and monoreactions on the same samples. Gruteke (Gruteke *et al.*, 2004) applied four multiplex reactions to detect 11 agents, Templeton (Templeton *et al.*, 2005) covered 15 agents by six multiplex real-time reactions and Gunson *et al.* (Gunson, Collins and Carman, 2005) targeted 12 agents through four real-time multiplex reactions.

Combined with traditional bacteriologic techniques to diagnose *Streptococcus pneumoniae* infections, only 24% of the infections remained etiologically undefined in the multiplex study by Templeton (Templeton *et al.*, 2005) and only 14% in the study by Gruteke (Gruteke *et al.*, 2004). All studies were limited in time and were pilot trials. More research is needed to identify those reactions that can be combined with a minimal loss in sensitivity.

The more than 100 rhinovirus types and their close relationship with enteroviruses constitute a special challenge. The judicious choice of primers and particularly of the hybridization probes should ensure a satisfactory coverage of the rhinovirus types as illustrated by the work of Loens (Loens *et al.*, 2003; Loens *et al.*, 2006): by the use of new primers, rhinoviruses were detected five times more frequently in clinical samples than traditional culture techniques and two to three times more than in studies using previously described primers.

As more epidemiological information on the role of a panel of respiratory viral pathogens becomes available, it is clear that screening for these viruses in specific patient populations such as immunocompromised patients, is desirable and preventive and therapeutic recommendations may take this information into account.

Bacterial respiratory infections

Besides the common respiratory pathogens, gram positive but a greater variety of opportunistic gram negative bacteria may cause respiratory infections in immunodeficient patients, such as Flavobacterium spp. (Manfredi *et al.*, 1999), *Serratia marcescens* (Manfredi *et al.*, 2000a), Pseudomonas spp. (Manfredi *et al.*, 2000b), Alcaligenes spp. (Manfredi *et al.*, 1997), *Stenotrophomonas maltophilia* (Calzo, Manfredi and Chiodo,

2003). The infections are frequently accompanied by septicemia. Viridans streptoccal shock syndrome may complicate HSCT particularly in children (Bochud, Candra and Francioli, 1994; Gassas *et al.*, 2004). Fever that continues after three to five days of broad spectrum antibiotic therapy is frequently due to fungal infections with *Candida* species as the primary infectious agents.

In the late post-transplantation phase (+100 days) sepsis is likely to be caused by encapsulated organisms such as *Streptococcus pneumoniae* and *Haemophilus influenzae*. Abnormalities of the pulmonary parenchyma are common after HSCT, and may result from the broadest range of infectious as well as noninfectious causes.

Diagnosis of bacterial respiratory infections

Bacterial infections, both the common etiologic respiratory agents as the opportunistic gram positives and gram negatives frequently detected in the immunocompromised patients, are diagnosed by both the conventional culture techniques, rapid techniques such as the immunochromatographic tests, urinary antigen tests and particularly the nucleic acid amplification tests (NAATs) in the most adequate clinical samples. These include either normally sterile samples such as blood cultures, pleural fluid, CT-guided fine-needle aspiration or open lung biopsy, or non sterile sampling sites. The first approach is generally by a BAL. The fluid obtained should be examined for an as wide as possible battery of tests to reveal bacteria and viruses (Cordonnier and Cunningham, 1998). The difficulty in establishing a laboratory diagnosis is identical to that for NTM and is frequently based on quantitative cultures of samples obtained by invasive techniques. These techniques have been described previously and will therefore not be discussed in this chapter (Ieven, 2007).

Fungal respiratory infections

Pneumonia due to *Pneumocystis jiroveci* occurs in up to 10% of HSCT recipients after nine weeks in the absence of specific prophylaxis (Nichols, 2003).

The incidence of fungal infections is high in transplant patients. They occur in 2–14% of infectious complications after kidney transplantation, in up to 3% of the pneumonias after liver transplantation, in 15–25% of patients after lung transplantation, in up to 20% of patients after bone marrow transplantation, and more after allogeneic than after autologous marrow transplantation (Nicod, Pache and Howarth, 2001).

Invasive aspergillosis is mainly due to *Aspergillus fumigatus* and *Aspergillus flavus*.

Mucormycosis is due to the genera *Mucor, Absidia* or *Rhizopus*. Rhinocerebral mucormycosis is best known in diabetic patients. Invasive fungal infections caused by unfamiliar species are increasingly being reported such as *Fusarium* and *Penicillium marneffei*. Disseminated candidiasis is a common opportunistic mycosis in severely immunocompromised patients, mostly following stem cell transplantation (Wheat, Goldman and Sarosi, 2002). Patients with AIDS and solid organ transplant recipients are at risk for endemic mycoses, histoplasmosis, coccidioidomycosis, blastomycosis and cryptococcosis.

Diagnosis of fungal infections is based on isolation of the organisms from normally sterile sites, however, disappointingly poor for aspergillosis (Reichenberger *et al.*, 1999), and in its absence the documentation of invasive disease by isolation of the fungi from the affected tissue or their presence in the tissues as evidenced by histopathology. Invasive disease by *Candida* in a patient with pulmonary infiltrates cannot be based on the sole isolation of the fungus from a sputum specimen, histologic confirmation of invasive disease is essential for diagnosis and the institution of aggressive antifungal therapy (Zamora, 2004). As a result of the inherent difficulties to document pulmonary aspergillosis the European Organization for the Research and Treatment of Cancer/Mycosis Group has proposed an algorithm for the diagnosis of aspergillosis (Ascioglu *et al.*, 2002).

Definite invasive pulmonary aspergillosis

1. Positive result of histological testing and positive result of culture from lung tissue obtained by biopsy or autopsy.

2. Positive result of culture of a specimen obtained from a normally sterile site by use of aseptic invasive technique.

Probable invasive pulmonary aspergillosis

1. *Aspergillus*-positive lower respiratory tract specimen culture.

2. Compatible signs and symptoms: fever refractory to at least three days of appropriate antibiotic therapy; recrudescent fever after a period of defervescence of at least 48 hours of antibiotics and without other apparent cause; pleuritic chest pain, pleuritic rub, dyspnoea, haemoptysis, worsening respiratory insufficiency in spite of appropriate antibiotic therapy and ventilatory support.

3. Abnormal medical imaging by portable chest X-ray or computerized tomography of the lungs.

4. Either:

    (a) host risk factors: one of the following conditions:

         • neutropenia (absolute neutrophil count less then 500/mm^3) preceding or at the time of ICU admission;

         • underlying haematological or oncological malignancy treated with cytotoxic agents;

         • glucocorticoid treatment (prednisone or equivalent, >20 mg/day);

         • congenital or acquired immunodeficiency.

    Or:

    (b) Semiquantitative *Aspergillus*-positive culture of BAL (+ or ++), without bacterial growth, together with a positive cytotological smear showing branching hyphae.

Aspergillus colonization

Not fulfilling the criteria for proven or probable invasive pulmonary aspergillosis.

Monitoring for *Aspergillus galactomannan* antigenemia assists in early diagnosis of invasive aspergillosis (Wheat, 2003). On this basis preemptive therapy of fungal infections can be considered (Maertens *et al.*, 2006).

The cut-off criterion for a positive test is 0.5. The highest sensitivity of the test is obtained by testing twice weekly. The sensitivity of the test using a 0.5 index cut-off is 59% but 89% in the subgroup not receiving mould-active antifungal therapy (Marr *et al.*, 2005). Some antibiotics, piperacillin-tazobactam and other β-lactam antibiotics are important causes of false positive results while antifungal agents reduce the sensitivity of galactomannan testing. Galactamanan detection in solid organ transplant patients and in BAL fluid requires further investigation.

$(1 \rightarrow 3)$-β-D-glucan assay yields results in a few hours, is negative in zygomycosis and cryptococcosis, and is reported to have a sensitivity in aspergillosis of 71–97% with a specificity of 54–93%. (Digby *et al.*, 2003; Odabasi *et al.*, 2004; Kawazu *et al.*, 2004 and Pazos, Panton and Del Palacio, 2005) The previous studies mention a sensitivity of 50–90% but false positive results are common.

PCR for invasive aspergillosis is not superior to galactonmannan testing (Donnelly, 2006). However, recent progress in PCR technology, such as automatic nucleic acid extraction and real-time PCR, have been insufficiently evaluated in this area.

2.6   Concluding remarks

With the armamentarium available it is, however, hard to conceive that every hospital laboratory would perform the broad spectrum of RT NAATs, even if standardized reagents at low cost become widely available. Strategies will have to be developed or adapted to the evolution of the technology of the NAATs, the population of patients served (children, elderly, immunocompromised patients) the resources available (infrastructure, staff, full-time service or service limited during some hours of the day, or some days of the week) and the number and nature of the agents that can be covered. Permanent consultation between laboratorians and clinicians is becoming more necessary than ever.

Practical issues in the laboratory may limit the theoretical possibilities of the rapid NAATs such as the necessity to handle specimens in batches, thereby losing some advantages of the rapidity of the tests. Moreover virology laboratories at present do not operate 24/7, but the situation may change as more molecular tests may be required as an emergency, perhaps outside the field of infectious diseases.

Laboratories might limit their initial investigations to the antibiotic treatable, bacterial infections and the most important viral infections such as influenza and RSV, avoiding unnecessary antibiotic treatment. For community-acquired bacterial pneumonia the Gram staining of a sputum specimen remains a fundamental and rapid low cost diagnostic procedure. It could be combined in a first approach with a multiplex NAAT for the diagnosis of the slowly growing, antibiotic sensitive bacteria, *Mycoplasma pneumoniae*, *Chlamydophila pneumoniae*, *Legionella pneumophila* *Bordetella pertussis*.

A positive result may lead to adaptation of antibiotic therapy, when these results are negative, tests for viral causes may be initiated, although at present most clinicians do not stop antibiotics in patients found negative for a bacterial cause. However, it is clear that screening for respiratory viruses in specific patient populations such as immuno-compromised patients, is desirable and preventive and therapeutic recommendations may take this information into account.

A closer collaboration between clinicians and the laboratory has a high priority.

Key learning points

Infections in immununodeficient patients are discussed mainly in HIV and transplant patients, similar infections occurring in cancer, during chemotherapy and in other conditions impairing the immune system. The main concern for the diagnosis of opportunistic infections is the differentiation between colonization and infection, the most important reliable criterium being the identification of an organism in normally sterile clinical specimens. Culture procedures in general lack sensitivity and are slow especially for the diagnosis of respiratory viral infections: the role of amplification techniques is therefore discussed. Rapid diagnostic methods, immunofluorescence on clinical specimens and nucleic acids amplification techniques, are also useful for monitoring transplant patients for viruses of the herpes virus group such as CMV and EBV. For the most important infections diagnostic guidelines have been proposed.

References

Afessa, B. and Peters, S.G. (2006) Major complications following hematopoietic stem cell transplantation, semin respir. *Critical Care Medicine*, **27**, 297–309.

Allander, T., Tammi, M.T., Eriksson, M. *et al.* (2005) Cloning of a human parvovirus by molecular screening of respiratory tract samples. *Proceedings of the National Academy of Sciences of the United States of America*, **102**, 12891–12896.

American Thoracic Society (2007) Diagnosis and treatment of disease caused by Nontuberculous Mycobacteria. *American Journal of Respiratory and Critical Care Medicine*, **156**, S1–S25.

Ascioglu, S., Rex, J.H., de Pauw, B. *et al.* (2002) Defining opportunistic invasive fungal infections in immunocompromised patients with cancer and hematopoietic stem cell transplants: an international consensus. *Clinical Infectious Diseases*, **34**, 7–14.

Baldanti, F., Grossi, P., Furione, M. *et al.* (2000) High levels of Epstein-Barr virus DNA in blood of solid-organ transplant recipients and their value in predicting posttransplant lymphoproliferative disorders. *Journal of Clinical Microbiology*, **38**, 613–619.

Barron, M.A. and Weinberg, A. (2005) Common viral infections in transplant recipients, Part 2. Respiratory viruses, polyomaviruses, and erythroviruses. *Clinical Microbiology Newsletter*, **27**, 115–122.

Bhorade, S.M., Sandesara, C., Garrity, E.R. *et al.* (2001) Quantification of cytomegalovirus (CMV) viral load by the hybrid capture assay allows for early detection of CMV disease in lung transplant recipients. *The Journal of Heart and Lung Transplantation*, **20**, 928–934.

Bochud, P.Y., Calandra, T. and Francioli, P. (1994) Bacteremia due to viridans streptococci in neutropenic patients: A review. *The American Journal of Medicine*, **97**, 256–264.

Boeckh, M., Huang, M., Ferrenberg, J. *et al.* (2004) Optimization of quantitative detection of cytomegalovirus DNA in plasma by real-time PCR. *Journal of Clinical Microbiology*, **42**, 1142–1148.

Boivin, G., De Serres, G., Hamelin, M.E. *et al.* (2007) An outbreak of severe respiratory tract infection due to human metapneumovirus in a long-term care facility. *Clinical Infectious Diseases*, **44** (9), 1152–1158. Epub 2007 Mar 28.

Boyton, R.J. (2005) Infectious lung complications in patients with HIV/AIDS. *Current Opinion in Pulmonary Medicine*, **11**, 203–207.

Brancart, F., Rodriguez-Villalobos, H., Fonteyne, P.A. *et al.* (2005) Quantitative TaqMan PCR for detection of Pneumocystis jiroveci. *Journal of Microbiological Methods*, **61**, 381–387.

Bruynseels, P., Jorens, P.G., Demey, H.E. *et al.* (2003) Herpes simplex virus in the respiratory tract of critical care patients: a prospective study. *Lancet*, **362**, 1536–1541.

Caliendo, A.M., Ingersoll, J., Fox-Canale, A.M. *et al.* (2007) Evaluation of real-time PCR laboratory-developed tests using analyte-specific reagents for cytomegalovirus quantification. *Journal of Clinical Microbiology*, **45**, 1723–1727.

Calzo, L., Manfredi, R. and Chiodo, F. (2003) Stenotrophomonas (Xanthomonas) maltophilia as an emerging opportunistic pathogen in association with HIV infection: a 10-year surveillance study. *Infection*, **31**, 155–161.

CDC (2000) Update: Nucleic acid amplification tests for tuberculosis. *Morbidity and Mortality Weekly Report*, **49**, 593–594.

Chakrabarti, S. (2007) Adenovirus infections after hematopoietic stem cell transplantation: still unravelling the story. *Clinical Infectious Diseases*, **45**, 066–968.

Chakrabarti, S., Mautner, V., Osman, H. *et al.* (2002) Adenovirus infections following allogeneic stem cell transplantation: incidence and outcome in relation to graft manipulation, immunosuppression and immune recovery. *Blood*, **100**, 1619–1627.

Chemaly, R.F., Ghosh, S., Bodey, G. *et al.* (2006) Respiratory viral infections in adults with hematologic malignancies and human stem cell transplantation recipients: a retrospective study at a major cancer center. *Medicine (Baltimore)*, **85**, 278–287.

Cohen, J.M., Cooper, N., Chakrabarti, S. *et al.* (2007) EBV-related disease following haematopoietic stem cell transplantation with reduced intensity conditioning. *Leukemia & Lymphoma*, **48**, 256–269.

Cordonnier, C. and Cunningham, I. (1998) Transplant Infections (eds R.A. Bowden, P. Ljungman and C.V. Paya), Lippincott-Raven, Philadelphia, USA, pp. 105–120.

Covalciuc, K.A., Webb, K.H. and Carlson, C.A. (1999) Comparison of four clinical specimen types for detection of influenza A and B viruses by optical immunoassay (FLU OIA test) and cell culture methods. *Journal of Clinical Microbiology*, **37**, 3971–3974.

Crump, J.A., Tanner, D.C., Mirrett, S. *et al.* (2003) Controlled comparison of BACTEC 13A, MYCO/F LYTIC, BacT/ALERT MB, and ISOLATOR 10 systems for detection of mycobacteremia. *Journal of Clinical Microbiology*, **41**, 1987–1990.

Cunha, B.A., Eisenstein, L.E., Dillard, T. and Krol, V. (2007) Herpes simplex virus (HSV) pneumonia in a heart transplant: diagnosis and therapy. *Heart Lung*, **36**, 72–78.

Daley, C.L., Small, P.M., Schecter, G.F. *et al.* (1992) An outbreak of tuberculosis with accelerated progression among persons infected with the human immunodeficiency virus. An analysis using restriction-fragment-length polymorphisms. *The New England Journal of Medicine*, **326**, 231–235.

Dare, R., Sanghavi, S., Bullotta, A. *et al.* (2007) Diagnosis of human metapneumovirus infection in immunosuppressed lung transplant recipients and children evaluated for pertussis. *Journal of Clinical Microbiology*, **45**, 48–52.

Di Perri, G., Cruciani, M., Danzi, M.C. *et al.* (1989) Nosocomial epidemic of active tuberculosis among HIV-infected patients. *Lancet*, **2**, 1502–1504.

Digby, J., Kalbfleisch, J., Glenn, A. *et al.* (2003) Serum glucan levels are not specific for presence of fungal infections in intensive care unit patients. *Clinical and Diagnostic Laboratory Immunology*, **10**, 882–885.

Dignan, F., Alvares, C., Riley, U. *et al.* (2006) Parainfluenza type 3 infection post stem cell transplant: high prevalence but low mortality. *The Journal of Hospital Infection*, **63**, 452–458.

Donnelly, J.P. (2006) Polymerase chain reaction for diagnosing invasive aspergillosis: getting closer but still a ways to go. *Clinical Infectious Diseases*, **42**, 487–489.

Dykewicz, C.A. (2001) Guidelines for preventing opportunistic infections among hematopoietic stem cell transplant recipients: focus on community respiratory virus infections. *Biology of Blood and Marrow Transplantation*, **7**, 19S–22S.

Elliott, A.M., Namaambo, K., Allen, B.W. *et al.* (1993) Negative sputum smear results in HIV-positive patients with pulmonary tuberculosis in Lusaka, Zambia. *Tubercle and Lung Disease*, **74**, 191–194.

Emery, V.C., Sabin, C.A., Cope, A.V. *et al.* (2000) Application of viral-load kinetics to identify patients who develop cytomegalovirus disease after transplantation. *Lancet*, **355**, 2032–2036.

Eng, R.H., Bishburg, E., Smith, S.M. and Mangia, A. (1989) Diagnosis of Mycobacterium bacteremia in patients with acquired immunodeficiency syndrome by direct examination of blood films. *Journal of Clinical Microbiology*, **27**, 768–769.

Enzensberger, R., Hunfeld, K.P., Krause, M. *et al.* (1999) Mycobacterium malmoense infections in immunocompetent patients. *European Journal of Clinical Microbiology & Infectious Diseases*, **18**, 579–581.

Feuchtinger, T., Lang, P. and Handgretinger, R. (2007) Adenovirus infection after allogeneic stem cell transplantation. *Leukemia & Lymphoma*, **48**, 244–255.

Fishman, J.A., Emery, V., Freeman, R. *et al.* (2007) Cytomegalovirus in transplantation–challenging the status quo. *Clinical Transplantation*, **21**, 149–158.

Gassas, A., Grant, R., Richardson, S. *et al.* (2004) Predictors of viridans streptococcal shock syndrome in bacteremic children with cancer and stem-cell transplant recipients. *Journal of Clinical Oncology*, **22**, 1222–1227.

Gentile, G., Picardi, A., Capobianchi, A. *et al.* (2006) A prospective study comparing quantitative Cytomegalovirus (CMV) polymerase chain reaction in plasma and pp65 antigenemia assay in monitoring patients after allogeneic stem cell transplantation. *BMC Infectious Diseases*, **6**, 167.

Getahun, H., Harrington, M., O'Brien, R. and Nunn, P. (2007) Diagnosis of smear-negative pulmonary tuberculosis in people with HIV infection or AIDS in resource-constrained settings: informing urgent policy changes. *Lancet*, **369**, 2042–2049.

Ghisetti, V., Barbui, A., Franchello, A. *et al.* (2004) Quantitation of cytomegalovirus DNA by the polymerase chain reaction as a predictor of disease in solid organ transplantation. *Journal of Medical Virology*, **73**, 223–229.

Gruteke, P., Glas, A.S., Dierdorp, M. *et al.* (2004) Practical implementation of a multiplex PCR for acute respiratory tract infections in children. *Journal of Clinical Microbiology*, **42**, 5596–5603.

Gunson, R.N., Collins, T.C. and Carman, W.F. (2005) Real-time RT-PCR detection of 12 respiratory viral infections in four triplex reactions. *Journal of Clinical Virology*, **33**, 341–344.

Haller, A., von Segesser, L., Baumann, P.C. and Krause, M. (1995) Severe respiratory insufficiency complicating Epstein-Barr virus infection: Case report and review. *Clinical Infectious Diseases*, **21**, 206–209.

Hanna, B.A., Walters, S.B., Bonk, S.J. and Tick, L.J. (1995) Recovery of mycobacteria from blood in mycobacteria growth indicator tube and Lowenstein-Jensen slant after lysis-centrifugation. *Journal of Clinical Microbiology*, **33**, 3315–3316.

Harries, A.D., Maher, D. and Nunn, P. (1998) An approach to the problems of diagnosing and treating adult smear-negative pulmonary tuberculosis in high-HIV-prevalence settings in sub-Saharan Africa. *Bulletin of the World Health Organization*, **76**, 651–662.

Henrickson, K.J. (2004) Advances in the laboratory diagnosis of viral respiratory disease. *The Pediatric Infectious Disease Journal*, **23**, S6–S10.

Henry, M.T., Inamdar, L., O'Riordain, D. *et al.* (2004) Nontuberculous mycobacteria in non-HIV patients: epidemiology, treatment and response. *The European Respiratory Journal*, **23**, 741–746.

Hughes, W.T. (1989) Current issues in the epidemiology, transmission, and reactivation of Pneumocystis carinii. *Semin Respir Infect*, **13**, 283–288.

Ieven, M. (2007) Microbiological diagnosis of community acquired pneumonia, in *Community Acquired Pneumonia* (ed. A. Torres), John Wiley and Sons Ltd, United Kingdom, 43–67.

Ison, M.G., Hayden, F.G., Kaiser, L. *et al.* (2003) Rhinovirus infections in hematopoietic stem cell transplant recipients with pneumoni. *Clinical Infectious Diseases*, **36**, 1139–1143.

Karstaedt, A.S., Jones, N., Khoosal, M. and Crewe-Brown, H.H. (1998) The bacteriology of pulmonary tuberculosis in a population with high human immunodeficiency virus seroprevalence. *International Journal of Tuberculosis and Lung Disease*, **2**, 312–316.

Kawazu, M., Kanda, Y., Nannya, Y. *et al.* (2004) Prospective comparison of the diagnostic potential of real-time PCR, double-sandwich enzyme-linked immunosorbent assay for galactomannan, and a $(1 \rightarrow 3)$-beta-D-glucan test in weekly screening for invasive aspergillosis in patients with hematological disorders. *Journal of Clinical Microbiology*, **42**, 2733–2741.

Kesebir, D., Vazquez, M., Weibel, C. *et al.* (2006) Human bocavirus infection in young children in the United States: molecular epidemiological profile and clinical characteristics of a newly emerging respiratory virus. *The Journal of Infectious Diseases*, **94**, 1276–1282.

Khushalani, N.I., Bakri, F.G., Wentling, D. *et al.* (2001) Respiratory syncytial virus infection in the late bone marrow transplant period: report of three cases and review. *Bone Marrow Transplantation*, **27**, 1071–1073.

Kleines, M., Scheithauer, S., Rackowitz, A. *et al.* (2007) High prevalence of human bocavirus detected in young children with severe acute lower respiratory tract disease by use of a standard PCR protocol and a novel real-time PCR protocol. *Journal of Clinical Microbiology*, **45**, 1032–1034.

Koetz, A., Nilsson, P., Linden, M. *et al.* (2006) Detection of human coronavirus NL63, human metapneumovirus and respiratory syncytial virus in children with respiratory tract infections in south-west Sweden. *Clinical Microbiology and Infection*, **12**, 1089–1096.

Kotloff, R.M., Ahya, V.N. and Crawford, S.W. (2004) Pulmonary complications of solid organ and hematopoietic stem cell transplantation. *American Journal of Respiratory and Critical Care Medicine*, **170**, 22–48.

Kupfer, B., Vehreschild, J., Cornely, O. *et al.* (2006) Severe pneumonia and human bocavirus in adult. *Emerging Infectious Diseases*, **12**, 1614–1616.

La Rosa, A.M., Champlin, R.E., Mirza, N. *et al.* (2001) Adenovirus infections in adult recipients of blood and marrow transplant. *Clinical Infectious Diseases*, **32**, 871–876.

Landry, M.L., Cohen, S. and Ferguson, D. (2000) Impact of sample type on rapid detection of influenza virus A by cytospin-enhanced immunofluorescence and membrane enzyme-linked immunosorbent assay. *Journal of Clinical Microbiology*, **38**, 429–430.

Lee, B.E., Robinson, J.L. and Khurana, V. (2006) Enhanced detection of viral and atypical bacterial pathogens in lower respiratory tract samples with nucleic acid amplification tests. *Journal of Medical Virology*, **78**, 702–710.

Li, C.R., Greenberg, P.D., Gilbert, M.J. *et al.* (1994) Recovery of HLA-restricted cytomegalovirus (CMV)-specific T-cell responses after allogeneic bone marrow transplant: correlation with CMVdisease and effect of ganciclovir prophylaxis. *Blood*, **83**, 1971–1979.

Ljungman, P. (2007) Respiratory virus infections in bone marrow transplant recipients: the European perspective. *The American Journal of Medicine*, **102**, 44–47.

Ljungman, P., Griffiths, P. and Paya, C. (2002) Definitions of cytomegalovirus infection and disease in transplant recipients. *Clinical Infectious Diseases*, **34**, 1094–1097.

Loens, K., Ieven, M., Ursi, D. *et al.* (2003) Improved detection of rhinoviruses by nucleic acid sequence-based amplification after nucleotide sequence determination of the 5' noncoding regions of additional rhinovirus strains. *Journal of Clinical Microbiology*, **41**, 1971–1976.

Loens, K., Goossens, H., De Laat, C. *et al.* (2006) Detection of rhinoviruses by tissue culture and two independent amplification techniques, nucleic acid sequence-based amplification and reverse transcription-PCR, in children with acute respiratory infections during a winter season. *Journal of Clinical Microbiology*, **44**, 166–171.

Lucas, K.G., Burton, R.L., Zimmerman, S.E. *et al.* (1998) Semiquantitative Epstein-Barr virus (EBV) polymerase chain reaction for the determination of patients at risk for EBV-induced lymphoproliferative disease after stem cell transplantation. *Blood*, **91**, 3654–3661.

Maertens, J., Deeren, D., Dierickx, D. and Theunissen, K. (2006) Pre-emptive antifungal therapy: still a way to go. *Current Opinion in Infectious Diseases*, **19**, 551–556.

Malcolm, E., Arruda, E., Hayden, F.G. and Kaiser, L. (2001) Clinical features of patients with acute respiratory illness and rhinovirus in their bronchoalveolar lavages. *Journal of Clinical Virology*, **21**, 9–16.

Manfredi, R., Nanetti, A., Ferri, M. and Chiodo, F. (1997) Bacteremia and respiratory involvement by Alcaligenes xylosoxidans in patients infected with the human immunodeficiency virus. *European Journal of Clinical Microbiology & Infectious Diseases*, **6**, 933–938 Review.

Manfredi, R., Nanetti, A., Ferri, M. *et al.* (1999) Flavobacterium spp. organisms as opportunistic bacterial pathogens during advanced HIV disease. *The Journal of Infection*, **39**, 146–152.

Manfredi, R., Nanetti, A., Ferri, M. and Chiodo, F. (2000a) Clinical and microbiological survey of Serratia marcescens infection during HIV disease. *European Journal of Clinical Microbiology & Infectious Diseases*, **19**, 248–253.

Manfredi, R., Nanetti, A., Ferri, M. and Chiodo, Fl. (2000b) Pseudomonas spp. complications in patients with HIV disease: an eight-year clinical and microbiological survey. *European Journal of Epidemiology*, **16**, 111–118.

Marr, K.A., Laverdiere, M., Gugel, A. and Leisenring, W. (2005) Antifungal therapy decreases sensitivity of the Aspergillus galactomannan enzyme immunoassay. *Clinical Infectious Diseases*, **40**, 1762–1769.

Martino, R., Porras, R.P., Rabella, N. *et al.* (2005) Prospective study of the incidence, clinical features, and outcome of symptomatic upper and lower respiratory tract infections by respiratory viruses in adult recipients of hematopoietic stem cell transplants for hematologic malignancies. *Biology of Blood and Marrow Transplantation*, **11**, 781–796.

Marty, F.M. and Rubin, R.H. (2006) The prevention of infection post-transplant: the role of prophylaxis, preemptive and empiric therapy. *Transplant International*, **19**, 2–11.

Matulis, M. and High, K.P. (2002) Immune reconstitution after hematopoietic stem-cell transplantation and its influence on respiratory infections. *Seminars in Respiratory Infections*, **17**, 130–139.

Mazzulli, T., Drew, L.W., Yen-Lieberman, B. *et al.* (1999) Multicenter comparison of the digene hybrid capture CMV DNA assay (version 2.0), the pp65 antigenemia assay, and cell culture for detection of cytomegalovirus viremia. *Journal of Clinical Microbiology*, **37**, 958–963.

McIntosh, K. (2006) Human bocavirus: Developing evidence for pathogenicity. *The Journal of Infectious Diseases*, **194**, 1197–1199.

Miguez-Burbano, M.J., Flores, M., Ashkin, D. *et al.* (2006) Non-tuberculous mycobacteria disease as a cause of hospitalization in HIV-infected subjects. *International Journal of Infectious Diseases*, **10**, 47–55.

Miller, R. and Huang, L. (2004) Pneumocystis jirovecii infection. *Thorax*, **59**, 731–733.

Morris, A., Kingsley, L.A., Groner, G. *et al.* (2004) Prevalence and clinical predictors of Pneumocystis colonization among HIV-infected men. *AIDS (London, England)*, **18**, 793–798.

Murray, J.F. (2005) Pulmonary complications of HIV-1 infection among adults living in Sub-Saharan Africa. *International Journal of Tuberculosis and Lung Disease*, **9**, 826–835.

Nichols, W.G. (2003) Management of infectious complications in the hematopoietic stem cell transplant recipient. *Journal of Intensive Care Medicine*, **18**, 295–312.

Nicod, L.P., Pache, J.C. and Howarth, N. (2001) Fungal infections in transplant recipients. *The European Respiratory Journal*, **17**, 133–140.

Nosari, A., Anghilieri, M., Carrafiello, G. *et al.* (2003) Utility of percutaneous lung biopsy for diagnosing filamentous fungal infections in hematologic malignancies. *Haematologica*, **88**, 1405–1409.

Odabasi, Z., Mattiuzzi, G., Estey, E. *et al.* (2004) Beta-D-glucan as a diagnostic adjunct for invasive fungal infections: validation, cutoff development, and performance in patients with acute myelogenous leukemia and myelodysplastic syndrome. *Clinical Infectious Diseases*, **39**, 199–205.

Ordas, J., Boga, J.A., Alvarez-Arguelles, M. *et al.* (2006) Role of metapneumovirus in viral respiratory infections in young children. *Journal of Clinical Microbiology*, **44**, 2739–2742.

Pazos, C., Ponton, J. and Del Palacio, A. (2005) Contribution of $(1 \rightarrow 3)$-beta-D-glucan chromogenic assay to diagnosis and therapeutic monitoring of invasive aspergillosis in neutropenic adult patients: a comparison with serial screening for circulating galactomannan. *Journal of Clinical Microbiology*, **43**, 299–305.

Razonable, R.R. and Emery, V.C. (2004) Management of CMV infection and disease in transplant patients. *Herpes*, **11**, 77–86.

Razonable, R.R. and Paya, C.V. (2003) Herpesvirus infections in transplant recipients: current challenges in the clinical management of cytomegalovirus and Epstein-Barr virus infections. *Herpes*, **10**, 60–65.

Razonable, R.R., Brown, R.A., Humar, A. *et al.* (2005) Herpesvirus infections in solid organ transplant patients at high risk of primary cytomegalovirus disease. *The Journal of Infectious Diseases*, **192**, 1331–1339.

Reichenberger, F., Habicht, J., Matt, P. *et al.* (1999) Diagnostic yield of bronchoscopy in histologically proven invasive aspergillosis. *Bone Marrow Transplantation*, **24**, 1195–1199.

Rowe, D.T., Qu, L., Reyes, J., Jabbour, N. *et al.* (1997) Use of quantitative competitive PCR to measure Epstein-Barr virus genome load in the peripheral blood of pediatric transplant patients with lymphoproliferative disorders. *Journal of Clinical Microbiology*, **35**, 1612–1615.

Rubin, R.H. (1996) Prevention of infection in the liver transplant recipient. *Liver Transplantation and Surgery*, *(*Suppl 1), 89–98.

Ruell, J., Barnes, C., Mutton, K. *et al.* (2007) Active CMV disease does not always correlate with viral load detection. *Bone Marrow Transplantation*, **40**, 55–61.

Sandherr, M., Einsele, H., Hebart, H. *et al.* (2006) Antiviral prophylaxis in patients with haematological malignancies and solid tumours: Guidelines of the Infectious Diseases Working Party (AGIHO) of the German Society for Hematology and Oncology (DGHO). *Annals of Oncology*, **17**, 1051–1059.

Sia, I.G. and Patel, R. (2000) New strategies for prevention and therapy of cytomegalovirus infection and disease in solid-organ transplant recipients. *Clinical Microbiology Reviews*, **13**, 83–121.

Steininger, C., Kundi, M., Aberle, S.W. *et al.* (2002) Effectiveness of reverse transcription-PCR, virus isolation, and enzyme-linked immunosorbent assay for diagnosis of influenza A virus infection in different age groups. *Journal of Clinical Microbiology*, **40**, 2051–2056.

Templeton, K.E., Scheltinga, S.A., Beersma, M.F. *et al.* (2004) Rapid and sensitive method using multiplex real-time PCR for diagnosis of infections by influenza A and influenza B viruses, respiratory syncytial virus, and parainfluenza viruses 1, 2, 3 and 4. *Journal of Clinical Microbiology*, **42**, 1564–1569.

Templeton, K.E., Scheltinga, S.A., van den Eeden, W.C. *et al.* (2005) Improved diagnosis of the etiology of community-acquired pneumonia with real-time polymerase chain reaction. *Clinical Infectious Diseases*, **41**, 345–351.

Thorne, L.B., Civalier, C., Booker, J. *et al.* (2007) Analytic validation of a quantitative real-time PCR assay to measure CMV viral load in whole blood. *Diagnostic Molecular Pathology: The American Journal of Surgical Pathology, Part B*, **16**, 73–80.

Tortoli, E., Piersimoni, C., Bartoloni, A. *et al.* (1997) Mycobacterium malmoense in Italy: the modern Norman invasion? *European Journal of Epidemiology*, **13**, 341–346.

Vabret, A., Dina, J., Gouarin, S. *et al.* (2006) Detection of the new human coronavirus HKU1: a report of 6 cases. *Clinical Infectious Diseases*, **42**, 34–39 Epub 2006 Jan 24.

van den Hoogen, B.G., de Jong, J.C., Groen, J. *et al.* (2001) A newly discovered human pneumovirus isolated from young children with respiratory tract disease. *Nature Medicine*, **7**, 719–724.

van Elden, L.J., van Loon, A.M., van der Beeck, M. *et al.* (2003) Applicability of real-time quantitative PCR assay for diagnosis of respiratory syncycial virus infection in immunocompromised patients. *Journal of Clinical Microbiology*, **41**, 5378–7381.

van Esser, J.W., Niesters, H.G., Thijsen, S.F. *et al.* (2001) Molecular quantification of viral load in plasma allows for fast and accurate prediction of response to therapy of Epstein-Barr virus-associated lymphoproliferative disease after allogeneic stem cell transplantation. *British Journal of Haematology*, **113**, 814–821.

van Esser, J.W., Niesters, H.G., van der Holt, B. *et al.* (2002) Prevention of Epstein-Barr virus-lymphoproliferative disease by molecular monitoring and preemptive rituximab in high-risk patients after allogeneic stem cell transplantation. *Blood*, **99**, 4364–4369.

Wakefeld, A.E., Pixley, F.J., Banerji, S. *et al.* (1990) Detection of Pneumocystis carinii with DNA detection. *Lancet*, **336**, 451–453.

Wang, J.Y., Chang, Y.L., Lee, L.N. *et al.* (2004) Diffuse pulmonary infiltrates after bone marrow transplantation: the role of open lung biopsy. *The Annals of Thoracic Surgery*, **78**, 267–272 Review.

Wheat, L.J. (2003) Rapid diagnosis of invasive aspergillosis by antigen detection. *Transplant Infectious Disease*, **5**, 158–166.

Wheat, L.J., Goldman, M. and Sarosi, G. (2002) State-of-the-art review of pulmonary fungal infections. *Seminars in Respiratory Infections*, **17**, 158–181.

Whimbey, E. and Bodey, G.P. (1992) Viral pneumonia in the immunocompromised adult with neoplastic disease: the role of common community respiratory viruses. *Seminars in Respiratory Infections*, **7**, 122–131.

Whimbey, E., Englund, J.A. and Couch, R.B. (1997) Community respiratory virus infections in immunocompromised patients with cancer. *The American Journal of Medicine*, **102**, 10–18.

Zamora, M.R. (2004) Cytomegalovirus and lung transplantation. *American Journal of Transplantation*, **8**, 1219–1226.

3

Diagnosis of pneumonia in immunocompromised patient

Robert P. Baughman and Elyse E. Lower
University of Cincinnati Medical Center, Cincinnati, USA

3.1 Introduction

Regardless of the underlying cause of immunosuppression, pneumonia remains one of the most common infections in immunocompromised patients. There is an increased mortality for inadequate treatment of pneumonia (Iregui *et al.*, 2002; Kollef and Ward, 1998). Because there is a vast array of possible pathogens responsible for the pneumonia (Baughman, 1999), broad spectrum antibiotics are frequently employed to cover all potential pathogens. This leads to increased antimicrobial resistance in the patient and in the hospital. In some cases, de-escalation of antibiotics after 3–5 days has become a recommended approach to reduce the rate of antimicrobial resistance (Anon, 2005). The use of diagnostic procedures can aid both initial therapy choice and subsequent treatment adjustments which are necessary for management of pneumonia in immunosuppressed patients. The large number of potential pathogens and the overall higher mortality in these patients supports an aggressive approach in most patients to make a specific diagnosis.

Over the years, many approaches have been evaluated to diagnose the cause of pneumonia in immunosuppressed patients. In this chapter, we will review the various techniques and their yield. There is no perfect method for diagnosing pneumonia. Several factors influence the decision about which technique to use, including the severity of illness of the patient, experience of the treatment team, available technology, and analysis methods.

Table 3.1 summarizes the techniques to be discussed including their relative diagnostic yield for certain key pathogens and the relative cost and safety. Although some techniques (for example, PCR) may enhance the sensitivity for a specific pathogen, that may not be readily available.

Pulmonary Infection in the Immunocompromised Patient, Edited by Carlos Agustí and Antoni Torres
© 2009 John Wiley & Sons, Ltd.

Table 3.1 Relative risk, cost and yield of diagnostic procedures to diagnose pneumonia.

Specimen	Risk	Cost	Bacteria	P. jiroveci	M. tuberculosis	C. neoformans[b]	CMV	Aspergillus
Clinical Assessment	None	Very low	+2[b]	+1	+1	+1	+1	0
Blood	Minimal	Low	+1	0	0	0	+1	0
Sputum	Minimal	Low	+3	+2	+3	+1	0	+1
Tracheal Aspirate[a]	Minimal	Low	+2	+2	+3	+1	0	+1
Protected Brush Specimen	Moderate	High	+4	0	0	0	0	0
Non Bronchoscopic BAL[a]	Mild	Moderate	+4	+2	+3	+1	0	+2
Bronchoscopic BAL	Moderate	Moderate	+4	+4	+4	+3	+3	+2
Transbronchial Biopsy	Moderate	High	0	+2	+3	+3	+3	+3
Surgical Lung Biopsy	High	Very high	0	+4	+4	+4	+4	+4

[a]Usually performed on intubated patient only.

[b]Range from 0 = no benefit, +1 = low sensitivity, good specificity, +2 = low sensitivity, low specificity, +3 = good sensitivity, good specificity, +4 = good sensitivity, high specificity, +5 = high specificity, high specificity. No test was +5.

3.2   Clinical assessment

The first step in diagnosing pneumonia is the clinical assessment. Perhaps the most important information to be obtained by the clinical evaluation is the assessment of immunosuppression. Not all immunosuppression is the same (Baughman, 1999). Some defects are associated with certain infectious complications. Table 3.2 lists the defects and the associated infections.

Immunoglobulin deficiency can range from mild to severe. Patients with common variable immune deficiency (CVID) lack all subclasses of IgG and are susceptible to acute as well as chronic respiratory infections (Aghamohammadi *et al.*, 2005; Cunningham-Rundles and Bodian, 1999). Immunoglobulin replacement can reduce the number of infections dramatically (Quinti *et al.*, 2007). Patients with IgG2 subclass and possible IgG4 subclass have this same problem, although usually not as severe as CVID (Kutukculer *et al.*, 2007). Multiple myeloma can lead to immunoglobulin deficits and increased risk for infection (Costa, Shin and Cooper, 2004; Schutt *et al.*, 2006). Patients with chronic lymphocytic leukemia (CLL) can also be immunoglobulin deficient and develop respiratory infections (Landgren *et al.*, 2007). Some evidence suggests that the pneumonia itself may cause an abnormal immune response leading to multiple myeloma or CLL (Ghiotto *et al.*, 2004; Landgren *et al.*, 2007; Landgren *et al.*, 2006).

While CVID is an IgG deficiency, these patients can have other immune deficiencies, including neutropenia and T cell defects. In one large survey, 40% of the patients with CVID had T-cell defects (Cunningham-Rundles and Bodian, 1999). Therefore patients

Table 3.2   Immune defects and associated pathogens and underlying cases.

Defect	Measure	Pulmonary pathogens	Underlying disease
Immunoglobulin defect	IgG <400 mg/dl	S. pneumoniae	Common variable immune deficiency
		H. influenzae	Multiple myeloma Chronic lymphocytic leukaemia
Neutropenia	Neutrophils <1000 cells/cu mm	S. aureus	Acute leukemias
		P. aeuriginosa	Chemotherapy induced neutropenia
		Aspergillus	Aplastic anemia Bone marrow/stem cell transplant
T-cell defect	CD4 <500 cells/cu mm	Cytomegalovirus	
		P. jiroveci M. tuberculosis C. neoformans H. capsulatum L. pneumophilia Nocardia	

with CVID can have other opportunistic infections causing pneumonia, including *P. jiroveci* (Aghamohammadi *et al.*, 2005). Likewise, patients with multiple myeloma often develop other immune deficiencies during treatment. High dose chemotherapy can be associated with severe CD4 depletion and the development of pneumocystis pneumonia (PcP) or disseminated varicella infection (Schutt *et al.*, 2006). In patients with advanced CLL, PcP has also been diagnosed (Otahbachi, Nugent and Buscemi, 2007; Vavricka *et al.*, 2004).

A reduction in neutrophil number or function can also cause immune defects. Corticosteroids cause neutrophil dysfunction (Tuckermann *et al.*, 2007; Vagaggini *et al.*, 2007) which persists for some time after exposure (Theogaraj *et al.*, 2006). In some studies, treatment with glucocorticoids has been identified as a risk factor for pneumonia (Agusti *et al.*, 2006; Bont *et al.*, 2007).

Absolute neutrophil deficiency is a specific risk for infection. The usual cut-off for neutropenia is between 500 and 1000 neutrophils per cu mm, and the lower the cell count, the higher the risk for infection (Jagarlamudi *et al.*, 2000). The duration of neutropenia is also important as more infections are encountered when neutropenia persists longer than 30 days (Afessa and Peters, 2006). Certainly prolonged neutropenia which accompanies bone marrow and stem cell transplant (SCT) is associated with a high infection rate; whereas transient neutropenia in an otherwise healthy individual may not be a risk factor for pneumonia (Alario and O'Shea, 1989).

Routine bacteria are the most commonly encountered pathogens in untreated neutropenic patients who acquire pneumonia. Severe infections with *S. pneumonia* can occur in this group (Engelhard *et al.*, 2002), even after pneumococcal vaccinations (Youssef *et al.*, 2007). However, empiric therapy is commonly used in this group. Because empiric therapy is often successful in treating most routine pathogens, such as *S. pneumoniae*, frequently opportunistic infections in these patients are multi drug resistant bacteria such as *P. aureginisa* and *S. aureus* (Attal *et al.*, 1991; Bohme *et al.*, 1995; Jagarlamudi *et al.*, 2000). Fungal pathogens are also a major problem in this group (Bohme *et al.*, 1995; Link *et al.*, 1994). This includes aspergillus species, often seen as a consequence of long term neutropenia and the use of broad spectrum antibiotics (Afessa and Peters, 2006; Heussel, Kauczor and Ullmann, 2004). Fungal pneumonias can also be seen after prolonged corticosteroid therapy (Agusti *et al.*, 2006).

T cell defects represent a broad form of immunosuppression, and several medical conditions cause T-cell defects including HIV infection and Hodgkin's and non-Hodgkin's lymphoma. In addition, immunosuppression for solid organ transplantation is associated with T cell defects (Olsen *et al.*, 1993). Other diseases treated with immunosuppressive agents can lead to opportunistic fungal infections (Baughman and Lower, 2005). The CD-4 cell is a useful marker for T cell defect where the lower the CD-4 count, the more severe the T cell defect. Mild CD-4 depletion leads to increased risk for *M. tuberculosis*, while a more severe defect (CD4 lymphocytes<250/cu mm) is associated with an increased risk for PcP, and a very severe depletion (CD4 lymphocytes<100/cu mm) increases the risk for mycobacterium avium complex (Masur *et al.*, 1989). While high activity anti retroviral therapy (HAART) has reduced the incidence of severe CD4 depletion in HIV infected patients, *P. jiroveci* and *M. tuberculosis* remain significant causes of pneumonia in HIV infected patients (Beck *et al.*, 2001).

The most common infections associated with CD4 depletion are *P. jiroveci*, *M. tuberculosis*, and CMV (Beck *et al.*, 2001). Fungal infections such as *C. neoformans*, *H. capsulatum*, *C. mycosis*, and *B. dermatides* have also been associated with CD-4 depletion (Baughman and Lower, 2005; Baughman *et al.*, 1992; Chang *et al.*, 2004; Ellis *et al.*, 1995; Velez *et al.*, 2007). Other infections associated with T cell defect include *L. pneumophila* (Beck *et al.*, 2001; Kirby *et al.*, 1980; Marshall, Foster and Winn, 1981) and Nocardia (Peleg *et al.*, 2007; Roberts *et al.*, 2000).

Despite the specific T cell defect seen in transplant patients and HIV infected patients, bacterial infection still represents the most common infection diagnosed in patients with pneumonia (Baughman, Dohn and Frame, 1994; Beck *et al.*, 2001). Figure 3.1 lists the pathogens identified as causing pneumonia in HIV infected and transplant patients from several large series. This figure includes two series from our institution, where the same diagnostic approach was used for HIV infected (Baughman, Dohn and Frame, 1994) and transplant patients (Sternberg *et al.*, 1993). Several factors can influence the proportion of different pathogens encountered. Prophylaxis therapy can modify the risk for some of these infections. The most effective prophylaxis therapy has been trimethoprim/ sulfamethoxazole which markedly reduces the risk of PcP (Hughes *et al.*, 1987; Lindemulder and Albano, 2007; Podzamczer *et al.*, 1995). A reduction in the rate of PcP in HIV has been reported in many centres (Gona *et al.*, 2006; Kohli *et al.*, 2006; Wallace *et al.*, 1997). However, da Silva reported many PcP cases in his Brazilian patients, many of whom were not receiving prophylaxis at the time of diagnosis

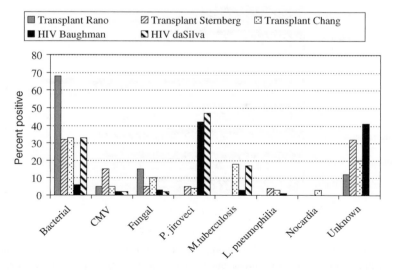

Figure 3.1   The proportion of specific causes for pneumonia in solid organ transplant patients as reported by (Rano *et al.*, 2001; Sternberg *et al.*, 1993; Chang *et al.*, 2004) versus HIV infected patients reported by (Baughman, Dohn and Frame, 1994; da Silva, Teixeira and Moreira, 2006).

(da Silva, Teixeira and Moreira, 2006). Prophylaxis will also reduce the risk for nocardia and toxoplasmosis (Fishman, 2007; Podzamczer *et al.*, 1995). While bacterial pneumonia remains a complication of HIV infection, HAART therapy with or without PcP prophylaxis also reduces the risk for bacterial pneumonia (Gona *et al.*, 2006; Kohli *et al.*, 2006; Wallace *et al.*, 1997). Patients on more than a year of HAART therapy experienced a significantly lower rate of bacterial pneumonia (Kohli *et al.*, 2006). Because patients may also develop multiple infections as the cause of pneumonia (Baughman, Dohn and Frame, 1994; Huang and Hopewell, 1998), specific diagnostic tests may be required.

Although the classic symptoms of pneumonia include fever, cough, dyspnea and purulent sputum, these symptoms may be suppressed or totally absent in the immuno-suppressed patient. For example, in a study of autopsy confirmed cases of pulmonary aspergillus, 41% of patients had no respiratory symptoms (Vaideeswar *et al.*, 2004). Therefore a high level of suspicion is required in managing these patients.

Figure 3.2 summarizes the most common symptoms and physical findings for 229 HIV infected patients with documented pneumonia (Selwyn *et al.*, 1998). The

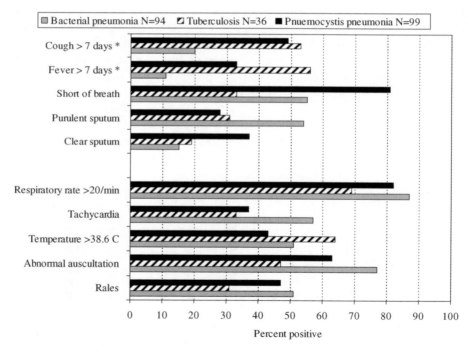

Figure 3.2   The prevalence of specific signs and symptoms for HIV infected patients diagnosed with either bacterial pneumonia, M. tuberculosis pneumonia, or pneumocystis pneumonia. The number of patients in each group (*N*) is indicated. Almost all patients experienced cough and fever. Patients with bacterial pneumonia tended to have these symptoms for a shorter time than those with M. tuberculosis or pneumonocystis pneumonia (PcP). Adapted from (Selwyn *et al.*, 1998).

frequency of some signs and symptoms depend on the causative agent. However, the differences were not distinct enough to lead to a specific diagnosis.

Fever and cough were noted in the majority of HIV infected patients. Figure 3.2 demonstrates that those with *M. tuberculosis* or *P. jiroveci* were more likely to have these symptoms for more than a week, compared to the patient with bacterial pneumonia. Patients with PcP tend to have a more insidious onset of symptoms over the course of weeks prior to diagnosis. In one series, the duration of symptoms prior to diagnosis was three weeks. At the time of diagnosis of *P. jiroveci*, these HIV infected patients usually develop fever (74%), cough (74%) and dyspnea (65%) (Fujii *et al.*, 2007). The persistence of symptoms prior to a final diagnosis has been noted as a feature for *P. jiroveci*, *M. tuberculosis*, and other opportunistic infections (Baughman, Dohn and Frame, 1994; da Silva, Teixeira and Moreira, 2006; Ewig *et al.*, 1995; Vaideeswar *et al.*, 2004).

Cough is a common complaint in pneumonia. In the study by Selmyn *et al.* (Figure 3.2), purulent sputum was more frequently reported in patients with bacterial pneumonia than PcP (Selwyn *et al.*, 1998). However, patients in all three groups had a non productive cough. In another study of HIV infected patients with pneumonia, 46% reported dry cough and only 14% noted any sputum production (da Silva, Teixeira and Moreira, 2006).

The chest roentgenogram is usually the determinant as to whether a patient has pneumonia or not. While some would argue that a normal chest roentgenogram rules out pneumonia, it is clear that the chest roentgenogram has its limitations even in the non immunocompromised patient (Wunderink, 2000; Wunderink *et al.*, 1992). In the immunocompromised patient, the chest roentgenogram fails to detect pulmonary infiltrates in patients with PcP in up to 10% of cases (Friedman *et al.*, 1975; Israel *et al.*, 1987; Opravil *et al.*, 1994). When the chest roentgenogram is abnormal in PcP, it tends to reveal a diffuse infiltrate, with upper lobes more prominently affected than the lower lobes (Baughman *et al.*, 1993).

For the immunosuppressed patient with an opportunistic infection, the infiltrates tend to be diffuse and interstitial or alveolar (da Silva, Teixeira and Moreira, 2006). However, localized infiltrates can be encountered. While localized infiltrates suggest a bacterial process, this pattern can be seen with CMV and *P. jiroveci* infection (Friedman *et al.*, 1975).

Computerized tomography (CT) scan is more sensitive than routine chest roentgenogram in assessing possible pneumonia. The findings on CT scan may suggest specific pathogens. In one study of liver transplant patients with clinical features consistent with pneumonia, several CT patterns were identified (Knollmann *et al.*, 2000). An interstitial pattern was identified in 13 of 20 patients found to have CMV. Five of eight patients with *P. jiroveci* pneumonia had peribronchovascular infiltrates. Of the 24 patients with bacterial pneumonia, bilateral effusions were seen in 14 and lobar consolidation in 13. Unfortunately, no pathogen was identified in 7/41 (17%) of patients with CT signs of pneumonia.

Heussel and coworkers compared the value of high resolution CT scanning to routine chest roentgenogram for immunosuppressed patients with possible pneumonia and fever for more than 48 hours despite empiric antibiotic therapy (Heussel *et al.*, 1999). All patients were neutropenic secondary to chemotherapy with or without transplant, with a clinical diagnosis of pneumonia but a normal chest roentgenogram. Of the 188 HRCT studies, 112 (60%) showed pneumonia and 76 were normal. Sensitivity of HRCT for pneumonia was 87% and specificity was 57%. Only seven patients with a normal initial HRCT subsequently had evidence for pneumonia. The investigators reported that even in patients who subsequently developed an infiltrate on chest roentgenogram, a time gain of five days was achieved by the use of HRCT when the presentation suggested pneumonia.

In patients with possible pneumonia, the chest roentgenogram remains the first imaging study. However, those patients with normal chest roentgenogram and a high index of suspicion, then the next step should be a CT scan of the chest. The CT scan may also suggest other potential causes for respiratory symptoms, including pulmonary edema or pulmonary embolism.

3.3   Blood cultures

While blood cultures remain part of the routine assessment of community acquired pneumonia, they appear to have limited utility in the assessment of pulmonary infiltrates in immunosuppressed patients. This may reflect the low dissemination of most pulmonary pathogens. In a study of non HIV immunosuppressed patients with pulmonary infiltrates, Rano *et al.* reported positive blood cultures in 30 out of 191 (16%); however, the blood culture results changed therapy in only four patients. Therefore, one can not assume that the patient has been adequately evaluated with only blood cultures.

3.4   Sputum

The sputum has been the classic sample to diagnose pneumonia. However, it is clear that sputum examination has its limitations (Barrett-Connor, 1971). For all respiratory samples, one has to assess the ability to detect a pathogen (sensitivity) and the probability of the organism detected as the cause of the pneumonia (specificity). Table 3.3 helps to

Table 3.3   Pathogen as a cause of pneumonia: relative risk.

Always a pathogen	Usually a pathogen	Can be a pathogen	Pathogen in immuno-suppressed patient	Rarely a pathogen in markedly immuno-suppressed patient
M. tuberculosis	S. pneumoniae	S. aureus	Cytomegalovirus	M. gordonae
P. jiroveci	C. neoformans	Aspergillus	M. avium	Candida
	Nocardia	P. aeruoginosa		
	Legionella			
Comments				
No need for more nformation	Clinical criteria of pneumonia	Clinical criteria of pneumonia; Quantitation of organisms	Pathologic changes; Clinical setting	Clinical setting

separate potential pulmonary pathogens. Some organisms are almost always pathogenic and their identification requires therapy. However, in other cases, the finding of a potential pathogen such as *S. pneumoniae* or *S. aureus* must be placed in clinical context, since these bacteria are known to colonize the upper airway. Other organisms may reside in the airway of healthy individuals, but can lead to disease in the immunosuppressed patient.

Obtaining adequate spontaneous sputum is often difficult in immunosuppressed patients. As shown in Figure 3.2, purulent sputum was frequently reported by patients with bacterial pneumonia than with other opportunistic infections. However, even in patients with bacterial pneumonia, less than 50% of patients in this study expectorated purulent sputum (Selwyn *et al.*, 1998). In another prospective study of HIV infected patients with community acquired pneumonia, only 15% had productive sputum (da Silva, Teixeira and Moreira, 2006).

If the patient is able to provide a sputum sample, the quality of the sputum should be assessed prior to processing (Murray and Washington, 1975). For diagnosing bacterial pneumonia, the specimen should contain inflammatory cells, not squamous epithelial cells from the oral cavity (Bartlett *et al.*, 1979; Heineman, Chawla and Lopton, 1977). However, detecting organisms that are always pathogens, such as *P. jiroveci* and *M. tuberculosis*, in an 'inadequate' sample should lead to further evaluation (Fischer *et al.*, 2001).

The number of organisms in the sputum is a reflection of the burden of infection in the chest. For many years, smear negative tuberculosis was recognized as a condition with lower infectivity, but still significant disease. Attempts to increase sensitivity with PCR and other techniques in these smear negative patients has led to earlier detection (Schluger, 2001). For PcP, the recognition that *P. jiroveci* could be identified in the sputum did not occur until the HIV epidemic. At that time, it became clear that HIV infected patients developed larger burdens of *P. jiroveci* compared to non-HIV infected patients with PcP (Limper *et al.*, 1989). This observation led to a series of papers reporting on the utility of examining sputum for *P. jiroveci* in HIV infected patients with possible PcP. These studies also demonstrated the value of using more sensitive techniques, such as immunoflourescence (Kovacs *et al.*, 1988).

Induced sputum, using ultrasonic saline, allows for a higher yield of adequate sample in the immunocompromised patient with possible pneumonia (Bigby *et al.*, 1986; Fishman *et al.*, 1994). It allows one to look for various pathogens, including *P. jiroveci* and *M. tuberculosis* (Fishman *et al.*, 1994) as well as bacterial pathogens, such as *S. pneumoniae*. Figure 3.3 demonstrates the yield of induced sputum versus bronchoscopy obtained samples in HIV infected patients. It was assumed that the bronchoscopy diagnosis was the 'gold standard' and the results of the induced sputum were compared to the bronchoscopy diagnosis (da Silva, Teixeira and Moreira, 2006).

3.5 Endotracheal aspirate

For the immunosuppressed patient who is intubated, the endotracheal aspirate can be obtained in all cases. This specimen can be analyzed like spontaneous sputum. The endotracheal aspirate is most commonly evaluated to diagnose bacterial pneumonia for

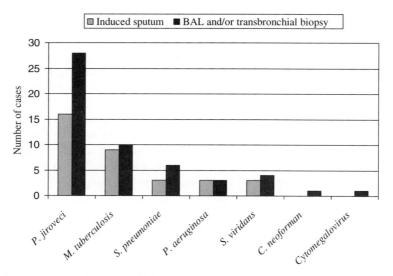

Figure 3.3 Comparison of yield for induced sputum versus bronchoscopy specimen (bronchoal-veolar lavage (BAL) or transbronchial biopsy) in 54 HIV positive patients with a bronchoscopy confirmed diagnosis of pneumonia and evaluated with both techniques. Adapted from (da Silva, Teixeira and Moreira, 2006).

ventilated patients (Baughman, 2003; Cook and Mandell, 2000); however, it has also been used to diagnose fungal infections in immunocompromised patients (Rano *et al.*, 2001).

A question remains as to whether semi-quantitative cultures of the bacterial samples from the specimen should be performed (Cook and Mandell, 2000; Fujitani and Yu, 2006). Controversy exists because the non quantitated samples have a sensitivity of greater than 95%, but a specificity of less than 40% (Lambert, Vereen and George, 1989), while using semi-quantitative cultures enhances specificity but reduces sensitivity to 60–70% (el Ebiary *et al.*, 1993; Marquette *et al.*, 1995). The recommendation that semi-quantitative cultures be used to assess samples seems reasonable (Cook and Mandell, 2000); however, it is associated with an increased cost as well as reduced sensitivity (Baughman, 2003; Fujitani and Yu, 2006).

The major advantage of endotracheal aspirate is the relative ease in which a sample can be obtained. This technique does not require highly trained personnel and the specimen can be sent at any time without waiting until equipment is available. The cost for acquiring the sample is low, but the cost can be markedly increased if additional testing is performed on the sample. Figure 3.4 illustrates the relative yield of endotracheal aspirate compared to other techniques of a study at one institution on 200 non-HIV immunosuppressed patients with possible pneumonia. Not all patients had all samples obtained, with only 55 patients having an endotracheal aspirate (Rano *et al.*, 2001). While other techniques, such as BAL, had a higher yield, the endotracheal aspirate was useful in detecting bacteria and fungi in this group of patients.

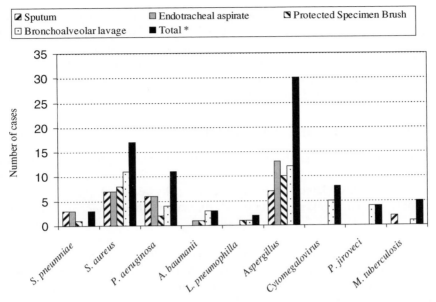

Figure 3.4 The yield of sputum ($N = 88$), endotracheal aspirate ($N = 55$), protected specimen brush ($N = 125$), and bronchoalveolar lavage ($N = 135$) obtained from 200 non HIV immunosuppressed patients with potential pneumonia. The yield for each technique was compared to various potential pathogens. More than one specimen could be positive for an organism and some organisms were detected by other techniques. Adapted from (Rano *et al.*, 2001).

3.6 Non bronchoscopic bronchoalveolar lavage

The non bronchoscopic BAL catheter, a disposable catheter used to obtain a clean sample from the lower respiratory tract, was originally developed to be passed through an endotracheal tube (Pugin *et al.*, 1991; Rouby *et al.*, 1989). It can be performed on non intubated patients (Bustamante and Levy, 1994; Caughey *et al.*, 1985).

It has equal sensitivity and specificity compared to a bronchoscopic BAL sample (Campbell, 2000) and it can also diagnose *P. jiroveci* as readily as a bronchoscopic BAL (Levy, 1994).

The advantage of non bronchoscopic BAL is that it can be obtained by non physicians (Kollef *et al.*, 1995). However, it still requires specific training and assessment of the sample (Baughman *et al.*, 2000). This attention to detail has proved to be useful. An aspirated sample that is more than 10% of the instilled volume and contains less than 5% bronchial epitheal cells was considered an adequate sample by one proposed guideline (Baughman *et al.*, 2000). Samples considered adequate were more likely to be diagnostic than inadequate samples (Baughman *et al.*, 2000). In general, the guideline for adequate samples are similar to that used for bronchoscopic BAL samples (Klech and Pohl, 1989).

The volume of sample is a major limitation of the non bronchoscopic BAL. Although the amount of aspirated fluid varies depending on the catheter, it is usually less than

10 ml (Campbell, 2000). One of the original catheters with a retrieved volume of less than 2 ml limited its utility to only bacterial sampling (Rouby *et al.*, 1992). Other catheters with larger diameters allow for larger instilled volumes (Levy, 1994). In one study, the recommended instilled volume was 60 ml and in the majority of cases, more than 6 ml was aspirated (Baughman *et al.*, 2000). This larger aspirated volume allows for additional analysis for tuberculosis, fungi, viral infection and even cytology.

3.7   Protected brush sample (PBS)

The PBS was originally described as a method to obtain relatively sterile samples from the lower respiratory tract in non intubated patients (Wimberly, Faling and Bartlett, 1979). It was quickly adapted for use on mechanically ventilated patients where it has been widely studied (Baughman, 2000). The brush is inside an inner and outer catheter and the outer catheter has a gelatin plug, which is pushed into an area which is not to be sampled. The brush is advanced through the inner catheter and the brush sample is obtained in the area of purulent material (Wimberly, Faling and Bartlett, 1979). The cut-off of 1000 colony forming units (cfu) of bateria/ml of specimen has been shown to be a reliable distinction between infection and colonization (Meduri *et al.*, 1992). The results are fairly reproducible, usually within a log on repeated testing (Marquette *et al.*, 1993). However, 1000 cfu of bacteria/ml have also been found in samples from patients with acute bronchitis (Baughman *et al.*, 2000; Cabello *et al.*, 1997; Monso *et al.*, 1995).

For the immunocompromised patient, the PBS has been used with some success (Xaubet *et al.*, 1989). Its major advantage is in the diagnosis of bacterial pathogens. However, it may also be useful in detecting fungal infections, such as Aspergillus (Figure 3.4) (Rano *et al.*, 2001). The PBS sample is resuspended in a total volume of 1 ml. However, this small volume of sample is usually inadequate for aliquots for viral or tuberculous cultures. In addition, cytology is not easily performed after the routine semi-quantitative cultures have been performed (Meduri *et al.*, 1992). Even with a routine cytologic brush sample, the yield of bronchoscopic brushing for *P. jiroveci* has been reported as less than 40% (Coleman *et al.*, 1983).

Therefore the PBS is a complimentary test in the evaluation of pneumonia in immunosuppressed patients. Figure 3.5 compares the yield of PBS to other diagnostic tests, including sputum, BAL and transbronchial biopsy from two large studies of immunosuppressed patients (Jain *et al.*, 2004; Rano *et al.*, 2001). The yield for PBS was lower than BAL. Of the 104 patients studied by Jain *et al.*, 51 had both a PBS and BAL performed. Three cases were identified in which the BAL was negative and the PBS provided a specific diagnosis (Jain *et al.*, 2004). In the Rano study of 55 of 200 patients with a PBS obtained, in only two cases were the results of the PBS the exclusive reason to change therapy (Rano *et al.*, 2001). Based on this information, it is not clear that PBS need be obtained on all immunosuppressed patients. However, obtaining an adequate sample is one of the difficulties with both bronchoscopic and non bronchoscopic BAL. In a patient in whom the amount of BAL fluid aspirated is inadequate for whatever reason, the PBS is a useful alternative to sample for potential bacterial pathogens.

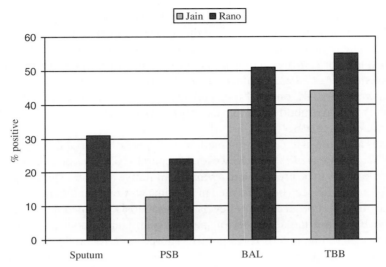

Figure 3.5 The overall % positive results for sputum, protected brush specimen (PBS), bronchoalveolar lavage (BAL), and transbronchial biopsy (TBB) from two large series of immunosuppressed patients (Jain *et al.*, 2004; Rano *et al.*, 2001).

3.8 Bronchoalveolar lavage (BAL)

During a bronchoscopy, normal saline can be introduced into the airways and then collected. The amount of fluid and the location of the bronchoscope can have a major impact on the contents of the lung fluid sampled. Bronchial washing is obtained by collecting fluid with the bronchoscope in a non wedged position. The bronchial wash is usually obtained throughout the entire bronchoscopy. The bronchoscope can be wedged by advancing as far as possible, often in a subsegment of the right middle lobe or lingula, and the fluid instilled and immediately aspirated (Baughman, 2003). If 10–20 ml of saline are introduced and then aspirated, this is a bronchial lavage (Rennard *et al.*, 1990). This fluid has a higher percentage of epithelial and other airway cells. Using an instilled volume of greater than 100 ml of saline, the aspirated fluid has features more consistent with an alveolar sample (Dohn and Baughman, 1985). Recommendations have been made suggesting that the minimal instilled volume for a BAL sample should be at least 100 ml (Klech and Pohl, 1989). The BAL technique is fairly safe and can be performed in patients with thrombocytopenia and/or hypoxia (Hohenadel *et al.*, 2001; Steinberg *et al.*, 1994).

The use of a fiberoptic bronchoscope to obtain a large volume washing of the alveolar space was introduced by (Reynolds and Newball, 1974). Although the technique was used initially as a research tool for healthy controls and patients with interstitial lung diseases such as sarcoidosis, the use of BAL to diagnose pneumonia in the immunosuppressed patient was reported ten years later (Stover *et al.*, 1984). Various sites adapted the technique for the diagnosis of infections that had previously required biopsy. The outbreak of PcP among HIV infected patients led to a large number of patients in whom the diagnosis with BAL could be easily made (Baughman, Dohn and Frame, 1994; Broaddus *et al.*, 1985), and the sensitivity of BAL to diagnose *P. jiroveci* was found to be higher than 95% (Golden *et al.*, 1986). The BAL sample has a higher diagnostic yield for *P. jiroveci* compared to bronchial washing alone (Baughman *et al.*, 1989; Coleman *et al.*, 1983; Golden *et al.*, 1986). In one study directly comparing bronchial wash to BAL, only 70% of patients with *P. jiroveci* identified in the BAL sample had a positive modified silver stain for *P. jiroveci* in their bronchial wash sample (Baughman *et al.*, 1989).

BAL was also shown to be a useful method to diagnose bacterial infection (Kahn and Jones, 1987; Thorpe *et al.*, 1987). However, to separate colonization from infection, the BAL sample needs to be processed in a semi-quantitative manner (Meduri *et al.*, 1992). The semi-quantitation can be performed in the same way one handles a urine culture. To determine the appropriate cut off levels for diagnosis of pneumonia, two studies performed BAL in a large number of patients with and without pneumonia. These are summarized in Figure 3.6. The report by Thorpe *et al.* found that patients could be categorized by the quantity of bacteria found per ml of BAL sample (Thorpe *et al.*, 1987). All 13 patients with more than 100 000 cfu/ml BAL had pneumonia and the BAL from the remaining two patients with a clinical diagnosis of pneumonia contained between 10 and 100 000 cfu of bacteria/ml of BAL. A subsequent study by Cantral *et al.* confirmed that the same general guidelines reporting the number of organisms could be used to distinguish between those with and without pneumonia (Cantral *et al.*, 1993). However, the authors identified a subgroup of patients without pneumonia whose BAL cultures grew more than 10 000 cfu/ml of BAL. In these subjects, the bacteria identified

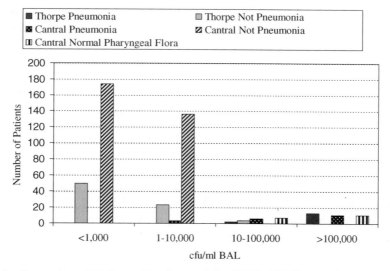

Figure 3.6   Comparison of the bacterial culture results of BAL fluid from patients with or without bacterial pneumonia from two studies of non intubated patients by (Thorpe *et al.*, 1987; Cantral *et al.*, 1993). Cantral *et al.* also described a group of healthy patients with BAL samples that grew normal pharyngeal flora in their BAL specimen but had no evidence of pneumonia.

were considered part of the normal pharyngeal flora (NPF), such as diptheroids. Because the authors felt this was a contamination that occurred as the result of the BAL procedure itself, the treating physician could discount the importance of these bacteria, and consider them part of NPF. Subsequent reports suggest that diptheroids, cultured at high concentrations in the BAL fluid, have been associated with pneumonia (Lambotte *et al.*, 2002). While colonization in the lower airways is more common in COPD and lung cancer patients, the proposed cut-offs of 10–100 000 are still useful (Baughman *et al.*, 2000; Cabello *et al.*, 1997).

The utility of BAL in diagnosing pneumonia has been most widely studied in ventilator associated pneumonia (VAP). Several studies have used BAL to diagnose ventilator associated pneumonia. In some cases, the BAL diagnosis is compared to immediate post mortem findings (Chastre *et al.*, 1988; Torres *et al.*, 1994). In other studies, clinical criteria were used to diagnose pneumonia (Guerra and Baughman, 1990). The overall sensitivity and specificity exceeded 80% for most of these studies. No difference was reported in the sensitivity and specificity for the clinical versus immediate post mortem studies (Torres and El-Ebiary, 2000). Other studies have demonstrated that failure to treat pathogens identified by BAL leads to a higher mortality (Luna *et al.*, 1997), supporting the diagnostic importance of BAL findings.

For fungal infections, a range of potential pathogens can be identified in the BAL sample of the immunosuppressed patient. Certain fungi including *C. neoformans*, *H. capsulatum*, *C. immitis*, and *B. dermatitidis* are always considered pathogenic in the immunosuppressed patient (Baughman *et al.*, 1991; Kerkering, Duma and Shadomy, 1981; Sobonya *et al.*, 1990). While these organisms have the potential to cause a self limited infection in the immunocompetent host, their discovery in the immunosuppressed patient usually leads to subsequent therapy. In one study of immunocompetent patients, *C. neoformans* pneumonia was self limiting, with resolution of their roentgenographic abnormalities within six months with or without therapy. Conversely, only 1 of 16 immunosuppressed patients had improvement in the chest roentgenogram after six months of therapy (Chang *et al.*, 2006). There is also a high risk for disseminated infection, including meningitis, in the immunosuppressed patient (Chang *et al.*, 2006; Kerkering, Duma and Shadomy, 1981). This same risk for dissemination in the immunosuppressed patient occurs with the endemic fungi *H. capsulatum*, *C. immitis*, and *B. dermatitidis*. The HIV infected patient with a low CD-4 count is at particularly high risk dissemination of endemic fungal infections (Conces, 1999; Sobonya *et al.*, 1990; Wheat *et al.*, 1990).

While culture remains the standard method for fungal infection identification, it often takes more than two weeks for the culture to become positive. Although less sensitive than culture, fungi can be identified by cytologic examination of the sample, usually with a modified silver stain (Baughman *et al.*, 1991). *C. neoformans* is associated with a large antigen load which has been detected in either serum or cerebral spinal fluid. In one retrospective study of previously frozen BAL specimens, a high degree of sensitivity and specificity for cryptococcal antigen in the BAL (Baughman *et al.*, 1992). However, this relatively simple test has been difficult to reproduce, and the routine measurement of fresh BAL samples for cryptococcal antigen using the latex agglutination test is no longer recommended (Kralovic and Rhodes, 1998). The test may still be useful when there is a high index of suspicion (Bottone, Sindone and Caraballo, 1998). *H. capsulatum* antigen has also been detected in the BAL of patients with histoplasmosis pneumonia (Wheat *et al.*, 1992). Second generation antigen testing appears to have enhanced both the sensitivity and specificity for the diagnosis of *H. capsulatum* and *B. dermatitidis* (Hage *et al.*, 2007).

Nocardia and Rhodococcus are rare, but serious pulmonary pathogens that can be identified in the BAL sample either by cytology or by routine fungal culture techniques (Baughman, Dohn and Frame, 1994; Forbes *et al.*, 1990; Munoz *et al.*, 2000). The radiologic appearance of these infections is usually nodular, and the diagnosis can be confirmed by needle aspiration (Forbes *et al.*, 1990; Mari *et al.*, 2001).

Aspergillus species can cause a wide range of pulmonary problems (Judson, 2004) including simple colonization, with or without associated asthmatic reaction, or the more severe asthmatic manifestation of allergic bronchopulmonary aspergillosis (ABPA). In both situations, the host's reaction, as measured by the IgE level, is the cause of the symptoms. Immunocompetent patients can also experience serious aspergillus infections such as a mycetoma, a fungal collection within a prior lung cavity. Mycetomas can become symptomatic due to local invasion and irritation, and on rare occasions hemoptysis can be fatal.

Because invasive aspergillosis is a well recognized cause of death in immunosuppressed patients (Kotloff, Ahya and Crawford, 2004; Lortholary *et al.*, 1993; Paterson and Singh, 1999), recognition of aspergillus infection as a pneumonia prior to dissemination may lead to reduced mortality (Kotloff, Ahya and Crawford, 2004). In one study of HIV infected patients, the median survival was only eight weeks once invasive aspergillosis was diagnosed (Lortholary *et al.*, 1993). The importance of finding aspergillus also depends on the immunosuppression of the host. Neutropenia and very low CD4 cell counts are associated with increased risk for severe aspergillosis in HIV infected patients (Wallace *et al.*, 1998). Aspergillus pneumonitis is a major complication after bone marrow transplantation (Huaringa *et al.*, 2000).

Culture is the most common method for the diagnosis of aspergillosis. However, since colonization can occur, the presence of compatible fungal forms seen in respiratory specimens makes the clinician more comfortable with the diagnosis. In a study of immunosuppressed patients with possible invasive aspergillosis, cytology and culture of bronchoscopic samples were compared (Levy *et al.*, 1992). Invasive pulmonary aspergillosis was identified in 21 patients, of whom 16 died. BAL cytology was positive for aspergillus in 19 specimens, including 16 specimens from patients with invasive aspergillosis. Although 41 specimens were culture positive, only 10 of these were from patients with invasive aspergillosis. While cytology was more specific, it failed to make the diagnosis in a significant number of cases. Unfortunately, the use of aspergillus antigen has not been useful in improving sensitivity. In one study, none of the 17 samples tested from patients with autopsy confirmed invasive aspergillosis was positive, while three of ten BAL samples from control patients were positive for aspergillus antigen (Rath *et al.*, 1996). Antigen detection may be more useful in examining bronchial wash samples (Seyfarth *et al.*, 2001). On the other hand, PCR may be more helpful as this technique can provide a more specific diagnosis and the ability to quantitate the burden of fungus (Raad *et al.*, 2002; Rantakokko-Jalava *et al.*, 2003). The use of BAL to diagnose aspergillus is comparable to other techniques including PBS (Boersma *et al.*, 2007).

Over the last few years, more fungi are being recognized as potential pulmonary pathogens in the immunosuppressed patients (Costa and Alexander, 2005; Wingard, 2005). The specific diagnosis of fungi requires final confirmation. However, cytologic appearance can often be helpful. The presence of any fungal elements in a respiratory sample should lead to consideration for therapy until final diagnosis can be made. Candida is a common colonizer of the lower respiratory tract, especially in a patient receiving prior antibiotics. Although it rarely causes pneumonia, candida pneumonia has been clearly documented in some patients (el Ebiary *et al.*, 1997).

Mycobacterial infections can be diagnosed by stain and culture of the BAL sample. For some groups, such as HIV infected patients, mycobacterial infections are a common reason for pneumonia (da Silva, Teixeira and Moreira, 2006; Joos *et al.*, 2007; Velez *et al.*, 2007). We have observed that *M. tuberculosis* is more likely to be identified in the bronchial wash over the BAL sample. The higher yield may simply be the wider sampling of various parts of the lung obtained during the bronchial wash. For tuberculosis, a combination of bronchoscopic samples enhances the diagnostic yield (Baughman *et al.*, 1991; Chan, Sun and Hoheisel, 1990).

Atypical mycobacteria are frequently diagnosed in immunosuppressed patients. These infections can be readily diagnosed by BAL (Sugihara *et al.*, 2003). Mycobacterium avium complex (MAC) was frequently encountered in severely immunosuppressed HIV infected patients. In many cases, the MAC appears to be a commensal infection not responsible for the pulmonary infiltrates (Raju and Schluger, 2000). Disseminated MAC is associated with very low CD4 counts (<100 cells/cu mm) (Chaisson *et al.*, 1992). When HIV patients have their immunodeficiency reversed by HAART, MAC can lead to a granulomatous reaction (Phillips *et al.*, 2005). This syndrome, called immune reconstitution syndrome, supports the concept that for many patients, the major clinical significance of MAC is the host's response to the organism.

Other mycobacteria such as *M. gordonae* and *M. xenopi* can lead to clinical important pneumonias in immunosuppressed patients (Bishburg *et al.*, 2004; Eckburg *et al.*, 2000; El-Solh *et al.*, 1998). The clinician therefore needs to be careful in not dismissing a mycobacterial culture that is PCR probe negative for *M. tuberculosis*.

Cytomegalovirus (CMV) can be a significant problem for immunosuppressed patients. For bone marrow transplant patients, CMV is one of the most common causes of pneumonia (Dunagan *et al.*, 1997; Huaringa *et al.*, 2000; Joos *et al.*, 2007) and it remains a major cause of morbidity and mortality in this group of patients (Afessa and Peters, 2006; Enright *et al.*, 1993). However, routine prophylaxis with anti-viral agents such as gancyclovir is effective in reducing the risk for CMV pneumonitis (Feinstein *et al.*, 2001; Schmidt *et al.*, 1991). However, pneumonia due to CMV is still encountered in the prophylactic era (da Silva, Teixeira and Moreira, 2006; Jain *et al.*, 2004; Velez *et al.*, 2007). Still pneumonia due to CMV is encountered in the prophylactic era (da Silva, Teixeira and Moreira, 2006; Jain *et al.*, 2004; Velez *et al.*, 2007).

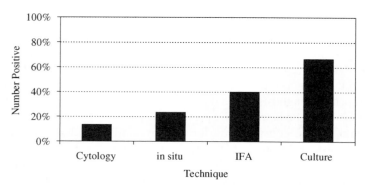

Figure 3.7   A comparison of the yield for CMV in 30 consecutive HIV infected patients studied at the University of Cincinnati. Less than 25% of the samples had cytologic evidence for CMV or evidence of CMV by in situ hybridization. On the other hand, over 60% of the samples were culture positive for CMV.

The presence of CMV in the lung can be detected by several methods including cytopathic changes in the cells retrieved in the BAL sample (Lemert *et al.*, 1996), *in situ* hybridization demonstrating evidence of CMV-DNA within respiratory cells (Hilborne *et al.*, 1987), immunoflourescent screening for early CMV antigen (Miles *et al.*, 1990; Weiss *et al.*, 1991), and direct culture of the BAL fluid for CMV (Miles *et al.*, 1990). Figure 3.7 compares these four techniques on 30 consecutive BAL samples obtained from HIV infected patients at our institution. Over 60% of the BAL samples were CMV positive, comparable to other studies at our institution (Hayner *et al.*, 1995; Miles *et al.*, 1990). Real time PCR can also be performed to detect CMV (Nitsche *et al.*, 2000). Overall, PCR and culture are more sensitive methods than cytology for detecting CMV infection (Goto *et al.*, 1996). However, it is unclear whether cytology is more specific for actual infection.

The importance of CMV in the lung of the immunosuppressed patient can be quite unclear. For the HIV infected patient, some authors have demonstrated that CMV in the BAL was not associated with clinical infection (Mann *et al.*, 1997). However, it has been demonstrated that CMV can be the sole pathogen causing pneumonia (Waxman *et al.*, 1997) and CMV pneumonia has been reported in an autopsy study of HIV infected patients (McKenzie *et al.*, 1991). In an observational study, the presence of CMV was associated with an increased three and six month mortality (Hayner *et al.*, 1995). Interestingly, there was no difference in those who were culture positive alone versus those who also had cytopathic changes in the BAL. While CMV in bone marrow transplant patient has been associated with increased mortality (Afessa and Peters, 2006; Enright *et al.*, 1993), some authors have reported asymptomatic colonization (Ruutu *et al.*, 1990).

These observations point out the difficulty the clinician encounters when interpreting the presence of CMV in a BAL sample. If the patient has evidence for pneumonia, CMV may be a cause for the pneumonia. In a patient with no alternative cause for pneumonia, CMV still needs to be considered the culprit for the pneumonia (Waxman *et al.*, 1997).

The presence of CMV can also be a risk factor for increased morbidity in patients with other causes for pneumonia, including PcP (Baughman, Dohn and Frame, 1994).

Virus other than CMV can also be diagnosed in immunocompromised patients. These include herpes simplex, adenovirus and influenza virus (Connolly *et al.*, 1994; Gona *et al.*, 2006). Herpes and adeno virus can be cultured using the same method to culture CMV (Connolly *et al.*, 1994) and the herpes virus can be detected in the lower respiratory tract of patients with acute respiratory distress syndrome (Schuller *et al.*, 1993; Tuxen *et al.*, 1982). In one study, herpes virus in the lung specimen was associated with a higher mortality for immunocompetent versus immunosuppressed mechanically ventilated patients (Schuller *et al.*, 1993). However, it is not clear that the herpes virus infection itself causes increased mortality or is just a marker for the underlying severity of disease (van den Brink *et al.*, 2004). In a randomized trial, although acyclovir prophylaxis prevented herpes infection compared to the placebo group, it did not change survival (Tuxen, Wilson and Cade, 1987).

Legionella can also be diagnosed by direct culture of the usually sterile BAL fluid (Kohorst *et al.*, 1983; Pereira Gomes *et al.*, 2000; Sternberg *et al.*, 1993). Other techniques have been developed to detect Legionella in BAL samples, including direct fluorescent antibody (Hayden *et al.*, 2001) and PCR (Hayden *et al.*, 2001; Hohenthal *et al.*, 2005; Wilson *et al.*, 2004). Although the PCR technique can be more rapidly applied than other techniques, PCR is species specific and may not detect all species of Legionella (Hayden *et al.*, 2001).

Noninfectious causes of pulmonary infiltrates can also be diagnosed by BAL. These include malignancy, either as the original cause of the immunosuppression or a complication of therapy (Pirozynski, 1992; Rennard and Schluger, 1990). Positive BAL can diagnose lymphangitic spread of tumor, which can have the clinical presentation of pneumonia (Lower and Baughman, 1992). Diffuse alveolar hemorrhage (DAH) can be diagnosed by BAL, based on a bloody return of the BAL fluid and the presence of hemosiderin laden macrophages (De Lassence *et al.*, 1995; Kahn, Jones and England, 1987). Although it is a common complication of bone marrow transplantation (Agusti *et al.*, 1995; Sisson *et al.*, 1992), it can be encountered in other immunosuppressed patients (De Lassence *et al.*, 1995; Jain *et al.*, 2004) with underlying thrombocytopenia or underlying coagulopathies.

BAL is one of the most commonly used methods to diagnose pneumonia in immunosuppressed patients. Table 3.4 summarizes the results of BAL in several large studies published in the past few years. BAL remains useful in diagnosing a range of pathogens in patients with various causes of immunosuppression.

3.9 Transbronchial biopsy (TBB)

Although transbronchial biopsy provides samples for histopathologic examination, it is also used to assess for infection and other causes of pulmonary infiltrates in immunocompromised patients (Broaddus *et al.*, 1985; Jain *et al.*, 2004). Because in many cases, transbronchial biopsy does not increase the yield over BAL, it has been recommended that only BAL be performed in high risk patients (Broaddus *et al.*, 1985). In one study

Table 3.4 Yield of BAL in diagnosis of pneumonia in immunosuppressed patients.

Author	Huaringa et al., 2000	Hohenadel et al., 2001	Jain et al., 2004	da Silva, Teixeira and Moreira, 2006	Velez et al., 2007[a]	Joos et al., 2007
Characteristics of immunosuppression	BMT	Hematologic abnormalities	non-HIV	HIV	80% HIV	Mixed
Number of studies	89	95	104	54	109	1066
Percent diagnostic	47%	65%	66%	NR	64%	85%
Infections[a]						
All bacteria	14.3%	57.2%	22.1%	37.0%	17.4%	33.6%
Mycobacteria	0.0%	6.6%	0.0%	18.5%	24.8%	6.0%
All fungal	14.3%	35.2%	9.6%	1.7%	13.5%	1.9%
Aspergillus	14.3%	7.7%	7.7%	0.0%	4.6%	1.9%
All viral	31.0%	1.1%	11.5%	1.7%	0.9%	29.6%
CMV	9.5%	1.1%	8.7%	1.7%	0.9%	7.8%
P. jiroveci	11.9%	0.0%	1.9%	46.7%	16.5%	14.6%
Other causes						
DAH	36%	NR	14.80%	NR	NR	NR

NR = Not reported; DAH = diffuse alveolar hemorrhage, CMV = cytomegalovirus.
[a]Unspecific airway inflammatory condition reported in 23.8%.

comparing PBS, BAL and TBB in 104 immunosuppressed patients, the biopsy was the exclusive diagnostic technique in 17 cases (Jain *et al.*, 2004). In all but two of these, the causes were noninfectious, such as malignancy.

Others have demonstrated an additional value for TBB in diagnosing infections. In a study of 31 HIV infected patients at risk for tuberculosis, an immediate diagnosis of *M. tuberculosis* was confirmed in 15, including 7 in whom the TBB was the only positive sample (Salzman *et al.*, 1992). Others have noted that TBB can enhance the yield for the diagnosis of aspergillus and *P. jiroveci* (Broaddus *et al.*, 1985; da Silva, Teixeira and Moreira, 2006).

Complications remain a major limitation of TBB. Pneumothorax can occur between 5 and 10% of cases (Broaddus *et al.*, 1985; Jain *et al.*, 2004). Bleeding from bronchoscopy is enhanced with biopsies and thrombocytopenia is a relative contraindication to biopsy.

3.10 Surgical lung biopsy (SLB)

The surgical lung biopsy has been considered the 'gold standard' for diagnosis of pneumonia. Since it provides a large sample for histologic evaluation, most clinicians feel a non diagnostic biopsy can be considered specific (Ellis *et al.*, 1995; White, Wong and Downey, 2000). For example, a 'negative' biopsy can confirm no further treatment required (Hall, Hutchins and Baker, 1987) and antibiotics can be withdrawn (White, Wong and Downey, 2000).

Currently, most surgical lung biopsy samples are obtained by the video assisted thorascopic surgery (VATS) technique. The results appear comparable to traditional open lung biopsies (White, Wong and Downey, 2000).

Infections can be diagnosed by SLB, including *P. jiroveci*, fungi, and CMV (Ellis *et al.*, 1995; White, Wong and Downey, 2000). In addition, nonspecific interstitial lung disease and alveolar hemorrhage may be diagnosed (Ellis *et al.*, 1995; White, Wong and Downey, 2000). The diagnosis of non specific interstitial lung disease requires specific pathologic changes which are not associated with any infection (Suffredini *et al.*, 1987).

Because the complication rate is high with SLB, risks versus benefits must be considered prior to the procedure. Table 3.5 compares five studies which evaluated surgical lung biopsy for the diagnosis of pulmonary infiltrates in immunosuppressed patients. Although all studies confirmed a specific diagnosis in most patients and therapy was often changed because of the SLB, the complication rate from the procedure ranged from 5 to 20% (Ellis *et al.*, 1995; Hayes-Jordan *et al.*, 2002; Robbins *et al.*, 1992; Wagner *et al.*, 1992; White, Wong and Downey, 2000). In fact, the one month mortality was higher than 10% in all series, with two series reporting a one month mortality rate of more than 60%. The high mortality was usually attributed to the patient's underlying co-morbidities, although in one study the post operative complications and need for mechanical ventilation decreased survival (Hayes-Jordan *et al.*, 2002). Delay in diagnosis is also important. Because most patients undergoing SLB have already failed empiric therapy, a delay in adequate therapy can be associated with increased mortality (Kollef *et al.*, 1999).

Table 3.5 Results of surgical lung biopsy in immunosuppressed patients with new pulmonary infiltrates.

	Number patients studied	Percent with diagnosis by SLB	Percent with change in therapy	One month mortality	Risk factors for increased mortality
Ellis *et al.*, 1995	13	92%	NS[a]	62%	NS
Hayes-Jordan *et al.*, 2002	19	89%	89%	37%	Mechanical ventilation, Post operative complications
Robbins *et al.*, 1992	74	42%	42%[b]	68%[c]	NS
Wagner *et al.*, 1992	50	58%	78%	14%	Respiratory failure
White, Wong and Downey, 2000	63	62%	57%	18%	Thrombocytopenia

[a]NS = not specified.
[b]Percent in whom infection was diagnosed.
[c]Survival of hospitalization.

3.11 Sample processing

In order to correctly interpret results, the respiratory samples obtained by the various techniques require careful handling and assessment. This applies for all samples, from the sputum to the surgical lung biopsy. Table 3.6 summarizes one approach to handling these samples and includes additional testing that can be performed. The indication for additional tests depends on the technology available as well as the particular concern for specific infection.

Sample assessment is an important part of result evaluation. Sputum needs to be assessed for quality, usually by determining whether the sample is adequately purulent and not contaminated with squamous epithelial cells, which indicates contamination by saliva (Heineman, Chawla and Lopton, 1977; Murray and Washington, 1975). Likewise, examination of the lower respiratory samples should assess for the absence of epithelial cells and also the presence of neutrophils. The BAL sample should have less than 10% epithelial cells to be considered an acceptable lower respiratory specimen (Baughman *et al.*, 2000; Klech and Pohl, 1989) and the BAL from patients with pneumonia should contain increased neutrophils and/or lymphocytes. For example, the BAL from most patients with bacterial pneumonia will have at least 30% neutrophils, whereas the normal value is less than 5% (Drent *et al.*, 2001). Lavage from patients with tuberculosis or PcP will contain increased lymphocytes, sometimes with no increase in neutrophils (Baughman, Dohn and Frame, 1991; Baughman *et al.*, 1991). Gram staining the PBS sample allows one to assure that the sample was from an area of infection (Marquette *et al.*, 1994). The transbronchial and surgical lung biopsy should also be assessed for the presence of alveolar tissue. In patients in whom no specific diagnosis can be made, the presence of adequate alveolar tissue allows the clinician to feel comfortable with the diagnosis of non specific interstitial pneumonia.

Table 3.6 Handling of specimens.

Specimen	Routine testing	Special tests	Quality assessment
Blood cultures	Aerobic and anaerobic testing	Fungal, AFB and virology cultures	Assess positive cultures for contamination
Sputum	Respiratory culture	AFB and fungal culture	Gram stain sputum to assess for purulence of sample
Tracheal aspirate	Respiratory culture	AFB and fungal culture	Gram stain sputum to assess for purulence of sample
Non bronchoscopic BAL sample	Semi-quantitative respiratory culture	AFB and fungal culture, Viral culture	Cytospin to assess that >90% of cells are alveolar, Record volume of aspirated fluid
Protected brush sample	Semi-quantitative respiratory culture		Gram stain to assess for purulence of sample
Bronchoscopic BAL	Semi-quantitative respiratory culture, Cytology including silver stain, Viral culture, AFB and fungal culture, Legionella culture	IFA for CMV, DFA for Legionella, PCR analysis, Fungal antigens	Cytospin to assess that >90% of cells are alveolar, Record volume of aspirated fluid
Bronchial wash	AFB and fungal culture, Cytology including silver stain	Bacterial culture, Viral culture	
Transbronchial biopsy	Histopathologic staining including silver stain	Bacterial culture, AFB and fungal culture, Viral culture	Alveolar tissue in sample
Surgical lung biopsy	Histopathologic staining including silver stain	Bacterial culture, AFB and fungal culture, Viral culture	Alveolar tissue in sample

Various techniques used to detect individual pathogens are summarized in Table 3.7. In general, immunofluorescence, antigen and PCR techniques are more sensitive than cytologic examination or culture. In some cases, the increased sensitivity may enhance diagnostic utility of a less sensitive sample. For example, the use of immunofluorescent staining enhances the diagnostic yield for induced sputum and bronchial wash to approximate the yield for BAL (Baughman *et al.*, 1989; Kovacs *et al.*, 1988). On the down side, increased sensitivity may lead to more detection of colonization. In one study of a commercially available antigen for aspergillus, ability to distinguish between colonization and infection was poor (Rath *et al.*, 1996).

Because PCR technique appears more sensitive and specific than routine culture techniques (Connolly *et al.*, 1994), this technique can increase the diagnostic yield of several different viruses (Garbino *et al.*, 2004). PCR has also been used to detect fastidious bacteria such as *M. pneumoniae* and *C. pneumoniae* (Garbino *et al.*, 2004). The use of PCR on the relatively sterile BAL sample should enhance both the sensitivity and specificity of these techniques.

However, PCR is not always the best technique. PCR can detect *P. jiroveci* (Sing *et al.*, 2000). This enhanced sensitivity has been used to diagnose PcP in mouth washings (Fischer *et al.*, 2001). However, in BAL samples, difficulty is encountered for distinguishing between colonization and infection (Maskell *et al.*, 2003; Sing *et al.*, 2000). In one study, quantitated PCR was useful in detecting invasive aspergillus infection (Rantakokko-Jalava *et al.*, 2003).

The use of the gamma interferon stimulation test to diagnose tuberculosis is highly specific and sensitive (Lee *et al.*, 2006), and it has been increasingly adopted for the rapid diagnosis of *M. tuberculosis* infection (Richeldi, 2006). In the immunosuppressed patient, the technique may detect latent infection (Matulis *et al.*, 2007), which does not seem related to false positives such as BCG inoculation (Soborg *et al.*, 2007). For immunosuppressed patients, the gamma interferon stimulation test will determine exposure, especially in patients who have a negative PPD due to immunosuppression or anergy (Matulis *et al.*, 2007). However, it does not separate latent from active disease.

3.12   Clinical approach to pulmonary infiltrates in immunosuppressed patient

The approach to the individual immunosuppressed patient must consider several factors including the level of illness and underlying illness. In all patients, the initial evaluation should include an assessment of the clinical status of the patient. The clinician needs to determine whether the patient could have pneumonia and the severity of the patient's illness.

The clinical symptoms of pneumonia including fever, increased dyspnea, new onset cough, and/or purulent sputum often lead to chest roentgenogram examination. If the chest roentgenogram is unrevealing, a CT scan may be useful. Regardless of whether the infiltrates are localized or diffuse, assessment of the level of illness is necessary. An immunosuppressed patient with a community acquired pneumonia is considered a case of health care associated pneumonia (Anon, 2005). The guidelines for hospitalization

Table 3.7 Evaluation for specific pathogens.

Pathogen	Smear	Culture	Immuno-fluorescent	Antigen	PCR	Other
P. jiroveci	Silver, Papinicolau, Wright-Giemsa	Not available	Both DFA and IFA (Baughman et al., 1989; Kovacs et al., 1988)	No	Yes (Maskell et al., 2003; Sing et al., 2000)	
M. tuberculosis	AFB smear	Yes	Auramine-Rhodamine (nonspecific)	Yes (Raja, Baughman and Daniel, 1988)	Yes	Gamma interferon (Lee et al., 2006)
C. neoformans	Silver, Mucicarmine	Yes	No	Yes	Yes (Takahashi et al., 2003)	
H. capsulatum	Silver	Yes	No	Yes (Hage et al., 2007; Wheat et al., 1992)		
B. dermatidides	Silver	Fungal	No	Yes (Hage et al., 2007)		
C. immites	Silver	Fungal	No	No		
Aspergillus	Silver	Fungal	No	Yes (Rath et al., 2002; Verweij et al., 1995)	Yes (Raad et al., 2002; Rantakokko-Jalava et al., 2003; Verweij et al., 1995)	Galactomannan (Nguyen et al., 2007)
CMV	Papanicolau	Viral culture	DFA (Miles et al., 1990)	No	Yes (Boivin et al., 1996)	RNA (Keightley et al., 2006)
Bacteria	Gram	Semi-quantitative	No	No	No	Specific bacteria by PCR (Garbino et al., 2004)

for community acquired pneumonia are a reasonable first step (Mandell *et al.*, 2007). However, for the immunocompromised patient factors associated with immuno-suppression including neutropenia and thrombocytopenia have to be considered.

The decision to perform bronchoscopy is a major component in the evaluation of the immunosuppressed patient. Advantages of the bronchoscopy include the larger samples associated with the BAL, disadvantages include the increased morbidity associated with the procedure as well as cost.

Although empiric therapy without bronchoscopy has its supporters, it is clear that BAL plays an important diagnostic role in many immunosuppressed patients. In a study by Rano *et al.*, BAL was associated with a highest likelihood of diagnosis and was the procedure most likely to change therapy (Rano *et al.*, 2001). It is a procedure associated with high yield even in patients who have received prior antibiotics. In a study of 95 immunocompromised patients with persistent signs or symptoms of pneumonia despite up to 10 days of antibiotics or antifungal therapy, BAL identified a pathogen in 65% of all cases. Furthermore, the BAL was the only positive sample in 29 of the 95 cases (Hohenadel *et al.*, 2001). In another series, patients hospitalized for pneumonia with persistent symptoms for more than 72 hours despite therapy underwent bronchoscopy with BAL. In 45 of 62 episodes, the BAL was positive for infection (Pereira Gomes *et al.*, 2000). Unfortunately, the overall mortality was 43%, pointing out the increased mortality seen with inadequate initial therapy.

Multiple studies reconfirm the observation of increased mortality for hospital acquired pneumonia (Kollef *et al.*, 1999; Luna *et al.*, 1997). In patients with persistent symptoms despite broad spectrum antibiotics, bronchoscopy with BAL (Hohenadel *et al.*, 2001) and SLB (Ellis *et al.*, 1995; Hayes-Jordan *et al.*, 2002; Robbins *et al.*, 1992) often identify a specific diagnosis. However, many studies report the 30 day mortality as greater than 30% for these patients. This may be due to inadequate initial therapy.

Figure 3.8 summarizes one approach to this problem which has been adapted from hospital acquired pneumonia guidelines (Anon, 2005). For the non hospitalized

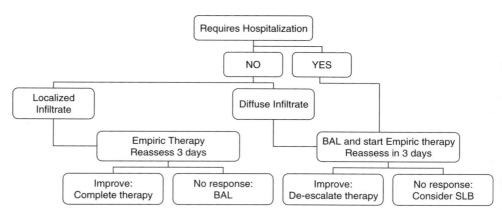

Figure 3.8   An approach to the immunosuppressed patient with possible pneumonia. Patients with diffuse infiltrates or those who require hospitalization for either localized or diffuse infiltrates should be considered for bronchoscopy with BAL. All patients will need empiric therapy pending results of diagnostic testing and clinical course.

patient with a localized infiltrate, empiric therapy for a bacterial pneumonia is reasonable. For the non hospitalized patient with diffuse infiltrates, a bronchoscopy with BAL should be considered. The procedure will have a high yield for routine as well as opportunistic infections. A hospitalized patient with either a localized or diffuse infiltrate is a candidate for a bronchoscopy with BAL provided the patient can tolerate the procedure. However, empiric therapy should be instituted immediately pending the results of the BAL.

Empiric therapy should be targeted to the underlying suspected pathogens which will depend on several factors, including underlying immunosuppression, institution and concurrent therapy. Prophylaxis against *P. jiroveci* and cytomegalovirus are quite effective and widely used. Figure 3.9 analyzes the frequency of different causes of pneumonia in two immunosuppressed groups (HIV and SCT). All patients were studied at one institution and BAL was the most common method of obtaining a final diagnosis (Joos *et al.*, 2007). As can be seen, there was a shift in potential pathogens as prophylaxis measures were frequently utilized in the later time period.

After three days of therapy, the clinical features of pneumonia should be reassessed. At that time, the initial diagnostic test results will be available. For routine bacterial pneumonia, clinical improvement should be noted if adequate therapy has been administered (Luna *et al.*, 2003; Singh *et al.*, 2000). However, some infections may require longer treatment. For immunosuppressed patients with Legionella, response to adequate therapy can require a week (Sopena *et al.*, 2002), and for patients with PcP, the delay in response can be masked by the use of corticosteroids.

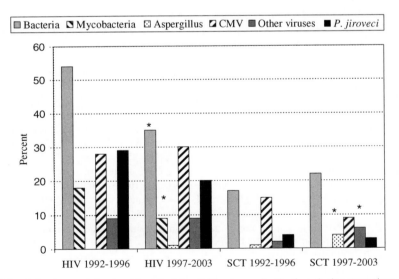

Figure 3.9 Infectious etiologies identified by BAL at one institution during two time periods: 1992–1996 versus 1997–2003. Immunosuppression due to HIV infection (420 studies) was compared to 374 studies in patients undergoing stem cell transplant and high-dose chemotherapy (SCT). There was significant difference in the frequency of infections between the two time periods (* $= p < 0.05$).

For those patients who are improving or in whom a specific diagnosis has been confirmed, de-escalation of empiric therapy is appropriate. The concept of de-escalation to avoid over use of broad spectrum antibiotics has become popular in treating ventilator associated pneumonia (Anon, 2005). However, the immunosuppressed patient is also at high risk for acquiring multi-resistant bacteria or fungal superinfection.

3.13   Conclusion

For the immunosuppressed patient with possible pneumonia, several diagnostic tests have been studied. These tests may not influence initial empiric therapy. However, these tests, when properly applied to the clinical response of the patient, may limit the overuse of antibiotics. The tests will also be useful in identifying patients who have a process other than infection, in whom no further antibiotics are needed.

References

Anon. Guidelines for the management of adults with hospital-acquired, ventilator-associated, and healthcare-associated pneumonia. *American Journal of Respiratory and Critical Care Medicine*, (2005) **171** (4), 388–416.

Afessa, B. and Peters, S.G. (2006) Major complications following hematopoietic stem cell transplantation. *Semin Respir Crit Care Med*, **27** (3), 297–309.

Aghamohammadi, A., Farhoudi, A., Moin, M., Rezaei, N., Kouhi, A., Pourpak, Z. *et al.* (2005) Clinical and immunological features of 65 Iranian patients with common variable immunodeficiency. *Clinical and Diagnostic Laboratory Immunology*, **12** (7), 825–832.

Agusti, C., Ramirez, J., Picado, C., Xaubet, A., Carreras, E., Ballester, E. *et al.* (1995) Diffuse alveolar hemorrhage in allogeneic bone marrow transplantation. A postmortem study. *American Journal of Respiratory and Critical Care Medicine*, **151** (4), 1006–1010.

Agusti, C., Rano, A., Aldabo, I. and Torres, A. (2006) Fungal pneumonia, chronic respiratory diseases and glucocorticoids. *Medical Mycology*, **44** (Suppl), 207–211.

Alario, A.J. and O'Shea, J.S. (1989) Risk of infectious complications in well-appearing children with transient neutropenia. *American Journal of Diseases of Children*, **143** (8), 973–976.

Attal, M., Schlaifer, D., Rubie, H., Huguet, F., Charlet, J.P., Bloom, E. *et al.* (1991) Prevention of gram-positive infections after bone marrow transplantation by systemic vancomycin: A prospective, randomized trial. *Journal of Clinical Oncology*, **9** (5), 865–870.

Barrett-Connor, E. (1971) The nonvalue of sputum culture in the diagnosis of pneumococcal pneumonia. *The American Review of Respiratory Disease*, **103** (6), 845–848.

Bartlett, R.C., Tetreault, J., Evers, J., Officer, J. and Derench, J. (1979) Quality assurance of gram-stained direct smears. *American Journal of Clinical Pathology*, **72** (6), 984–989.

Baughman, R.P. (1999) The lung in the immunocompromised patient: Infectious complications Part 1. *Respiration; International Review of Thoracic Diseases*, **66**, 95–109.

Baughman, R.P. (2000) Protected-specimen brush technique in the diagnosis of ventilator-associated pneumonia. *Chest*, **117**, 203S–206S.

Baughman, R.P. (2003) How I do bronchoalveolar lavage. *Journal of Bronchology*, **10** (4), 309–314.

Baughman, R.P. (2003) Nonbronchoscopic evaluation of ventilator-associated pneumonia. *Seminars in Respiratory Infections*, **18** (2), 95–102.

Baughman, R.P., Daunt, S.R., Kleykamp, B.A. and Staneck, J. (2000) Evaluation of various bronchoscopic techniques to diagnose the cause of an acute exacerbation of chronic bronchitis. *Journal of Bronchology*, **7**, 221–225.

Baughman, R.P., Dohn, M.N. and Frame, P.T. (1991) Generalized immune response to Pneumocystis carinii infection in the lung. *The Journal of Protozoology*, **38** (6), 187S–188S.

Baughman, R.P., Dohn, M.N. and Frame, P.T. (1994) The continuing utility of bronchoalveolar lavage to diagnose opportunistic infection in AIDS patients. *The American Journal of Medicine*, **97** (6), 515–522.

Baughman, R.P., Dohn, M.N., Loudon, R.G. and Frame, P.T. (1991) Bronchoscopy with bronchoalveolar lavage in tuberculosis and fungal infections. *Chest*, **99** (1), 92–97.

Baughman, R.P., Dohn, M.N., Shipley, R., Buchsbaum, J.A. and Frame, P.T. (1993) Increased Pneumocystis carinii recovery from the upper lobes in Pneumocystis pneumonia. The effect of aerosol pentamidine prophylaxis. *Chest*, **103** (2), 426–432.

Baughman, R.P. and Lower, E.E. (2005) Fungal infections as a complication of therapy for sarcoidosis. *QJM: Monthly Journal of the Association of Physicians*, **98**, 451–456.

Baughman, R.P., Rhodes, J.C., Dohn, M.N., Henderson, H. and Frame, P.T. (1992) Detection of cryptococcal antigen in bronchoalveolar lavage fluid: A prospective study of diagnostic utility. *The American Review of Respiratory Disease*, **145** (5), 1226–1229.

Baughman, R.P., Spencer, R.E., Kleykamp, B.O., Rashkin, M.C. and Douthit, M.M. (2000) Ventilator associated pneumonia: Quality of nonbronchoscopic bronchoalveolar lavage sample affects diagnostic yield. *The European Respiratory Journal*, **16**, 1152–1157.

Baughman, R.P., Strohofer, S.S., Clinton, B.A., Nickol, A.D. and Frame, P.T. (1989) The use of an indirect fluorescent antibody test for detecting Pneumocystis carinii. *Archives of Pathology and Laboratory Medicine*, **113** (9), 1062–1065.

Beck, J.M., Rosen, M.J. and Peavy, H.H. (2001) Pulmonary complications of HIV infection. Report of the Fourth NHLBI Workshop. *American Journal of Respiratory and Critical Care Medicine*, **164** (11), 2120–2126.

Bigby, T.D., Margolskee, D., Curtis, J.L., Michael, P.F., Sheppard, D., Hadley, W.K. *et al.* (1986) The usefulness of induced sputum in the diagnosis of Pneumocystis carinii pneumonia in patients with the acquired immunodeficiency syndrome. *The American Review of Respiratory Disease*, **133** (4), 515–518.

Bishburg, E., Zucker, M.J., Baran, D.A. and Arroyo, L.H. (2004) Mycobacterium xenopi infection after heart transplantation: An unreported pathogen. *Transplantation Proceedings*, **36** (9), 2834–2836.

Boersma, W.G., Erjavec, Z., van der Werf, T.S., de Vries-Hosper, H.G., Gouw, A.S. and Manson, W.L. (2007) Bronchoscopic diagnosis of pulmonary infiltrates in granulocytopenic patients with hematologic malignancies: BAL versus PSB and PBAL. *Respiratory Medicine*, **101** (2), 317–325.

Bohme, A., Just-Nubling, G., Bergmann, L., Shah, P.M., Stille, W. and Hoelzer, D. (1995) A randomized study of imipenem compared to cefotaxime plus piperacillin as initial therapy of infections in granulocytopenic patients. *Infection*, **23** (6), 349–355.

Boivin, G., Olson, C.A., Quirk, M.R., Kringstad, B., Hertz, M.I. and Jordan, M.C. (1996) Quantitation of cytomegalovirus DNA and characterization of viral gene expression in bronchoalveolar cells of infected patients with and without pneumonitis. *The Journal of Infectious Diseases*, **173** (6), 1304–1312.

Bont, J., Hak, E., Hoes, A.W., Schipper, M., Schellevis, F.G. and Verheij, T.J. (2007) A prediction rule for elderly primary-care patients with lower respiratory tract infections. *The European Respiratory Journal*, **29** (5), 969–975.

Bottone, E.J., Sindone, M. and Caraballo, V. (1998) Value of assessing cryptococcal antigen in bronchoalveolar lavage and sputum specimens from patients with AIDS. *The Mount Sinai Journal of Medicine, New York*, **65** (5–6), 422–425.

Broaddus, C., Dake, M.D., Stulbarg, M.S., Blumenfeld, W., Hadley, W.K., Golden, J.A. *et al.* (1985) Bronchoalveolar lavage and transbronchial biopsy for the diagnosis of pulmonary infections in the acquired immunodeficiency syndrome. *Annals of Internal Medicine*, **102** (6), 747–752.

Bustamante, E.A. and Levy, H. (1994) Sputum induction compared with bronchoalveolar lavage by Ballard catheter to diagnose Pneumocystis carinii pneumonia. *Chest*, **105** (3), 816–822.

Cabello, H., Torres, A., Celis, R., El-Ebiary, M., de la Bellacasa, J.P., Xaubet, A. *et al.* (1997) Bacterial colonization of distal airways in healthy subjects and chronic lung disease: A bronchoscopic study. *The European Respiratory Journal*, **10**, 1137–1144.

Campbell, G.D. (2000) Blinded invasive diagnostic procedures in ventilator-associated pneumonia. *Chest*, **117**, 207S–211S.

Cantral, D.E., Tape, T.G., Reed, E.C., Spurzem, J.R., Rennard, S.I. and Thompson, A.B. (1993) Quantitative culture of bronchoalveolar lavage fluid for the diagnosis of bacterial pneumonia. *The American Journal of Medicine*, **95**, 601–607.

Caughey, G., Wong, H., Gamsu, G. and Golden, J. (1985) Nonbronchoscopic bronchoalveolar lavage for the diagnosis for Pneumocystis carinii pneumonia in the acquired immunodeficiency syndrome. *Chest*, **88** (5), 659–662.

Chaisson, R.E., Moore, R.D., Richman, D.D., Keruly, J. and Creagh, T. (1992) Incidence and natural history of Mycobacterium avium-complex infections in patients with advanced human immuno-deficiency virus disease treated with zidovudine. The Zidovudine Epidemiology Study Group. *The American Review of Respiratory Disease*, **146** (2), 285–289.

Chan, H.S., Sun, A.J. and Hoheisel, G.B. (1990) Bronchoscopic aspiration and bronchoalveolar lavage in the diagnosis of sputum smear-negative pulmonary tuberculosis. *Lung*, **168** (4), 215–220.

Chang, G.C., Wu, C.L., Pan, S.H., Yang, T.Y., Chin, C.S., Yang, Y.C. *et al.* (2004) The diagnosis of pneumonia in renal transplant recipients using invasive and noninvasive procedures. *Chest*, **125** (2), 541–547.

Chang, W.C., Tzao, C., Hsu, H.H., Lee, S.C., Huang, K.L., Tung, H.J. *et al.* (2006) Pulmonary cryptococcosis: Comparison of clinical and radiographic characteristics in immunocompetent and immunocompromised patients. *Chest*, **129** (2), 333–340.

Chastre, J., Fagon, J.Y., Soler, P., Bornet, M., Domart, Y., Trouillet, J.L. *et al.* (1988) Diagnosis of nosocomial bacterial pneumonia in intubated patients undergoing ventilation: Comparison of the usefulness of bronchoalveolar lavage and the protected specimen brush. *The American Journal of Medicine*, **85**, 499–506.

Coleman, D.L., Dodek, P.M., Luce, J.M., Golden, J.A., Gold, W.M. and Murray, J.F. (1983) Diagnostic utility of fiberoptic bronchoscopy in patients with Pneumocystis carinii pneumonia and the acquired immune deficiency syndrome. *The American Review of Respiratory Disease*, **128** (5), 795–799.

Conces, D.J., Jr (1999) Endemic fungal pneumonia in immunocompromised patients. *Journal of Thoracic Imaging*, **14** (1), 1–8.

Connolly, M.G.J., Baughman, R.P., Dohn, M.N. and Linnemann, C.C.J. (1994) Recovery of viruses other than cytomegalovirus from bronchoalveolar lavage fluid. *Chest*, **105**, 1775–1781.

Cook, D.J. and Mandell, L.A. (2000) Diagnosis of ventilator associated pneumonia: A systematic review of endotracheal aspirates. *Chest*, **117**, 195S–197S.

Costa, D.B., Shin, B. and Cooper, D.L. (2004) Pneumococcemia as the presenting feature of multiple myeloma. *American Journal of Hematology*, **77** (3), 277–281.

Costa, S.F. and Alexander, B.D. (2005) Non-Aspergillus fungal pneumonia in transplant recipients. *Clinics in Chest Medicine*, **26** (4), 675–690 vii.

Cunningham-Rundles, C. and Bodian, C. (1999) Common variable immunodeficiency: Clinical and immunological features of 248 patients. *Clinical Immunology (Orlando, Fla)*, **92** (1), 34–48.

da Silva, R.M., Teixeira, P.J. and Moreira, J.S. (2006) The clinical utility of induced sputum for the diagnosis of bacterial community-acquired pneumonia in HIV-infected patients: A prospective cross-sectional study. *The Brazilian Journal of Infectious Diseases*, **10** (2), 89–93.

De Lassence, A., Fleury-Feith, J., Escudier, E., Beaune, J., Bernaudin, J.F. and Cordonnier, C. (1995) Alveolar hemorrhage. Diagnostic criteria and results in 194 immunocompromised hosts. *American Journal of Respiratory and Critical Care Medicine*, **151** (1), 157–163.

Dohn, M.N. and Baughman, R.P. (1985) Effect of changing instilled volume for bronchoalveolar lavage in patients with interstitial lung disease. *The American Review of Respiratory Disease*, **132**, 390–392.

Drent, M., Jacobs, J.A., Cobben, N.A., Costabel, U., Wouters, E.F. and Mulder, P.G. (2001) Computer program supporting the diagnostic accuracy of cellular BALF analysis: A new release. *Respiratory Medicine*, **95** (10), 781–786.

Dunagan, D.P., Baker, A.M., Hurd, D.D. and Haponik, E.F. (1997) Bronchoscopic evaluation of pulmonary infiltrates following bone marrow transplantation. *Chest*, **111** (1), 135–141.

Eckburg, P.B., Buadu, E.O., Stark, P., Sarinas, P.S., Chitkara, R.K. and Kuschner, W.G. (2000) Clinical and chest radiographic findings among persons with sputum culture positive for Mycobacterium gordonae: A review of 19 cases. *Chest*, **117** (1), 96–102.

el Ebiary, M., Torres, A., Fabregas, N., de la Bellacasa, J.P., Gonzalez, J., Ramirez, J. *et al.* (1997) Significance of the isolation of Candida species from respiratory samples in critically ill, non-neutropenic patients. An immediate postmortem histologic study. *American Journal of Respiratory and Critical Care Medicine*, **156** (2 Pt 1), 583–590.

el Ebiary, M., Torres, A., Gonzalez, J., de la Bellacasa, J.P., Garcia, C., Jimenez de Anta, M.T. *et al.* (1993) Quantitative cultures of endotracheal aspirates for the diagnosis of ventilator-associated pneumonia. *The American Review of Respiratory Disease*, **148** (6 Pt 1), 1552–1557.

El-Solh, A.A., Nopper, J., bdul-Khoudoud, M.R., Sherif, S.M., Aquilina, A.T. and Grant, B.J. (1998) Clinical and radiographic manifestations of uncommon pulmonary nontuberculous mycobacterial disease in AIDS patients. *Chest*, **114** (1), 138–145.

Ellis, M.E., Spence, D., Bouchama, A., Antonius, J., Bazarbashi, M., Khougeer, F. *et al.* (1995) Open lung biopsy provides a higher and more specific diagnostic yield compared to broncho-alveolar lavage in immunocompromised patients. Fungal Study Group. *Scandinavian Journal of Infectious Diseases*, **27** (2), 157–162.

Engelhard, D., Cordonnier, C., Shaw, P.J., Parkalli, T., Guenther, C., Martino, R. *et al.* (2002) Early and late invasive pneumococcal infection following stem cell transplantation: A European Bone Marrow Transplantation survey. *British Journal of Haematology*, **117** (2), 444–450.

Enright, H., Haake, R., Weisdorf, D., Ramsay, N., McGlave, P., Kersey, J. *et al.* (1993) Cytomegalovirus pneumonia after bone marrow transplantation. Risk factors and response to therapy. *Transplantation*, **55** (6), 1339–1346.

Ewig, S., Bauer, T., Schneider, C., Pickenhain, A., Pizzulli, L., Loos, U. *et al.* (1995) Clinical characteristics and outcome of Pneumocystis carinii pneumonia in HIV-infected and otherwise immunosuppressed patients. *The European Respiratory Journal*, **8** (9), 1548–1553.

Feinstein, M.B., Mokhtari, M., Ferreiro, R., Stover, D.E. and Jakubowski, A. (2001) Fiberoptic bronchoscopy in allogeneic bone marrow transplantation: Findings in the era of serum cytomegalovirus antigen surveillance. *Chest*, **120** (4), 1094–1100.

Fischer, S., Gill, V.J., Kovacs, J., Miele, P., Keary, J., Silcott, V. *et al.* (2001) The use of oral washes to diagnose Pneumocystis carinii pneumonia: A blinded prospective study using a polymerase chain reaction-based detection system. *The Journal of Infectious Diseases*, **184** (11), 1485–1488.

Fishman, J.A. (2007) Infection in renal transplant recipients. *Seminars in Nephrology*, **27** (4), 445–461.

Fishman, J.A., Roth, R.S., Zanzot, E., Enos, E.J. and Ferraro, M.J. (1994) Use of induced sputum specimens for microbiologic diagnosis of infections due to organisms other than Pneumocystis carinii. *Journal of Clinical Microbiology*, **32** (1), 131–134.

Forbes, G.M., Harvey, F.A., Philpott-Howard, J.N., O'Grady, J.G., Jensen, R.D., Sahathevan, M. *et al.* (1990) Nocardiosis in liver transplantation: Variation in presentation, diagnosis and therapy. *TheJournal of Infection*, **20** (1), 11–19.

Friedman, B.A., Wenglin, B.D., Hyland, R.N. and Rifkind, D. (1975) Roentgenographically atypical Pneumocystis carinii pneumonia. *The American Review of Respiratory Disease*, **111** (1), 89–96.

Fujii, T., Nakamura, T. and Iwamoto, A. (2007) Pneumocystis pneumonia in patients with HIV infection: Clinical manifestations, laboratory findings, and radiological features. *Journal of Infection and Chemotherapy*, **13** (1), 1–7.

Fujitani, S. and Yu, V.L. (2006) Diagnosis of ventilator-associated pneumonia: Focus on nonbroncho-scopic techniques (nonbronchoscopic bronchoalveolar lavage, including mini-BAL, blinded protected specimen brush, and blinded bronchial sampling) and endotracheal aspirates. *Journal of Intensive Care Medicine*, **21** (1), 17–21.

Garbino, J., Gerbase, M.W., Wunderli, W., Deffernez, C., Thomas, Y., Rochat, T. *et al.* (2004) Lower respiratory viral illnesses: Improved diagnosis by molecular methods and clinical impact. *American Journal of Respiratory and Critical Care Medicine*, **170** (11), 1197–1203.

Ghiotto, F., Fais, F., Valetto, A., Albesiano, E., Hashimoto, S., Dono, M. *et al.* (2004) Remarkably similar antigen receptors among a subset of patients with chronic lymphocytic leukemia. *The Journal of Clinical Investigation*, **113** (7), 1008–1016.

Golden, J.A., Hollander, H., Stulbarg, M.S. and Gamsu, G. (1986) Bronchoalveolar lavage as the exclusive diagnostic modality for Pneumocystis carinii pneumonia. A prospective study among patients with acquired immunodeficiency syndrome. *Chest*, **90** (1), 18–22.

Gona, P., Van Dyke, R.B., Williams, P.L., Dankner, W.M., Chernoff, M.C., Nachman, S.A. *et al.* (2006) Incidence of opportunistic and other infections in HIV-infected children in the HAART era. *The Journal of the American Medical Association*, **296** (3), 292–300.

Goto, H., Yuasa, K., Sakamaki, H., Nakata, K., Komuro, I., Iguchi, M. *et al.* (1996) Rapid detection cytomegalovirus pneumonia in recipients of bone marrow transplant: Evaluation and comparison of five survey methods for bronchoalveolar lavage fluid. *Bone Marrow Transplantation*, **17** (5), 855–860.

Guerra, L.F. and Baughman, R.P. (1990) Use of bronchoalveolar lavage to diagnose bacterial pneumonia in mechanically ventilated patients. *Critical Care Medicine*, **18**, 169–173.

Hage, C.A., Davis, T.E., Egan, L., Parker, M., Fuller, D., Lemonte, A.M. *et al.* (2007) Diagnosis of pulmonary histoplasmosis and blastomycosis by detection of antigen in bronchoalveolar lavage fluid using an improved second-generation enzyme-linked immunoassay. *Respiratory Medicine*, **101** (1), 43–47.

Hall, T.S., Hutchins, G.M. and Baker, R.R. (1987) A critical review of the use of open lung biopsy in the management of the oncologic patient with acute pulmonary infiltrates. *American Journal of Clinical Oncology*, **10** (3), 249–252.

Hayden, R.T., Uhl, J.R., Qian, X., Hopkins, M.K., Aubry, M.C., Limper, A.H. *et al.* (2001) Direct detection of Legionella species from bronchoalveolar lavage and open lung biopsy specimens: Comparison of LightCycler PCR, in situ hybridization, direct fluorescence antigen detection, and culture. *Journal of Clinical Microbiology*, **39** (7), 2618–2626.

Hayes-Jordan, A., Benaim, E., Richardson, S., Joglar, J., Srivastava, D.K., Bowman, L. *et al.* (2002) Open lung biopsy in pediatric bone marrow transplant patients. *Journal of Pediatric Surgery,* **37** (3), 446–452.

Hayner, C.E., Baughman, R.P., Linnemann, C.C.J. and Dohn, M.N. (1995) The relationship between cytomegalovirus retrieved by bronchoalveolar lavage and mortality in patients with HIV. *Chest,* **107**, 735–740.

Heineman, H.S., Chawla, J.K. and Lopton, W.M. (1977) Misinformation from sputum cultures without microscopic examination. *Journal of Clinical Microbiology,* **6** (5), 518–527.

Heussel, C.P., Kauczor, H.U., Heussel, G.E., Fischer, B., Begrich, M., Mildenberger, P. *et al.* (1999) Pneumonia in febrile neutropenic patients and in bone marrow and blood stem-cell transplant recipients: Use of high-resolution computed tomography. *Journal of Clinical Oncology,* **17** (3), 796–805.

Heussel, C.P., Kauczor, H.U. and Ullmann, A.J. (2004) Pneumonia in neutropenic patients. *European Radiology,* **14** (2), 256–271.

Hilborne, L.H., Nieberg, R.K., Cheng, L. and Lewin, K.J. (1987) Direct in situ hybridization for rapid detection of cytomegalovirus in bronchoalveolar lavage. *American Journal of Clinical Pathology,* **87** (6), 766–769.

Hohenadel, I.A., Kiworr, M., Genitsariotis, R., Zeidler, D. and Lorenz, J. (2001) Role of broncho-alveolar lavage in immunocompromised patients with pneumonia treated with a broad spectrum antibiotic and antifungal regimen. *Thorax,* **56** (2), 115–120.

Hohenthal, U., Itala, M., Salonen, J., Sipila, J., Rantakokko-Jalava, K., Meurman, O. *et al.* (2005) Bronchoalveolar lavage in immunocompromised patients with haematological malignancy–value of new microbiological methods. *European Journal of Haematology,* **74** (3), 203–211.

Huang, L. and Hopewell, P.C. (1998) Bronchoscopy versus sputum induction as the initial procedure for the diagnosis of Pneumocystis carinii pneumonia in paitents with HIV. Pro sputum induction. *Journal of Bronchology,* **5**, 163–168.

Huaringa, A.J., Leyva, F.J., Signes-Costa, J., Morice, R.C., Raad, I., Darwish, A.A. *et al.* (2000) Bronchoalveolar lavage in the diagnosis of pulmonary complications of bone marrow transplant patients. *Bone Marrow Transplantation,* **25** (9), 975–979.

Hughes, W.T., Rivera, G.K., Schell, M.J., Thornton, D. and Lott, L. (1987) Successful intermittent chemoprophylaxis for Pneumocystis carinii pneumonitis. *The New England Journal of Medicine,* **316** (26), 1627–1632.

Iregui, M., Ward, S., Sherman, G., Fraser, V.J. and Kollef, M.H. (2002) Clinical importance of delays in the initiation of appropriate antibiotic treatment for ventilator-associated pneumonia. *Chest,* **122** (1), 262–268.

Israel, H.L., Gottlieb, J.E. and Schulman, E.S. (1987) Hypoxemia with normal chest roentgenogram due to Pneumocystis carinii pneumonia. Diagnostic errors due to low suspicion of AIDS. *Chest,* **92** (5), 857–859.

Jagarlamudi, R., Kumar, L., Kochupillai, V., Kapil, A., Banerjee, U. and Thulkar, S. (2000) Infections in acute leukemia: An analysis of 240 febrile episodes. *Medical Oncology (Northwood, London, England),* **17** (2), 111–116.

Jain, P., Sandur, S., Meli, Y., Arroliga, A.C., Stoller, J.K. and Mehta, A.C. (2004) Role of flexible bronchoscopy in immunocompromised patients with lung infiltrates. *Chest,* **125** (2), 712–722.

Joos, L., Chhajed, P.N., Wallner, J., Battegay, M., Steiger, J., Gratwohl, A. *et al.* (2007) Pulmonary infections diagnosed by BAL: A 12-year experience in 1066 immunocompromised patients. *Respiratory Medicine,* **101** (1), 93–97.

Judson, M.A. (2004) Noninvasive Aspergillus pulmonary disease. *Semin Respir Crit Care Med,* **25** (2), 203–219.

Kahn, F.W. and Jones, J.M. (1987) Diagnosing bacterial respiratory infection by bronchoalveolar lavage. *Journal Infectious Disease,* **155**, 862–869.

Kahn, F.W., Jones, J.M. and England, D.M. (1987) Diagnosis of pulmonary hemorrhage in the immunocompromised host. *The American Review of Respiratory Disease*, **136** (1), 155–160.

Keightley, M.C., Rinaldo, C., Bullotta, A., Dauber, J. and St, G.K. (2006) Clinical utility of CMV early and late transcript detection with NASBA in bronchoalveolar lavages. *Journal of Clinical Virology*, **37** (4), 258–264.

Kerkering, T.M., Duma, R.J. and Shadomy, S. (1981) The evolution of pulmonary cryptococcosis: Clinical implications from a study of 41 patients with and without compromising host factors. *Annals of Internal Medicine*, **94** (5), 611–616.

Kirby, B.D., Snyder, K.M., Meyer, R.D. and Finegold, S.M. (1980) Legionnaires' disease: Report of sixty-five nosocomially acquired cases of review of the literature. *Medicine (Baltimore)*, **59** (3), 188–205.

Klech, H. and Pohl, W. (1989) Technical recommendations and guidelines for bronchoalveolar lavage (BAL). *The European Respiratory Journal*, **2**, 561–585.

Knollmann, F.D., Maurer, J., Bechstein, W.O., Vogl, T.J., Neuhaus, P. and Felix, R. (2000) Pulmonary disease in liver transplant recipients. Spectrum of CT features. *Acta Radiologica*, **41** (3), 230–236.

Kohli, R., Lo, Y., Homel, P., Flanigan, T.P., Gardner, L.I., Howard, A.A. *et al.* (2006) Bacterial pneumonia, HIV therapy, and disease progression among HIV-infected women in the HIV epidemiologic research (HER) study. *Clinical Infectious Diseases*, **43** (1), 90–98.

Kohorst, W.R., Schonfeld, S.A., Macklin, J.E. and Whitcomb, M.E. (1983) Rapid diagnosis of Legionnaires' disease by bronchoalveolar lavage. *Chest*, **84** (2), 186–190.

Kollef, M.H., Bock, K.R., Richards, R.D. and Hearns, M.L. (1995) The safety and diagnostic accuracy of minibronchoalveolar lavage in patients with suspected ventilator-associated pneumonia. *Annals of Internal Medicine*, **122** (10), 743–748.

Kollef, M.H., Sherman, G., Ward, S. and Fraser, V.J. (1999) Inadequate antimicrobial treatment of infections: A risk factor for hospital mortality among critically ill patients. *Chest*, **115** (2), 462–474.

Kollef, M.H. and Ward, S. (1998) The influence of mini-BAL cultures on patient outcomes: Implications for the antibiotic management of ventilator-associated pneumonia. *Chest*, **113**, 412–420.

Kotloff, R.M., Ahya, V.N. and Crawford, S.W. (2004) Pulmonary complications of solid organ and hematopoietic stem cell transplantation. *American Journal of Respiratory and Critical Care Medicine*, **170** (1), 22–48.

Kovacs, J.A., Ng, V.L., Masur, H., Leoung, G., Hadley, W.K., Evans, G. *et al.* (1988) Diagnosis of Pneumocystis carinii pneumonia: Improved detection in sputum with use of monoclonal antibodies. *The New England Journal of Medicine*, **318** (10), 589–593.

Kralovic, S.M. and Rhodes, J.C. (1998) Utility of routine testing of bronchoalveolar lavage fluid for cryptococcal antigen. *Journal of Clinical Microbiology*, **36** (10), 3088–3089.

Kutukculer, N., Karaca, N.E., Demircioglu, O. and Aksu, G. (2007) Increases in serum immunoglobulins to age-related normal levels in children with IgA and/or IgG subclass deficiency. *Pediatric Allergy and Immunology*, **18** (2), 167–173.

Lambert, R.S., Vereen, L.E. and George, R.B. (1989) Comparison of tracheal aspirates and protected brush catheter specimens for identifying pathogenic bacteria in mechanically ventilated patients. *The American Journal of the Medical Sciences*, **297** (6), 377–382.

Lambotte, O., Timsit, J.F., Garrouste-Org, M., Misset, B., Benali, A. and Carlet, J. (2002) The significance of distal bronchial samples with commensals in ventilator-associated pneumonia: Colonizer or pathogen? *Chest*, **122** (4), 1389–1399.

Landgren, O., Rapkin, J.S., Caporaso, N.E., Mellemkjaer, L., Gridley, G., Goldin, L.R. *et al.* (2007) Respiratory tract infections and subsequent risk of chronic lymphocytic leukemia. *Blood*, **109** (5), 2198–2201.

Landgren, O., Rapkin, J.S., Mellemkjaer, L., Gridley, G., Goldin, L.R. and Engels, E.A. (2006) Respiratory tract infections in the pathway to multiple myeloma: A population-based study in Scandinavia. *Haematologica*, **91** (12), 1697–1700.

Lee, J.Y., Choi, H.J., Park, I.N., Hong, S.B., Oh, Y.M., Lim, C.M. *et al.* (2006) Comparison of two commercial interferon-gamma assays for diagnosing Mycobacterium tuberculosis infection. *The European Respiratory Journal*, **28** (1), 24–30.

Lemert, C.M., Baughman, R.P., Hayner, C.E. and Nestok, B.R. (1996) Relationship between cytomegalovirus cells and survival in acquired immunodeficiency syndrome patients. *Acta Cytologica*, **40** (2), 205–210.

Levy, H. (1994) Comparison of Ballard catheter bronchoalveolar lavage with bronchoscopic bronchoalveolar lavage. *Chest*, **106** (6), 1753–1756.

Levy, H., Horak, D.A., Tegtmeier, B.R., Yokota, S.B. and Forman, S.J. (1992) The value of bronchoalveolar lavage and bronchial washings in the diagnosis of invasive pulmonary aspergillosis. *Respiratory Medicine*, **86** (3), 243–248.

Limper, A.H., Offord, K.P., Smith, T.F. and Martin, W.J. (1989) Pneumocystis carinii pneumonia. Differences in lung parasite number and inflammation in patients with and without AIDS. *The American Review of Respiratory Disease*, **140** (5), 1204–1209.

Lindemulder, S. and Albano, E. (2007) Successful intermittent prophylaxis with trimethoprim/sulfamethoxazole 2 days per week for Pneumocystis carinii (jiroveci) pneumonia in pediatric oncology patients. *Pediatrics*, **120** (1), e47–e51

Link, H., Maschmeyer, G., Meyer, P., Hiddemann, W., Stille, W., Helmerking, M. *et al.* (1994) Interventional antimicrobial therapy in febrile neutropenic patients. Study group of the Paul Ehrlich Society for Chemotherapy. *Annals of Hematology*, **69** (5), 231–243.

Lortholary, O., Meyohas, M.C., Dupont, B., Cadranel, J., Salmon-Ceron, D., Peyramond, D. *et al.* (1993) Invasive aspergillosis in patients with acquired immunodeficiency syndrome: Report of 33 cases. French cooperative study group on aspergillosis in AIDS. *The American Journal of Medicine*, **95** (2), 177–187.

Lower, E.E. and Baughman, R.P. (1992) Pulmonary lymphangitic metastasis from breast cancer. Lymphocytic alveolitis is associated with favorable prognosis. *Chest*, **102**, 1113–1117.

Luna, C.M., Blanzaco, D., Niederman, M.S., Matarucco, W., Baredes, N.C., Desmery, P. *et al.* (2003) Resolution of ventilator-associated pneumonia: Prospective evaluation of the clinical pulmonary infection score as an early clinical predictor of outcome. *Critical Care Medicine*, **31** (3), 676–682.

Luna, C.M., Vujacich, P., Niederman, M.S., Vay, C., Gherardi, C., Matera, J. *et al.* (1997) Impact of BAL data on the therapy and outcome of ventilator- associated pneumonia. *Chest*, **111** (3), 676–685.

Mandell, L.A., Wunderink, R.G., Anzueto, A., Bartlett, J.G., Campbell, G.D., Dean, N.C. *et al.* (2007) Infectious Diseases Society of America/American Thoracic Society consensus guidelines on the management of community-acquired pneumonia in adults. *Clinical Infectious Diseases*, **44** (Suppl 2), S27–S32

Mann, M., Shelhamer, J.H., Masur, H., Gill, V.J., Travis, W., Solomon, D. *et al.* (1997) Lack of clinical utility of bronchoalveolar lavage cultures for cytomegalovirus in HIV infection. *American Journal of Respiratory and Critical Care Medicine*, **155**, 1723–1728.

Mari, B., Monton, C., Mariscal, D., Lujan, M., Sala, M. and Domingo, C. (2001) Pulmonary nocardiosis: Clinical experience in ten cases. *Respiration; International Review of Thoracic Diseases*, **68** (4), 382–388.

Marquette, C.H., Copin, M.C., Wallet, F., Neviere, R., Saulnier, F., Mathieu, D. *et al.* (1995) Diagnostic tests for pneumonia in ventilated patients: Prospective evaluation of diagnostic accuracy using histology as a diagnostic gold standard. *American Journal of Respiratory and Critical Care Medicine*, **151** (6), 1878–1888.

Marquette, C.H., Herengt, F., Mathieu, D., Saulnier, F., Courcol, R. and Ramon, P. (1993) Diagnosis of pneumonia in mechanically ventilated patients. Repeatability of the protected specimen brush. *The American Review of Respiratory Disease*, **147**, 211–214.

Marquette, C.H., Wallet, F., Neviere, R., Copin, M.C., Saulnier, F., Drault, J.N. *et al.* (1994) Diagnostic value of direct examination of the protected specimen brush in ventilator-associated pneumonia. *The European Respiratory Journal*, **7** (1), 105–113.

Marshall, W., Foster, R.S., Jr and Winn, W. (1981) Legionnaires' disease in renal transplant patients. *American Journal of Surgery*, **141** (4), 423–429.

Maskell, N.A., Waine, D.J., Lindley, A., Pepperell, J.C., Wakefield, A.E., Miller, R.F. *et al.* (2003) Asymptomatic carriage of Pneumocystis jiroveci in subjects undergoing bronchoscopy: A prospective study. *Thorax*, **58** (7), 594–597.

Masur, H., Ognibene, F.P., Yarchoan, R., Shelhamer, J.H., Baird, B.F., Travis, W. *et al.* (1989) CD4 counts as predictors of opportunistic pneumonias in human immunodeficiency virus (HIV) infection. *Annals of Internal Medicine*, **111** (3), 223–231.

Matulis, G., Juni, P., Villiger, P.M. and Gadola, S.D. (2008) Detection of latent tuberculosis in immunosuppressed patients with autoimmune diseases performance of a mycobacterium tuberculosis antigen specific IFN-gamma assay. *Annals of the Rheumatic Diseases*, **67**, 84–90.

McKenzie, R., Travis, W.D., Dolan, S.A., Pittaluga, S., Feuerstein, I.M., Shelhamer, J. *et al.* (1991) The causes of death in patients with human immunodeficiency virus infection: A clinical and pathologic study with emphasis on the role of pulmonary diseases. *Medicine (Baltimore)*, **70** (5), 326–343.

Meduri, G.U. and Chastre, J. (1992) The standardization of bronchoscopic techniques for ventilator-associated pneumonia. *Chest*, **102** (5 Suppl 1), 557S–564.

Miles, P.R., Baughman, R.P. and Linnemann, C.C.J. (1990) Cytomegalovirus in the bronchoalveolar lavage fluid of patients with AIDS. *Chest*, **97**, 1072–1076.

Monso, E., Ruiz, J., Rosell, A., Manterola, J., Fiz, J., Morera, J. *et al.* (1995) Bacterial infection in chronic obstructive pulmonary disease. A study of stable and exacerbated outpatients using the protected specimen brush. *American Journal of Respiratory and Critical Care Medicine*, **152** (4 Pt 1), 1316–1320.

Munoz, P., Palomo, J., Guembe, P., Rodriguez-Creixems, M., Gijon, P. and Bouza, E. (2000) Lung nodular lesions in heart transplant recipients. *The Journal of Heart and Lung Transplantation*, **19** (7), 660–667.

Murray, P.R. and Washington, J.A. (1975) Microscopic and bacteriologic analysis of sputum. *Mayo Clinic Proceedings*, **50**, 339–344.

Nguyen, M.H., Jaber, R., Leather, H.L., Wingard, J.R., Staley, B., Wheat, L.J. *et al.* (2007) Bronchoalveolar lavage (BAL) galactomannan in the diagnosis of pulmonary aspergillosis among non-immunocompromised hosts. *Journal of Clinical Microbiology*, **45**, 2787–2792.

Nitsche, A., Steuer, N., Schmidt, C.A., Landt, O., Ellerbrok, H., Pauli, G. *et al.* (2000) Detection of human cytomegalovirus DNA by real-time quantitative PCR. *Journal of Clinical Microbiology*, **38** (7), 2734–2737.

Olsen, S.L., Renlund, D.G., O'Connell, J.B., Taylor, D.O., Lassetter, J.E., Eastburn, T.E. *et al.* (1993) Prevention of Pneumocystis carinii pneumonia in cardiac transplant recipients by trimethoprim sulfamethoxazole. *Transplantation*, **56** (2), 359–362.

Opravil, M., Marincek, B., Fuchs, W.A., Weber, R., Speich, R., Battegay, M. *et al.* (1994) Shortcomings of chest radiography in detecting Pneumocystis carinii pneumonia. *Journal of Acquired Immune Deficiency Syndromes*, **7** (1), 39–45.

Otahbachi, M., Nugent, K. and Buscemi, D. (2007) Granulomatous Pneumocystis jiroveci Pneumonia in a patient with chronic lymphocytic leukemia: A literature review and hypothesis on pathogenesis. *The American Journal of the Medical Sciences*, **333** (2), 131–135.

Paterson, D.L. and Singh, N. (1999) Invasive aspergillosis in transplant recipients. *Medicine (Baltimore)*, **78** (2), 123–138.

Peleg, A.Y., Husain, S., Qureshi, Z.A., Silveira, F.P., Sarumi, M., Shutt, K.A. *et al.* (2007) Risk factors, clinical characteristics, and outcome of Nocardia infection in organ transplant recipients: A matched case-control study. *Clinical Infectious Diseases*, **44** (10), 1307–1314.

Pereira Gomes, J.C., Pedreira, J.W., Jr, Araujo, E.M., Soriano, F.G., Negri, E.M., Antonangelo, L. *et al.* (2000) Impact of BAL in the management of pneumonia with treatment failure: Positivity of BAL culture under antibiotic therapy. *Chest*, **118** (6), 1739–1746.

Phillips, P., Bonner, S., Gataric, N., Bai, T., Wilcox, P., Hogg, R. *et al.* (2005) Nontuberculous mycobacterial immune reconstitution syndrome in HIV-infected patients: Spectrum of disease and long-term follow-up. *Clinical Infectious Diseases*, **41** (10), 1483–1497.

Pirozynski, M. (1992) Bronchoalveolar lavage in the diagnosis of peripheral, primary lung cancer. *Chest*, **102** (2), 372–374.

Podzamczer, D., Salazar, A., Jimenez, J., Consiglio, E., Santin, M., Casanova, A. *et al.* (1995) Intermittent trimethoprim-sulfamethoxazole compared with dapsone-pyrimethamine for the simultaneous primary prophylaxis of Pneumocystis pneumonia and toxoplasmosis in patients infected with HIV. *Annals of Internal Medicine*, **122** (10), 755–761.

Pugin, J., Auckenthaler, R., Mili, N., Janssens, J.P., Lew, P.D. and Suter, P.M. (1991) Diagnosis of ventilator-associated pneumonia by bacteriologic analysis of bronchoscopic and nonbronchoscopic 'blind' bronchoalveolar lavage fluid. *The American Review of Respiratory Disease*, **143** (5 Pt 1), 1121–1129.

Quinti, I., Soresina, A., Spadaro, G., Martino, S., Donnanno, S., Agostini, C. *et al.* (2007) Long-term follow-up and outcome of a large cohort of patients with common variable immunodeficiency. *Journal of Clinical Immunology*, **27** (3), 308–316.

Raad, I., Hanna, H., Huaringa, A., Sumoza, D., Hachem, R. and Albitar, M. (2002) Diagnosis of invasive pulmonary aspergillosis using polymerase chain reaction-based detection of aspergillus in BAL. *Chest*, **121** (4), 1171–1176.

Raja, A., Baughman, R.P. and Daniel, T.M. (1988) The detection by immunoassay of antibody to mycobacterial antigens and mycobacterial antigens in bronchoalveolar lavage fluid from patients with tuberculosis and control subjects. *Chest*, **94**, 133–137.

Raju, B. and Schluger, N.W. (2000) Significance of respiratory isolates of Mycobacterium avium complex in HIV-positive and HIV-negative patients. *International Journal of Infectious Diseases*, **4** (3), 134–139.

Rano, A., Agusti, C., Jimenez, P., Angril, J., Benito, N., Danes, C. *et al.* (2001) Pulmonary infiltrates in non-HIV immunocompromised patients: A diagnostic approach using non-invasive and broncho-scopic procedures. *Thorax*, **56**, 379–387.

Rantakokko-Jalava, K., Laaksonen, S., Issakainen, J., Vauras, J., Nikoskelainen, J., Viljanen, M.K. *et al.* (2003) Semiquantitative detection by real-time PCR of Aspergillus fumigatus in bronch-oalveolar lavage fluids and tissue biopsy specimens from patients with invasive aspergillosis. *Journal of Clinical Microbiology*, **41** (9), 4304–4311.

Rath, P.M., Oeffelke, R., Muller, K.D. and Ansorg, R. (1996) Non-value of Aspergillus antigen detection in bronchoalveolar lavage fluids of patients undergoing bone marrow transplantation. *Mycoses*, **39** (9–10), 367–370.

Rennard, S.I. (1990) Bronchoalveolar lavage in the diagnosis of cancer. *Lung*, **168** (Suppl), 1035–1040.

Rennard, S.I., Ghafouri, M., Thompson, A.B., Linder, J., Vaughan, W., Jones, K. *et al.* (1990) Fractional processing of sequential bronchoalveolar lavage to separate bronchial and alveolar samples. *The American Review of Respiratory Disease*, **141**, 208–217.

Reynolds, H.Y. and Newball, H.H. (1974) Analysis of proteins and respiratory cells obtained from human lungs by bronchial lavage. *The Journal of Laboratory and Clinical Medicine*, **84** (4), 559–573.

Richeldi, L. (2006) An update on the diagnosis of tuberculosis infection. *American Journal of Respiratory and Critical Care Medicine*, **174** (7), 736–742.

Robbins, B.E., Steiger, Z., Wilson, R.F., Ratanath, V., Karanes, C., Bander, J. *et al.* (1992) Diagnosis of acute diffuse pulmonary infiltrates in immunosuppressed patients by open biopsy of the lung. *Surgery Gynecology and Obstetrics*, **175** (1), 8–12.

Roberts, S.A., Franklin, J.C., Mijch, A. and Spelman, D. (2000) Nocardia infection in heart-lung transplant recipients at Alfred Hospital, Melbourne, Australia, 1989–1998. *Clinical Infectious Diseases*, **31** (4), 968–972.

Rouby, J.J., Martin De Lassale, E., Poete, P., Nicolas, M.H., Bodin, L., Jarlier, V. *et al.* (1992) Nosocomial bronchopneumonia in the critically ill. Histologic and bacteriologic aspects. *The American Review of Respiratory Disease*, **146** (4), 1059–1066.

Rouby, J.J., Rossignon, M.D., Nicolas, M.H., Martin De Lassale, E., Cristin, S., Grosset, J. *et al.* (1989) A prospective study of protected bronchoalveolar lavage in the diagnosis of nosocomial pneumonia. *Anesthesiology*, **71** (5), 679–685.

Ruutu, P., Ruutu, T., Volin, L., Tukiainen, P., Ukkonen, P. and Hovi, T. (1990) Cytomegalovirus is frequently isolated in bronchoalveolar lavage fluid of bone marrow transplant recipients without pneumonia. *Annals of Internal Medicine*, **112** (12), 913–916.

Salzman, S.H., Schindel, M.L., Aranda, C.P., Smith, R.L. and Lewis, M.L. (1992) The role of bronchoscopy in the diagnosis of pulmonary tuberculosis in patients at risk for HIV infection. *Chest*, **102** (1), 143–146.

Schluger, N.W. (2001) Changing approaches to the diagnosis of tuberculosis. *American Journal of Respiratory and Critical Care Medicine*, **164** (11), 2020–2024.

Schmidt, G.M., Horak, D.A., Niland, J.C., Duncan, S.R., Forman, S.J. and Zaia, J.A. (1991) A randomized, controlled trial of prophylactic ganciclovir for cytomegalovirus pulmonary infection in recipients of allogeneic bone marrow transplants; The City of Hope-Stanford-Syntex CMV Study Group. *The New England Journal of Medicine*, **324** (15), 1005–1011.

Schuller, D., Spessert, C., Fraser, V.J. and Goodenberger, D.M. (1993) Herpes simplex virus from respiratory tract secretions: Epidemiology, clinical characteristics, and outcome in immunocompromised and nonimmunocompromised hosts. *The American Journal of Medicine*, **94** (1), 29–33.

Schutt, P., Brandhorst, D., Stellberg, W., Poser, M., Ebeling, P., Muller, S. *et al.* (2006) Immune parameters in multiple myeloma patients: Influence of treatment and correlation with opportunistic infections. *Leukemia and Lymphoma*, **47** (8), 1570–1582.

Selwyn, P.A., Pumerantz, A.S., Durante, A., Alcabes, P.G., Gourevitch, M.N., Boiselle, P.M. *et al.* (1998) Clinical predictors of Pneumocystis carinii pneumonia, bacterial pneumonia and tuberculosis in HIV-infected patients. *AIDS (London, England)*, **12** (8), 885–893.

Seyfarth, H.J., Nenoff, P., Winkler, J., Krahl, R., Haustein, U.F. and Schauer, J. (2001) Aspergillus detection in bronchoscopically acquired material. Significance and interpretation. *Mycoses*, **44** (9–10), 356–360.

Sing, A., Trebesius, K., Roggenkamp, A., Russmann, H., Tybus, K., Pfaff, F. *et al.* (2000) Evaluation of diagnostic value and epidemiological implications of PCR for Pneumocystis carinii in different immunosuppressed and immunocompetent patient groups. *Journal of Clinical Microbiology*, **38** (4), 1461–1467.

Singh, N., Rogers, P., Atwood, C.W., Wagener, M.M. and Yu, V.L. (2000) Short-course empiric antibiotic therapy for patients with pulmonary infiltrates in the intensive care unit. A proposed solution for indiscriminate antibiotic prescription. *American Journal of Respiratory and Critical Care Medicine*, **162** (2 Pt 1), 505–511.

Sisson, J.H., Thompson, A.B., Anderson, J.R., Robbins, R.A., Spurzem, J.R., Spence, P.R. *et al.* (1992) Airway inflammation predicts diffuse alveolar hemorrhage during bone marrow transplantation in patients with Hodgkin disease. *The American Review of Respiratory Disease*, **146** (2), 439–443.

Sobonya, R.E., Barbee, R.A., Wiens, J. and Trego, D. (1990) Detection of fungi and other pathogens in immunocompromised patients by bronchoalveolar lavage in an area endemic for coccidioido-mycosis. *Chest*, **97** (6), 1349–1355.

Soborg, B., Andersen, A.B., Larsen, H.K., Weldingh, K., Andersen, P., Kofoed, K. *et al.* (2007) Detecting a low prevalence of latent tuberculosis among health care workers in Denmark detected by *M. tuberculosis* specific IFN-gamma whole-blood test. *Scandinavian Journal of Infectious Diseases*, **39** (6), 554–559.

Sopena, N., Sabria, M., Pedro-Botet, M.L., Reynaga, E., Garcia-Nunez, M., Dominguez, J. *et al.* (2002) Factors related to persistence of Legionella urinary antigen excretion in patients with legionnaires' disease. *European Journal of Clinical Microbiology and Infectious Diseases*, **21** (12), 845–848.

Steinberg, K.P., Milberg, J.A., Martin, T.R., Maunder, R.J., Cockrill, B.A. and Hudson, L.D. (1994) Evolution of bronchoalveolar cell populations in the adult respiratory distress syndrome. *American Journal of Respiratory and Critical Care Medicine*, **150**, 113–122.

Sternberg, R.I., Baughman, R.P., Dohn, M.N. and First, M.R. (1993) Utility of bronchoalveolar lavage in assessing pneumonia in immunosuppressed renal transplant recipients. *The American Journal of Medicine*, **95**, 358–364.

Stover, D.E., Zaman, M.B., Hajdu, S.I. *et al.* (1984) Role of bronchoalveolar lavage in the diagnosis of diffuse pulmonary infiltrates in the immunosuppressed host. *Annals of Internal Medicine*, **101**, 1–7.

Suffredini, A.F., Ognibene, F.P., Lack, E.E., Simmons, J.T., Brenner, M., Gill, V.J. *et al.* (1987) Nonspecific interstitial pneumonitis: A common cause of pulmonary disease in the acquired immunodeficiency syndrome. *Annals of Internal Medicine*, **107** (1), 7–13.

Sugihara, E., Hirota, N., Niizeki, T., Tanaka, R., Nagafuchi, M., Koyanagi, T. *et al.* (2003) Usefulness of bronchial lavage for the diagnosis of pulmonary disease caused by Mycobacterium avium-intracellulare complex (MAC) infection. *Journal of Infection and Chemotherapy*, **9** (4), 328–332.

Takahashi, T., Goto, M., Kanda, T. and Iwamoto, A. (2003) Utility of testing bronchoalveolar lavage fluid for cryptococcal ribosomal DNA. *The Journal of International Medical Research*, **31** (4), 324–329.

Theogaraj, E., John, C.D., Dewar, A., Buckingham, J.C. and Smith, S.F. (2006) The long-term effects of perinatal glucocorticoid exposure on the host defence system of the respiratory tract. *The Journal of Pathology*, **210** (1), 85–93.

Thorpe, J.E., Baughman, R.P., Frame, P.T., Wesseler, T.A. and Staneck, J.L. (1987) Bronchoalveolar lavage for diagnosing acute bacterial pneumonia. *The Journal of Infectious Diseases*, **155**, 855–861.

Torres, A., el Ebiary, M., Padro, L., Gonzalez, J., de la Bellacasa, J.P., Ramirez, J. *et al.* (1994) Validation of different techniques for the diagnosis of ventilator-associated pneumonia. Comparison with immediate postmortem pulmonary biopsy. *American Journal of Respiratory and Critical Care Medicine*, **149** (2 Pt 1), 324–331.

Torres, A. and El-Ebiary, M. (2000) Bronchoscopic BAL in the diagnosis of venntilator-associated pneumonia. *Chest*, **117**, 198S–202S.

Tuckermann, J.P., Kleiman, A., Moriggl, R., Spanbroek, R., Neumann, A., Illing, A. *et al.* (2007) Macrophages and neutrophils are the targets for immune suppression by glucocorticoids in contact allergy. *The Journal of Clinical Investigation*, **117** (5), 1381–1390.

Tuxen, D.V., Cade, J.F., McDonald, M.I., Buchanan, M.R., Clark, R.J. and Pain, M.C. (1982) Herpes simplex virus from the lower respiratory tract in adult respiratory distress syndrome. *The American Review of Respiratory Disease*, **126** (3), 416–419.

Tuxen, D.V., Wilson, J.W. and Cade, J.F. (1987) Prevention of lower respiratory herpes simplex virus infection with acyclovir in patients with the adult respiratory distress syndrome. *The American Review of Respiratory Disease*, **136** (2), 402–405.

Vagaggini, B., Cianchetti, S., Bartoli, M., Ricci, M., Bacci, E., Dente, F.L. *et al.* (2007) Prednisone blunts airway neutrophilic inflammatory response due to ozone exposure in asthmatic subjects. *Respiration; International Review of Thoracic Diseases*, **74** (1), 61–68.

Vaideeswar, P., Prasad, S., Deshpande, J.R. and Pandit, S.P. (2004) Invasive pulmonary aspergillosis: A study of 39 cases at autopsy. *Journal of Postgraduate Medicine*, **50** (1), 21–26.

van den Brink, J.W., Simoons-Smit, A.M., Beishuizen, A., Girbes, A.R., Strack van Schijndel, R.J. and Groeneveld, A.B. (2004) Respiratory herpes simplex virus type 1 infection/colonisation in the critically ill: Marker or mediator? *Journal of Clinical Virology*, **30** (1), 68–72.

Vavricka, S.R., Halter, J., Hechelhammer, L. and Himmelmann, A. (2004) Pneumocystis carinii pneumonia in chronic lymphocytic leukaemia. *Postgraduate Medical Journal*, **80** (942), 236–238.

Velez, L., Correa, L.T., Maya, M.A., Mejia, P., Ortega, J., Bedoya, V. *et al.* (2007) Diagnostic accuracy of bronchoalveolar lavage samples in immunosuppressed patients with suspected pneumonia: Analysis of a protocol. *Respiratory Medicine*, **101**, 2160–2167.

Verweij, P.E., Latge, J.P., Rijs, A.J., Melchers, W.J., De Pauw, B.E., Hoogkamp-Korstanje, J.A. *et al.* (1995) Comparison of antigen detection and PCR assay using bronchoalveolar lavage fluid for diagnosing invasive pulmonary aspergillosis in patients receiving treatment for hematological malignancies. *Journal of Clinical Microbiology*, **33** (12), 3150–3153.

Wagner, J.D., Stahler, C., Knox, S., Brinton, M. and Knecht, B. (1992) Clinical utility of open lung biopsy for undiagnosed pulmonary infiltrates. *American Journal of Surgery*, **164** (2), 104–107.

Wallace, J.M., Hansen, N.I., Lavange, L., Glassroth, J., Browdy, B.L., Rosen, M.J. *et al.* (1997) Respiratory disease trends in the Pulmonary Complications of HIV Infection Study cohort. Pulmonary Complications of HIV Infection Study Group. *American Journal of Respiratory and Critical Care Medicine*, **155** (1), 72–80.

Wallace, J.M., Lim, R., Browdy, B.L., Hopewell, P.C., Glassroth, J., Rosen, M.J. *et al.* (1998) Risk factors and outcomes associated with identification of Aspergillus in respiratory specimens from persons with HIV disease. Pulmonary complications of HIV infection study group. *Chest*, **114** (1), 131–137.

Waxman, A.B., Goldie, S.J., Brett-Smith, H. and Matthay, R.A. (1997) Cytomegalovirus as a primary pulmonary pathogen in AIDS. *Chest*, **111** (1), 128–134.

Weiss, R.L., Snow, G.W., Schumann, G.B. and Hammond, M.E. (1991) Diagnosis of cytomegalovirus pneumonitis on bronchoalveolar lavage fluid: Comparison of cytology, immunofluorescence, and in situ hybridization with viral isolation. *Diagn Cytopathol*, **7** (3), 243–247.

Wheat, L.J., Connolly-Stringfield, P., Williams, B., Connolly, K., Blair, R., Bartlett, M. *et al.* (1992) Diagnosis of histoplasmosis in patients with the acquired immunodeficiency syndrome by detection of Histoplasma capsulatum polysaccharide antigen in bronchoalveolar lavage fluid. *The American Review of Respiratory Disease*, **145** (6), 1421–1424.

Wheat, L.J., Connolly-Stringfield, P.A., Baker, R.L., Curfman, M.F., Eads, M.E., Israel, K.S. *et al.* (1990) Disseminated histoplasmosis in the acquired immune deficiency syndrome: Clinical findings, diagnosis and treatment, and review of the literature. *Medicine (Baltimore)*, **69** (6), 361–374.

White, D.A., Wong, P.W. and Downey, R. (2000) The utility of open lung biopsy in patients with hematologic malignancies. *American Journal of Respiratory and Critical Care Medicine*, **161** (3 Pt 1), 723–729.

Wilson, D., Yen-Lieberman, B., Reischl, U., Warshawsky, I. and Procop, G.W. (2004) Comparison of five methods for extraction of Legionella pneumophila from respiratory specimens. *Journal of Clinical Microbiology*, **42** (12), 5913–5916.

Wimberly, N., Faling, L.J. and Bartlett, J.G. (1979) A fiberoptic bronchoscopy technique to obtain uncontaminated lower airway secretions for bacterial culture. *The American Review of Respiratory Disease*, **119**, 337–343.

Wingard, J.R. (2005) The changing face of invasive fungal infections in hematopoietic cell transplant recipients. *Current Opinion in Oncology*, **17** (2), 89–92.

Wunderink, R.G. (2000) Radiologic diagnosis of ventilator-associated pneumonia. *Chest*, **117**, 188S–190S.

Wunderink, R.G., Woldenberg, L.S., Zeiss, J., Day, C.M., Ciemins, J. and Lacher, D.A. (1992) The radiologic diagnosis of autopsy-proven ventilator-associated pneumonia. *Chest*, **101** (2), 458–463.

Xaubet, A., Torres, A., Marco, F., Puig-De la Bellacasa, J., Faus, R. and Agusti-Vidal, A. (1989) Pulmonary infiltrates in immunocompromised patients. Diagnostic value of telescoping plugged catheter and bronchoalveolar lavage. *Chest*, **95**, 130–135.

Youssef, S., Rodriguez, G., Rolston, K.V., Champlin, R.E., Raad, I.I. and Safdar, A. (2007) Streptococcus pneumoniae infections in 47 hematopoietic stem cell transplantation recipients: Clinical characteristics of infections and vaccine-breakthrough infections, 1989–2005. *Medicine (Baltimore)*, **86** (2), 69–77.

4

Pulmonary imaging in immunocompromised patients

Tomás Franquet

*Thoracic Imaging Section, Department of Radiology, Hospital de Sant Pau,
Universitat Autónoma of Barcelona, Barcelona, Spain*

Immunocompromised patients can be divided into two major groups, those with AIDS and those patients who are immunocompromised for other reasons such as hematologic malignancies, recipients of hematopoietic stem cell and solid-organ transplantation, and patients under treatment with cytotoxic drugs or with high-dose corticosteroids.

Although imaging evaluation of lower respiratory infections is essentially confined to chest radiography and computed tomography (CT), there is considerable overlap in the imaging appearances of many of the infectious diseases found in immunocompromised patients (Brown, Miller and Muller, 1994). In this chapter, we discuss and illustrate the role of imaging in the diagnosis and management of respiratory infections in immuno-compromised patients.

4.1   Pulmonary infections in immunocompromised patient

Diagnosis of pulmonary infections requires clinical acumen, appropriate microbiologic tests, and imaging. Pneumonia should be suspected in a febrile patient with cough and crackles. The infection may be caused by a variety of different organisms that may present with similar clinical symptoms and signs and result in similar radiographic manifestations. Furthermore, the radiographic manifestations of a given organism may be variable depending on the immunologic status of the patient and the presence of pre- or coexisting lung disease.

The number of immunocompromised patients has increased considerably in the last three decades because of three main phenomena: the AIDS epidemic, advances in cancer chemotherapy, and expanding solid organ and hematopoietic stem cell trans-plantation (HSCT). At the onset of the AIDS epidemic, in the early and mid-1980s, there was 50–80% mortality for each episode of *Pneumocystis* pneumonia (PCP). Since

Pulmonary Infection in the Immunocompromised Patient, Edited by Carlos Agustí and Antoni Torres
© 2009 John Wiley & Sons, Ltd.

routine prophylaxis was instituted in 1989, there has been a declining incidence of PCP in the AIDS population (Moe and Hardy, 1994; Murray and Mills, 1990b; Murray and Mills, 1990a) and a decrease in mortality in mild to moderate cases (Lyon *et al.*, 1996). However, other infections including bacterial pneumonia, fungal infection, Cytomegalovirus (CMV), *Mycobacterium Avium-Complex* (MAC), and tuberculosis remain a significant cause of morbidity and mortality in these patients (Lyon *et al.*, 1996; Moe and Hardy, 1994; Murray and Mills, 1990b; Murray and Mills, 1990a).

A clinico-radiologic approach

In symptomatic patients it is important to determine whether the cause of symptoms is infectious or non-infectious. Differentiating immunosuppression-related disease from infectious-related respiratory disease is difficult and distinction of localized pneumonia from other pulmonary processes cannot be made with certainty on radiological grounds (Boiselle *et al.*, 1997; Janzen *et al.*, 1993). Diagnosis is equally difficult when pneumonia appears as a diffuse pulmonary abnormality. In the absence of clinical information, radiologists cannot reliably distinguish between bronchopneumonia and other pulmonary processes such as hydrostatic pulmonary edema, acute respiratory distress syndrome (ARDS), or diffuse pulmonary haemorrhage (Chastre *et al.*, 1998; Niederman and Fein, 1990; Seidenfeld *et al.*, 1986; Primack and Muller, 1994).

Imaging examinations should always be interpreted with awareness of the clinical findings including duration of symptoms, presence of fever, cough, dyspnea, presence or not of leukocytosis, and the immune status of the patient (Shah *et al.*, 1997; Hanson *et al.*, 1995). Furthermore, the clinical data and radiographic findings often fail to lead to a definitive diagnosis of pneumonia because there is an extensive number of noninfectious processes associated with febrile pneumonitis, including drug-induced pulmonary disease, acute eosinophilic pneumonia, organizing pneumonia (bronchiolitis obliterans organizing pneumonia, BOOP), and pulmonary vasculitis, that may mimic pulmonary infection (Boiselle *et al.*, 1997).

The role of imaging is to identify the presence, location and extent of pulmonary abnormalities, the course and evolution of pneumonia, the presence of associated complications, and detection of additional or alternative diagnosis (Franquet, 2001). Chest radiography must be routinely undertaken in patients with 'presumptive' pneumonia to make the diagnosis. The American Thoracic Society (ATS) guidelines recommend that posteroanterior (PA) (and lateral when possible) chest radiographs be obtained whenever pneumonia is suspected in adults (Boiselle, Crans and Kaplan, 1999).

In most cases the radiographic findings are suggestive or consistent with the diagnosis of pneumonia and sufficiently specific in the proper clinical context to preclude the need for additional imaging (Franquet, 2001; Gharib and Stern, 2001; Tarver *et al.*, 2005; Vilar *et al.*, 2004). However, a normal chest radiograph should not exclude the diagnosis of pneumonia because the radiograph can lag behind the clinical findings by several days. In a study of 87 consecutive patients with febrile neutropenia, the CT scan revealed a pulmonary lesion not seen on the radiograph in 50% of subjects (Heussel *et al.*, 1999).

Radiologic patterns

Chest radiographs and CT demonstrate different radiographic patterns depending on the state and type of immunosuppression associated. The most usual patterns seen at CT are airspace consolidation, nodules, ground-glass attenuation and tree-in-bud appearance.

Airspace consolidation, defined as a localized increase in lung attenuation that obscures the underlying vascular structures, may be seen in association with bacterial, fungal and viral infections. This is the commonest radiographic manifestation of pneumonia in the vast majority of cases. The usual imaging findings comprise an air-space consolidation limited by the pleural surfaces with visible air-bronchogram (Figure 4.1). Bronchopneumonia results from infection of the airways with an infectious agent, with subsequent airway obstruction and spread to airspaces; this pattern may not be distinguished from air-space consolidation if the radiograph is obtained later in the course. On the chest radiograph there is a prominence of the bronchovascular markings and later, multiple ill-defined nodular opacities coalescing to air-space consolidation.

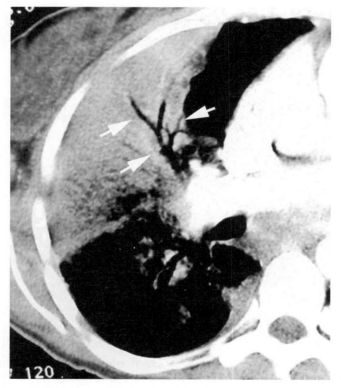

Figure 4.1 Segmental consolidation (pneumonia). Close-up view from CT image shows a segmental area of air-space consolidation in the right upper lobe. Air-bronchogram is nicely seen within the consolidation (arrows).

Computed tomography (CT) is a useful adjunct to conventional radiography and should be used in unresolved cases or when complications of pneumonia are suspected (Brown, Miller and Muller, 1994; Janzen *et al.*, 1993; Primack and Muller, 1994; Tomiyama *et al.*, 2000). Optimal assessment of the parenchyma is obtained with the use of high-resolution CT (HRCT) which allows assessment of pattern and distribution of abnormalities down to the level of the secondary pulmonary lobule (Brown, Miller and Muller, 1994).

Airspace nodules measure 6–10 mm in diameter and usually reflect the presence of peribronchiolar consolidation, and therefore are centrilobular in distribution. They are best appreciated in early disease and best seen at the edge of the pathologic process where consolidation is incomplete. In some circumstances, nodules may be associated with a 'halo' of ground-glass attenuation (Figure 4.2). In severely neutropenic patients this 'halo' sign is highly suggestive of angioinvasive aspergillosis (Kuhlman, Fishman and Siegelman, 1985). However, a similar appearance has been described in other conditions including infection by nontuberculous mycobacteria, Mucorales, Candida, Herpes simplex virus, cytomegalovirus, Wegener's granulomatosis, Kaposi's sarcoma and hemorrhagic metastases (Primack *et al.*, 1994).

Ground-glass opacification is a nonspecific finding on thin-section CT. It is defined as hazy increased lung opacity that does not obscure the underlying vascular structures. Ground-glass opacities may result from changes in the airspaces or interstitial tissues in

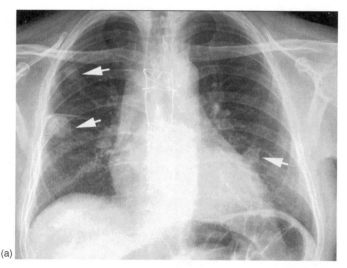

(a)

Figure 4.2   Angioinvasive aspergillosis. (a) Anteroposterior chest radiograph shows multiple bilateral ill-defined nodules (arrows). (b) HRCT scan (1.0-mm collimation) at the level of the carina shows a nodule in the right upper lobe surrounded by a halo of ground-glass attenuation ('halo sign') (arrow). The patient was a 68-year-old man with heart transplant.

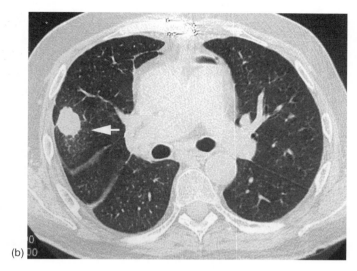

(b)

Figure 4.2   (*Continued*)

acute or chronic infiltrative lung disease. Infections that typically present with bilateral ground-glass opacities are *Pneumocystis* and cytomegalovirus pneumonia (Figure 4.3). In AIDS patients the presence of extensive bilateral ground-glass opacities is highly suggestive of PCP. In immunocompromised non-AIDS patients the differential diagnosis includes cytomegalovirus pneumonia, drug-induced lung disease, pulmonary hemorrhage and organizing pneumonia (Worthy, Flint and Muller, 1997).

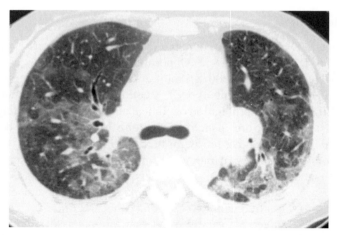

Figure 4.3   CMV pneumonitis. HRCT scan (1-mm collimation) at the level of the carina in a 25-year-old man with acute myeloid leukemia and bone marrow transplant shows a typical pattern of 'mosaic attenuation'. Note multiple areas of 'ground-glass' attenuation in a patchy distribution.

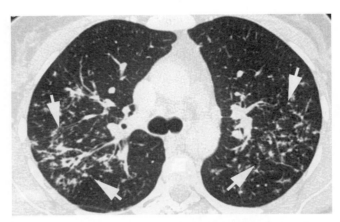

Figure 4.4   Tuberculosis. HRCT image (2-mm collimation) shows bilateral multiple branching opacities ('tree-in-bud') in a centrilobular distribution (arrows). Sputum cultures grew *Mycobacterium tuberculosis*.

A 'tree-in-bud' pattern is a characteristic, high-resolution CT manifestation of infectious bronchiolitis. It consists of centrilobular branching tubular and nodular structures and reflects the presence of bronchiolar inflammation and filling of the lumen by inflammatory material or mucus (Im *et al.*, 1995). This pattern may be seen in a variety of bacterial, mycobacterial, fungal and viral infections (Figure 4.4) (Im *et al.*, 1995; Aquino *et al.*, 1996).

4.2   Respiratory infections

Bacterial infections

In AIDS patients, CD4 lymphocyte count is a valuable measure for assessing the degree of impairment of the immune system. Opportunistic lung infections usually occur in patients with CD4 counts below 200 cell/mm^3, meanwhile typical bacterial pneumonia is more associated with CD4 counts above 500 cell/mm^3. So it is important to know the CD4 count for the correct interpretation of clinical and radiological findings (Franquet, 2004). In the last decade the prevalence of opportunistic infections have decreased with the introduction of highly active retroviral therapy (HAART).

The most common etiology of pulmonary infection in AIDS patients is bacterial pneumonia (Hirschtick *et al.*, 1995), usually caused by typical agents as *Streptococcus pneumoniae*, *Haemophilus influenzae*, *Pseudomonas aeruginosa* and *Staphylococcus aureus* (Figure 4.5). Less frequently, *Rochamilacea sp* and *Rhodococcus equi* may be the cause of bacterial infection, usually seen as pneumonia associated with cavitation (Padley and King, 1999). The classic radiological presentation is as single or multiple areas of focal distribution, although differentiation from the atypical patterns associated with opportunistic infections may be difficult on the basis of radiographic images, being necessary to perform more invasive techniques for etiologic diagnosis (Franquet, 2004).

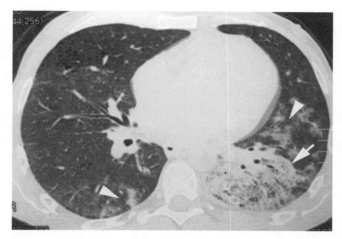

Figure 4.5 Pneumoccocal bronchopneumonia. CT image (5-mm collimation) in a 53-year-old man shows a segmental homogeneous consolidation in the left lower lobe (arrow). Note the presence of air-bronchogram within the consolidation. Bilateral lobular areas of 'ground-glass' attenuation are also seen in the lower lobes (arrowheads). Sputum culture produced a heavy growth of *S. pneumoniae*.

Pulmonary complications following HSCT are common, occurring in 40–60% of patients. These include infectious and noninfectious pneumonitis, graft-vs-host disease (GVHD), bronchiolitis obliterans, diffuse alveolar hemorrhage, pulmonary edema, and pulmonary vascular abnormalities.

Fungi (mainly *Aspergillus* species) are the common cause of pulmonary infection during the neutropenic phase (up to three weeks after transplantation), meanwhile cytomegalovirus (CMV) pneumonia is typical three weeks to 100 days after transplantation (Sable and Donowitz, 1994).

Following solid organ transplantation, infection during the first month may result from a pre-existing infection in the donor or recipient, or from the surgical wound, endotracheal tube, vascular access or drainage. During one to six months after transplantation, viruses attack and, with sustained immunosuppression, make opportunistic infections possible. Beyond six months after transplantation, the 80% of patients with good result from the transplant are at risk primarily for community-acquired microbes. In solid organ transplantation, bacterial pneumonia is the most common respiratory infectious complication; CMV infection usually occurs within the first three months after transplantation (Ettinger and Trulock, 1991).

Nocardiosis (mainly caused by *Nocardia asteroides*) is relatively common in organ transplants, patients with hematologic diseases and patients with systemic lupus erythematosus receiving high-dose corticosteroids. Radiological findings are solitary or multiple masses or areas of nodular air-space consolidations, usually homogeneous and nonsegmental (Yoon *et al.*, 1995) (Figure 4.6). Several reports have highlighted the increasing role of non-*Legionella pneumophila* spp. as pulmonary pathogens in immunosuppressed patients. *L. micdadei* and *L. bozemanii* are the most frequently

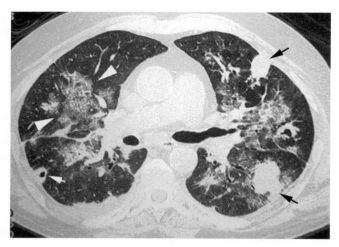

Figure 4.6   Nocardiosis. HRCT image (2-mm collimation) shows multiple bilateral nodules of variable size (arrows). One of the nodules is cavitated (small arrow). Also noted are patchy bilateral ground-glass opacities (arrowheads).

reported species after L. pneumophila as causes of infection in transplant patients (Muder and Yu, 2002; Singh *et al.*, 1993).

Mycobacterial infections

It is estimated that between 1997 and 2020 approximately 1 billion people will acquire the infection and 70 million people will die of TB (Dye *et al.*, 1999; Leung, 1999). The main factors that have contributed to the reappearance of TB include infection in HIV+ patients and the appearance of multi drug-resistant TB (Harisinghani *et al.*, 2000; Barber, Craven and Mccabe, 1990). The HIV/AIDS epidemic has been important in the re-emergence of tuberculosis in last decades. Its risk is 200–500 times higher in AIDS patients than in the general population (Leung, 1999).

Mycobacterial infections are not only caused by *Mycobacterium tuberculosis*, but also nontuberculous (atypical) mycobacteria such as *Mycobacterium avium intracellulare* (MAI) are frequently causing opportunistic infections in AIDS. The immunosuppresed state associated with AIDS predisposes to the reactivation of latent tuberculosis, meanwhile MAI infection occurs in advanced stages of AIDS, when CD4 count is lower than 50 cells/mm^3 (Kotloff, 1993).

The spectrum of radiographic findings in tuberculosis and non-tuberculous infections is so variable that diagnosis may be difficult (Harisinghani *et al.*, 2000; Leung, 1999). In immunocompromised patients, radiological findings are very similar to those in immunocompetent patients, although mediastinal lymph node and bronchogenic spread forms occur more frequently in HIV-infected patients (Figure 4.7) (Leung, 1999).

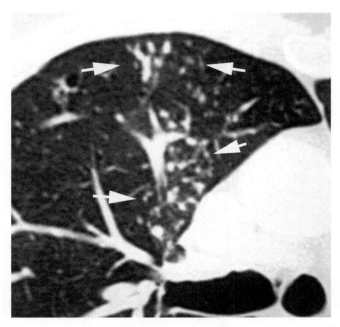

Figure 4.7   Endobronchial spread of tuberculosis. Close-up view from HRCT image (1.0-mm collimation) at the level of the carina shows multiple branching linear opacities combined with centrilobular nodules (arrows) in the anterior segment of the right upper lobe. The combination of branching linear opacities and centrilobular nodules gives the characteristic 'tree-in-bud' appearance. The patient was a 45-year-old male HIV-positive.

Primary tuberculosis

Primary tuberculosis represents about 23–34% of all adult cases of tuberculosis (Miller and Miller, 1993). Although primary tuberculosis typically presents with radiographic manifestations, a chest radiograph may be normal in 15% of cases (Miller and Miller, 1993). The most frequent manifestations of primary tuberculosis are parenchymal disease, lymphadenopathy, pleural effusion, miliary disease or atelectasis (Harisinghani *et al.*, 2000) (Figure 4.8). On CT imaging, the presence of centrilobular nodules and a 'tree-in-bud' appearance in the area nearby to the consolidation is typical of pulmonary tuberculosis. Tuberculous mediastinal lymphadenitis is a common manifestation of primary tuberculosis, especially in pubertal and young adult women, the elderly and HIV-patients (Hopewell, 1995). Indeed, lymph nodes characteristically present with a low attenuation, necrotic or caseous centre and a hyper-vascularised periphery that enhances following intra-venous contrast (Im *et al.*, 1987). Although cavitary lesions are present in up to 29% of patients with primary tuberculosis, they are more frequently associated with post-primary tuberculosis (Choyke *et al.*, 1983).

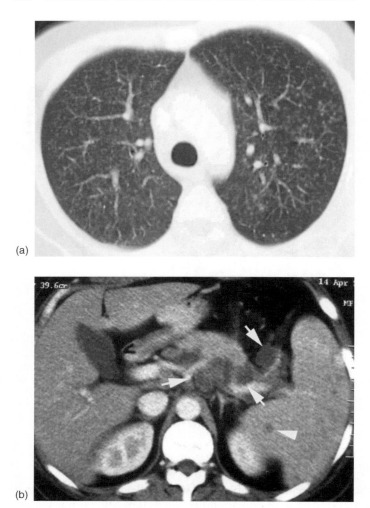

Figure 4.8 Miliary pulmonary tuberculosis with abdominal lymphadenitis. (a) CT image (5.0-mm collimation) shows multiple miliary nodules of different sizes in a random distribution throughout both lungs. (b) Multiple peri-pancreatic lymph nodes are visible on contrast-enhanced CT. Lymph nodes show typical central low attenuation and a rim enhancement after intravenous contrast administration (arrows). A hypodense splenic nodule is also seen (arrowhead). The patient was a 42-year-old male with AIDS.

Post-primary tuberculosis

The radiological manifestations may overlap with those of primary tuberculosis, but the absence of lymphadenopathy, more frequent cavitation and a predilection for the upper lobes, are more typical of post-primary tuberculosis (Ellis, 2004).

Cavitation indicates active disease; communication with bronchi enables the expectoration of tubercle bacilli and endobronchial spread, leading to the appearance of the typical images of 'tree-in-bud'.

Sequelae and complications may present in pulmonary or extrapulmonary portions of the thorax, as a consequence of the progression of pulmonary tuberculosis.

Residual thin-walled cavities may be present in both active and inactive disease. After antituberculous treatment, cavities may disappear, but occasionally, the wall becomes paper-thin and air-filled cystic space remains (Kim *et al.*, 2001).

Pulmonary non-tuberculous mycobacteria (NTMB)

Pulmonary non-tuberculous mycobacteria (NTMB) infection is progressively increasing in prevalence, mainly due to *Mycobacterium avium-intracellulare* and *M. kansasii*. The severity of the disease depends on the presence of underlying lung disease and the status of immunocompetence (Woodring and Vandiviere, 1990).

The most typical form of pulmonary NTMB infection is frequently associated with elderly men with underlying lung disease. Radiological manifestations are very similar to post-primary tuberculosis, although in NMTB infection the progression is slower than tuberculosis (Figure 4.9).

Other forms of pulmonary NTMB infection affect elderly white women without underlying lung disease. Radiological findings consist of mild to moderate cylindrical bronchiectasis and multiple 1–3 mm diameter centrilobular nodules (Hartman, Swensen and Williams, 1993; Miller, 1994). Cavitation, ground-glass areas, volume loss and adenopathy do not usually present in nonclassic infection. In some cases, infection presents with solitary or multiples nodules, which are usually incidentally detected in asymptomatic patients and may represent the initial manifestation of pulmonary infection (Miller, 1994).

Viral infections

Cytomegalovirus infection is commonly seen in immunocompromised patients. In AIDS, CMV pneumonia usually occurs in patients with a CD4 count below 50 cells/mm³. The radiographic findings are unpredictable and may consist of a reticular or reticulonodular pattern, ground-glass opacities, air-space consolidation or a combination of these findings (Olliff and Williams, 1989; Schulman, 1987). Consolidation and masses are more typical of AIDS patients compared to immunocompromised non-AIDS patients (Franquet, Lee and Muller, 2003; Moon *et al.*, 2000).

CMV pneumonia has been reported especially in hematopoietic stem cell transplantation (HSCT) during the post-engraftment period (30–100 days after transplantation). Although mortality is high (85%), the main determinant of prognosis is the early diagnosis. The most typical radiographic findings consisted of pulmonary consolidation and multiple nodules smaller than 55 mm in diameter (Leung *et al.*, 1999). In solid-organ transplantation, CMV pneumonia usually occurs with a normal chest radiograph, although in some cases may demonstrate alveolar or interstitial infiltrates, being necessary thin-section CT to clarify radiological diagnosis.

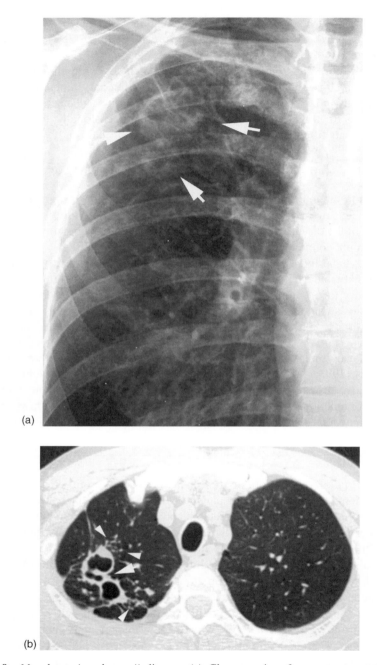

Figure 4.9 *Mycobacterium kansasii* disease. (a) Close-up view from a posteroanterior chest radiograph shows ill-defined rounded opacities in the right upper lobe (arrows). (b) HRCT image (2.0-mm collimation) at the level of the upper lobes shows two cavities (arrows) surrounded by numerous small nodules in a centrilobular distribution (arrowheads). The patient was a 53-year-old male.

Community respiratory viruses (CRVs) such as influenza, parainfluenza, respiratory syncytial virus (RSV), and human metapneumovirus infections, have been recognized as a possible cause of pneumonia and death in patients undergoing hematopoietic stem cell transplantation (HSCT) (Chemaly *et al.*, 2006). CT features are non-specific and consist of solitary or multiple areas of ground-glass attenuation, multiple nodules surrounded by a halo of ground-glass attenuation (halo sign) and areas of consolidation (Figure 4.10) (Franquet *et al.*, 2006; Franquet *et al.*, 2005). An absolute lymphocyte

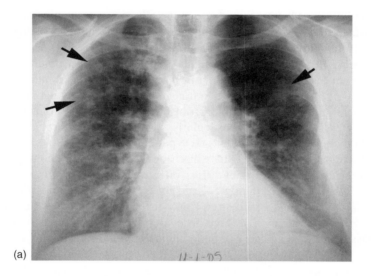

(a)

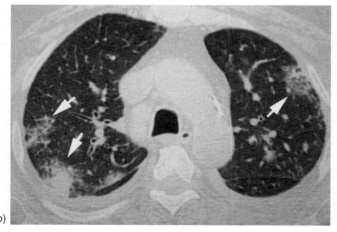

(b)

Figure 4.10 Acute pneumonia caused by *RSV*. (a) Posteroanterior chest radiograph shows numerous ill-defined nodules in the upper lobes (arrows). (b) HRCT scan (1-mm collimation; lung window) at the level of the aortic arch shows bilateral ill-defined areas of 'ground-glass' attenuation (arrows). The patient was a 38-year-old man after allogeneic hematopoietic stem cell transplant.

count of greater than 200 cells/mL, which may reflect the severe immunosuppressive status of the patient at the time of diagnosis with CRV infection, is an independent predictor of fatal outcome in patients with influenza pneumonia (Chemaly *et al.*, 2006).

Fungal infections

Fungi involved in pulmonary infections are either pathogenic fungi, which can infect any host, or saprophytic fungi, which infect only immunocompromised hosts. Pathogenic fungi include coccidioidomycosis, blastomycosis and histoplasmosis. Saprophytes include Candidiasis, Mucormycosis and Aspergillosis. Pulmonary fungal infections may be difficult to diagnose and a definitive diagnosis of pulmonary fungal infections is made by isolating the fungus from tissue specimen.

Pneumocystis jiroveci (formerly *Pneumocystis carinii*) is a unique opportunistic fungal pathogen that causes pneumonia in immunocompromised individuals such as patients with AIDS, patients with organ transplants, and patients with hematologic or solid organ malignancies who are undergoing chemotherapy-and in patients receiving immune-suppressive treatments, particularly systemic corticosteroids. *Pneumocystis jiroveci* pneumonia (PCP) is typical in AIDS patients with CD4 counts below 100 cells/mm^3. In 90% of patients with PCP there has been reported chest radiograph abnormalities, mainly the classical findings of diffuse bilateral interstitial infiltrates in a perihilar distribution, although normal radiographs do not exclude the diagnosis (Franquet, 2004; Hidalgo *et al.*, 2003). In these patients, CT may be helpful in confirming the diagnosis of PCP when clinical suspicion is high, showing typical images including perihilar ground-glass opacity, in a patchy or geographical distribution (Figure 4.11) (Primack and Muller, 1994; Hidalgo *et al.*, 2003). In AIDS patients receiving prophylaxis with aerosolized pentamidine and trimethroprim-sulfamethoxazole (TMP-SMX), there has been reported a cystic form of *P. jiroveci* pneumonia, associated with increased risk of spontaneous pneumothorax. The risk of *Pneumocystis jiroveci* infection has been substantially lowered in recent years in transplant patients by the prophylactic use of TMP-SMX.

Aspergillosis is a fungal disease caused by *Aspergillus* species, usually *A. fumigatus*. There are different patterns of aspergillosis as follows: angioinvasive aspergillosis, bronchial invasive aspergillosis, pseudomembranous necrotizing tracheobronchial aspergillosis, obstructing bronchial aspergillosis and chronic cavitary forms. Bronchial invasive aspergillosis is associated to patients with severe neutropenia and in patients with AIDS. The clinical and radiological manifestations include acute tracheobronchitis, bronchiolitis and bronchopneumonia (Franquet, 2004). Obstructing bronchopulmonary aspergillosis (OBA) is a non-invasive form of aspergillosis characterized by massive intraluminal overgrowth of *Aspergillus sp*. The characteristic CT findings consist of bilateral bronchial and bronchiolar dilatations, large mucoid impactions and postobstructive atelectasis (Franquet *et al.*, 2004). Angioinvasive aspergillosis is almost exclusively seen in patients with severe neutropenia (Worthy, Flint and Muller, 1997; Kuhlman *et al.*, 1987; Kuhlman, Fishman and Siegelman, 1985). This form is characterized by invasion and occlusion of small to medium pulmonary arteries,

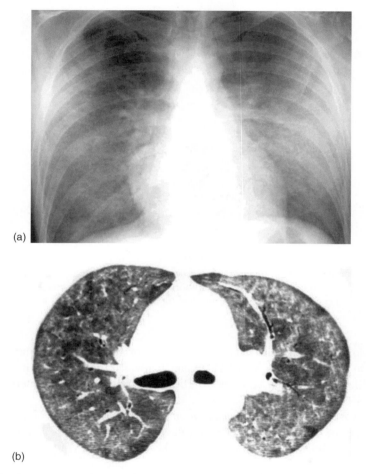

(a)

(b)

Figure 4.11   *Pneumocystis* pneumonia. (a) Posteroanterior chest radiograph shows bilateral hazy ground-glass opacities. (b) HRCT at the level of the carina (2.0-mm collimation; lung window) shows diffuse bilateral areas of 'ground-glass' attenuation. The patient was a 43-year-old man with AIDS.

developing necrotic hemorrhagic nodules or infarcts. The most common pattern seen in CT consists of multiple nodules surrounded by a halo of ground-glass attenuation (halo sign) or pleural-based wedge-shaped areas of consolidation (Figure 4.12). In mildly immunocompromised patients such as those with chronic illness, diabetes mellitus, malnutrition, alcoholism, advanced age, prolonged corticosteroid administration and chronic obstructive disease there have been described an aspegillosis form named semi-invasive or chronic necrotizing aspergillosis. Radiological findings consist of unilateral or bilateral segmental areas of consolidation with or without cavitation and/or adjacent pleural thickening and multiple nodular opacities (Franquet *et al.*, 2000).

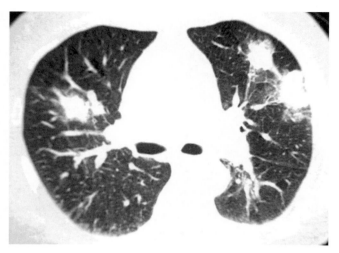

Figure 4.12   Angioinvasive aspergillosis. HRCT scan (2-mm collimation) at the level of the carina shows multiple bilateral nodules with a surrounding halo of ground-glass attenuation. These findings correspond to a nodular area of infarction surrounded by haemorrhage. The patient was a 47-year-old woman after allogeneic bone marrow transplantation.

Cryptococcal pneumonia (*Cryptococcus neoformans*) is a common pulmonary infection in AIDS patients with CD4 count below $100\,cells/mm^3$. The most typical radiographic manifestation consists of reticular or reticulonodular interstitial pattern (Stansell, 1991) (Figure 4.13).

Histoplasmosis (*Histoplasma capsulatum*) is an endemic infection of areas such Ohio-Missisipi and St Lawrence River valleys (North America). The most common radiographic findings consist of diffuse nodular opacities of 3 mm or less in diameter, nodules greater than 3 mm in diameter, small linear opacities and focal or patchy areas of consolidation, although these findings are not seen in chest radiograph in approximately 40% of patients with pulmonary histoplasmosis, even with the help of CT (Conces *et al.*, 1993).

Mucormycosis is an opportunistic fungal infection of the order Mucorales, characterized by broad, nonseptated hyphae that randomly branch at right angles (McAdams *et al.*, 1997). The most common radiographic findings consist of lobar or multilobar areas of consolidation and solitary or multiple pulmonary nodules and masses; associated cavitation is found in 26–40% of cases (Figure 4.14). An air-crescent sign, highly suggestive of an invasive fungal infection, can be identified in 5–12.5% of cases (McAdams *et al.*, 1997). CT features are non-specific and consist of solitary or multiple areas of consolidation and solitary or multiple nodules surrounded by a halo of ground-glass attenuation (halo sign) and areas. Although the CT halo sign may be seen in a number of other conditions, including other infections, in the setting of patients with severe neutropenia, it is highly diagnostic of an angioinvasive fungal pneumonia (Kuhlman, Fishman and Siegelman, 1985).

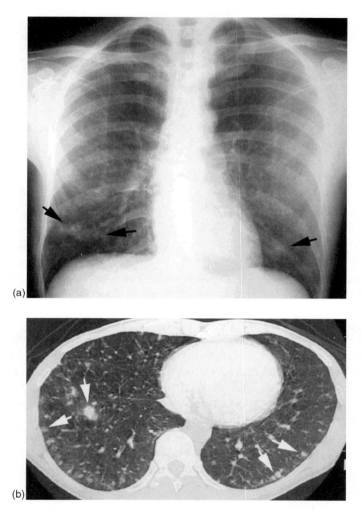

Figure 4.13   Cryptoccocal pneumonia. (a) Posteroanterior chest radiograph shows bilateral ill-defined nodules in the lower lobes (arrows). (b) HRCT scan (2-mm collimation) at the level of lung bases shows multiple bilateral ill-defined nodules in a predominant subpleural distribution (arrows). Note a nodule with a surrounding halo of ground-glass attenuation (arrowhead).

4.3   Interventional procedures in patients with pneumonia

Identifying the etiologic agent(s) responsible for pneumonia remains a challenge, primarily because of difficulty in obtaining adequate samples for culture and in differentiating infection from colonization and lack of reliable diagnostic methods. The only definitive way to reach a specific diagnosis is through demonstration of the organism that is by examination of stained smears of sputum, pleural fluid or other biologic material, by culture of respiratory secretions and blood, or by other interventional

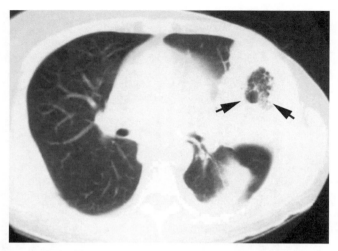

Figure 4.14   Mucormycosis CT scan at the level of the bronchus intermedius shows an air-space cavitated consolidation in the left upper lobe (arrows). A zone of consolidation is also visible in the apical segment of the left lower lobe (arrowhead) (Courtesy Nestor L. Müller MD, Vancouver).

procedures such as transthoracic fine needle aspiration or biopsy under fluoroscopy or CT guidance. Non-invasive and bronchoscopic procedures are useful techniques for the diagnosis of pulmonary infiltrates in immunocompromised patients. Bronchial aspirates (FBAS and TBAS) and BAL have the highest diagnostic yield and impact on therapeutic decisions (Rano *et al.*, 2001). However, in most large series of pneumonia a causative organism cannot be identified in 33–45% of patients, even when extensive diagnostic tests are undertaken. In certain circumstances, the lack of specific organism requires a more aggressive approach in order to obtain histopathologic and cultural identification of the cause of the pulmonary infection.

Flexible fibreoptic bronchoscopy with lung biopsy

Fibreoptic bronchoscopy (FOB) is increasingly used and has supplanted open lung biopsy as the diagnostic procedure of choice in the diagnosis of pulmonary infection. Fibreoptic bronchoscopy with bronchoalveolar lavage (BAL) and protected specimen brushing (PSB) may provide a diagnosis in 50–80% of BMT patients with pulmonary infiltrates (Jolis *et al.*, 1996; Campbell *et al.*, 1993). This method has proved particularly useful in the diagnosis of *Pneumocystis* pneumonia in AIDS patients providing an etiologic diagnosis in about 95% of cases. In the special setting of a serious pulmonary process and lack of definable cause with noninvasive methods, fibreoptic bronchoscopy in conjunction with transbronchial lung biopsy is indicated.

Although self-limiting bleeding has been reported, BAL is a relatively safe procedure even for patients with a low platelet count when compared with the risk of untreated or unsuccessfully treated pneumonia in patients with neutropenia (Hohenadel *et al.*, 2001).

Transthoracic needle aspiration

Although the reported results in the diagnosis of pulmonary infection are variable, percutaneous fine needle aspiration is an alternative method used to identify causative pathogens in selected patients with pneumonia (Haverkos *et al.*, 1983; Hwang *et al.*, 2000; Johnston, 1984; Perlmutt, Johnston and Dunnick, 1989). Transthoracic needle aspiration should be considered for patients who have not responded to initial therapy or in whom tuberculosis is suspected but has not been confirmed by examination of the sputum or gastric lavage.

4.4 Summary

In summary, chest radiography is recommended in all patients with suspected pulmonary infection in order to confirm or exclude the presence of pulmonary abnormalities.

Management of immunocompromised patients is challenging and difficult because of the diversity of causative organisms. In this group of patients, high-resolution CT and invasive procedures are commonly required. High-resolution CT can be useful in patients who have respiratory symptoms but normal or questionable radiographic findings, depicting abnormalities not evident on the radiograph and the presence of complications and concurrent parenchymal, mediastinal or pleural disease.

Diagnostic information may also be obtained by means of bronchoalveolar lavage and transbronchial needle aspiration. Under these circumstances, CT is useful as a road-map to direct fibreoptic bronchoscopy toward the region most likely to yield the diagnosis.

References

Aquino, S.L., Gamsu, G., Webb, W.R. and Kee, S.T. (1996) Tree-in-bud pattern: frequency and significance on thin section CT. *Journal of Computer Assisted Tomography*, **20**, 594–599.

Barber, T.W., Craven, D.E. and Mccabe, W.R. (1990) Bacteremia due to Mycobacterium tuberculosis in patients with human immunodeficiency virus infection. A report of 9 cases and a review of the literature. *Medicine (Baltimore)*, **69**, 375–383.

Boiselle, P.M., Crans, C.A., Jr and Kaplan, M.A. (1999) The changing face of Pneumocystis carinii pneumonia in AIDS patients. *American Journal of Roentgenology*, **172**, 1301–1309.

Boiselle, P.M., Tocino, I., Hooley, R.J., Pumerantz, A.S., Selwyn, P.A., Neklesa, V.P. and Lange, R.C. (1997) Chest radiograph interpretation of Pneumocystis carinii pneumonia, bacterial pneumonia, and pulmonary tuberculosis in HIV-positive patients: accuracy, distinguishing features, and mimics. *Journal of Thoracic Imaging*, **12**, 47–53.

Brown, M.J., Miller, R.R. and Muller, N.L. (1994) Acute lung disease in the immunocompromised host: CT and pathologic examination findings. *Radiology*, **190**, 247–254.

Campbell, J.H., Blessing, N., Burnett, A.K. and Stevenson, R.D. (1993) Investigation and management of pulmonary infiltrates following bone marrow transplantation: an eight year review. *Thorax*, **48**, 1248–1251.

Chastre, J., Trouillet, J.L., Vuagnat, A., Joly-Guillou, M.L., Clavier, H., Dombret, M.C. and Gibert, C. (1998) Nosocomial pneumonia in patients with acute respiratory distress syndrome. *American Journal of Respiratory and Critical Care Medicine*, **157**, 1165–1172.

Chemaly, R.F., Ghosh, S., Bodey, G.P., Rohatgi, N., Safdar, A., Keating, M.J., Champlin, R.E., Aguilera, E.A., Tarrand, J.J. and Raad, I.I. (2006) Respiratory viral infections in adults with hematologic malignancies and human stem cell transplantation recipients: a retrospective study at a major cancer center. *Medicine (Baltimore)*, **85**, 278–287.

Choyke, P.L., Sostman, H.D., Curtis, A.M., Ravin, C.E., Chen, J.T., Godwin, J.D. and Putman, C.E. (1983) Adult-onset pulmonary tuberculosis. *Radiology*, **148**, 357–362.

Conces, D.J., Jr, Stockberger, S.M., Tarver, R.D. and Wheat, L.J. (1993) Disseminated histoplasmosis in AIDS: findings on chest radiographs. *American Journal of Roentgenology*, **160**, 15–19.

Dye, C., Scheele, S., Dolin, P., Pathania, V. and Raviglione, M.C. (1999) Consensus statement. Global burden of tuberculosis: estimated incidence, prevalence, and mortality by country. WHO Global Surveillance and Monitoring Project. *The Journal of the American Medical Association*, **282**, 677–686.

Ellis, S.M. (2004) The spectrum of tuberculosis and non-tuberculous mycobacterial infection. *European Radiology*, **14** (Suppl 3), E34–E42.

Ettinger, N.A. and Trulock, E.P. (1991) Pulmonary considerations of organ transplantation. Part 2. *The American Review of Respiratory Disease*, **144**, 213–223.

Franquet, T. (2001) Imaging of pneumonia: trends and algorithms. *The European Respiratory Journal*, **18**, 196–208.

Franquet, T. (2004) Respiratory infection in the AIDS and immunocompromised patient. *European Radiology*, **14** (Suppl 3), E21–E23.

Franquet, T., Lee, K.S. and Muller, N.L. (2003) Thin-section CT findings in 32 immunocompromised patients with cytomegalovirus pneumonia who do not have AIDS. *American Journal of Roentgenology*, **181**, 1059–1063.

Franquet, T., Muller, N.L., Gimenez, A., Domingo, P., Plaza, V. and Bordes, R. (2000) Semiinvasive pulmonary aspergillosis in chronic obstructive pulmonary disease: radiologic and pathologic findings in nine patients. *American Journal of Roentgenology*, **174**, 51–56.

Franquet, T., Muller, N.L., Oikonomou, A. and Flint, J.D. (2004) Aspergillus infection of the airways: computed tomography and pathologic findings. *Journal of Computer Assisted Tomography*, **28**, 10–16.

Franquet, T., Rodriguez, S., Martino, R., Gimenez, A., Salinas, T. and Hidalgo, A. (2006) Thin-section CT findings in hematopoietic stem cell transplantation recipients with respiratory virus pneumonia. *American Journal of Roentgenology*, **187**, 1085–1090.

Franquet, T., Rodriguez, S., Martino, R., Salinas, T., Gimenez, A. and Hidalgo, A. (2005) Human metapneumovirus infection in hematopoietic stem cell transplant recipients: high-resolution computed tomography findings. *Journal of Computer Assisted Tomography*, **29**, 223–227.

Gharib, A.M. and Stern, E.J. (2001) Radiology of pneumonia. *Medical Clinics of North America*, **85**, 1461–1491.

Hanson, D.L., Chu, S.Y., Farizo, K.M. and Ward, J.W. (1995) Distribution of CD4+ T lymphocytes at diagnosis of acquired immunodeficiency syndrome-defining and other human immunodeficiency virus-related illnesses. The Adult and Adolescent Spectrum of HIV Disease Project Group. *Archives of Internal Medicine*, **155**, 1537–1542.

Harisinghani, M.G., Mcloud, T.C., Shepard, J.A., Ko, J.P., Shroff, M.M. and Mueller, P.R. (2000) Tuberculosis from head to toe. *Radiographics*, **20**, 449–470; quiz 528–529, 532.

Hartman, T.E., Swensen, S.J. and Williams, D.E. (1993) Mycobacterium avium-intracellulare complex: evaluation with CT. *Radiology*, **187**, 23–26.

Haverkos, H.W., Dowling, J.N., Pasculle, A.W., Myerowitz, R.L., Lerberg, D.B. and Hakala, T.R. (1983) Diagnosis of pneumonitis in immunocompromised patients by open lung biopsy. *Cancer*, **52**, 1093–1097.

Heussel, C.P., Kauczor, H.U., Heussel, G.E., Fischer, B., Begrich, M., Mildenberger, P. and Thelen, M. (1999) Pneumonia in febrile neutropenic patients and in bone marrow and blood stem-cell transplant recipients: use of high-resolution computed tomography. *Journal of Clinical Oncology*, **17**, 796–805.

Hidalgo, A., Falco, V., Mauleon, S., Andreu, J., Crespo, M., Ribera, E., Pahissa, A. and Caceres, J. (2003) Accuracy of high-resolution CT in distinguishing between Pneumocystis carinii pneumonia and non-Pneumocystis carinii pneumonia in AIDS patients. *European Radiology*, **13**, 1179–1184.

Hirschtick, R.E., Glassroth, J., Jordan, M.C., Wilcosky, T.C., Wallace, J.M., Kvale, P.A., Markowitz, N., Rosen, M.J., Mangura, B.T. and Hopewell, P.C. (1995) Bacterial pneumonia in persons infected with the human immunodeficiency virus. Pulmonary Complications of HIV Infection Study Group. *The New England Journal of Medicine*, **333**, 845–851.

Hohenadel, I.A., Kiworr, M., Genitsariotis, R., Zeidler, D. and Lorenz, J. (2001) Role of bronchoalveolar lavage in immunocompromised patients with pneumonia treated with a broad spectrum antibiotic and antifungal regimen. *Thorax*, **56**, 115–120.

Hopewell, P.C. (1995) A clinical view of tuberculosis. *Radiologic Clinics of North America*, **33**, 641–653.

Hwang, S.S., Kim, H.H., Park, S.H., Jung, J.I. and Jang, H.S. (2000) The value of CT-guided percutaneous needle aspiration in immunocompromised patients with suspected pulmonary infection. *American Journal of Roentgenology*, **175**, 235–238.

Im, J.G., Itoh, H., Lee, K.S. and Han, M.C. (1995) CT-pathology correlation of pulmonary tuberculosis. *Critical Reviews in Diagnostic Imaging*, **36**, 227–285.

Im, J.G., Song, K.S., Kang, H.S., Park, J.H., Yeon, K.M., Han, M.C. and Kim, C.W. (1987) Mediastinal tuberculous lymphadenitis: CT manifestations. *Radiology*, **164**, 115–119.

Janzen, D.L., Padley, S.P., Adler, B.D. and Muller, N.L. (1993) Acute pulmonary complications in immunocompromised non-AIDS patients: comparison of diagnostic accuracy of CT and chest radiography. *Clinical Radiology*, **47**, 159–165.

Johnston, W.W. (1984) Percutaneous fine needle aspiration biopsy of the lung. A study of 1,015 patients. *Acta Cytologica*, **28**, 218–224.

Jolis, R., Castella, J., Puzo, C., Coll, P. and Abeledo, C. (1996) Diagnostic value of protected BAL in diagnosing pulmonary infections in immunocompromised patients. *Chest*, **109**, 601–607.

Kim, H.Y., Song, K.S., Goo, J.M., Lee, J.S., Lee, K.S. and Lim, T.H. (2001) Thoracic sequelae and complications of tuberculosis. *Radiographics*, **21**, 839–858 discussion 859–860.

Kotloff, R.M. (1993) Infection caused by nontuberculous mycobacteria: clinical aspects. *Seminars in Roentgenology*, **28**, 131–138.

Kuhlman, J.E., Fishman, E.K., Burch, P.A., Karp, J.E., Zerhouni, E.A. and Siegelman, S.S. (1987) Invasive pulmonary aspergillosis in acute leukaemia. The contribution of CT to early diagnosis and aggressive management. *Chest*, **92**, 95–99.

Kuhlman, J.E., Fishman, E.K. and Siegelman, S.S. (1985) Invasive pulmonary aspergillosis in acute leukemia: characteristic findings on CT, the CT halo sign, and the role of CT in early diagnosis. *Radiology*, **157**, 611–614.

Leung, A.N. (1999) Pulmonary tuberculosis: the essentials. *Radiology*, **210**, 307–322.

Leung, A.N., Gosselin, M.V., Napper, C.H., Braun, S.G., Hu, W.W., Wong, R.M. and Gasman, J. (1999) Pulmonary infections after bone marrow transplantation: clinical and radiographic findings. *Radiology*, **210**, 699–710.

Lyon, R., Haque, A.K., Asmuth, D.M. and Woods, G.L. (1996) Changing patterns of infections in patients with AIDS: a study of 279 autopsies of prison inmates and nonincarcerated patients at a university hospital in eastern Texas, 1984–1993. *Clinical Infectious Diseases*, **23**, 241–247.

Mcadams, H.P., Rosado De Christenson, M., Strollo, D.C. and Patz, E.F., Jr (1997) Pulmonary mucormycosis: radiologic findings in 32 cases. *American Journal of Roentgenology*, **168**, 1541–1548.

Miller, W.T., Jr (1994) Spectrum of pulmonary nontuberculous mycobacterial infection. *Radiology*, **191**, 343–350.

Miller, W.T. and Miller, W.T., Jr (1993) Tuberculosis in the normal host: radiological findings. *Seminars in Roentgenology*, **28**, 109–118.

Moe, A.A. and Hardy, W.D. (1994) Pneumocystis carinii infection in the HIV-seropositive patient. *Infectious Disease Clinics of North America*, **8**, 331–364.

Moon, J.H., Kim, E.A., Lee, K.S., Kim, T.S., Jung, K.J. and Song, J.H. (2000) Cytomegalovirus pneumonia: high-resolution CT findings in ten non-AIDS immunocompromised patients. *Korean Journal of Radiology*, **1**, 73–78.

Muder, R.R. and Yu, V.L. (2002) Infection due to Legionella species other than L. pneumophila. *Clinical Infectious Diseases*, **35**, 990–998.

Murray, J.F. and Mills, J. (1990a) Pulmonary infectious complications of human immunodeficiency virus infection. Part I. *The American Review of Respiratory Disease*, **141**, 1356–1372.

Murray, J.F. and Mills, J. (1990b) Pulmonary infectious complications of human immunodeficiency virus infection. Part II. *The American Review of Respiratory Disease*, **141**, 1582–1598.

Niederman, M.S. and Fein, A.M. (1990) Sepsis syndrome, the adult respiratory distress syndrome, and nosocomial pneumonia. A common clinical sequence. *Clinics in Chest Medicine*, **11**, 633–656.

Olliff, J.F. and Williams, M.P. (1989) Radiological appearances of cytomegalovirus infections. *Clinical Radiology*, **40**, 463–467.

Padley, S.P. and King, L.J. (1999) Computed tomography of the thorax in HIV disease. *European Radiology*, **9**, 1556–1569.

Perlmutt, L.M., Johnston, W.W. and Dunnick, N.R. (1989) Percutaneous transthoracic needle aspiration: a review. *American Journal of Roentgenology*, **152**, 451–455.

Primack, S.L., Hartman, T.E., Lee, K.S. and Muller, N.L. (1994) Pulmonary nodules and the CT halo sign. *Radiology*, **190**, 513–515.

Primack, S.L. and Muller, N.L. (1994) High-resolution computed tomography in acute diffuse lung disease in the immunocompromised patient. *Radiologic Clinics of North America*, **32**, 731–744.

Rano, A., Agusti, C., Jimenez, P., Angrill, J., Benito, N., Danes, C., Gonzalez, J., Rovira, M., Pumarola, T., Moreno, A. and Torres, A. (2001) Pulmonary infiltrates in non-HIV immunocompromised patients: a diagnostic approach using non-invasive and bronchoscopic procedures. *Thorax*, **56**, 379–387.

Sable, C.A. and Donowitz, G.R. (1994) Infections in bone marrow transplant recipients. *Clinical Infectious Diseases*, **18**, 273–281 quiz 282–284.

Schulman, L.L. (1987) Cytomegalovirus pneumonitis and lobar consolidation. *Chest*, **91**, 558–561.

Seidenfeld, J.J., Pohl, D.F., Bell, R.C., Harris, G.D. and Johanson, W.G., Jr (1986) Incidence, site, and outcome of infections in patients with the adult respiratory distress syndrome. *The American Review of Respiratory Disease*, **134**, 12–16.

Shah, R.M., Kaji, A.V., Ostrum, B.J. and Friedman, A.C. (1997) Interpretation of chest radiographs in AIDS patients: usefulness of CD4 lymphocyte counts. *Radiographics*, **17**, 47–58; discussion 59–61.

Singh, N., Muder, R.R., Yu, V.L. and Gayowski, T. (1993) Legionella infection in liver transplant recipients: implications for management. *Transplantation*, **56**, 1549–1551.

Stansell, J.D. (1991) Fungal disease in HIV-infected persons: cryptococcosis, histoplasmosis, and coccidioidomycosis. *Journal of Thoracic Imaging*, **6**, 28–35.

Tarver, R.D., Teague, S.D., Heitkamp, D.E. and Conces, D.J. Jr. (2005) Radiology of community-acquired pneumonia. *Radiologic Clinics of North America*, **43**, 497–512, viii.

Tomiyama, N., Muller, N.L., Johkoh, T., Honda, O., Mihara, N., Kozuka, T., Hamada, S., Nakamura, H., Akira, M. and Ichikado, K. (2000) Acute parenchymal lung disease in immunocompetent patients: diagnostic accuracy of high-resolution CT. *American Journal of Roentgenology*, **174**, 1745–1750.

Vilar, J., Domingo, M.L., Soto, C. and Cogollos, J. (2004) Radiology of bacterial pneumonia. *European Journal of Radiology*, **51**, 102–113.

Woodring, J.H. and Vandiviere, H.M. (1990) Pulmonary disease caused by nontuberculous mycobacteria. *Journal of Thoracic Imaging*, **5**, 64–76.

Worthy, S.A., Flint, J.D. and Muller, N.L. (1997) Pulmonary complications after bone marrow transplantation: high-resolution CT and pathologic findings. *Radiographics*, **17**, 1359–1371.

Yoon, H.K., Im, J.G., Ahn, J.M. and Han, M.C. (1995) Pulmonary nocardiosis: CT findings. *Journal of Computer Assisted Tomography*, **19**, 52–55.

5

Pulmonary infections in HIV patients in the highly active antiretroviral therapy era

Natividad Benito[1] and Asunción Moreno-Camacho[2]

[1]Infectious Diseases Unit (Internal Medicine Service), Hospital de la Santa Creu i Sant Pau, Barcelona [2]Infectious Diseases Service, Hospital Clínic de Barcelona – IDIBAPS, Barcelona, Spain

5.1 Introduction

Importance of the problem

The first published reports of acquired immunodeficiency syndrome (AIDS) in the United States appeared in the *Morbidity and Mortality Weekly Report* in June 1981, when five homosexual men in Los Angeles were diagnosed with *Pneumocystis carinii* pneumonia (currently *Pneumocystis jiroveci*) (Centers of Diseases Control and Prevention [CDC], 1981; Stringer *et al.*, 2000). Since then, HIV infection has become a widespread epidemic and continues to expand (Centers for Disease Control and Prevention, 2001a, 2001b). Overall, the HIV incidence rate (the proportion of people who have become infected with HIV) is believed to have peaked in the late 1990s and subsequently to have stabilized, notwithstanding increasing incidence in several countries. However, the number of people living with HIV continues to grow, as does the number of deaths due to AIDS. A total of 39.5 million [34.1–47.1 million] people were living with HIV in 2006, 2.6 million more than in 2004 (UNAIDS, 2006). This figure includes the estimated 4.3 million (3.6–6.6 million) adults and children who were newly infected with HIV in 2006, which is about 400 000 more than in 2004. There were 2.9 million (2.5–3.5 million) AIDS deaths in 2006 (UNAIDS, 2006).

The AIDS epidemic remains one of the most important global health problems of the twenty-first century, despite the substantial advancements in therapy achieved over the past 20 years. The first effective medication against the HIV virus was introduced in 1987, and combination therapy with multiple agents, currently known as highly active antiretroviral therapy (HAART) became widely used between 1996 and 1997.

Pulmonary Infection in the Immunocompromised Patient, Edited by Carlos Agustí and Antoni Torres
© 2009 John Wiley & Sons, Ltd.

Since then, the incidence of AIDS-related opportunistic infections and AIDS in HIV-positive patients has dramatically decreased in the United States and Europe. Despite these gains, pulmonary disease remains a leading cause of morbidity and mortality.

From the first descriptions of HIV/AIDS, the respiratory tract has been the site most frequently affected by the disease (Murray *et al.*, 1984, 1987; Stover *et al.*, 1985; Meduri *et al.*, 1992). Up to 70% of HIV patients have a pulmonary complication during the evolution of the disease, mainly of infectious etiology (Miller *et al.*, 1996). According to results of autopsy findings, the lung is the organ most frequently affected by HIV-related processes, with an incidence ranging from 100% in the early period of the epidemic to 70% in the HAART era (Afessa *et al.*, 1992; Masliah *et al.*, 2000). In the USA and Europe as well as Africa, lower-respiratory-tract infections are 25-fold more common in patients with HIV than in the general community, occurring at rates up to 90 cases per 1000 person/years (Feikin *et al.*, 2004). Pulmonary infections remain a frequent cause of morbidity and hospital admission of HIV infected patients in the HAART era. In recent studies an incidence of approximately 20–25 episodes per 100 hospital admission/years has been observed (Benito *et al.*, 2001, 2004). These numbers give an idea of the magnitude of the problem of pulmonary infections in HIV patients. Moreover, it has been suggested that *Pneumocystis* pneumonia (PCP), tuberculosis and bacterial pneumonia are associated with a significantly worse subsequent HIV disease course (Whalen *et al.*, 1995; Osmond *et al.*, 1999; Kaplan, Janoff and Masur, 1999; Shaunak, Veryard and Javan, 2001), although not all studies agree with these findings (Del Amo *et al.*, 2003). Pulmonary infection usually appears as pulmonary infiltrates on chest radiographs and is frequently – but not always- associated with clinical respiratory symptoms (Gold *et al.*, 2002).

5.2   Epidemology and etiology

Few studies have systematically described the full spectrum of pulmonary disorders associated with HIV infection (Wallace *et al.*, 1993, 1997). Most investigators have focused on pneumonias of specific etiologies such as those caused by *Pneumocystis jirovecii* or bacterial pneumonias. Therefore, there is no consensus on any diagnostic algorithm of pulmonary infections in HIV patients. The diagnostic decision could be different depending on the epidemiological features in a specific geographic area (Daley *et al.*, 1996; Salzman, 1998). Thus, the incidence of tuberculosis in HIV patients ranges considerably in different geographical areas, depending on the prevalence of disease in the general population. In Africa, tuberculosis is the most common pulmonary complication of HIV (Daley *et al.*, 1996; Murray, 2005); second among HIV-associated pulmonary infections is community-acquired pneumonia, most commonly caused by *Streptococcus pneumoniae* (Murray, 2005). On the other hand, PCP is uncommon compared with the incidence of pulmonary tuberculosis and bacterial pneumonia, with rates in persons with CD4 counts <200/mm^3, clearly lower than in the United States before the introduction of routine trimethoprim-sulfamethoxazole prophylaxis and HAART (Lucas *et al.*, 1989; Mcleod *et al.*, 1989; Carme *et al.*, 1991; Kamanfu *et al.*, 1993; Batungwanayo *et al.*, 1994; Daley *et al.*, 1996; van Oosterhout *et al.*, 2007). Nevertheless, the prevalence of PCP pneumonia in Sub-Saharan Africa is increasing (Murray, 2005). In Western Europe, in the 1990s, PCP was the commonest AIDS-defining illness whereas pulmonary tuberculosis was more common in Eastern Europe. In addition, within Western Europe, tuberculosis was more common in the south than in the north and increased steadily over time (Serraino *et al.*, 2003).

The epidemiology of pulmonary infections in HIV has notably changed in the last decades. There have been several reasons to explain these changes. General prescription of PCP primary prophylaxis since 1989 is one of the main causes (Centers for Disease Control and Prevention, 1989), and the use of HAART since 1996 is the other underlying explanation. Some studies have suggested that *P. jiroveci* prophylaxis with trimethoprim-sulfamethoxazole (TMP-SMX) could have decreased the incidence of bacterial infections, including pneumonias in HIV patients with less than 200 lymphocytes CD4/mm^3, however, not all studies agree with this statement (Cohn, 1991; Hardy *et al.*, 1992; Hirschtick *et al.*, 1995; Edge and Rimland, 1996; Tabet *et al.*, 1997). More recently, the introduction and generalized use of HAART has decreased the incidence of opportunistic infections and the number of hospital infections increasing the life expectancy of HIV patients (Torres and Barr, 1997; Palella *et al.*, 1998; Michelet *et al.*, 1998; Moore and Chaisson, 1999; Sullivan *et al.*, 2000; Mönkemüller *et al.*, 2000). Nevertheless, its influence on the incidence, etiology and prognosis of pulmonary complications, mainly on non-opportunistic infections, remains unknown.

In summary, bacterial pneumonia is the most frequent cause of pulmonary infection in HIV patients all over the world, followed by PCP and tuberculosis with different incidences depending on the geographical area (Benito-Hernández, Moreno-Camacho, Gatell-Artigas, 2005).

Pneumocystis pneumonia

In early studies in the United States, PCP was the most frequent cause of pulmonary infections in HIV patients, accounting for 85% of cases (Murray *et al.*, 1984; Stover *et al.*, 1985). The majority of these were AIDS patients. It was estimated that 75% of HIV-infected persons would develop PCP during their lifetime (Huang *et al.*, 2006).

The rate of PCP greatly decreased as a result of *P. jiroveci* primary prophylaxis (Centers for Disease Control, 1989). Thus, the incidence of PCP rose steeply until 1987 but has declined significantly since then, while the other AIDS-defining conditions showed significant upward trends (Muñoz *et al.*, 1993). In a study from January 1988, PCP was not the leading cause of death in HIV patients (Stein *et al.*, 1992). *Pneumocystis* pneumonia was the first cause of hospital admissions in patients with HIV infection before the widespread use of PCP prophylaxis. However, during the post-prophylaxis period, there was a significant decrease in the number of PCP admissions (Chien *et al.*, 1992). In Europe in the 1980s, 30–50% of patients had a PCP at the time of their diagnosis while only 10–20% of patients had a PCP at the time of their diagnosis in the 1990s (Lungdren *et al.*, 1994; Lungdren *et al.*, 1997). These figures are similar to those observed in the USA and Australia after the generalized use of PCP prophylaxis (Hoover *et al.*, 1993; Muñoz *et al.*, 1993; Montaner *et al.*, 1994; Dore *et al.*, 1997). More recently, the widespread administration of HAART has been associated with a reduction of PCP incidence as well as other opportunistic infections (Palella *et al.*, 1998; Moore *et al.*, 1999; Masur, 2000; Wolff and O'Donnell, 2001).

Despite the declining incidence of PCP, it remains the most common AIDS defining indicator condition and the most frequent opportunistic infection in North America and Europe in HIV patients in the last years (Blaxhult *et al.*, 2000; Dore *et al.*, 2002; Serraino *et al.*, 2003; Thomas and Limper, 2004) However, *P. jiroveci* pneumonia has become a complication for those patients who are not receiving HAART and for those who are not receiving anti-PCP prophylaxis since a significant percentage of these patients (up to 50%) are not known to be infected with HIV (Smith and Orholm, 1994; Pradier *et al.*, 1997; Stoehr *et al.*, 1999; Edge and Rimland, 1999; Benito *et al.*, 2001; Pulvirenti *et al.*, 2003; Benito *et al.*, 2004). This situation emphasizes the importance of performing an early diagnosis of HIV infection, especially in patients at risk (Pulvirenti *et al.*, 2003).

There is a strong correlation between the incidence of PCP and the number of CD4 cells in the peripheral blood of individuals infected with HIV. *Pneumocystis* pneumonia develops predominantly in patients whose CD4 cell count is less than 200 cells/ml (Phair *et al.*, 1990). Patients in whom the CD4 count is less than 200 cells/μL and who are not receiving prophylaxis are nine times more likely to develop PCP within six months than individuals on therapy (Stansell *et al.*, 1997). The median CD4 count in patients with PCP is 20 cells/mm^3, and the plasma viral load of HIV is usually greater than 10 000 copies/ml; no cases generally occur among patients with less than 200 copies/ml (Benito *et al.*, 2001).

The *clinical presentation* of PCP in HIV-infected people differs from the presentation in the other immunocompromised patients. In general, HIV patients have a sub-acute course and longer symptoms duration than the other immunocompromised patients (Thomas and Limper, 2004). In the HIV infection setting, the clinical presentation of PCP is similar to that in the pre-HAART era and consists of nonproductive cough, bilateral interstitial infiltrates and high alveolar-arterial gradients. The most common findings on physical examination are fever and tachypnea. Chest radiographs are initially normal in up to one-fourth of patients with PCP. High resolution computed tomography (HRCT) has a high sensitivity for PCP (100%) and a specificity of 89% (Hartman *et al.*, 1994; Gruden *et al.*, 1997; Hidalgo *et al.*, 2003). A negative HRCT may allow exclusion of PCP. The most common abnormal laboratory value associated with PCP in HIV-infected patients is an elevated lactate deshydrogenase level (LDH), present in 90% of patients and with a prognostic significance (Zaman and White, 1988; Phair *et al.*, 1990; Butt, Michaels and Kissinger, 2002). Moreover, a rising LDH level despite appropriate treatment portends a poor prognosis. Although PCP can be suspected based upon clinical and radiological findings, the diagnosis should usually be pursued.

Specific *diagnosis* of PCP requires documentation of the organism by means of the microscopic visualization of the characteristic cysts and/or trophic forms on stained respiratory specimens. It is usually performed by bronchoalveolar lavage (BAL), induced sputum, and in rare occasions surgical lung biopsy (Lazarous and O'Donnell, 2007). Bronchoscopy with BAL is the preferred diagnostic procedure for PCP, with reported sensitivity ranging from 89% to more than 98% (Broaddus *et al.*, 1985; Huang *et al.*, 1995). The most rapid and least invasive method of diagnostic is by analysis of sputum induced by the inhalation of hypertonic saline. While the specificity of this method approaches 100%, the sensitivity ranges from 55 to 92% (Zaman *et al.*, 1988; Cruciani *et al.*, 2002). This variability is especially related to the skills of the team inducing the sputum. Thus, in select institutions, sputum induction is performed as the initial diagnostic procedure, thereby decreasing the need for bronchoscopy (Ng *et al.*, 1989; Huang *et al.*, 1995). Several PCR assays have been developed for the diagnosis of PCP (Alvarez-Martínez *et al.*, 2006). The assays have been tested on BAL, induced sputum, and non-invasive oral wash specimens. In general, PCR assays have been more sensitive but also less specific for diagnosis of *Pneumocystis* pneumonia compared to traditional microscopic methods.

Trimethoprim-sulfamethoxazole (TMP-SMX) remains the drug of choice for the *treatment and prevention* of this infection, but the best choice of alternative agents has not been established. Corticosteroids given in conjunction with anti-*Pneumocystis* therapy decrease the incidence of mortality and respiratory failure associated with severe PCP, particularly in those patients with abnormalities in oxygen exchange at the time of presentation (Briel *et al.*, 2006). Certain strains of *Pneumocystis jiroveci* have mutations in the dihydropteroate synthase (DHPS) gene, an essential enzyme that is inhibited by sulfonamides. The DHPS mutation is associated with the use and duration of TMP-SMX prophylaxis, but it is not definitely clear if these mutations only reflect exposure to the drug or if they are related to a possible failure of TMP-SMX treatment and a worst prognosis (Beck *et al.*, 2001; Valerio *et al.*, 2007). Once immunologic response is documented with the use of HAART (CD4 cells count increase by more than 200 cells/ml for at least three months), primary PCP prophylaxis may be discontinued. Additionally, secondary prophylaxis may be discontinued safely provided the response to HAART is sustained (Lopez Bernaldo de Quirós *et al.*, 2001; Ledergerber *et al.*, 2001).

Bacterial pulmonary infections

Bacterial pulmonary infection is currently the most frequent infection in HIV patients, as well as the most common admission diagnosis in this population. (Hirschtick *et al.*, 1995; Benito *et al.*, 2001, 2004; Wallace *et al.*, 1993; Paul *et al.*, 1999; Altés *et al.*, 1999). HIV infection is associated with a greater than 10-fold increased incidence of bacterial pneumonia in both industrialized and poor countries (Feikin *et al.*, 2004). Although bacterial pneumonia can occur throughout the course of HIV infection, it tends to develop more frequently in individuals with advanced immunosuppression (Hirschtick *et al.*, 1995; Wallace *et al.*, 1997). Thus, a direct relation between the CD4 count and the incidence of bacterial pneumonia has been demonstrated. Intravenous drugs and smoking (cigarettes and illicit drugs, as cocaine, crack or marijuana) are other risk factors for the development of bacterial pneumonia in this group of patients.

The benefits of HAART on reducing opportunistic infections and mortality among HIV-infected people have been well documented, but relatively few reports have characterized the impact of HAART on bacterial pneumonia (Wolff and O'Donnell, 2001; De Gaetano Donati et al., 2000; Sullivan et al., 2000; Serraino et al., 2003). Moreover, none of the published reports was designed to directly assess this effect. Most observational studies have shown that HAART could decrease the incidence of bacterial pneumonia or pneumococcal disease in HIV infected adults (Paul et al., 1999; Nuorti et al., 2000; Sullivan et al., 2000; De Gaetano Donati et al., 2000; Dworkin et al., 2001). In one of these reports, performed in patients with less than 200 CD4 lymphocytes/mm^3; the incidence of bacterial pneumonia decreased from 22.7 episodes/100 persons-year in 1993 to 12.3 episodes/100 persons-year in 1996 and 9.1 episodes in 1997 (Sullivan et al., 2000). A further study investigating the impact of the introduction of HAART on the incidence of bacterial pneumonia noted a statistically significant decrease from 13.1 to 8.5 episodes per 100 persons (De Gaetano Donati et al., 2000). The incidence of community-acquired bacterial pneumonia decreased from 10.7 to 7.7, while that of nosocomial episodes decreased from 2.4 to 0.8 episodes. An additional study of this group showed that the greatest impact of introducing HAART was on nosocomial infections rather than community acquired infections. Although community-acquired pneumonias were noted to decrease over the time period, this did not reach statistical significance (De Gaetano Donati et al., 2003). An important decline in the rate of hospital admission due to bacterial pneumonia was observed in another study between 1995 and 1997 (8.0 per 100 patient-years in 1995 versus 3.6 per 100 patient/years in 1997) (Paul et al., 1999). In population-based studies, invasive pneumococcal disease in AIDS patients has been significantly lower since 1996 (Nuorti et al., 2000; Dworkin et al., 2001). However, a recent study showed a decrease in the tendency for the incidence of invasive pneumococcal disease during the first two years after the introduction of HAART, but this tendency was not apparent from 1999 onward (Jordano et al., 2004).

Bacterial pneumonia has increased as a proportion of diagnosed pulmonary infections despite an overall decrease in the number of cases. In one study, bacterial pneumonia proportion was greater in patients receiving HAART than in the pre-HAART era among patients referred to a Pulmonary and Critical Care Medicine Service (Wolff and O'Donnell, 2001). In another study, bacterial pneumonia was the cause of almost 50% of pulmonary infiltrates in HIV patients (Benito et al., 2004) without differences between patients receiving or not HAART (Benito et al., 2001). This percentage is higher than that observed in studies performed at the end of the 1980s (20–45%) (Magnenat et al., 1991; Ferrer et al., 1992) and specially in the first series which included AIDS patients (2–10%) (Murray et al., 1984; Stover et al., 1985; Polski et al., 1986). This increase in the proportion of bacterial pneumonia could reflect greater declines in other opportunistic infections rather than a direct increase in the number of bacterial pneumonias. In summary, most observational studies showed that HAART could be associated with a decrease in the incidence of bacterial pneumonias. In patients with less than 200 CD4/mm^3, this decline could have been most important (Sullivan et al., 2000). Moreover, the greatest impact of HAART could be on nosocomial infections rather than community-acquired infections (De Gaetano Donati *et al.*, 2000).

In HIV-infected individuals, the most consistent risk factor for bacterial pneumonia is the stage of HIV disease. Although bacterial pneumonia tends to occur earlier in the course of HIV than other opportunistic infections, the incidence increases as *CD4 cell numbers* decline and is consistently highest in individuals with fewer than 200 CD4/ mm^3 lymphocytes (Hirschtick *et al.*, 1995; Wallace *et al.*, 1997). Eighty per cent of cases of bacterial pneumonia occur with a CD4 count lower than 400 CD4/mm^3, and recurrent pneumonia with less than 300 CD4/mm^3 (Hanson *et al.*, 1995). Based upon these observations, the CDC added recurrent bacterial pneumonia as an AIDS-defining condition in 1992 (CDC, 1992). Median of CD4 lymphocyte count in cases of bacterial pneumonia is 200 cells/mm^3, significantly higher than median of CD4 lymphocyte in tuberculosis or *Pneumocystis* pneumonia (Benito *et al.*, 2001). Moreover, median of HIV viral load is lower in bacterial pneumonia than in tuberculosis or PCP (Benito *et al.*, 2001).

The most common *cause of bacterial pneumonia* is *Streptococcus pneumoniae* followed by *Haemophylus influenzae* (Magnenat *et al.*, 1991; Baril *et al.*, 1998; De Gaetano Donati *et al.*, 2000; Boschini *et al.*, 1996; Witt, Craven and McCabe, 1987; Rimland *et al.*, 2002).

As in the general population, *S. pneumoniae* is consistently the most common bacterial cause of community-acquired pneumonia among HIV-infected adults, implicated in approximately 20% of all bacterial pneumonias, 40% of those for which a specific diagnosis is made, and 70% of bacteremic pneumonias. Many studies have described the high incidence of pneumococcal pneumonia and its epidemiologic and clinical characteristics in this population (Janoff *et al.*, 1992; Feldman *et al.*, 1999; Nuorti *et al.*, 2000; Dworkin *et al.*, 2001; Queralt *et al.*, 2004). It is worth noting the increased rate of bacteremia complicating pneumococcal pneumonia among HIV infected people (more than 50% in some studies), and the high rates of recurrent pneumococcal pneumonia (10–25%) (Redd *et al.*, 1990; Falcó *et al.*, 1994; Afessa *et al.*, 2000; French *et al.*, 2000). Data regarding the effectiveness of pneumococcal vaccination in HIV-positive patients has been evaluated in several studies, but it is still inconclusive (Feikin *et al.*, 2004; French *et al.*, 1998; French *et al.*, 2000; Breiman *et al.*, 2000; Spoulou, Gilgk and Ioannidis, 2002; Tasker *et al.*, 2002; López-Palomo *et al.*, 2004; Hung *et al.*, 2004). Cumulative results from USA observational studies provide support for a modest efficacy of the 23-valent polysaccharide vaccine in selected HIV infected adults, particularly those with higher CD4 T cells/mm^3 and laboratory-confirmed pneumococcal disease (Gebo *et al.*, 1996; Guerrero *et al.*, 1999; Dworkin *et al.*, 2001). In East Africa, a well-designed randomized, double-blind placebo-controlled trial showed no protective effect of the polysaccharide vaccine among patients at any clinical or immunological stage (French *et al.*, 2000). A more recent observational study from Taiwan documented that the vaccine and administration of HAART were associated with a reduced risk of pneumococcal disease (Hung *et al.*, 2004). However, results from other observational study do not support an important additional protective effect of 23-valent pneumococcal vaccine in HIV-patients with immunological response to HAART (López-Palomo *et al.*, 2004). In 1999 the Centre for Disease Control (CDC) and the Infectious Disease Society of America (IDSA) (CDC/ IDSA, 1999) guidelines recommended that a single dose of polysaccharide vaccine should be given as soon as possible after the diagnosis of HIV infection to adults and adolescents who have a CD4 T cell count higher than 200 cells/mm^3 and who have not had one during the previous five years. Despite these recommendations, pneumococcal polysaccharide vaccine has tended to be underused in HIV-infected adults.

Haemophilus influenzae is associated with 10–15% of cases, including 5% of bacteremias. Recently, the epidemiological, clinical and radiological characteristics and outcome of pneumonia caused by *H. influenzae* in this group of patients has been described (Cordero *et al.*, 2000). It affects mainly patients with advanced HIV disease, and a subacute clinical presentation has been observed in almost 30% of cases. Bilateral lung infiltrates are noted radiographically in more than a half of patients. The mortality rate associated is not higher than that occurring in the general population (Cordero *et al.*, 2000).

Nosocomial pneumonia in HIV-infected patients is most commonly caused by gram-negative organisms, including *Pseudomonas aeruginosa*, *Klebsiella pneumoniae*, and *Enterobacter* spp. *Sthaphylococcus aureus* is also a common cause of bacterial pneumonia (Cohn, 1991; Benito *et al.*, 2001, 2004; Boschini *et al.*, 1996; Levine, White and Fels, 1990). These infections usually occur late in the course of HIV infection and in patients with additional factors predisposing to bacterial infections, such as neutropenia. Although *Pseudomonas aeruginosa* was frequently found as an etiologic agent of bacterial pneumonia (Hirschtick *et al.*, 1995; Baril *et al.*, 1998; Nuorti *et al.*, 2000; Afessa and Green, 2000) in early studies, currently only a few episodes are caused by this microorganism (Benito *et al.*, 2001, 2004). *P. aeruginosa* was the most frequent causal microorganism isolated in studies performed in the pre-HAART era, in which there was a higher incidence of nosocomial pneumonia in HIV-infected patients. (Tumbarello *et al.*, 2001). Moreover, bronchopulmonary infections due to *P. aeruginosa* were common in patients with a very advanced immunosuppression state (median CD4 lymphocytes 11/mm^3). After the introduction of HAART, patients remained in this state of severe immunosuppression for a shorter period of time, and the infections caused by these microorganisms are infrequent (Santín Cerezales *et al.*, 1996).

Legionella infection is uncommon, but some studies suggest that it occurs up 40 times more frequently in patients with AIDS than in the general population (Pedro-Botet *et al.*, 2003, 2004; Marston *et al.*, 1994). Some authors have described a worse prognosis in HIV patients with *Legionella* pneumonia, with a higher number of complications; however, other studies comparing the clinical features of Legionnaires diseases in HIV-seropositive and HIV-seronegative patients showed few significant differences (Pedro-Botet *et al.*, 2003, 2004; Blatt *et al.*, 1994; Gutiérrez Rodero *et al.*, 1995; Sene *et al.*, 2002). Other uncommon infections include nocardia and rhodococcus.

The *clinical presentation* of bacterial pneumonia in the HIV-seropositive patients is similar to that of patients not infected with HIV. Most patients have an abrupt onset of fever, chills, cough with sputum production, dyspnea and pleuritic chest pain (Janoff *et al.*, 1992). The leukocyte count is generally elevated except in advanced immunosuppression. Bacteremia is frequently associated with bacterial pneumonia, with rates of up to 75% with *S. pneumoniae* infection. The most common chest roentgenographic manifestation of bacterial pneumonia in the HIV-infected patients is segmental or lobar consolidation, although diffuse reticulonodular infiltrates and patchy lobar infiltrates may also be seen (Polsky *et al.*, 1986; Magnenat *et al.*, 1991).

Treatment. Initial antibiotic regimen will be directed at the most common community-acquired or nosocomial pathogens. Treatment is similar in patients with the same diagnosis without HIV infection.

Tuberculosis

The coincidence of tuberculosis (TB) and HIV epidemics has created a devastating international public health crisis. Millions of people are infected with both HIV and tuberculosis, especially in underdeveloped countries.

In the USA, a decline in the incidence of tuberculosis was observed from 1992 in spite of an increase of the number of AIDS cases (CDC, 1996). In a cohort of HIV-infected patients recruited between 1988 and 1990, and controlled during a median of 53 months, the incidence of tuberculosis was 0.7 cases per 100 person/years (Markowitz *et al.*, 1997). Similarly, in Europe, the incidence of tuberculosis in HIV-infected patients in the period from 1994 to1999 was 0.8 case per 100 person/years of follow-up (Kirk *et al.*, 2000), which is lower than the incidence in the 1980s (three cases per 100 person-years) (Sudre *et al.*, 1996). This marked decrease in Europe seems to be associated with the introduction of HAART. However, remarkable regional differences are observed (Kirk *et al.*, 2000): the incidence of tuberculosis is 3.1 cases per 100 person/years in southwest Europe, which is four to seven times higher than in other regions (Kirk *et al.*, 2000). In Africa, tuberculosis is the most common pulmonary complication of HIV, and at least one-third of all cases occur in HIV-infected patients.

Co-infection with TB and HIV alters the natural history of both diseases. HIV-infected persons are at increased risk of developing active TB from both reactivated latent and exogenous infection (Quelar *et al.*, 1993). HIV seropositivity status is also a risk factor for accelerated progression of TB. HIV-associated tuberculosis is most common among intravenous drug users. The use of HAART has been found to be associated with a notable reduction in the risk of TB.

In a recent study in an endemic area in southern Europe, mycobacteriosis was the third cause of pulmonary infection in HIV patients (Benito *et al.*, 2004). This high rate, together with the frequent association of mycobacteriosis with other pulmonary infections, supports the performance of routine *Mycobacterium* cultures in all HIV patients with pulmonary infections. Additionally, pulmonary infections due to *Mycobacterium* species other than tuberculosis (*Mycobacterium kansasii*, *Mycobacterium avium* complex, *Mycobacterium fortuitum* and *Mycobacterium xenopi*), and which require specific treatments, are not infrequent (Benito *et al.*, 2004). Moreover, species such as *Mycobacterium xenopi* are considered emerging microorganisms causing pulmonary infections in HIV patients (Juffermans *et al.*, 1998).

Concurrent *treatment* of both tuberculosis and HIV is challenging. Complex drug interactions between anti-TB drugs (primarily rifamycins) and antiretroviral agents (both protease inhibitors and non-nucleoside reverse transcriptase inhibitors) have led to the treatment of many patients with a variety of unproven combinations of anti-TB and antiretroviral regimens.

Rifampicin may interact pharmacokinetically with protease inhibitors, accelerating their metabolism through the induction of P450 cytochrome oxidase, which may result in sub-therapeutic serum levels of these drugs. In addition, protease inhibitors retard the metabolism of rifabutin, resulting in increased serum levels of rifabutin and an increased likelihood of drug toxicity (CDC, 1998).

For patients with CD4 counts less than 100 cells/mm^3, antiretroviral therapy should be started early, because delaying HAART in such TB patients may increase the risk of death or HIV progression. For patients with higher CD4 counts, HAART may be delayed until the continuation phase (after two months of anti-TB therapy), or until the end of anti-TB therapy (Dean *et al.*, 2002; Hung and Chang, 2004).

Fungal infections

The effect of HAART on *endemic fungal infections* of the lung is hard to elucidate, as the incidence of this infection in HIV patients has never been fully determined. The three major endemic fungi are *Histoplasma capsulatum*, *Coccidiodes inmitis* and *Blastomyces dermatitidis* (Sarosi and Davies, 1996). They are acquired by inhalation into the lung. Disease can represent primary infection caused by exogenous exposure or reactivation of a latent focus. Infections in AIDS patients who reside outside endemic regions generally represent reactivation of latent foci of infection from previous residence in these areas (Benito *et al.*, 1998). Endemic areas include the southwestern United States, Northern Mexico and parts of Central and South America.

Histoplasmosis and coccidioidomicosis can occur in up to 27% of HIV-positive patients living in endemic areas. Blastomycosis is an uncommon, but serious complication in HIV patients. Histoplasmosis generally occurs with CD4 lymphocyte counts below 100 cells/mm^3. Coccidioidomycosis and blastomycosis rarely occur in patients with CD4 lymphocyte counts above 200 cells/mm^3. All of them have a wide spectrum of manifestations in HIV-infected patients with frequent lung involvement.

Current recommendations are to continue lifelong suppressive therapy for histoplasmosis, coccidioidomycosis and blastomycosis (CDC, 2002).

The presentation of pulmonary *cryptococcosis* in HIV-infected persons appears to be more acute than in other patient groups. The severity of symptoms and extent of dissemination are inversely proportional to the CD4 lymphocyte count, with most symptomatic cases occurring in patients with less than 100/mm^3. Chest radiographs usually show interstitial infiltrates. Expectorated sputum samples can be positive, but higher yields are obtained using bronchoscopic sampling (Malabonga *et al.*, 1991). The serum cryptococcal antigen is positive in virtually all patients with HIV infection and disseminated crytococcosis. Pulmonary cryptococcosys has also been diagnosed as a co-infection with pathogens such as *P. jirovecii*, *Mycobacterium avium* complex, *M. tuberculosis*, cytomegalovirus, and *H. capsulatum* (Cameron *et al.*, 1991). Secondary prophylaxis can be discontinued for cryptococcosis when there is a sustained increase (for example, longer than six months) of CD4 lymphocyte counts higher than 100– 200 cells/mm^3 after HAART (CDC, 2002).

Invasive *aspergillosis* is a relatively uncommon infection in patients with AIDS compared with other immunocompromised hosts with an overall incidence of approximately 1% (Miller *et al.*, 1994). *Aspergillus* infections most often occur late in the course of HIV immunosuppression and in AIDS patients with identified risk factors for the development of invasive disease, such as neutropenia or corticosteroid use (Denning *et al.*, 1991; Minamoto *et al.*, 1992). The lung is the most common site of *Aspergillus* infection in patients with AIDS. Two forms of pulmonary disease have been described in these patients: invasive pulmonary disease, which accounts for more than 80% of cases, and tracheobronchial disease (Minamoto *et al.*, 1992).

Viral infections

Viral pathogens also contribute to the burden of pulmonary diseases in patients infected with HIV. Viruses can produce clinical pneumonia and may be cofactors in producing other patterns of disease, including neoplasms. However, the incidence of viral infections of the lung is not known.

The clinical significance of isolating *cytomegalovirus* (*CMV*) from respiratory secretions is an area of particular controversy (Uberti-Foppa *et al.*, 1998). CMV as a sole cause of pneumonia is not common, at least until the late stages of HIV disease. A particular problem is posed by the coexistence of CMV with other pathogens found in BAL fluid, particularly *Pneumocystis jiroveci*, and it is not clear that clinical sequelae can be attributed to the presence of CMV. Treatment of CMV could be recommended in the presence of symptomatic pulmonary disease, evidence of CMV in the lung, and the absence of other treatable pulmonary infections.

Parasitic infections

Parasitic infections result in substantial morbidity and mortality among this population worldwide. Responsible organisms include *Toxoplama gondii*, *Strongyloides stercoralis*, *Cryptosporidium* and *Microsporidium*.

Most active cases of *T. gondii* disease are due to reactivation of latent infection. Although encephalitis is overwhelmingly the most common manifestation of *T. gondii* in AIDS patients, pneumonitis has become its second most common presentation (Gadea *et al.*, 1995; Derouin *et al.*, 1990). Active pulmonary toxoplasmosis does not usually occur in HIV-infected patients until the CD4 count falls bellow 100 cells/mm^3. Pulmonary toxoplasmosis may be clinically indistinguishable from PCP, tuberculosis, cryptococcosis, or histoplasmosis. Bronchoscopy with BAL is the preferred method for diagnosis, but its sensitivity and specificity are unknown.

S. stercoralis is an intestinal parasite, but some patients, particularly those who are immunosuppressed, can develop systemic strongyloidiasis. However, there have only been scattered cases of systemic strongyloidiasis in HIV infected patients.

Cryptosporidium and *Microsporidium* are causative agents of gastrointestinal disease in HIV patients. There are a few case reports of pulmonary disease due to these organisms, which occur in the setting of disseminated infection.

Polimicrobial etiology

Pulmonary infections with more than one pathogen are not unusual in HIV infected patients. In one study, a polimicrobial etiology was identified in 9% of all pulmonary infections (Benito *et al.*, 2001). Several studies have shown that frequently one of the etiologic microorganisms identified was not initially suspected (Benito *et al.*, 2001; Orlovic *et al.*, 2001; Schleicher and Feldman, 2003).

5.3   Diagnosis

There is no consensus on a diagnostic algorithm of pulmonary infections in HIV patients. Some investigators have recommended an empiric approach based on clinical features and local epidemiology. They have also suggested that diagnostic techniques should only be considered for patients in whom empiric therapy fails (Daley *et al.*, 1996; Msur and Shelhamer, 1996). Other authors think that a definitive diagnosis should be achieved initially by means of non-invasive specimens, followed by invasive techniques if these specimens are non-diagnostic (Salzman, 1998). A study showed that not having an etiologic diagnosis was associated with increased mortality (Benito *et al.*, 2001). Moreover, the frequency of polimicrobial etiology in patients whose etiologic microorganisms was not initially suspected supports the last approach (Benito *et al.*, 2001).

The initial approach to any patient includes an adequate clinical history and physical examination; the same is true for patients diagnosed with HIV infection.

Epidemiologic and environmental considerations

HIV-infected intravenous drug users are at an increased risk for the development of bacterial pneumonia and tuberculosis.

A detailed assessment of any possible exposure to active tuberculosis is an important part of the medical history. Many cases of tuberculosis in HIV-infected patients represent newly acquired infection, rather than reactivation of old disease. Healthcare facilities, prisons and homeless shelters are potential sources for transmission of tuberculosis.

There is an increased incidence of pulmonary histoplasmosis and coccidioidomycosis in patients who live or travel in endemic areas (the Mississippi River Valley and the southwest United States, respectively, as well as in several South American countries). Reactivation can occur especially in histoplasmosis; thus, patients who resided or spent time in endemic areas earlier in their lives are at risk for overt disease, as they become more immunosuppressed (Benito *et al.*, 1998).

Patients receiving HAART may develop recrudescence of diseases that have been dormant. As an example, patients with latent mycobacterial disease may develop fever, lymphadenopathy and pulmonary opacities following immune restoration.

CD4 count

In patients with HIV, the occurrence of specific infections is closely correlated with the degree of impairment of host defences. The sequence of pulmonary infections occurring in HIV-infected individuals parallels the depletion of CD4 lymphocytes. As a result, the CD4 count can provide information about the type of pulmonary infection to which the patient is susceptible.

Bacterial pneumonia and TB can occur early in the course of HIV infection, when the CD4 count is greater than 500 cells/mm^3 and before opportunistic infections occur. However, both occur more frequently as immune function declines.

PCP, disseminated fungal disease and CMV infections almost always occur when the CD4 counts are very low, usually below 200 cells/mm^3.

Specific diagnostic tests

The overall yield of the non-invasive sputum sample microbiology in pulmonary infections (more than 50%) is worthy of mention. In the case of bacterial pneumonia the yield of sputum culture ranges from 35 to 60% (Benito *et al.*, 2001; Cordero *et al.*, 2002). Additionally, its availability and ease of performance, as well as its good correlation with the culture of sterile samples, emphasize the usefulness of this technique in HIV-infected patients (Cordero *et al.*, 2002). On the other hand, as it has been mentioned, it should be considered the need of performing sputum cultures for mycobacteria systematically in these patients. A sputum sample for mycobacterial smear and culture is the best technique for diagnosing pulmonary TB. While induced sputum is not superior to a good expectorated sample, it is helpful in patients who are suspected to have TB but who are unable to produce sputum.

Antigen and antibody testing are generally of little value in the diagnosis of acute infections in the HIV-infected host. Notable exceptions include assays designed to detect *Histoplasma* polysaccharide antigen (HPA) and cryptococcal antigen. HPA can be detected in the urine of 90% of patients with disseminated infections, and 75% of those with diffuse acute pulmonary histoplasmosis (Wheat, 1997).The sensitivity of antigen detection is highest when urine and serum are tested. Cryptococcal antigen is less likely to be positive in localized cryptococcal pneumonia compared to disseminated cryptococcosis. Its presence is useful in confirming the diagnosis because the assay has excellent specificity. Following titers of HPA and cryptococcal antigen may also be helpful in evaluating response or therapy.

Another non-invasive technique which probably could have an important diagnostic role of bacterial pneumonia in HIV patients is the detection of pneumococcal antigen in urine, since *S. pneumoniae* is the most frequent cause of bacterial pneumonia in this group. There are no specific studies in HIV-infected patients, but the good results obtained in the general population suggest probable usefulness in this group (Gutiérrez *et al.*, 2003).

The absence of diagnosis of atypical pneumonias (different from *Legionella pneumophila*) in different series suggests that the routinely serologic analysis for diagnosis of these etiologic agents is probably not necessary in the majority of cases. However, the role of atypical pathogens such as *Mycoplasma* or *Chlamydia* has not been studied systematically (Benito *et al.*, 2001, 2004; Rimland *et al.*, 2002; Mundy *et al.*, 1995).

The major invasive tests that are used to diagnose pulmonary disease in HIV-infected patients include fibreoptic bronchoscopy, computed tomographic (CT)-guided trans-thoracic needle aspiration (TTNA), and surgical lung biopsy using either video-assisted thoracoscopic surgery (VATS) or open thoracotomy.

Because of its high yield and low complication rate, fibreoptic bronchoscopy remains the procedure of choice for diagnosing many pulmonary diseases in HIV-infected patients. In a recent study this technique achieved the etiologic diagnostic in 56% of cases of pulmonary infiltrates (Benito *et al.*, 2001). These results agree with those from previous studies showing a similar yield as well as the diagnostic importance of bronchoscopy in this group of patients (Ferrer *et al.*, 1992; Villuendas *et al.*, 1996; Narayanswami and Salzman, 2003). The disorders most commonly diagnosed using bronchoscopy include infections caused by *P. jirovecii*, fungal, mycobacterial and viral pathogens. Fibreoptic bronchoscopy is rarely performed in HIV-infected patients for the diagnosis of bacterial infection. Occasionally, an HIV-infected patient with nosocomial pneumonia will undergo bronchoscopy. To circum-vent contamination from the upper airways, a double lumen catheter system or a protected BAL is recommended. Semi-quantitative cultures of the collected speci-mens should be performed. Any antibiotic usage before the bronchoscopic procedure markedly decreases its sensitivity.

TTNA using CT guidance has a high yield in diagnosing the cause of peripheral nodules and localized infiltrates; the yield is much lower in patients with diffuse disease.

Surgical lung biopsy, performed by means of thoracotomy or VATS, remains the procedure with the greatest sensitivity in the diagnosis of parenchymal lung disease.

The initial evaluation of an HIV-infected patient with suspected pulmonary infection should include a chest radiograph, sputum examination, white blood cell count and blood cultures. Expectorated sputum should be sent for gram stain examination, acid-fast bacilli smear, and bacterial and mycobacterial culture. Urinary antigen for *S. pneumoniae* and *Legionella* should also be considered. If the patient is at risk for *P. jiroveci* and/or if TB is suspected, but the patient is unable to produce sputum, induced sputum should also be requested; and, if induced sputum is not conclusive, bronchoalveolar lavage should be performed. More rarely, TTNA using CT guidance or surgical lung biopsy are needed to obtain an etiologic diagnosis in particular cases.

More studies are needed in order to establish the best diagnostic algorithm for HIV-infected patients with pulmonary infections, which should take into account geographic differences in epidemiology.

5.4 Prognosis

Overall studies analyzing prognostic factors of pulmonary infections in HIV patients are scarce. In a previous series of HIV patients with pulmonary infections requiring intensive care hospitalization, PCP and mechanical ventilation were factors associated with higher mortality (Torres *et al.*, 1995). In a study on HIV patients with pulmonary infections, not having an etiologic diagnosis was an independent factor associated with higher mortality (Benito *et al.*, 2001). This is a factor of special concern, because it focuses on the need for an improvement in the diagnostic yield of techniques and optimizing the diagnostic algorithm.

Most investigations have focused on PCP, and 10–30% mortality has been reported (Fernández *et al.*, 1995; Azoulay *et al.*, 1999; Fernández Cruz *et al.*, 2002; Pulvirenti *et al.*, 2003; Benito *et al.*, 2001, 2004; Calderon *et al.*, 2004). In PCP, factors such as respiratory impairment and mechanical ventilation have consistently been related to fatal outcome (Fernández *et al.*, 1995; Azoulay *et al.*, 1999; Fernández Cruz *et al.*, 2002); others factors include age greater than 45 years, high lactate dehydrogenase levels (>800 IU/L), marked neutrophilia in BAL, malnourishment and CD4 count <50 cells/mm^3 (Azoulay *et al.*, 1999; Fernández Cruz *et al.*, 2002; Calderon *et al.*, 2004; Wachter *et al.*, 1995). A study suggests that HAART started either before or during hospitalization is associated with a decrease in the mortality related to severe PCP (defined as that requiring admission to an intensive care unit [ICU]) (Morris *et al.*, 2003). However, other studies suggests that recent improved survival in patients admitted to the ICU with PCP is independent of HAART therapy; it would be reflecting general improvements in ICU management of acute respiratory failure requiring mechanical ventilation (Miller *et al.*, 2006). In any case, PCP requiring admission to the ICU still carries a grim prognosis, with mortality rates ranging from 35 to 55% after 1996 (Morris *et al.*, 2003; Miller *et al.*, 2006).

Previous studies have indicated a variable mortality (5–30%) for HIV-associated bacterial pneumonia, although most of them range from 10 to 15% (Feikin *et al.*, 2004; Hirschtick *et al.*, 1995; Polsky *et al.*, 1986; Baril *et al.*, 1998). Predicting factors of higher mortality are neutropenia, pO2 < 70 mmHg, and a Karnofsky score less than or equal to 50 (Tumbarello *et al.*, 1998). Despite of the increased incidence of bacterial pneumonia, rates of associated mortality, although substantial, are not typically increased in HIV-infected patients compared with those in community control subjects (Feikin *et al.*, 2004). These case-fatality proportions are difficult to compare, since pneumonia in the absence of HIV infection often occurs in adults significantly older than those with HIV infection. However, mortality with pneumococcal bacteremia in age-matched adults is similar, but may be increased in older HIV-infected adults and in patients with AIDS (Pesola and Charles, 1992; Janoff and Rubins, 1997; Hibbs *et al.*, 1997; Feikin *et al.*, 2004). The rate of associated mortality in a recent series was of 3.4%;

it would be related to a low incidence of pneumonia caused by enterobacteriaceae and *Pseudomonas aeruginosa*, which are associated with a higher mortality in previous studies (Benito *et al.*, 2001, 2004).

5.5 Conclusions

Pulmonary infections are still an important problem in HIV-infected patients and are the first cause of hospital admission in these patients. Most of these patients develop a pulmonary infection during the history of HIV infection. Since earlier studies, important changes in the epidemiology of HIV-related pulmonary infections have occurred. Overall, prescription of PCP prophylaxis and, more recently the introduction of HAART, are the main causes. Currently the most frequent diagnosis is bacterial pneumonia, especially pneumococcal pneumonia; the second most frequent cause is PCP and the third cause is mycobacteriosis, particularly *Mycobacterium tuberculosis* infection. Achieving an etiologic diagnosis of pulmonary infection is important due to its prognostic consequences.

References

Afessa, B., Greaves, W., Gren, W., Oloponeic, L., Saxinger, C. and Frederick, W. (1992) Autopsy findings in HIV-infected inner city patients. *Journal of Acquired Immunedeficiency Syndrome*, **5**, 132–136.

Afessa, B. and Green, B. (2000) Bacterial pneumonia in hospitalized patients with HIV infection. The pulmonary complications, ICU support, and prognostic factors of hospitalized patients with HIV (PIP) study. *Chest*, **117**, 1017–1022.

Altés, J., Guadarrama, M., Force, L. *et al.* (1999) The impact of highly active antirretroviral therapy on HIV-related hospitalizations in 17 county hospitals in Catalonia, Spain. *AIDS (London, England)*, **13**, 1418–1419.

Alvarez-Martínez, M., Miró, J. Valls, M. *et al.* (2006) Sensitivity and specificity of nested and real-time PCR for the detection of *Pneumocystis jiroveci* in clinical specimens. *Diagnostic Microbiology and Infectious Diseases*, **56**, 153–160.

Azoulay, E., Parrot, A., Flahault, A. *et al.* (1999) AIDS-related *Pneumocystis carinii* pneumonia in the era of adjunctive steroids. Implication of BAL neutrophilia. *American Journal of Respiratory and Critical Care Medicine*, **160**, 493–499.

Baril, L., Astagneau, P., Nguyen, J. *et al.* (1998) Pyogenic bacterial pneumonia in human immunodeficiency virus-infected inpatients: a clinical, radiological, microbiological and epidemiological study. *Clinical Infectious Diseases*, **26**, 964–971.

Batungwanayo, J., Taelman, H., Lucas, S., Bogaerts, J., Alard, D., Kagame, A. *et al.* (1994) Pulmonary disease associated with the human immunodeficiency virus in Kigali, Rwanda. *American Journal of Respiratory and Critical Care Medicine*, **149**, 1591–1596.

Beck, J.M., Rosen, M.J. and Peavy, H.H. (2001) Pulmonary complications of HIV infection. Report of the Fourth NHLBI Workshop. *American Journal of Respiratory and Critical Care Medicine*, **11**, 2120–2126.

Benito, N., Garcia Vazquez, E., Blanco, A. *et al.* (1998) Disseminated histoplasmosis in AIDS patients. A study of 2 cases and review of the Spanish literature. *Enfermades Infecciosas y Microbiología Cínica*, **7**, 316–321.

Benito, N., Moreno, A., Filella, X. *et al.* (2004) Inflammatory responses in blood samples of human immunodeficiency virus-infected patients with pulmonary infections. *Clinical and Diagnostic Laboratory Immunology*, **11**, 608–614.

Benito, N., Rañó, A., Moreno, A. *et al.* (2001) Pulmonary infiltrates in HIV-infected patients in the highly active antiretroviral therapy in Spain. *Journal of Acquired Immune Deficiency Syndrome*, **27**, 35–43.

Benito-Hernández, N., Moreno-Camacho, A. and Gatell-Artigas, J.M. (2005) Complicaciones infecciosas pulmonares en los pacientes con infección por el virus de la inmunodeficiencia humana en la era del tratamiento antirretroviral de gran actividad en Españo. *Medicina Clínica (Barcelona)*, **125**, 548–555.

Blatt, S.P., Dolan, M.J., Hendrix, C.W. and Melcher, G.P. (1994) Legionnaires' disease in human immunodeficiency virus-infected patients: eight cases and review. *Clinical Infectious Diseases*, **18**, 227–232.

Blaxhult, A., Kirk, O., Pedersen, C. *et al.* (2000) Regional differences in presentation of AIDS in Europe. *Epidemiology and Infection*, **125**, 143–151.

Boschini, A., Smacchia, C., Di Fine, M. *et al.* (1996) Community-acquired pneumonia in a cohort of former injection drug users with and without human immunodeficiency virus infection: incidence, etiologies, and clinical aspects. *Clinical Infectious Diseases*, **23**, 107–113.

Breiman, R.F., Keller, D.W., Phelan, M.A. *et al.* (2000) Evaluation of effectiveness of the 23-valent pneumococcal capsular polysaccharide vaccine for HIV-infected patients. *Archives Internal Medicine*, **160**, 2633–2638.

Briel, M., Bucher, H., Boscacci, R. and Furrer, H. (2006) Adjunctive corticosteroids for *Pneumocystis jiroveci* pneumonia in patients with HIV-infection. *Cochrane Database of Systematic Reviews*, **3**, CD006150.

Broaddus, C., Dake, M.D., Stulbarg, M.S. *et al.* (1985) Bronchoalveolar lavage and transbronchial biopsy for the diagnosis of pulmonary infections in the acquired immunodeficiency syndrome. *Annals of Internal Medicine*, **102**, 747–752.

Butt, A.A., Michaels, S. and Kissinger, P. (2002) The association of serum lactate dehydrogenase level with selected opportunistic infections and HIV progression. *International Journal of Infectious Diseases*, **6**, 178–181.

Calderon, E.J., Varela, J.M., Medrano, F.J., Nieto, V., González-Becerra, C., Respaldiza, N. *et al.* (2004) Epidemiology of *Pneumocystis carinii* pneumonia in southern Spain. *Clinical Microbiology and Infection*, **10**, 673–676.

Cameron, M.L., Barlett, J.A., Gallis, H.A. and Waskin, H.A. (1991) Manifestations of pulmonary cryptococcosis in patients with acquired immunodeficiency syndrome. *Review of Infectious Diseases*, **13**, 64–67.

Carme, B., Mboussa, J., Andzin, M., Mbouni, E., Mpele, P. and Datry, A. (1991) *Pneumocystis carinii* is rare in AIDS in Central Africa. *Transactions of the Royal Society of Tropical Hygiene*, **85**, 80.

CDC/IDSA (1999) USPHS/IDSA guidelines for the prevention of opportunistic infections in people infected with human immunodeficiency virus. *Morbidity and Mortality Weekly Report*, **48**, 1–66.

Centers for Disease Control and Prevention (1981) *Pneumocystis carinii* pneumonia-Los Angeles. *Morbidity and Mortality Weekly Report*, **30**, 250–252.

Centers for Disease Control and Prevention (1989) Guidelines for prophylaxis against *Pneumocystis carinii* pneumonia for persons infected with human immunodeficiency virus. *Morbidity and Mortality Weekly Report*, **38** (Suppl 5), 1–9.

Centers for Disease Control and Prevention (1992) 1993 revised classification system for HIV infection and expanded surveillance case definition for AIDS among adolescent and adults. *Morbidity and Mortality Weekly Report*, **41**, (RR-17), 1–19.

Centers for Disease control and Prevention (1996) Tuberculosis morbidity – United States. *Morbidity and Mortality Weekly Report*, **45**, 365–370.

Centers for Disease Control and Prevention (1998) Prevention and treatment of tuberculosis among patients infected with human immunodeficiency virus: principles of therapy and revised recommendations. *Morbidity and Mortality Weekly Report*, **47**, 1–58.

Centers for Disease Control and Prevention (2001a) HIV and AIDS-United States, 1981–2000. *Morbidity and Mortality Weekly Report*, **50**, 430–434.

Centers for Disease Control and Prevention (2001b) The global HIV and AIDS epidemic, 2001. *Morbidity and Mortality Weekly Report*, **50**, 434–439.

Centers for Disease Control and Prevention (2002) Guidelines for preventing opportunistic infections among HIV-Infected persons. Recommendations of the U.S. public health service and the infectious diseases society of America. *Morbidity and Mortality Weekly Report*, **51**, 1–46.

Chien, S.M., Rawji, M., Mintz, S., Rachils, A. and Chan, C.K. (1992) Changes in hospital admissions pattern in patients with human immunodeficiency virus infection in the era of *Pneumocystis carinii* prophilaxis. *Chest*, **102**, 1035–1039.

Cohn, D.L. (1991) Bacterial pneumonia in the HIV-infected patient. *Infection Diseases Clinics of North America*, **5**, 485–507.

Cordero, E., Pachón, J., Rivero, A. *et al.* (2000) *Haemophilus influenzae* pneumonia in human immunodeficiency virus-infected patients. *Clinical Infectious Diseases*, **30**, 461–465.

Cordero, E., Pachon, J., Rivero, A., Girón-González, J.A. *et al.* (2002) Usefulness of sputum culture for diagnosis of bacterial pneumonia in HIV-infected patients. *European Journal of Clinical Microbiology and Infectious, Diseases*, **21**, 362–367.

Cruciani, M., Marcati, P., Malena, M. *et al.* (2002) Meta-analysis of diagnostic procedures for *Pneumocystis carinii* pneumonia in HIV-1-infected patients. *European Respiratory Journal*, **20**, 982–989.

Daley, C.L., Mugusi, F., Chen, L.L., Schmidt, D.M., Small, P.M. and Bearer, E. *et al.* (1996) Pulmonary complications of HIV infection in Dar es Salaam, Tanzania. Role of bronchoscopy and bronchoalveolar lavage. *American Journal of Respiratory and Critical Care, Medicine*, **154**, 105–110.

De Gaetano Donati, K., Bertagnolio, S. *et al.* (2000) Effect of highly active antiretroviral therapy on the incidence of bacterial pneumonia in HIV-infected subjects. *International Journal of Antimicrobial Agents*, **16**, 357–360.

De Gaetano Donati, K., Tumbarello, M., Tacconelli, E. *et al.* (2003) Impact of highly active antiretroviral therapy (HAART) on the incidence of bacterial infections in HIV infected subjects. *Journal of Chemotherapy*, **16**, 60–65.

Dean, G.L., Edwards, S.G., Ives, N.J. *et al.* (2002) Treatment of tuberculosis in HIV-infected patients in HIV-infected persons in the era of highly active antiretroviral therapy. *AIDS (London, England)*, **16**, 75–83.

Del Amo, J., Perez-Hoyos, S., Hernández Aguado, I. *et al.* (2003) Impact of tuberculosis on HIV disease progression in persons with well-documented time of HIV seroconversion. *Journal of Acquired Immunodeficiency Syndrome*, **33**, 184–190.

Denning, D.W., Follansbee, S.E., Scolaro, M. *et al.* (1991) Pulmonary aspergillosis in the acquired immunodeficiency syndrome. *The New England Journal of Medicine*, **324**, 654–662.

Derouin, F., Sarfati, C., Beauvais, B. *et al.* (1990) Prevalence of pulmonary toxoplasmosis in HIV-infected patients. *AIDS (London, England)*, **4**, 1036.

Dore, G.J., Hoy, J.F., Mallal, S.A. *et al.* (1997) Trends in incidence of AIDS illnesses in Australia from 1983 to 1994: the Australian AIDS cohort. *Journal of Acquired Immune Deficiency Syndromes and, Human Retrovirology*, **16**, 39–43.

Dore, G.J., Li, Y., McDonald, A., Ree, H. and Kaldo, J.M. (2002) Impact of higly active antiretroviral therapy on individual AIDS-defininig illness incidence and survival in Australia. *Journal of Acquired Immune Deficiency Syndromes*, **29**, 388–395.

Dworkin, M.S., Ward, J.W., Hanson, D.L. *et al.* (2001) Pneumoccal disease among human immuno-deficiency virus-infected persons: incidence, risk factors, and impact of vaccination. *Clinical Infectious Diseases*, **32**, 794–800.

Edge, M.D. and Rimland, D. (1996) Community-acquired bacteremia in HIV-positive patients: protective benefit of co-trimoxazole. *AIDS (London, England)*, **10**, 1635–1639.

Edge, M.D. and Rimland, D. (1999) Reasons for failure of prophylaxis for Pneumocystis carinii pneumonia: a retrospective study and review. *AIDS (London, England)*, **13**, 991–992.

Falcó, V., de Sevilla, T., Alegre, J. *et al.* (1994) Bacterial pneumonia in HIV-infected patients: a prospective study of 68 episodes. *European Respiratory Journal*, **7**, 235–239.

Feikin, D.R., Feldman, C., Schuchat, A. and Janoff, E.N. (2004) Global strategies to prevent bacterial pneumonia in adults with HIV disease. *The Lancet Infectious Diseases*, **4**, 445–455.

Feldman, C., Glatthaar, M., Morar, R. *et al.* (1999) Bacteriemic pneumococcal pneumonia in HIV-seropositive and HIV-seronegative adults. *Chest*, **116**, 107–114.

Fernández Cruz, A., Pulido Ortega, F., Peña Sánchez de Rivera, J.M., Sanz García, M., Lorenzo Hernández, F., González García, J. *et al.* (2002) Factores pronósticos de mortalidad durante el episodio de neumonía por *Pneumocystis carinii* en pacientes con infección por VIH. *Revista Clínica Española*, **202**, 418–422.

Fernández, P., Torres, A., Miró, J.M. *et al.* (1995) Prognostic factors influencing the outcome in *Pneumocystis carinii pneumonia* in patients with AIDS. *Thorax*, **50**, 668–671.

Ferrer, M., Torres, A., Xaubet, A. *et al.* (1992) Diagnostic value of telescoping plugged catheters in HIV-infected patients with pulmonary infiltrates. *Chest*, **102**, 76–83.

French, N., Gilks, C.F., Mujugira, A., Fasching, C., O'Brien, J. and Janoff, E.N. (1998) Pneumococcal vaccination in HIV-infected adults in Uganda: humonal response and two vaccine failures. *AIDS (London, England)*, **12**, 1683–1689.

French, N., Nakiyingi, J., Carpenter, L.M. *et al.* (2000) 23-valent pneumococcal polysaccharide vaccine in HIV-1-infected Ugandan adults: double-blind, randomised and placebo controlled trial. *Lancet*, **355**, 2106–2111.

Gadea, I., Cuenca, M., Benito, N. *et al.* (1995) Bronchoalveolar lavage for the diagnosis of disseminated toxoplasmosis in AIDS patients. *Diagnostic Microbiology and Infectious Diseases*, **22**, 339–341.

Gebo, K.A., Moore, R.D., Keruly, J.C. and Chaisson, R.E. (1996) Risk factors for pneumococcal disease in human immunodeficiency virus-infected patients. *Journal of Infectious Diseases*, **173**, 857–862.

Gold, J.A., Rom, W.N. and Harkin, T.J. (2002) Significance of abnormal chest radiograph findings in patients with HIV-1 infection without respiratory simptoms. *Chest*, **121**, 1472–1477.

Gruden, J.F., Huang, L., Turner, J. *et al.* (1997) High-resolution CT in the evaluation of clinically suspected *Pneumocystis carinii* pneumonia in AIDS patients with normal, equivocal or non-specific radiographic findings. *American Journal of Roengenology*, **169**, 967–975.

Guelar, A., Gatell, J.M., Verdejo, J. *et al.* (1993) A prospective study of the risk of tuberculosis among HIV-infected patients. *AIDS (London, England)*, **7**, 1345–1349.

Guerrero, M., Kruguer, S., Saitoh, A. *et al.* (1999) Pneumonia in HIV – infected patients: a case-control study of factors involved in risk and prevention. *AIDS (London, England)*, **13**, 1971–1975.

Gutiérrez, F., Masiá, M., Carlos Rodríguez, J. *et al.* (2003) Evaluation of the immunochromatographic binax NOW assay for detection of *Streptococcus pneumoniae* urinary antigen in a prospective study of community-acquired pneumonia in Spain. *Clinical Infectious Diseases*, **36**, 286–292.

Gutiérrez Rodero, F., Ortiz de la Tabla, V., Martínez, C. *et al.* (1995) Legionnaires' disease in patients infected with human immunodeficiency virus. *Clinical Infectious Diseases*, **21**, 712–713.

Hanson, D.L., Chu, S.Y., Farizo, K.M. and Ward, J.W., and the Adult and Adolescent Spectrum of HIV Disease Study Group (1995) Distribution of CD4+ lymphocytes at diagnosis of acquired immunodeficiency syndrome-defining and other human immunodeficiency virus-related illnesses. *Archives of Internal Medicine*, **155**, 1537–1542.

Hardy, W.D., Feinberg, J., Finkelstein, D.M. *et al.* (1992) A controlled trial of trimethoprim-sulfamethoxazole or aerosolized pentamidine for secondary prophylaxis of *Pneumocystis carinii* pneumonia in patients with the acquired immunodeficiency syndrome. AIDS Clinical Trials Group Protocol 021. *The New England Journal of Medicine*, **327**, 1842–1848.

Hartman, T.E., Primack, S.L., Muller, N.L. and Staples, C.A. (1994) Diagnosis of thoracic complications in AIDS: accuracy of CT. *American Journal of Roengenology*, **162**, 547–553.

Hibbs, J.R., Douglas, J.M., Jr, Judson, F.N. *et al.* (1997) Prevalence of human immunodeficiency virus infection, mortality rate, and serogroup distribution among patients with pneumococcal bacteriemia at Denver General Hospital, 1984–1994. *Clinical Infectious Diseases*, **25**, 195–199.

Hidalgo, A., Falco, V., Mauleon, S. *et al.* (2003) Accuracy of high-resolution CT in distinguishing between *Pneumocistis carinii* pneumonia an non-*Pneumocystis cariniii* pneumonia in AIDS patients. *European Radiology*, **13**, 1179–1184.

Hirschtick, R.E., Glassroth, J., Jordan, M.C. (1995) *et al.* Bacterial pneumonia in persons infected with the human immunodeficiency virus. *The New England Journal of Medicine*, **333**, 845–851.

Hoover, D.R., Saah, A.J., Bacellar, H. *et al.* (1993) Clinical manifestations of AIDS in the era of Pneumocystis prophylaxis. *The New England Journal of Medicine*, **329**, 1922–1926.

Huang, L., Hecht, F.M., Stansell, J.D. *et al.* (1995) Suspected *Pneumocystis carinii* pneumonia with a negative induced sputum examination: is early bronchoscopy useful? *American Journal of Respiratory and Critical Care Medicine*, **151**, 1866–1871.

Huang, L., Morris, A., Limper, A.H. and Beck, J.M., ATS Pneumocystis Workshop Participants. (2006) An Official ATS Workshop Summary: Recent advances and future directions in pneumocystis pneumonia (PCP). *Proceeding of the American Thoracic Society*, **8**, 655–664.

Hung, C. and Chang, S. (2004) Impact of highly active antiretroviral therapy on incidence and management of human immunodeficiency virus-related opportunistic infections. *Journal of Antimicrobial Chemotherapy*, **54**, 849–853.

Hung, C.C., Chen, M.Y., Hsieh, S.M., Hsiao, C.F., Sheng, W.H. and Chang, S.C. (2004) Clinical experience of the 23-valent capsular polysaccharide pneumococcal vaccination in HIV-1-infected patients receiving highly active antiretroviral therapy: a prospective observational study. *Vaccine*, **22**, 2006–2012.

Janoff, E.N., Breiman, R.F., Daley, C.L. and Hopewell, P.C. (1992) Pneumococcal disease during HIV infection. Epidemiologic, clinical and immunologic perspectives. *Annals Internal Medicine*, **117**, 314–324.

Janoff, E.N. and Rubins, J.B. (1997) Invasive pneumococcal disease in the immunocompromised host. *Microbial Drug Resistance*, **3**, 215–232.

Jordano, Q., Falcó, V., Almirante, B., Planes, A.M., del Valle, O., Ribera, E., Len, O. *et al.* (2004) Invasive pneumococcal disease in patients infected with HIV: still a threat in the era of highly active antiretroviral therapy. *Clinical Infectious Diseases*, **38**, 1623–1628.

Juffermans, N.P., Verbon, A., Danner, S.A., Kuijper, E.J. and Speelman, P. (1998) *Mycobacterium xenopi* in HIV-infected patients: an emerging pathogen. *AIDS (London, England)*, **12**, 1661–1666.

Kamanfu, G., Mlika-Cabanne, N., Girard, P.M., Nimubona, S., Mpfizi, B., Cishako, A. *et al.* (1993) Pulmonary complications of human immunodeficiency virus infection in Bujumbura, Burundi. *American Review of Respiratory Diseases*, **147**, 658–663.

Kaplan, J.E., Janoff, E.N. and Masur, H. (1999) Do bacterial pneumonia and *Pneumocystis carinii* pneumonia accelerate progression of human immunodeficiency virus disease? *Clinical Infectious Diseases*, **29**, 544–546.

Kirk, O., Gatell, J.M., Mocroft, A. *et al.* (2000) Infections with *Mycobacterium tuberculosis* and *Mycobacterium avium* among HIV-patients after the introduction of highly active antiretroviral therapy. *American Journal of Respiratory and Critical Care Medicine*, **162**, 865–872.

Lazarous, D.G., O'donnell, A.E. (2007) Pulmonary infections in the HIV-infected patient in the era of highly active antiretroviral therapy: an update. *Current Infection Disease Reports*, **3**, 228–232.

Ledergerber, B., Morcroft, A., Reiss, P. *et al.* (2001) Discontinuation of secondary prophylaxis against *Pneumocystis carinii* pneumonia in patients with HIV infection who have a response to antiretroviral therapy. *The New England Journal of Medicine*, **344**, 168–174.

Levine, S.J., White, D.A. and Fels, A.D. (1990) The incidence and significance of *Staphylococcus aureus* in respiratory cultures from patients infected with the human immunodeficiency virus. *American Review of Respiratory Diseases*, **141**, 89–93.

Lopez Bernaldo de Quirós, J.C., Miró, J.M., Pena, J.M. *et al.* (2001) A randomized trial of the discontinuation of primary and secondary prophylaxis against *Pneumocystis carinii* pneumonia after highly active antiretroviral therapy in patients with HIV infection. Grupo de Estudio del SIDA 04/98. *The New England Journal of Medicine*, **344**, 159–167.

López-Palomo, C., Martín-Zamorano, M., Benítez, E. *et al.* (2004) Pneumonia in HIV-infected patients in the HAART era: incidence, risk, and impact of the pneumococcal vaccination. *Journal of Medical Virologie*, **72**, 517–524.

Lucas, S., Goodgame, R., Kocjan, G. and Serwadda, D. (1989) Absence of pneumocystosis in Ugandan AIDS patients. *AIDS (London, England)*, **3**, 47–48.

Lungdren, J.D., Pedersen, C., Clumeck, N. *et al.* (1994) Survival differences in European AIDS patients 1979–1989. AIDS in Europe Study Group. *British Medical Journal*, **308**, 1068–1073.

Lungdren, J.D., Philips, A.N., Vella, S. *et al.* (1997) Regional differences in use of antiretrovirals and primary prophylaxis in 3122 European HIV-infected patients. EuroSIDA Study Group. *Journal of Acquired Immune Deficiency Syndromes*, **16**, 93–99.

Magnenat, J.L., Nicod, L.P., Auckenthaler, R. and Junod, A.F. (1991) Mode of presentation and diagnosis of bacterial pneumonia in human immunodeficiency virus-infected patients. *The American Review of Respiratory Disease*, **144**, 917–922.

Malabonga, V.M., Basti, J. and Kamholz, S.L. (1991) Utility of bronchoscopic sampling techniques for cryptococcal disease in AIDS. *Chest*, **99**, 370–372.

Markowitz, N., Hansen, N., Hopewell, P.C. *et al.* (1997) Incidence of tuberculosis in the United States among HIV-infected persons. *Annals of Internal Medicine*, **126**, 123–132.

Marston, B.J., Lipman, H.B. and Breiman, R.F. (1994) Surveillance for Legionnaires' disease. Risk factors for morbidity and mortality. *Archives of Internal Medicine*, **154**, 2417–2422.

Masliah, E., DeTeresa, R.M., Mallory, M.E. and Hansen, L.A. (2000) Changes in pathological findings at autopsy in AIDS cases for the last 15 years. *AIDS (London, England)*, **14**, 69–74.

Masur, H. (2000) Human Immunodeficiency virus-related opportunistic infections in the era of highly active antiretroviral therapy, in *Emerging Infections* 4 (eds W.M. Scheld, W.A. Craig and J.M. Hughes), ASM Press, Washington, pp. 165–186.

Mcleod, D.T., Neill, P., Robertson, V.J., Latif, A.S., Emmanuel, J.C., Els, J.E. *et al.* (1989) Pulmonary diseases in patients in patients infected with the human immunodeficiency virus in Zimbabwe, Central Africa. *Transactions of the Royal Society of Tropical Hygiene*, **83**, 694–697.

Meduri, G.U. and Stein, D.S. (1992) Pulmonary manifestations of acquired immunodeficiency syndrome. *Clinical Infectious Diseases*, **14**, 98–113.

Michelet, C., Arvieux, C., François, C. *et al.* (1998) Opportunistic infections occurring during highly active antiretroviral treatment. *AIDS (London, England)*, **12**, 1815–1822.

Miller, R. (1996) HIV-associated respiratory diseases. *The Lancet*, **348**, 307–312.

Miller, W.T., Jr, Sais, G.J., Frank, I. *et al.* (1994) Pulmonary aspergillosis in patients with AIDS. Clinical and radiographic correlations. *Chest*, **105**, 37–44.

Miller, R.F., Allen, E., Copas, A., Singer, M. and Edwards, S.G. (2006) Improved survival for HIV infected patients with severe pneumocystis jirovecii pneumonia is independent of highly active antiretroviral therapy. *Thorax*, **61**, 716–721.

Minamoto, G.Y., Barlam, T.F. and Armstrong, D. (1992) Invasive aspergillosis in patients with AIDS. *Clinical Infectious Diseases*, **14**, 66–74.

Mönkemüller, K.E., Call, S.A., Lazenby, A.J. and Wilcox, C.M. (2000) Declining prevalence of opportunistic gastrointestinal disease in the era of combination antiretroviral therapy. *The American Journal of Gastroenterology*, **95**, 457–462.

Montaner, J.S., Le, T., Hogg, R. *et al.* (1994) The changing spectrum of AIDS index diseases in Canada. *AIDS (London, England)*, **8**, 693–696.

Moore, R.D. and Chaisson, R.E. (1999) Natural history of HIV infection in the era of combination antiretroviral therapy. *AIDS (London, England)*, **13**, 1933–1942.

Morris, A., Wachter, R.M., Luce, J., Turner, J. and Huang, L. (2003) Improved survival with highly active antiretroviral therapy in HIV-infected patients with severe *Pneumocystis carinii* pneumonia. *AIDS (London, England)*, **17**, 73–80.

Msur, H. and Shelhamer, J. (1996) Empiric outpatient management of HIV-related pneumonia: economical or unwise? *Annals of Internal Medicine*, **124**, 451–453.

Mundy, L.M., Autwaerter, P.G., Oldach, D. *et al.* (1995) Community acquired pneumonia: impact of immune status. *American Journal of Respiratory and Critical Care Medicine*, **152**, 1309–1315.

Muñoz, A., Schager, L.K., Bacellar, H. *et al.* (1993) Trends in the incidence and outcomes defining acquired immunodeficiency syndrome (AIDS) in the multicenter AIDS cohort study: 1985–1999. *American Journal of Epidemiology*, **137**, 423–428.

Muñoz, A., Schrager, L.K., Bacellar, H. *et al.* (1993) Trends in the incidence of outcomes defining acquired immunodeficiency syndrome (AIDS) in the Multicenter AIDS Cohort Study: 1985–1991. *American Journal of Epidemiology*, **137**, 1985–1991.

Murray, J.F., Felton, C.P., Garay, S.M. *et al.* (1984) Pulmonary complications of the acquired immunodeficiency syndrome: report of a National Heart, Lung, and Blood Institute workshop. *New England Journal of Medicine*, **310**, 1682–1688.

Murray, F. (2005) Pulmonary complications of HIV-1 infection among adults living in Sub-Saharan Africa. *International Journal of Tuberculosis Lung Diseases*, **9**, 826–835.

Murray, J.F., Garay, S.M., Hopewell, P.C., Mills, J., Snider, G.L. and Stover, D.E. (1987) NHLBI workshop summary. Pulmonary complications of the acquired syndrome: an update. *American Review of Respiratory Diseases*, **135**, 504–509.

Narayanswami, G. and Salzman, S.H. (2003) Bronchoscopy in the human immunodeficiency virus-infected patient. *Seminars of Respiratory Infections*, **18**, 80–86.

Ng, V.L., Gartner, I., Weymouth, L.A. *et al.* (1989) The use of mucolysed induced sputum for the identification of pulmonary pathogens associated with human immunodeficiency virus infection. *Archives of Pathology and Laboratory Medicine*, **113**, 488–493.

Nuorti, J.P., Butler, J.C., Gelling, L. *et al.* (2000) Epidemiologic relation between HIV and invasive pneumococcal disease in San Francisco County. *California. Annals of Internal Medicine*, **132**, 82–90.

Orlovic, D., Kularatne, R., Ferraz, V. and Smego, R.A. (2001) Dual pulmonary infection with *Mycobacterium tuberculosis* and *Pneumocystis carinii* in patients with human immunodeficiency virus. *Clinical Infectious Diseases*, **32**, 289–294.

Osmond, D.H., Chin, D.P., Glassroth, J. *et al.* (1999) Impact of bacterial pneumonia and *Pneumocystis carinii* pneumonia on human immunodeficiency virus disease progression. *Clinical Infectious Diseases*, **29**, 536–543.

Palella, F.J., Delaneu, K.M., Moorman, A.C. *et al.* (1998) Declining morbidity and mortality among patients with advanced human immunodeficiency virus infection. *The New England Journal of Medicine*, **338**, 853–860.

Paul, S., Gilbert, H.M., Ziecheck, W. *et al.* (1999) The impact of potent antirretroviral therapy on the characteristics of hospitalized patients with HIV infection. *AIDS (London, England)*, **13**, 415–418.

Pedro-Botet, M.L., García Cruz, A., Sopena, N. *et al.* (2004) Legionelosis e infección por el virus de la inmunodeficiencia humana: e infección oportunista? *Medicina Clínica (Barcelona)*, **123**, 582–584.

Pedro-Botet, M.L., Sabrià, M., Sopena, N. *et al.* (2003) Legionnaires diseases and HIV infection. *Chest*, **124**, 543–547.

Pesola, G.R. and Charles, A. (1992) Pneumococcal bacteremia with pneumonia: mortality in acquired immunodeficiency syndrome. *Chest*, **101**, 150–155.

Phair, J., Muñoz, A., Detels, R. *et al.* (1990) The risk of *Pneumocystis carinii* pneumonia among men infected with human immunodeficiency virus type 1. *The New England Journal of Medicine*, **322**, 161–165.

Polsky, B., Gold, J.W., Whimbey, E., Dryjanski, J., Brown, A.E., Schiffman, G. *et al.* (1986) Bacterial pneumonia in patients with the acquired immunodeficiency syndrome. *Annals of Internal Medicine*, **104**, 38–41.

Pradier, C., Pesce, A., Taillan, B., Roger, P.M., Bentz, L. and Dellamonica, P. (1997) Reducing the incidence of Pneumocystis carinii pneumonia: a persisting challenge. *AIDS (London, England)*, **11**, 832–833.

Pulvirenti, J., Herrera, P., Venkataraman, P. and Ahmed, N. (2003) *Pneumocystis carinii* pneumonia in HIV-infected patients in the HAART era. *AIDS Patient Care STDs*, **17**, 261–265.

Queralt, J., Falcó, V., Almirante, B. *et al.* (2004) Invasive pneumococcal disease in patients infected with HIV: still a threat in the era of highly active antirretroviral therapy. *Clinical Infectious Diseases*, **38**, 1623–1628.

Redd, S.C., Rutherford, G.W., Sande, M.A. *et al.* (1990) The role of humna immunodeficiency virus in pneumococcccal bacteremia in San Francisco residents. *Journal of Infectious Diseases*, **162**, 1012–1017.

Rimland, D., Navin, T.R., Lennox, J.L. *et al.* (2002) Prospective study of etiologic agents of community acquired pneumonia in patients with HIV infection. *AIDS (London, England)*, **16**, 85–95.

Salzman, S.H. (1998) Bronchoscopic and other invasive sampling techniques in the diagnosis of pulmonary complications of HIV infection, in *Human Immunodeficiency Virus and the Lung* (eds M.J. Rosen and J.M. Beck), Marcel Dekker, New York, pp. 95–227.

Santín Cerezales, M., Aranda Sánchez, M., Podzamcer Palter, D. *et al.* (1996) Espectro de la infección broncopulmonar por *Pseumomonas aeruginosa* en pacientes infectados por el virus de la inmunodeficiencia humana. *Revista Clínica Española*, **196**, 692–697.

Sarosi, G.A. and Davies, S.F. (1996) Endemic mycosis complicating human immunodeficiency virus infection. *Western Journal of Medicine*, **164**, 335–340.

Schleicher, G.K. and Feldman, C. (2003) Dual infection with *Streptococcus pneumoniae* and *Mycobacterium tuberculosis* in HIV-seropositive patients with community acquired pneumonia. *International Journal of Tuberculosis and Lung Diseases*, **7**, 1207–1208.

Sene, D., Bossi, P., Thomas, L., Ghosn, J., Zeller, V., Caumes, E. *et al.* (2002) Legionellosis in HIV-1 infected patients: 4 cases reports. *La Presse Medicale*, **31**, 356–358.

Serraino, D., Puro, V., Boumis, E. *et al.* (2003) Epidemiological aspects of major opportunistic infections of the respiratory tract in persons with AIDS: Europe, 1993–2000. *AIDS (London, England)*, **17**, 2109–2116.

Shaunak, S., Veryard, C. and Javan, C. (2001) Severe *Pneumocystis carinii* pneumonia increases the infectious titre of HIV-1 in blood and can promote the expansion of viral chemokine co-receptor tropism. *Journal of Infection*, **43**, 3–6.

Smith, E. and Orholm, M.K. (1994) Danish AIDS patients 1988–1993: a recent decline in *Pneumocystis carinii* pneumonia as AIDS-defining disease related to the period of known HIV positivity. *Scandinavian Journal of Infectious Diseases*, **26**, 517–522.

Spoulou, V., Gilks, C.F. and Ioannidis, J.P.A. (2002) Protein conjugate pneumococcal vaccines. Offer new opportunities for high risk individuals but skill lacks robust evidence. *British Medical Journal*, **324**, 750–751.

Stansell, J.D., Osmond, D.H., Charlebois, E. *et al.* (1997) Predictors of *Pneumocystis carinii* pneumonia in HIV-infected persons. Pulmonary Complications of HIV Infection Study Group. *American Journal of Respiratory and Critical Care Medicine*, **155**, 60–66.

Stein, M., O'Sullivan, P., Wachtel, T. *et al.* (1992) Causes of death in persons with human immunodeficiency virus infection. *The American Journal of Medicine*, **93**, 387–390.

Stoehr, A., Arasteh, K., Staszewski, S. *et al.* (1999) *Pneumocystis carinii pneumonia* in the Federal Republic of Germany in the era of changing antiretroviral therapy – IDKF 13 – German AIDS Study Group (GASG/IdKF). *European Journal of Medical Research*, **27**, 131–134.

Stover, D.E., White, D.A., Romano, P.A., Gellenee, R.A. and Robeson, W.A. (1985) Spectrum of pulmonary diseases associated with the acquired immune deficiency syndrome. *American Journal of Medicine*, **78**, 429–437.

Stringer, J.R., Beard, C.B., Miller, R.F. and Wakefield, A.E. (2002) A new name (*Pneumocystis jiroveci*) for pneumocystis from humans. *Emerging Infectious Diseases*, **8**, 891–896.

Sudre, P., Hirschel, B.J., Gatell, J.M. *et al.* (1996) Tuberculosis among European patients with the acquired immune deficiency syndrome: The AIDS in Europe Study Group. *Tuberculosis and Lung Diseases*, **77**, 322–328.

Sullivan, J.H., Moore, R.D., Keruly, J.C. and Chaisson, R.E. (2000) Effect of antiretroviral therapy on the incidence of bacterial pneumonia in patients with advanced HIV infection. *American Journal of Respiratory and Critical Care Medicine*, **162**, 64–67.

Sullivan, J.H., Moore, R.D., Keruly, J.C. and Chaisson, R.E. (2000) Epidemiology of human immunodeficiency virus-associated opportunistic infections in the United States in the era of highly active antiretroviral therapy. *Clinical Infectious Diseases*, **30**, S5–S14.

Tabet, S.R., Krone, M.R., Hooton, T.M., Koutsky, L.A. and Holmes, K.K. (1997) Bacterial infections in adult patients hospitalized with AIDS: case-control study of prophylactic efficacy of trimethoprim-sulfamethoxazole versus aerosolized pentamidine. *International Journal of STD & AIDS*, **8**, 563–569.

Tasker, S.A., Wallace, M.R., Rubins, J.B. *et al.* (2002) Reimmunization with 23-valent pneumococcal vaccine for patients infected with human immunodeficiency virus type 1: clinical, immunologic, and virologic responses. *Clinical Infectious Diseases*, **34**, 813–821.

Thomas, C.F. and Limper, A.H. (2004) *Pneumocystis pneumonia. The New England Journal of Medicine*, **50**, 2487–2498.

Torres, A., El-Ebiary, M., Marrades, R. *et al.* (1995) Aetiology and prognosis factors of patients with AIDS presenting life-threatening acute respiratory failure. *European Respiratory Journal*, **8**, 1922–1928.

Torres, R.A. and Barr, M. (1997) Impact of combination therapy for HIV infection on inpatient census. *The New England Journal of Medicine*, **33**, 1531–1532.

Tumbarello, M., Tacconelli, E., de Gaetano Doneti, K. *et al.* (2001) Nosocomial bacterial pneumonia in human immunodeficiency virus infected subjects: incidence, risk factors and outcome. *European Respiratory Journal*, **17**, 636–640.

Tumbarello, M., Tacconelli, E., de Gaetano, K. *et al.* (1998) Bacterial pneumonia in HIV-infected patients. Analysis of risk factors and prognosis indicators. *Journal of Acquired Immunodeficiency Syndrome and, Human Retrovirology*, **16**, 39–45.

Uberti-Foppa, C., Lillo, F., Terreni, M.R. *et al.* (1998) Cytomegalovirus pneumonia in AIDS patients: value of cytomegalovirus culture from BAL fluid and correlation with lung disease. *Chest*, **113**, 919–923.

UNAIDS/WHO (2006) AIDS epidemic update: special report on HIV/AIDS: December 2006. UNAIDS, Geneva. (Switzerland).

Valerio, A., Tronconi, E., Mazza, F., Fantoni, G., Atzori, C., Tartarone, F. *et al.* (2007) Genotyping of Pneumocystis jiroveci pneumonia in Italian AIDS patients. Clinical outcome is influenced by dihydropteroate synthase and not by internal transcribed spacer genotype. *Journal of Acquired Immunodeficiency Syndrome*, **45**, 521–528.

van Oosterhout, J.J.G., Laufer, M.K., Perez, M.A. *et al.* (2007) *Pneumocystis* pneumonia in HIV-positive adults. *Malawi. Emerging Infectious Diseases*, **13**, 325–328.

Villuendas, M.C., Remacha, M.A., Echávarri, B. *et al.* (1996) Neumonías diagnosticadas por broncoscopia en pacientes VIH-positivos. *Enfermedades Infecciosas y Microbiología Clínica*, **14**, 314–316.

Wachter, R.M., Luce, J.M., Safrin, S., Berrios, D.C. *et al.* (1995) Cost and outcome of intensive care for patients with AIDS. Pneumocystis cainii pneumonia and severe respiratory failure. *The Journal of the American Medical Association*, **273**, 230–235.

Wallace, J.M., Hansen, N.I., Lavange, L., Glassroth, J., Browdy, B.L., Rosen, M.J. *et al.* (1997) Respiratory disease trends in the pulmonary complications of HIV infection study cohort. *American Journal of Respiratory and Critical Care Medicine*, **155**, 72–80.

Wallace, J.M., Rao, A.V., Glassroth, J. *et al.* (1993) Respiratory illness in persons with human immunodeficiency virus infection. *The American Review of Respiratory Disease*, **148**, 1523–1529.

Whalen, C., Horsburgh, C.R., Hom, D. *et al.* (1995) Accelerated course of human immunodeficiency virus infection after tuberculosis. *American Journal of Critical Care Medicine*, **151**, 129–135.

Wheat, J. (1997) Histoplasmosis. Experience during outbreaks in Indianapolis and review of the literature. *Medicine (Baltimore)*, **76**, 339–354.

Witt, D.J., Craven, D.E. and McCabe, W.R. (1987) Bacterial infections in adult patients with the acquired immune deficiency syndrome (AIDS) and AIDS-related complex. *American Journal of Medicine*, **82**, 900–906.

Wolff, A.J. and O'Donnell, A.E. (2001) Pulmonary manifestations of HIV infection in the era of highly active antiretroviral therapy. *Chest*, **120**, 1888–1893.

Zaman, M.K. and White, D.A. (1988) Serum lactate dehydrogenase levels and *Pneumocystis carinii* pneumonia: diagnostic and prognostic significance. *American Review of Respiratory Diseases*, **137**, 796–800.

Zaman, M.K., Wooten, O.J., Suprahmanya, B. *et al.* (1988) Rapid non-invasive diagnosis of *Pneumocystis carinii* from induced liquefied sputum. *Annals of Internal Medicine*, **109**, 7–10.

6

Neutropenia

Maria J. Rüping,[1] Jörg J. Vehreschild,[1] Santiago Ewig[2]
and Oliver A. Cornely[1]

[1]Uniklinik Köln, Klinik I für Innere Medizin, Klinisches Studienzentrum, Schwerpunkt
Infektiologie II, Köln, Germany [2]Thoraxzentrum Ruhrgebiet, Kliniken für Pneumologie
und Infektiologie, Evangelisches Krankenhaus Herne und Augusta-Kranken-Anstalt,
Bochum, Germany

6.1   Introduction

Increasing prevalence of neutropenic patients

For over 60 years, antineoplastic chemotherapy has been used for treating a great variety
of malignancies (Goodman *et al.*, 1984). While chemotherapeutic treatment has
changed the face of many formerly incurable diseases like acute leukaemia or
aggressive lymphomas, the majority of cancers remain refractory to treatment with
chemotherapy alone or show a high rate of relapse. Increasing understanding of tumour-
cell biology, insights into the toxicology of chemotherapeutic drug regimens, and
marked improvements in supportive therapy have led to new treatment strategies.
Polychemotherapy allows highly active cancer treatment while reducing organ toxicity
at the same time – at the cost of a prolonged neutropenia. Improvements in antiemetic
and analgetic therapy as well as new strategies and treatment options for preventing and
treating opportunistic infections also have allowed intensifying chemotherapeutic
treatment efforts. At the same time, numbers of autologous and allogeneic stem cell
transplantations have been on the rise for the last two decades (Gratwohl *et al.*, 2007).
The latter also account for an increased prevalence of immunosuppressed patients as a
result of long-term prophylaxis against graft-versus-host disease.

Effect of steroids and chemotherapy on specific defence mechanisms of the lung

The pulmonary immune response is a complex process in which cytokines, macrophages, polymorphonuclear leukocytes and cell-mediated immunity play a crucial role.
Once a potential pathogen reaches the terminal airways, it is phagocytosed and

Pulmonary Infection in the Immunocompromised Patient, Edited by Carlos Agustí and Antoni Torres
© 2009 John Wiley & Sons, Ltd.

processed by alveolar macrophages. Antigen presentation and consecutive activation of B and T lymphocytes in the bronchus-associated lymphoid tissues (BALT) follow. If quantity or virulence of the intruding pathogen exceeds the macrophages' phagocytic capacities, neutrophil recruitment is initiated by cytokine excretion (TNFα, IL-1, IL-8 and others). These physiological mechanisms of immunity may be modulated by glucocorticoids or chemotherapeutic agents.

Glucocorticoids are the most important endogenous modulators of immune response. They act by binding to cytosolic glucocorticoid receptors and subsequent translocation of these receptor-ligand complexes into the cell nucleus where they activate or suppress gene transcription. As a result, the synthesis of almost all known cytokines and a variety of other anti-inflammatory gene products is down regulated, leading to reduced synthesis of prostaglandins and leukotrienes by cyclooxygenase-2, as well as impaired activity of cells involved in immune response.

Leukocytosis may ensue due to peripheral mobilization, but neutrophil trafficking to the sites of inflammation is inhibited. Similarly, tissue accumulation, antigen presentation and phagocytic activity of macrophages decrease. The number of circulating T-cells is rapidly depleted due to reduced mobilization from lymphoid tissues, induction of apoptosis of immature (CD4+/CD8+) thymocytes, increased emigration from the vascular system and reduced synthesis of IL-2 and the IL-2 receptor. The effect of glucocorticoids on the B lymphocyte population is less evident. Their numbers are not significally altered and short-term administration of glucocorticoids does not significantly impair antibody synthesis. Long-term administration over years may, however, result in decreased IgA and IgG levels.

The classical chemotherapeutic agents act by targeting fast-dividing cells, including bone marrow stem cells, leading to a dose-dependent degree of neutropenia. In contrast, the more recently introduced monoclonal antibodies, for example, rituximab or alemtuzumab, selectively bind to B- or T-lymphocytes, inducing their destruction via multiple mechanisms.

The depletion or functional inhibition of certain cell lines predisposes to different kinds of infections, mostly caused by atypical or opportunistic pathogens. The extensive interaction of glucocorticoids with granulocytes, macrophages and lymphocytes is associated with a dose-dependent increase in cryptococcal (Pappas et al., 2001) and Pneumocystis jiroveci pneumonia (Abernathy-Carver et al., 1994), as well as reactivation of tuberculosis (Guidelines, 2000b). The average dose necessary to significantly increase infection rates has been defined at prednisone 10 mg qd or at a cumulative dose of more than 700 mg (Ginzler et al., 1978; Stuck et al., 1989). Alternate-day dosage regimens can be used to minimize infectious complications (Fauci et al., 1976).

The neutropenic patient (ANC <500/µl) is prone to infection with pyogenic and enteric bacteria, as well as certain fungi. Relative frequencies of gram positive, gram negative and polymicrobial bacteremias are 57, 34 and 10% (Klastersky et al., 2007).

Selected lymphocyte suppression, particularly of T-lymphocytes, results in increased predisposition to viral disease, for example, CMV pneumonia (Cornely et al., 2004).

Definition of neutropenia and selective risk profiles of different therapeutic agents

While neutropenia is usually simply defined as a neutrophil count below 500/µl, the actual risk of contracting severe opportunistic infections varies hugely amongst patients. The expected length of neutropenia has probably the most important and most obvious impact on the actual risk of infection. Many clinical trials differentiate between neutropenic episodes of up to 10 days and those of more than 10 days. It is also known that certain diseases like most invasive fungal infections rarely develop in patients with short-term neutropenia (Gerson *et al.*, 1984).

Another important factor for the actual risk of infection is the underlying disease. Some malignancies impair the immune function more than others. Patients suffering from haematological malignancies, especially leukaemia, often have a severely disturbed haematopoiesis and should be considered neutropenic until a lasting remission has been achieved.

Some therapeutic regimens include treatments that impair the host defence mechanisms beyond the actual neutropenic episodes. The nucleoside analogue fludarabine is known to cause severe T-cell depletion, sometimes still detectable even 24 months after treatment (Bergmann *et al.*, 1993). Antibodies like rituximab and alemtuzumab have a long half-life and may impair immune reconstitution after recovery from neutropenia (Frampton and Wagstaff, 2003; Regazzi *et al.*, 2005). Administration of corticosteroids, calcineurin inhibitors and other immunosuppressive drugs in the aftermath of allogeneic stem cell transplantations paves the way for opportunistic infections even after neutrophil regeneration.

For these reasons, in-depth knowledge of a patient's medical history is imperative when assessing the individual risk factors for any neutropenic patient.

Haematopoietic stem cell transplantation

Patients with haematopoietic stem cell transplantation exert some characteristics which should be taken into account. During the pre-engraftment phase (0–30 days after transplant), the most prevalent pathogens causing infection are bacteria and *Candida* spp. and, if the neutropenia persists, *Aspergillus* spp. In the early post-engraftment phase (30–100 days), *cytomegalovirus* (CMV), *Pneumocystis jiroveci* and *Aspergillus* spp are the pathogens most frequently encountered. During the late posttransplant phase (>100 days), allogeneic HSCT recipients are at risk for *CMV*, community-acquired respiratory virus, and encapsulated bacterial infections. Diffuse alveolar haemorrhage (DAH) and peri-engraftment respiratory distress syndrome occurs in both allogeneic and autologous HSCT recipients, usually during the first 30 days. Bronchiolitis obliterans occurs exclusively in allogeneic HSCT recipients with graft versus host disease. Idiopathic pneumonia syndrome occurs at any time following transplant (Afessa *et al.*, 2006).

Bone marrow transplantation

Pulmonary complications occur in 40–60% of recipients of bone marrow transplants and account for more than 90% of mortality. The time-table of possible complications differs somewhat from that of stem cell transplantation. Phase 1 (days 1–30) includes pulmonary oedema; diffuse alveolar haemorrhage; and various bacterial, fungal and viral infections. Phase 2 (days 31–100) usually requires a distinction between cytomegalovirus pneumonitis and idiopathic pneumonia syndrome. After day 100, complications due to chronic graft-versus-host disease and associated bronchiolitis obliterans predominate. Overall, the spectrum of pulmonary complications has been influenced by changes in transplantation technique, prophylactic treatment for infections, and the use of new chemotherapeutic agents that contribute to lung injury (Yen *et al.*, 2004).

Clinical peculiarities of the neutropenic patient

Neutrophils pose the first and most efficient line of defence against many pathogens, foremost bacteria and fungi (Bodey *et al.*, 1966). Neutropenia not only causes a higher risk of contracting infections, but may also markedly change the clinical course of infections. Typical signs and symptoms of infections are often caused not by the pathogen itself but by the host response. Without neutrophils, the specific symptoms like tissue swelling, tenderness, redness, or warmth may be missing or replaced by more general symptoms like fever, headache and hypotension. It may be hypothesized that symptoms appear later in the neutropenic patient than they usually would. Without a functioning immune system, pathogens quickly proliferate and may cause overwhelming disease. In particular, sepsis by gram-negative bacteria like *Pseudo-monas aeruginosa* is associated with an unfavourable outcome and should be treated in the early stage of disease (Elting *et al.*, 1997).

   For these reasons, every sign or symptom of infection in the neutropenic patient must be taken seriously and comprehensively followed up. Broad spectrum antimicrobial treatment should be initiated immediately within the first two hours after onset of fever. Efforts should be made to determine the nature and site of infection by diagnostic imaging and microbiological sampling of blood and other tissues.

Overview: Pathogens and disease transmission in neutropenic patients

Like most immunocompromised patients, neutropenic patients are not only at risk of contracting opportunistic infections (that is, infections not occurring in immunocompetent hosts), but also bear a markedly higher risk to acquire common nosocomial infections like pneumonia or sepsis (see Table 6.1).

Bacterial infections

Most bacterial infections in the neutropenic patient are probably caused by bacteria of the upper respiratory and gastrointestinal tract. A major predisposing factor is mucositis

Table 6.1 Infectious agents of pulmonary disease in neutropenic patients.

Agent	Mode of infection	Patients at risk
Gramnegative, gram-positive bacteria, *Candida* spp.	Transmission from alimentary/ upper respiratory tract (secondary, septic)	All, especially in combination with severe mucositis
	Transmission from skin via indwelling catheters, prosthetic devices (secondary, septic)	All
S. pneumoniae *Mycoplasma pneumoniae* *Legionella* spp.	Human-to-human transmission, environmental contamination (primary)	All, especially ambulatory patients
Aspergillus spp.	Inhalation of ubiquitous fungal spores (primary)	Neutropenia >10 d, previous allogeneic PBSCT[a], high-dose corticosteroids, dust exposure
Pneumocystis jiroveci	Unknown (activation of latent infection, human-to-human transmission)	Neutropenia >10 d, impaired cellular immunity (esp. HIV)
Cytomegalovirus, *varizella zoster virus*	Reactivation of latent infection	Impaired cellular immunity (esp. HIV, previous allogeneic PBSCT[a])
Respiratory viruses (*respiratory syncytial virus, influenza virus, parainfluenza virus, adenovirus, et al.*)	Human-to-human transmission	Unknown
Toxoplasma gondii	Reactivation of latent infection	Impaired cellular immunity (esp. HIV, previous allogeneic PBSCT[a])

[a]PBSCT = peripheral blood stem cell transplantation.

impairing the physical barrier of the intestinal mucosa. Gram negative (that is, *Escherichia coli*, *Klebsiella* spp. and *Pseudomonas aeruginosa*) as well as gram positive bacteria (that is, *Enterococcus* spp. and viridans streptococci) are among the frequent causes of bacteremia attributed to colonizing bacteria (Marron *et al.*, 2000; Ramphal, 2004). Another frequent source of bacterial infection is intravascular catheters. While coagulase-negative staphylococci are the most commonly isolated species, other gram-positive bacteria as well as gram-negative enterobacteriaceae, *Pseudomonas* spp., *Stenotrophomonas* spp. may also be encountered (Krause *et al.*, 2004; Lorente *et al.*, 2005).

Pulmonary bacterial infections in the neutropenic patient often develop as a complication of bacteremia. However, primary infections by pathogens typically involved in community acquired pneumonia such as *S. pneumoniae*, *Legionella* spp.,

Mycoplasma pneumonia may also occur and thus remain important differential diagnoses of any unclear pulmonary infiltrate. Immunosuppression may also cause reactivation of tuberculosis, especially in lung cancer patients and/or patients from countries with a high prevalence of tuberculosis (Karnak *et al.*, 2002).

Fungal infections

Invasive pulmonary aspergillosis (IPA) is the most common nosocomial fungal infection in neutropenic patients (Rotstein *et al.*, 1999; Winston *et al.*, 1993; Klimowski *et al.*, 1989; Denning, 1998). It is caused by ubiquitious fungal spores penetrating deep into the lung upon inhalation. As fungal disease needs several days to establish, the IPA is rare in patients with neutropenia of less than 10 days (Gerson *et al.*, 1984). While candidaemia is less common in neutropenic patients, it may occur in the context of risk factors like central venous catheters, intensive care treatment, and long-term exposure to antimicrobial agents. Though *Candida* spp. usually do not cause pneumonia upon aspiration or inhalation, candidaemia may cause severe pulmonary disease. Another fungal agent of pneumonia in patients with impaired cellular immunity or prolonged neutropenia is *Pneumocystis jiroveci*.

Although the incidence of *Pneumocystis jiroveci* pneumonia (PCP) has been on the decline in Western countries since the introduction of highly active antiretroviral treatment and PCP prophylaxis, it remains a common and often fatal disease in cancer patients (Torres *et al.*, 2006). There is an ongoing discussion on the means of disease transmission and development. There have been reports of patient-to-patient transmission; however, reactivation of latent infection seems to be the primary mode of infection (Morris *et al.*, 2004).

Viral infections

Systemic or pulmonary viral infections are remarkably rare in neutropenic patients, but may pose a threat to patients with long-term impairment of cellular immunity. In these patients, virus reactivation (CMV, VZV) may cause severe pulmonary disease. Otherwise community acquired viruses like RSV, adenovirus, influenza virus, or parainfluenza virus, are also encountered, though their prevalence remains yet to be defined (Chong *et al.*, 2006; Gasparetto *et al.*, 2004).

Parasitic and protozoan infections

Although neutropenia puts patients into an overall predisposition for contracting infections, *de novo* infections with these agents are scarce. This circumstance may primarily be attributed to the lack of exposure in the hospital environment. However, disease reactivation may occur in patients with previous symptomatic or latent disease. *Toxoplasma gondii* is known to reactivate in patients with compromised cellular immunity and may cause severe infections of brains, eyes and lungs (Bretagne *et al.*, 2000; Leal *et al.*, 2007).

6.2   Management of the neutropenic patient

Monitoring infectious diseases

Signs and symptoms of infectious disease in the neutropenic patient may become apparent late in the course and frequently have an uncharacteristic pattern. However, early and targeted antiinfective treatment is associated with reduced morbidity and a better outcome. Monitoring aims at early detection and identification of disease in patients at risk. However, injudicious use of diagnostic tests may lead to false positive results, and consequently, patient harm by overtreatment.

Clinical and laboratory monitoring

Besides routine clinical diagnostic measures like breathing frequency, pulse and temperature measurement, routine blood sampling often reveals ongoing infections before they become clinically apparent. Levels of C-reactive protein (CRP) and interleukin-6 often increase before fever onset. However, CRP is also responsive to noninfective causes of inflammation and unspecific causes of the infectious agent. Procalcitonin seems to be more specific of bacterial disease (especially bacteremia and pneumonia), and sometimes may help distinguishing probable infection sources (Dornbusch *et al.*, 2005; Petrikkos *et al.*, 2005; Simon *et al.*, 2004; Toikka *et al.*, 2000). Hepatosplenic candidiasis is often associated with an increase of alkaline phosphatase (Pagano *et al.*, 2002), while an elevated lactate dehydrogenase may be indicative of *Pneumocystis jiroveci* pneumonia (Quist and Hill, 1995).

Specific monitoring

Many infectious agents can be detected from the bloodstream via polymerase chain reaction, culture and/or serology, including antigen tests (see Table 6.2). Close monitoring of all conceivable infections would cause considerable cost and a high rate of false positive results. Hence disease monitoring should be based on the actual risk profile of the individual patient.

Bacterial infections

Any incidence of fever in neutropenic patients should entail antimicrobial treatment. Effective bacterial disease monitoring would need to either identify the bacterial species allowing targeted antimicrobial treatment and/or enable diagnosis before onset of fever. The use of surveillance cultures from several sites (including blood, oral cavity, sputum and faeces) in predicting infection and infectious agents has been discussed (Penack *et al.*, 2005; Daw *et al.*, 1988; Cohen *et al.*, 1983). Clinical data on this approach are scarce. As of yet, there are no prospective randomized trials showing a beneficial effect (that is, reduced morbidity/mortality) of cultural surveillance in neutropenic patients.

Table 6.2   Monitoring infectious diseases from blood samples.

Test	Monitoring for	Candidates	Suggested interval
Surveillance blood cultures	Bacteraemia, candidaemia	—	(not suggested)
Galactomannan	*Aspergillus* spp.	Neutropenia >10 d, patients undergoing allogeneic PBSCT[a]	Three times weekly
$(1 \rightarrow 3)\beta$-D-glucan	*Aspergillus* spp., *Candida* spp.	—	(not suggested)
Fungal PCR[†]	Invasive fungal infections (specific PCRs for various species are available)	—	(not suggested)
CMV-PCR[†], CMV antigen (pp65, pp67)	Cytomegalovirus reactivation	Patients undergoing allogeneic PBSCT[a], after treatment with alemtuzumab	Twice weekly

[a]PBSCT = peripheral blood stem cell transplantation.

Fungal infections

Early treatment of invasive fungal infection (IFI) may improve the outcome of this often fatal disease. However, diagnosis of fungal infection remains difficult and in most cases, treatment is initiated based on incomplete evidence of infection. Hence, effectively monitoring markers of fungal infections is important in patients at risk. Sampling galactomannan, a membrane component of *Aspergillus* spp., from patient blood may reveal invasive aspergillosis. Due to a lack of specificity, two consecutive blood samples must turn positive for making a confident diagnosis. A meta-analysis has shown a sensitivity of 71% and a specificity of 89% for proven invasive pulmonary aspergillosis by galactomannan detection (Pfeiffer *et al.*, 2006b). Other methods detecting 1,3-β-D-glucan or fungal DNA have demonstrated promising results in diagnosing IFI, but lack sufficiently powered prospective studies (Odabasi *et al.*, 2004; Pazos *et al.*, 2005; Ferns, 2006; Florent *et al.*, 2006).

Viral infections

While viral infections are rare in the neutropenic patient, they may occur in patients with an additional impairment of cellular immunity. Neutropenic patients with additional immunosuppression after allogeneic stem cell transplantation or treated with T cell depleting drugs like alemtuzumab or purine analogues may profit from monitoring cytomegalovirus by PCR or antigen (pp65, pp67) testing (Onishi *et al.*, 2006; Skapova *et al.*, 2005).

Pneumonia prophylaxis in neutropenic patients

Preventing pneumonia by application of an effective prophylaxis seems a promising means of reducing patient morbidity and mortality. Prophylaxis automatically means treating patients who would never have contracted an infection. Since neutropenic patients are almost always subject to a certain degree of morbidity, the most important endpoints for prophylaxis studies are attributable and overall mortality.

Prophylaxis does not exclusively mean technical appliances and drug treatment. It starts with basic measures like patient motivation and mobilization. For example, all patients at high risk should perform respiratory exercises, receive physiotherapy, and be motivated to leave bed as often as possible.

Air filtration

Reducing exposure of high-risk patients to fungal spores and other airborne pathogens by air filtration is a popular attempt for prevention of pulmonary infections. Air filtration is efficacious in reducing detectable fungal spores, even under adverse conditions like nearby construction activity (Kruger et al., 2003). However, a recent systematic review on the efficiency of high-efficiency particulate air (HEPA) filtration showed no significant survival advantage in the 16 trials analyzed (Eckmanns et al., 2006). Although the efficacy of air filtration may be questionable, it remains a safe way of reducing microbial exposure of high-risk patients.

Selective digestive decontamination (SDD)

There have been numerous attempts performing SDD to reduce incidence of infection, pneumonia and/or mortality in patients with neutropenia, receiving allogeneic stem cells, or requiring mechanical ventilation. While SDD has caused a pathogen-shift from gram-negative to gram-positive bacteria in neutropenic patients, no reduction in mortality attributable to bloodstream infections or overall mortality was seen (Lee et al., 2002; Daxboeck et al., 2004; Verhoef et al., 1993).

Neutropenic diet

Cancer patients are often provided with low microbial diets while neutropenic. They are also frequently advised to stick to a rigorous nutritional regimen. There is no convincing evidence for a reduced morbidity or mortality by any nutritional behaviour (Moody et al., 2006). Indeed, unnecessary dietary restrictions may cause significant cost, morbidity and negative impact on quality of life (Moody et al., 2002).

Antiinfective prophylaxis

An overview of antiinfective prophylaxis is given in Table 6.3.

Antibacterial prophylaxis

A vast number of trials have been conducted to test for the efficacy of antibiotic prophylaxis in neutropenic patients. Most trials used a fluoroquinolone or TMP-SMX as

Table 6.3 Antiinfective prophylaxis.

Prophylaxis	Pathogens	Candidates
TMP-SMX 160/800 mg three times weekly	*Pneumocystis jiroveci*	• Allogeneic stem cell recipients before transplantation and after engraftment
	Toxoplasma spp.	• Acute leukaemia patients receiving chemotherapy
	Other bacterial infections	• Moderate risk for patients receiving T cell depleting drugs (purine analogues, alemtuzumab), autologous stem cell transplantation, or high-dose corticosteroids
Posaconazole 200 mg three times daily	Invasive fungal infections, mainly by *Aspergillus* and *Candida* spp.	• Allogeneic stem cell recipients in need of immunosuppressive therapy for graft-versus-host disease
		• Acute leukaemia patients receiving remission-induction chemotherapy with a presumed duration of neutropenia ≥ 10 d
Fluoroquinolone	Bacterial infections	• Moderate evidence for patients with deep neutropenia of ≥ 10 d

prophylactic agent. In a recent systemic review on antibiotic prophylaxis a distinct survival advantage for fluoroquinolone prophylaxis with a number needed to treat of 20 was shown (Gafter-Gvili *et al.*, 2005). In particular, high-risk patients with deep and/or prolonged neutropenia may benefit from prophylactic fluoroquinolone treatment (Pascoe and Cullen, 2006).

Antifungal prophylaxis

Numerous studies have tried to prove efficacy of antifungal prophylaxis for neutropenic patients, but did not show a marked advantage over placebo (Cornely *et al.*, 2003; Hughes *et al.*, 2002; Kern *et al.*, 2000; Vardakas *et al.*, 2005). Fluconazole was shown to significantly reduce morbidity and mortality of patients after haematopoietic stem-cell transplantation (Goodman *et al.*, 1992; Slavin *et al.*, 1995). This situation has changed with the availability of posaconazole, a new azole antifungal with a broad spectrum of activity against most clinically important yeasts and moulds (Hof, 2006). It has a favourable toxicity profile and the oral solution is well absorbed. Two landmark trials have shown marked efficacy of posaconazole for antifungal prophylaxis. One trial demonstrated a highly significant reduction of all-cause mortality, attributable mortality, and invasive fungal infections compared to other systemic triazoles in patients with acute leukaemia suffering from neutropenia ≥ 10 days after remission induction chemotherapy (Cornely *et al.*, 2007b). The other trial demonstrated reduction of invasive aspergillosis and attributable mortality by posaconazole compared to fluconazole in patients receiving immunsuppressive treatment for graft-versus-host disease after allogeneic stem cell transplantation (Ullmann *et al.*, 2007). Administration of posaconazole 200 mg TID is recommended in these patient groups.

Of note, PCP is not covered by triazole prophylaxis. While prospective randomized trials are lacking, prophylaxis is highly advised for high-risk patients with acute leukaemia or undergoing allogeneic stem cell transplantation. Use of TMP-SMX three times weekly is efficacious and tolerable (Hughes *et al.*, 1987). Other treatment options are atovaquone, dapsone (El-Sadr *et al.*, 1998) and – though less efficacious – aerosolized pentamidin (Vasconcelles *et al.*, 2000).

Antiviral prophylaxis

The role of respiratory viruses in neutropenic patients is still under investigation and remains elusive. Acyclovir prophylaxis is recommended for seropositive stem cell recipients to prevent HSV/VZV reactivation. CMV reactivation may cause severe pneumonia. However, prophylaxis against CMV is toxic and pre-emptive treatment strategies are preferred (Boeckh *et al.*, 1996a).

Diagnostic procedures and differential diagnosis

Figure 6.1 shows an algorithm for the clinical management of patients with profound neutropenia, fever and pulmonary infiltrates.

Radiology: Limitation of chest radiography

The mainstay of the diagnosis of pneumonia usually is the detection of a new or persistent infiltrate in chest radiography, usually p.a. and lateral in upright position. In patients with neutropenia, an infiltrate in chest radiography is only present in less than 10% of patients with persistent fever despite empiric antibacterial treatment. However, a simultaneous CT scan of the chest will reveal a pathological lung finding in up to 50% of these patients. Thus, pulmonary infiltrates, mostly pneumonia, have to be suspected and evaluated in any patient with fever of unknown origin despite an apparently normal chest radiograph.

Radiology: Importance of CT scanning

More recent research has shown that the early and concomitant use of CT scans markedly improves the detection of pulmonary infiltrates. Heussel and coworkers could demonstrate that in patients with febrile neutropenia that persisted for more than two days despite empiric antimicrobial treatment, in 70 (48%) of 146 cases findings on chest radiographs were normal, whereas findings on thin-section CT scans were suggestive of pneumonia. Pathogens were detected in 30 of these 70 cases. It appeared that 19 of 30 cases were not optimally treated before CT. Thus, thin-section CT scans showed

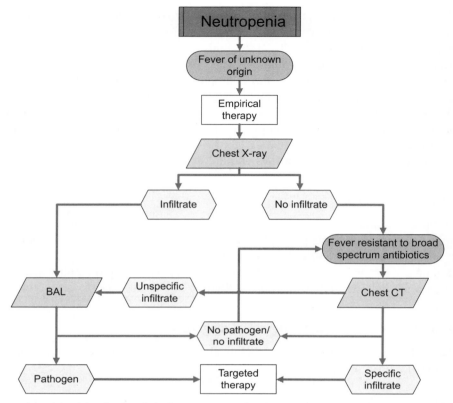

Figure 6.1   Algorithm for the clinical management of patients with profound neutropenia, fever and pulmonary infiltrates.

findings suggestive of pneumonia about five days earlier than chest radiographs showed suggestive findings. Interestingly, when thin-section CT scans show findings suggestive of pneumonia, the probability of pneumonia being detected on chest radiographs during the seven-day follow-up was 31%, whereas the probability was only 5% when the findings on the prior thin-section CT scan were normal (Heussel *et al.*, 1999). An early diagnosis seems to be of particular importance with regard to the generally difficult to treat fungal infections. Thus, it has become standard practice to incorporate CT scans, nowadays thin section multislice CT, early in the evaluation of a patient with febrile neutropenia.

Radiology: How to assess the lung as possible origin of febrile neutropenia

Neutropenic patients who develop fever ($\geq$38.3 °C or persistent 38 °C) should be always evaluated for pulmonary infiltrates by chest radiography. In selected patients at particular risk for fungal infections, CT scanning in the case of a negative chest radiograph may be considered. In patients not responding to empirical antibacterial

Table 6.4 Non-infectious causes of pulmonary infiltrates in neutropenic patients.

Fluid lung as a result of:
   Congestive heart failure
   Renal heart failure
   ARDS

Atelectasis
Drug-induced alveolitis
Pulmonary haemorrhage
Diffuse alveolar damage (DAD)
Leucocytostatic infiltrates
Graft versus host-disease

---

treatment after 72 hours (either with fever of unknown origin or documented infections other than the lungs), a repeated chest radiography should be performed. Those patients with infiltrates may be subjected to an additional CT scan in order to characterize the infiltrates which may be of help in the selection of secondary empirical treatment. All patients with normal chest radiography should undergo CT scan. The same is true for patients still not responding to the secondary empirical antimicrobial treatment. Finally, the evaluation of treatment response by CT is also mandatory prior to the next aggressive chemotherapy.

Differential diagnosis

It is important to recognize that pulmonary infiltrates in patients with neutropenia do not necessarily represent infectious pneumonia. Instead, there is a wide spectrum of non-infectious conditions which may lead to pulmonary infiltrates (see Table 6.4).

CT scanning and bronchoscopy are the major tools which help in clarifying the etiology also of non-infectious pulmonary infiltrates.

Non-invasive investigations

In all febrile patients two pairs of blood cultures should be obtained. Sputum may be sampled in selected patients with productive cough. Serological investigations include the detection of galactomannan antigen or β-Glucan. In patients at risk of viral pneumonia, detection of viral antigen or nucleic acid should be included. CMV may be investigated by CMV matrix protein pp65 (van der Bij *et al.*, 1988), CMV DNA PCR assays (Schulenburg *et al.*, 2001; Boivin *et al.*, 2000; Masaoka *et al.*, 2001; Sia *et al.*, 2000) or Hybrid Capture CMV DNA assay (Ho *et al.*, 2000; Mazzulli *et al.*, 1999). Influenza viruses may be detected by rapid bedside tests.

Bronchoscopy: Indications

Bronchoscopy is of great help in establishing a microbiological diagnosis. However, several limitations of invasive testing should not be ignored. First, several patients suffer from respiratory failure which may be worsened by invasive procedures, particularly bronchoalveolar lavage. Second, the yield of bronchoscopy varies considerably dependent on the site, extension and kind of infection. In any case, regardless of the results of non invasive and invasive testing, immediate initiation of empiric antimicrobial treatment is mandatory even before retrieval of diagnostic samples.

Bronchoscopy: How to use it appropriately

Bronchoscopy should be performed by physicians experienced in the diagnosis of pulmonary infections. Relevant information may be already gained by visualization of the bronchial tree. Important examples are apparent purulent secretions, bronchial obstruction by mucous plugs resulting in atelectasis, signs of diffuse bleeding, and mucosal pseudomembranes as hallmarks of fungal infections, particularly aspergillosis. Bronchoalveolar lavage should be performed according to standards given in Table 6.5. Throughout the investigation, the patient must be closely monitored for respiratory and

Table 6.5   Methodology of bronchoscopic sampling in spontaneously breathing and in ventilated patients.

Non-ventilated patients
    Patient preparation:
        oxygen insufflation through nasal sprongs until oxygen saturation >90%
        sedation with midazolam (1–5 mg i.v.) and propofol (0.5–1 mg/kg i.v. mg)

Ventilated patients
    Patient preparation:
        set oxygen supply at 100% until oxygen saturation 100%
        sedation with boli of e.g. midazolam or propofol
        aspirate and discard all secretions along the tracheal tube

All patients
    Do not aspirate through the channel of the bronchoscope prior to sampling
    Limit local anaesthetics on trachea and bronchi to a minimum
    Wedge bronchoscope in the orifice
        of the radiologically most prominently affected segment (localized infiltrates)
        of a standard segment, i.e. middle lobe or lingula (diffuse infiltrates)
    Instill 6 × 20 mL (up to 10 × 20 mL) of sterile and warm isotonic NaCL solution and
        gently reaspirate fluid
    Discard first portion recovered

Pool all following portions
    Divide in several aliquots for:
        giemsa stain
        gram stain
        quantitative bacterial culture
        mycobacterial culture
        fungal culture
        additional studies (CMV, Pneumocystis jiroveci etc.)

haemodynamic stability. It is extremely important to establish safe pathways for the rapid and adequate processing of the samples obtained.

In contrast to the investigation of patients with nosocomial pneumonia, the quantitative bacterial culture technique has not received any remarkable attention in neutropenic patients. Therefore, recommendations for patients with neutropenia can only be derived from the experience made in the investigation of nosocomial pneumonia. Although quantitative cultures cannot be regarded as independent predictors for the presence of bacterial pneumonia, they are of help in establishing the diagnosis and the causative pathogen when the bacterial load exceeds predefined thresholds. However, at least in patients with ventilator-associated pneumonia, survival rates seem to depend on immediate initiation of adequate antimicrobial treatment rather than the method of microbial investigation applied (Canadian Clinical Trials Group, 2006).

Bronchial, transbronchial, percutaneous or VATS-assisted biopsy: Indications and prerequisites

The performance of bronchial or transbronchial biopsies is not part of usual bronchoscopic investigation but may be indicated in selected cases, particularly in the case of treatment failure and a persistent life-threatening condition. Alternatively, ultrasound or CT-guided transthoracic needle aspiration may be considered. In these patients, it is mandatory to achieve a platelet count of at least 50.000/µl and a partial thromboplastin time of at least <60 s. Lung biopsy via video-assisted thoracoscopy (VATS) is another approach to obtain lung specimens but is not generally available in all institutions.

Diagnostic yield of systematic diagnostic investigation

Several investigators have reported recent data on pathogen patterns in neutropenic patients. The reported results are extremely difficult to compare due to differences in patient selection, timing of bronchoscopic investigation, pre-treatment regimen, and methodology of bronchoscopic sampling. In fact, to our knowledge, to date there is no single study addressing the diagnostic yield of microbial investigation in a relevant number of consecutive well-defined, treatment-naive neutropenic hemato-oncologic patients with pulmonary infiltrates.

In the most recent comprehensive study to date including 200 immunosuppressed patients, an etiological diagnosis was obtained in 162/200 (81%) of cases. The etiology was found to be infectious in 125 (77%) and non-infectious in 37 (23%) of cases. The remaining 19% remained undiagnosed. Non-invasive techniques led to the diagnosis of pulmonary infiltrates in 41% of the cases in which they were used; specifically, the diagnostic yield of blood cultures was 30/191 (16%); sputum cultures 27/88 (31%); nasopharyngeal wash 9/50 (18%); and tracheobronchial aspirates (TBAS) 35/55 (65%). Bronchoscopic techniques led to the diagnosis of pulmonary infiltrates in 59% of the cases in which they were used: fibrobronchial aspirate (FBAS) 16/28 (57%), BAL 68/135 (51%) and PSB 30/125 (24%) (Rañó et al., 2001). Such high yields of diagnostic investigation are unique, however, and probably due to the extensive diagnostic protocol applied systematically. For bronchoscopy alone, other authors reported yields ranging from 49 to 65% (Hohenadel *et al.*, 2001; Jain *et al.*, 2004; Peikert *et al.*, 2005) which are comparable with the study by Rañó *et al.*, 2001. However, there are also studies reporting much lower yields (<30%) (Boersma *et al.*, 2007).

Obviously, there is no specific advantage to applying a specific sampling technique such as protected specimen brush (PSB) or protected bronchoalveolar lavage (PBAL) as compared to standard bronchoalveolar lavage (BAL) (Jain *et al.*, 2004; Boersma *et al.*, 2007). In contrast, the additional contribution of transbronchial biopsies (TBB) was found to be significant in at least one recent study (Jain *et al.*, 2004). Whereas the diagnostic yields of BAL (38%) and TBB (38%) were similar, the combined diagnostic yield of BAL and TBB (70%) was significantly higher than that of BAL alone. Again, other authors did not find TBB to contribute significantly to the results of BAL (Peikert *et al.*, 2005; Patel *et al.*, 2005).

Whereas a high diagnostic yield is apparently desirable, a more important question is whether it contributes to better outcomes. In the study by Rañó *et al.*, 2001, the diagnostic results led to a change in antimicrobial treatment in 93 cases (46%). Although changes in treatment did not have an impact on the overall mortality, patients with pulmonary infiltrates of an infectious etiology in whom the change was made during the first seven days had a better outcome (29% mortality) than those in whom treatment was changed later (71% mortality; $p = 0.001$). These results hint at a limited but relevant contribution of diagnostic investigation and informed treatment policies to better outcomes. However, in the ICU setting, such effects seem to be very hard to demonstrate. Although BAL had an acceptable overall diagnostic yield (49%), it infrequently led to treatment changes and was not associated with improved patient survival (Gruson *et al.*, 2000). A recent study involving exclusively adult autologous and allogeneic bone marrow transplant patients could also not demonstrate a benefit of bronchoscopic evaluation, regardless of the establishment of a specific diagnosis (Patel *et al.*, 2005).

Considerations for the treatment course

Relevant evidence on the importance of early CT scanning in febrile neutropenic patients has led to significant alterations in diagnostic algorithms aiming at prompt detection and treatment of pulmonary infiltrates. Similarly structured recommendations for monitoring the transformation of these infiltrates through the course of treatment cannot be pronounced, since the interaction of different factors, including the type of infectious agent and the patient's immune status, call for an individual approach. Some general rules regarding the short and long term follow up of pulmonary infiltrates, should, however, be known and respected.

During the entire follow up period, the size of bacterial and fungal lung infiltrates is modulated by the neutrophil count. A patient recovering from neutropenia may display an increase in infiltrate size that should not be interpreted as lack of response to antiinfective treatment.

The radiographic response shortly after initiation of antiinfective treatment has been well documented for invasive pulmonary aspergillosis in the neutropenic patient and may serve as an orientation. Even under adequate antifungal treatment, infiltrates may continue to increase substantially until day seven and remain stable until day 14. Only thereafter, regression ensues (Caillot *et al.*, 2001). Consequently, a follow up CT after week one only serves to document the definite extension of infiltrates, but should have little influence on decisions concerning changes in the therapeutic approach. During this period, clinical signs and symptoms, as well as laboratory markers of inflammation (for example, CRP, IL-6, procalcitonin) are of higher informational content and spare the patient unnecessary radiation exposure. A CT follow up after week two is warranted, because the correlation of an improving clinical condition and stable infiltrates hints at an adequate choice of therapeutic measures.

After week two, the behaviour of pulmonary infiltrates is highly variable and may be influenced by several factors: While most bacterial infiltrates resolve more rapidly once normal neutrophil counts are reached, infiltrates of fungal origin are associated with delayed and often incomplete remission. Therefore, CT follow-ups should be repeated until complete regression of infiltrates. If such frequent assessment is not possible, a control CT should at least be carried out before predictable episodes of immunosuppression, such as consecutive cycles of chemotherapy, in order to assess the necessity of adequate secondary prophylaxis during this high risk situation.

Empirical treatment

Febrile neutropenic patients with unspecific lung infiltrates need empiric antiinfective treatment. In this population halo and air crescent signs in CT scans are typical for filamentous fungal infection, and do not represent an empiric treatment situation.

Since unspecific lung infiltrates may be caused by bacteria, fungi, or viruses, treatment is usually polypragmatic and driven by local epidemiology, patient risk and prognostic factors. Furthermore, the temporal relation between detection of pulmonary infiltrates, onset of fever and onset of neutropenia can be insightful. If pulmonary infiltrates emerge at the onset of fever, infection with an opportunistic agent typical of the neutropenic patient (*S. aureus*, *Klebsiella spp.*, *Pseudomonas aeruginosa*) is likely. Breakthrough infections, in patients already receiving broad spectrum antimicrobial therapy, point at the presence of fungi, resistant gram negative rods, and in rare cases, *Legionella spp.* Adequate diagnostic measures and antiinfective coverage of these agents will be discussed in depth in the corresponding sections of Chapter 3. Acute respiratory distress syndrome accompanied by septic shock is often associated with viridians streptococcal bacteremia. Potential or witnessed aspiration bears a high risk for anaerobic infection. In outpatients, the most common pathogens of community acquired pneumonia (*Streptococcus pneumoniae*, *Mycoplasma pneumoniae*, *Legionella spp.*, *Influenzaviruses*) should be considered.

With regards to the high mortality rate of invasive pulmonary aspergillosis (IPA), patients with acute leukemia and other aggressive haematological malignancies, presenting with fever and unspecific lung infiltrates, should be promptly treated with an antipseudomonal beta-lactam antibiotic plus an antifungal active against *Aspergillus* spp. The additional empirical use of antiviral drugs, aminoglycosides, glycopeptides or macrolide antibiotics is not recommended.

Treatment should be continued until resolution of neutropenia to 500/μl, clinical improvement and regression of radiological signs are achieved. Meanwhile, the diagnostic armamentarium should be fully exploited, in order to initiate selective treatment in the case of successful pathogen identification. If invasive fungal pneumonia can be proven by invasive diagnostic techniques and/or if a complete regression of suspect radiological signs cannot be achieved before the patient's discharge from hospital, therapy should be continued with oral antifungals, for example, voriconazole or posaconazole until demonstration of complete remission on control CT scans.

If fever persists, other antiinfective agents must be considered. Second line treatment options should always be chosen with respect to the possibility of an IPA. Voriconazole at 6 mg/kg bid iv loading dose and 4 mg/kg bid iv maintenance as well as liposomal amphotericin B 3 mg/kg qd can be considered (Cornely et al., 2007a; Herbrecht et al., 2002). Multiresistant bacterial pathogens to be taken into consideration include *Pseudomonas aeruginosa* and other gram negative rods (*Klebsiella* sp., *Serratia* sp. and *Enterobacter* sp.). These agents may be covered with meropenem at 1 g tid iv or imipenem plus cilastatin at 1 g tid iv.

Since patients after high dose chemotherapy and autologous peripheral stem cell transplantation are at low risk of pulmonary fungal infection (Reich et al., 2001), empirical antifungal treatment is rarely indicated. After autologous bone marrow transplantation or CD34-selected stem cell transplantation (Holmberg et al., 1999), CMV pneumonitis should be ruled out by bronchoalveolar lavage.

6.3   Specific infectious diseases

Bacterial pneumonia

Bacterial pneumonia is one of the most frequent causes of pulmonary infiltrates in neutropenic patients. The whole gram-positive and gram-negative spectrum of bacterial pathogens has to be taken into account. Clinical hints may arrive from the early time-point of appearance during neutropenia, the unilateral affection in chest radiograph, and the presentation with severe sepsis and/or septic shock. Non-invasive and invasive bronchoscopic evaluation help to establish etiology. Diagnostic results should primarily be regarded as a means to treat pathogens not covered by initial empiric antimicrobial treatment. Severe bacterial pneumonia is still associated with high mortality rates. Non-invasive ventilation has been shown to improve the outcomes of acute respiratory failure.

Pneumonia acquired in the community

Since by definition all patients with neutropenia are immunocompromised, they do not share the typical pathogen patterns characteristic for patients with community acquired pneumonia. Although this issue has not been thoroughly addressed in the literature, it may be useful to consider community acquired pathogens as well as the spectrum of pathogens described above.

Pneumonia acquired in the hospital

Accordingly, pneumonia developing during hospitalization differs considerably as compared to nosocomial pneumonia in the non-neutropenic host. Additional pathogens have to be kept in mind, for example, β-hemolytic streptococci are important pathogens in neutropenic patients, but rarely in non-neutropenic hosts. The same is true for many fungi and viruses.

Pathogen patterns

As stated above, the data available in the literature are highly variable in terms of patient populations studied and methods applied. Nevertheless, it seems useful to report examples of two large recent series indicating the pathogen patterns found in more detail.

In a German retrospective study in neutropenic patients already treated with a broad spectrum antibacterial and antifungal regimen, respiratory pathogens were detected in 29/95 (31%) patients, including 35% gram-positive and 40% gram-negative species, but also 11% mycobacteria, 11% fungi and 3% CMV (Hohenadel *et al.*, 2001).

In a comprehensive prospective Spanish study including mainly haemato- oncologic patients with neutropenia, infectious etiologies were identified in 77% of cases. Of these, the main etiologies included bacterial (24%), fungal (17%) and viral (10%) infections. The most frequent pathogens were Aspergillus fumigatus ($n = 29$), Staphylococcus aureus ($n = 17$), and Pseudomonas aeruginosa ($n = 12$) (Rañó *et al.*, 2001).

In view of the large and heterogeneous microbial spectrum reported, it is imperative to establish a dedicated diagnostic protocol for neutropenic patients presenting with pulmonary infiltrates. The institutional epidemiology must be continuously monitored.

Clinical presentation

Bacterial pneumonia in neutropenic patients does not exert specific symptoms or signs. Hints at a bacterial etiology mainly derive from the time point of infection – usually first infectious complication during neutropenia – as well as a unilateral, usually consolidating or bronchopneumonic affection in chest radiography. Severe bacterial pneumonia may present together with severe sepsis or even septic shock, a feature which is rarely present in fungal and viral pneumonia.

Targeted treatment

Antimicrobial treatment is always administered empirically and should cover a broad spectrum of gram-positive and gram-negative bacterial pathogens. Febrile neutropenic patients are at high risk for death in case of discordant treatment. Therefore, although the importance of mixed infections is not known, deescalation after identification of a pathogen should only be performed in stable and afebrile patients. On the other hand, it may be mandatory to change initial treatment in order to cover specific bacterial

Table 6.6 Directed treatment of important specific bacterial pathogens of pneumonia in neutropenic patients.

Pathogen	Directed treatment	Dosage (i.v.)
Streptococcus pneumoniae and other streptococci	Penicillin G	4×5 Mio Units
Resistant Streptococcus pneumoniae (MIC $\geq 2 \mu g/L$)	Ceftriaxone	1×2 g
	Levofloxacin	1×500–750 mg
	Moxifloxacin	1×400 mg
Staphylococcus aureus	Oxacillin	6×2 g
MRSA	Vancomycin + Rifampicin	2×1 g + 1×600 mg
	Linezolid	2×600 mg
Klebsiella pneumonia, ESBL	Imipenem/Cilastatin	3×1 g
	Meropenem	3×1 g
Pseudomonas aeruginosa	Piperacillin/Tazobactam + Ciprofloxacin or	3×4 g + 3×400 mg
	Piperacillin/Tazobactam + Meropenem	3×4 g + 3×1 g
Acinetobacter spp.	Imipenem/Cilastatin	3×1 g
	Ampicillin/Sulbactam	3×3 g
Legionella spp.	Levofloxacin	1×750 mg

pathogens or resistances. Important tools of directed antimicrobial treatment are summarized in Table 6.6. Treatment duration should be at least seven days, after recovery from neutropenia (neutrophils >500/μL) and including at least two days of stable defervescence.

Non-invasive ventilation

Immunosuppressed patients with pneumonia and acute respiratory (type I hypoxemic) failure have been shown to profit from noninvasive respiratory support by face mask ventilation. In a landmark study including 52 immunosuppressed patients (each group of 26 patients including 15 patients with hematologic cancer and neutropenia) with pulmonary infiltrates, fever and an early stage of hypoxemic acute respiratory failure, intermittent noninvasive ventilation was compared with standard treatment. Periods of noninvasive ventilation delivered through a face mask were alternated every three hours with periods of spontaneous breathing with supplemental oxygen. The ventilation periods lasted at least 45 minutes. Fewer patients in the noninvasive-ventilation group than in the standard-treatment group required intubation (12 vs. 20, $p = 0.03$), had serious complications (13 vs. 21, $p = 0.02$), died in the intensive care unit (10 vs. 18, $p = 0.03$), or died in the hospital (13 vs. 21, $p = 0.02$). The authors concluded that in selected immunosuppressed patients with infiltrates and acute respiratory failure, early initiation of noninvasive ventilation is feasible and associated with an improved likelihood of survival to hospital discharge (Hilbert, 2001). More recently, it could be shown that the use of NPPV delivered via helmet was as effective as NPPV delivered via face mask in avoiding endotracheal intubations (intubation rate, 37% vs 47%, respectively; $p = 0.37$) and improving gas exchange. Moreover, the patients receiving ventilation via helmet required significantly less NPPV discontinuations in the first 24 h of application ($p < 0.001$) than patients receiving ventilation via face mask (Rocco *et al.*, 2004). Accordingly, it could be shown that early nCPAP with helmet improved oxygenation in selected immunosuppressed patients with hypoxemic acute respiratory failure. The tolerance of helmet nCPAP seemed better than that of nCPAP delivered by mask. nCPAP could be applied continuously for an about four times longer time period in the helmet group, and whereas several patients were intolerant to face mask ventilation, no one was in the helmet group (Principi *et al.*, 2004).

Therefore, it might be justified to start a trial of noninvasive ventilation in these patients, probably preferably using a helmet rather than a face mask. However, strict adherence to exclusion criteria such as hemodynamic instability and impaired consciousness as well as to predefined criteria for intubation during a trial of noninvasive ventilation is mandatory.

Outcome

The outcome of patients with pulmonary infiltrates due to bacterial pneumonia strongly depends on initial severity and the duration of neutropenia. Patients with severe pneumonia requiring mechanical ventilation or presenting with septic shock as well as those with prolonged neutropenia have a dismal prognosis with mortality rates reaching 90–100%. Otherwise, rapid initiation of adequate broad-spectrum empirical antimicrobial treatment and early administration of non-invasive ventilation is effective in improving outcomes.

Invasive pulmonary aspergillosis

Invasive pulmonary aspergillosis (IPA) in the neutropenic patient is associated with high morbidity and mortality. Early diagnosis is crucial and relies mainly on the results of HRCT, galactomannan detection and PCR. First line treatment: voriconazole or L-AmB. Second line treatment: caspofungin, posaconazole or L-AmB. Prophylaxis in AML and after HSCT: posaconazole.

Etiology

IPA is the most common manifestation of invasive aspergillosis (IA) (Maschmeyer *et al.*, 2007) and represents a major cause of morbidity and mortality in neutropenic patients. *Aspergillus fumigatus* has been identified as the causative agent of 50–60% of all IA infections, followed by *A. flavus*, *A. niger* and *A. terreus* (10–15% each). *A. nidulans*, *A. ustus* and other rare *Aspergillus* spp. account for only 2% of all cases (Sutton *et al.*, 2004; Marr *et al.*, 2002; Patterson *et al.*, 2000; Maschmeyer *et al.*, 2007).

Pathogenesis

Aspergillus grows at a wide range of temperatures, including 37 °C, and is found ubiquitously in the indoor and outdoor environment where its conidia are permanently inhaled. Usually, this poses no threat to the immunocompetent individual, because ciliary clearance and ingestion by macrophages and polymorphonuclear leukocytes readily remove the organism from the airways. In the immunocompromised host, however, conidiae are allowed to germinate and transform into hyphae, capable of vascular invasion with subsequent occlusion, ischemic necrosis and disseminated infection. Neutropenia of greater than 100/µL for more than 10 days is considered the most important risk factor for IPA (Muhlemann *et al.*, 2005; Gerson *et al.*, 1984). Additional risk factors include T-cell suppression (Marr *et al.*, 2002; Martino *et al.*, 2006), long-term prophylaxis with fluconazole (Kontoyiannis, 2002; van Burik *et al.*, 1998) or ganciclovir (Einsele *et al.*, 2000), bacteremia during hematopoietic stem cell transplantation (HSCT) (Sparrelid *et al.*, 1998) and renal or hepatic impairment after solid organ transplantation (Singh *et al.*, 2003).

Clinical presentation

Pathognomonic symptoms of IPA do not exist. Cough, chest pain, haemoptysis, dyspnea, hypoxia and prolonged fever, even under broad spectrum antibiosis, are unspecific symptoms, which may present less intense and delayed in the immunocompromised patient. Under these circumstances, the diagnosis of IPA depends largely on alternative criteria.

Diagnosis

Due to current international consensus (Ascioglu *et al.*, 2002), IA can only be reliably proven by tissue biopsy showing hyphae and associated tissue damage or by a positive culture from usually sterile sites obtained using aseptic techniques. In clinical practice, however, these criteria are of limited use. *Aspergillus* growth from blood cultures is extremely rare, and taking lung biopsies from thrombocytopenic patients – as it is usually the case in leukaemia and allogeneic transplantation – bears a considerable risk. Likewise, sputum or BAL (bronchoalveolar lavage) samples are of limited value since accidental contamination during handling cannot be ruled out and the yield is limited anyway. Therefore, the diagnosis of IPA relies heavily on imaging and antigen detection techniques.

   HRCT (high resolution CT) is the imaging technique of choice, because pulmonary aspergillosis can be detected about five days earlier than in plain chest radiographs (Heussel *et al.*, 1999). Lesions usually acquire their maximum extension on day seven and remain stable until day 14. The presence of a 'halo' or an 'air crescent sign' is highly suggestive of IPA, the former being an early and the latter a late marker of infection (Figures 6.2 and 6.3) (Greene *et al.*, 2003; Caillot *et al.*, 2001). Histopathologically, the halo represents an outer area of haemorrhage and oedema, whereas the air crescent sign

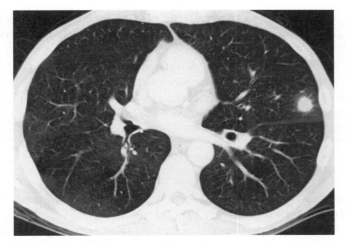

Figure 6.2   Halo sign: nodular lesion surrounded by low attenuation.

represents cavitation. Additional features are nodular and peripheral patchy densities. Hilar and mediastinal lymph node enlargements as well as pleural affection have also been described. Although 'halo' and 'air crescent' signs are suggestive, they are no proof of aspergillosis. Differential diagnoses include other fungal infections, herpes viral infections, legionellosis, Kaposi's sarcoma, metastatic angiosarcoma as well as Wegener's granulomatosis. Considering the dynamic nature of radiological IPA signs, repetition of CT scans is warranted.

A sandwich enzyme-linked immunosorbent assay (ELISA) using a monoclonal antibody to *Aspergillus* galactomannan (sensitivity 71%, specificity 89% in patients with proven IA (Pfeiffer *et al.*, 2006a), has been widely used. A paradoxical increase just after the initiation of treatment – due to antigen release after fungal cell destruction

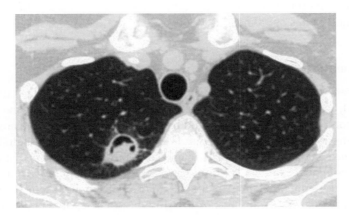

Figure 6.3   Air crescent sign: cavitation of a nodular lesion.

(Klont *et al.*, 2006) – can occasionally be observed. Galactomannan detection in BAL fluid, cerebrospinal fluid or urine appears promising, but remains investigational.

β-glucan, another fungal marker, detects infections with *Candida*, *Aspergillus*, *Fusarium*, *Cryptococcus* and *Trichosporon* with high sensitivity and specificity (Obayashi *et al.*, 1995; Ostrosky-Zeichner *et al.*, 2005), but does not differentiate between them. While the use of PCR assays has yielded promising results, it still lacks standardization.

Treatment

Independent of the chosen antifungal therapy, early initiation of treatment has been associated with a significant increase in survival rates.

First choice in the treatment of IPA is voriconazole at 6 mg/kg bid iv loading dose and 4 mg/kg bid iv maintenance (Herbrecht *et al.*, 2002). Alternatively, liposomal amphotericin B can be administered at 3 mg/kg qd iv. (Cornely *et al.*, 2007a) As second line treatment options, caspofungin (70 mg single loading dose iv and 50 mg qd iv maintenance) or posaconazole (400 mg bid po or 200 mg qid po) should be considered (Maertens *et al.*, 2004; Walsh *et al.*, 2007).

In the prophylaxis of IPA, posaconazole at 200 mg tid po has produced significant improval in the survival rates of patients with acute myelogenous leukaemia (AML) and myelodysplastic syndrome (MDS), as well as a reduction in the incidence of IA in patients with graft-versus-host-disease after HSCT (Cornely *et al.*, 2007b; Ullmann *et al.*, 2007). Strict reverse isolation is seen as an effective measure for patients undergoing allogeneic HSCT and for AML patients receiving aggressive chemotherapy. Unfortunately, there are no results from clinical trials corroborating this hypothesis.

Outcome

If left untreated, mortality in IPA reaches almost 100%. Even with antifungal treatment, overall mortality rates are almost up to 60%.

Other filamentous fungal diseases

Certain zygomycetes and Fusarium spp. have emerged as important pathogens in patients with haematological cancer and recipients of haematopoietic stem cell transplantation (HSCT). Organisms of both groups are angiotropic and angioinvasive, causing haemorrhage and tissue necrosis. Typical clinical symptoms include fever, dry cough, dyspnea and haemoptysis. The diagnosis is based on CT scans, blood cultures and histopathological examination of biopsy species. Differentiation from *Aspergillus* spp. is often difficult. First line treatment: liposomal amphotericin B. Second line treatment: voriconazole or posaconazole. Mortality rates approach 39 and 100% in invasive zygomycosis and fusariosis, respectively.

Epidemiology and etiology

Certain zygomycetes (Kontoyiannis *et al.*, 2005; Siwek *et al.*, 2004) and *Fusarium* spp. (Lionakis and Kontoyiannis, 2004; Nucci *et al.*, 2004) have emerged as important pathogens of invasive pulmonary infection in patients with haematological malignancies and recipients of haematopoietic stem cell transplantation.

Rhizopus and *Rhizomucor* spp., both of the order mucorales and with a worldwide distribution pattern, are the most common pathogens of invasive zygomycosis. In the neutropenic patient, zygomycosis usually presents as pulmonary or disseminated disease. Infection is contracted via inhalation of spores. Additional risk factors include diabetes (Chayakulkeeree *et al.*, 2006; Roden *et al.*, 2005), free serum iron (Gonzalez *et al.*, 2002), and voriconazole therapy (Kontoyiannis *et al.*, 2005).

Fusarium solani (causes approximately 50% of cases), *Fusarium oxysporum*, *Fusarium moniliforme*, *Fusarium verticillioides*, *Fusarium dimerum*, and *Fusarium proliferatum* account for most cases of human invasive fusariosis (Lionakis and Kontoyiannis, 2004). While 50–80% of all cases are reported from the United States, lower incidence rates have been registered in France, Italy and Brazil (Torres *et al.*, 2003). Pulmonary involvement may be primary or as a consequence of haematogenous dissemination. Infection by ingestion, skin traumas (Guarro and Gene, 1995) and colonization of central venous catheters (Ammari *et al.*, 1993) has been reported.

Pathogenesis

Members of the order mucorales, as well as *Fusarium* spp. are both angiotropic and angioinvasive moulds that produce haemorrhagic infarction and low tissue perfusion, resulting in thrombosis and tissue necrosis (Chayakulkeeree *et al.*, 2006; Gonzalez *et al.*, 2002; Lionakis and Kontoyiannis, 2004).

Clinical presentation

Clinical differentiation of invasive pulmonary aspergillosis from zygomycosis or fusariosis remains an enigma, particularly since it afflicts the same group of patients. Initially, patients present with fever despite coverage with broad-spectrum antibiotics, followed by dry cough and dyspnea. As angioinvasion and tissue necrosis set in, haemoptysis or full-blown haemorrhage may develop. Pulmonary fusariosis, zygomycosis and aspergillosis may all lead to secondary cutaneous involvement due to haematogenous dissemination. In this case, raised, painful erythematous lesions with a varying degree of central necrosis can be found.

Diagnosis

Although sensitivity of CT for detection of pulmonary fungal lesions is much higher than that of chest radiographs (Ascioglu *et al.*, 2002), it does not allow for reliable distinction of the different filamentous fungi. Aspergillus and zygomycetes present as multiple, bilateral nodular opacities with a peripheral distribution. Small (<1 cm) multiple nodules (≥10) suggest infection with a zygomycete rather than with Aspergillus. Air-space consolidation, cavitary lesions, the halo and air crescent sign, as well as pleural effusions are occasionally observed (Kontoyiannis *et al.*, 2005). Data on the radiological appearance of pulmonary fusariosis are scarce.

Blood cultures are positive in about 50% of infections with *Fusarium* spp. (Boutati and Anaissie, 1997), while agents of zygomycosis can rarely be isolated. Alternatively, suspect lesions may be biopsied and submitted to culture and histopathological examination. Zygomycetes have a distinct appearance, but *Aspergillus* and *Fusarium* spp. may be confounded, since their hyphae are both thin, hyaline, regularly shaped and with a frequent branching pattern.

Treatment

Before initiation of antifungal therapy, the impact of metabolic and immunosuppressive risk factors should be minimized. Surgical debridement of necrotic tissue should be attempted if no limitations due to neutropenia and thrombocytopenia exist. Lipid formulations of amphotericin B remain the treatment of choice (Perfect, 2005; Spellberg *et al.*, 2005; Paphitou *et al.*, 2002), but alternative antifungal agents are subject to clinical trials. Voriconazole is not active against zygomycetes (Kontoyiannis *et al.*, 2005), but can be used as second line therapy of invasive fusariosis (Perfect *et al.*, 2003). The clinical efficacy of posaconazole oral solution as salvage therapy in fusariosis, zygomycosis and aspergillosis has been shown in non-randomized trials. An intravenous formulation is being developed and might permit the use of posaconazole in the initial treatment of invasive fungal infections.

Outcome

Using lipid formulations of amphotericin B, invasive zygomycosis has been associated with mortality rates of 39% (Roden *et al.*, 2005). Invasive fusariosis reaches mortality rates of up to 100%, particularly if neutropenia does not resolve (Lionakis and Kontoyiannis, 2004; Nucci *et al.*, 2004).

Pneumocystis jiroveci (PCP)

Pneumocystis jiroveci pneumonia is a severe interstitial pneumonia caused by ubiquitous fungal pathogen in immunocompromised patients. It often presents with a triad of dry cough, fever and dyspnoea, but sometimes may present atypically or asymptomatic. While early treatment is imperative, bronchoalveolar lavage should be performed to confirm diagnosis. The role of PCR remains unclear and immunofluorescence microscopy should be performed. First line treatment: intravenous trimethoprim and sulfamethoxazole (TMP-SMX). Second line treatment: pentamidine. Adjunctive glucocorticoids in non-AIDS patients have not yet been evaluated. Prognosis depends on timely treatment onset and mortality may reach 40% in non-AIDS patients.

Etiology

Pneumocystis jiroveci is an ubiquitous fungal pathogen. It is highly host specific and cannot infect other mammals than humans. Infection is probably caused upon inhalation of trophic forms deep into the alveolar system. More than 85% of children are seropositive when they are 30 months old. There is an ongoing debate on the role of human to human transmission or environmental contamination. Isolation measures for infected patients are currently not recommended. Additionally, it remains uncertain whether infection occurs by reactivation of colonizing pathogens or by *de novo* infection. The incidence of PCP among non-AIDS patients has not yet been investigated. However, series of PCP in leukemia patients with long-term neutropenia after remission induction chemotherapy have been reported and there are numerous well documented cases in patients with other kinds of immunosuppression, most notably enduring and high-dosed treatment with glucocorticosteroids, but also at only 15 mg QD for 8 weeks.

Pathogenesis

After invading the alveolar system via the airways, the trophic form of the fungus attaches to alveolar macrophages type I. There it starts taking up nutrients from the host environment. Pneumocystis jiroveci reproduces itself by binary fission (asexual growth) or by conjugation forming a cyst with subsequent meiosis and mitosis ultimately producing eight trophic forms. In the later course of the infection, abundant pathogen loads fill the alveolar lumen and cause severe local inflammation typically presenting hyaline membranes, interstitial fibrosis, and oedema in histopathology. Inflammation and fungal burden reduce diffusion capacity, compliance and vital capacity, thus causing severe hypoxemia.

Clinical presentation

Signs and symptoms of PCP are well known in non-AIDS patients, but PCP may have a more rapid course in neutropenic patients. The classical triad is high fever, dry cough and dyspnoea. Sputum and crackles are much less frequent. Often, exertional dyspnoea may be the first and only clinical indicator of PCP.

Diagnosis

As *Pneumocystis jiroveci* is an ubiquitous pathogen, only patients at risk should be diagnosed to avoid false positive results. After clinical suspicion, a chest X-ray (sensitivity 75%) should be performed (DeLorenzo *et al.*, 1987). Typical presentation of PCP is a bilateral diffuse alveolar or interstitial infiltrate setting off from the lung hilus. Spiral and high resolution CT (HRCT) of the lung reach a sensitivity of almost 100% and often show the classical bilateral patchy ground glass opacities declining from the hilus to the periphery (see Figures 6.4 and 6.5) (Hidalgo *et al.*, 2003).

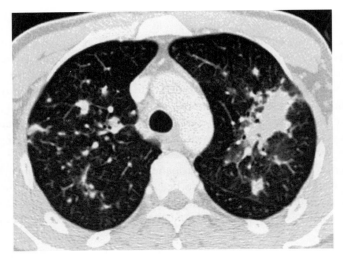

Figure 6.4   Nodular and patchy infiltrates caused by PCP in a neutropenic patient.

While imaging studies have high sensitivity, specificity is low in cancer patients undergoing chemotherapy, as numerous other conditions and diseases may cause similar lung infiltrates. Diagnosis should always be confirmed by bronchoalveolar lavage (or endotracheal aspirate from intubated patients) with immunofluorescence staining (Willocks *et al.*, 1993). If microbial results are negative but clinical suspicion is high, transbronchial or fine-needle biopsies should be obtained. The value of the PCR in the diagnosis of PCP has not yet been established. PCR often fails to differentiate between contamination, harmless colonization and actual infection. Positive PCR results must be interpreted cautiously to avoid over treatment.

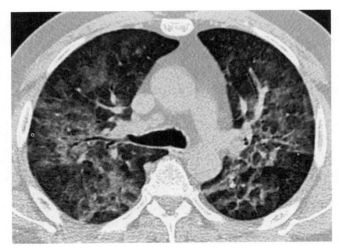

Figure 6.5   Patchy infiltrates and ground glass opacities starting at the lung hilus in a neutropenic patient with PCP.

Treatment

Standard treatment for PCP in non-AIDS patients remains intravenous TMP-SMX with trimethoprim 20 mg/kg plus sulfamethoxazole 100 mg/kg TID (Warren *et al.*, 1997). Treatment response usually occurs within the first seven days after treatment initiation. However, especially in patients with a high burden of disease, respiratory distress may worsen after two to three days of treatment. Adjunctive corticosteroids may play a minor role compared to AIDS patients, but may be considered in patients with severe infection (Pareja *et al.*, 1998). Initial dose should be 40 mg prednisone BID. After five days, dose may be reduced to 40 mg QD and finally, after 10 days, to 20 mg QD for the remainder of the therapy. Treatment duration is 14– 21 days, depending on treatment response and immunological status of the patient. Patients recovering from PCP should receive oral TMP-SMX in all future episodes at risk, usually 160 mg TMP with 800 mg SMX QD or three times weekly.

Oral treatment has not been evaluated in non-AIDS patients. As burden of disease is often higher in non-AIDS patients, oral and/or outpatient treatment is not recommended. In patients intolerant of or refractory to high-dosed TMP-SMX, intravenous pentamidine 4 mg/kg QD should be considered (Klein *et al.*, 1992; Siegel *et al.*, 1984; Hughes *et al.*, 1978). Because of frequent adverse events, patients should be monitored for hypotension and hypoglycaemia.

Outcome

Mortality of PCP usually is around 10%; however, figures up to 40% have been reported in non-AIDS patients (Mansharamani *et al.*, 2000).

Disseminated candidiasis

Neutropenic patients are at high risk for invasive candidiasis. Within the clinical pattern of acute (ADC) or chronic (CDC) disseminated candidiasis, secondary *Candida* pneumonia may develop. Primary pulmonary infection by *Candida* spp. is rare. Symptoms of disseminated infection usually mask respiratory symptoms. The definite diagnosis of invasive candidiasis is made by cultures or cyto- or histopathological examination of biopsies. Currently available treatment options include polyenes, azoles and echinocandins.

Etiology and epidemiology

Patients with haematological malignancies bear a high risk for invasive *Candida* spp. infection (Hajjeh *et al.*, 2004; Chen *et al.*, 2006). During febrile neutropenia, 3–5% of all blood cultures are positive for *Candida* spp. (Marr *et al.*, 2000; Pfaller *et al.*, 1998a; Pfaller *et al.*, 1998b). Additional risk factors include central venous catheters, total parenteral nutrition, broad-spectrum antibiosis, high APACHE II scores, renal failure and gastrointestinal surgery (Chen *et al.*, 2006; Marr *et al.*, 2000; Viscoli *et al.*, 1999).

Although more than 50% of all Candida infections are still caused by *C. albicans*, a recent increase in the incidence of non-*Candida albicans* infections, especially *C. tropicalis* and *C. parapsilosis* has been observed (Pfaller *et al.*, 2007).

While candidemia is the most common type of invasive candidiasis, progression to acute or chronic disseminated candidiasis may ensue. Both entities share fever refractory to antibiotic treatment as their principal symptom. Acute invasive candidiasis presents during the neutropenic phase whereas chronic disseminated candidiasis develops only after recovery from neutropenia (Bodey and Luna, 1998). In both clinical entities, secondary *Candida* pneumonia may occur and is associated with a high mortality rate (Bodey *et al.*, 1992; Hughes, 1982).

Pathogenesis

Candida spp. are part of the normal intestinal flora, and haematogenous dissemination in the neutropenic patient usually occurs by penetration of the gastrointestinal tract wall. Other possible routes of infection include indwelling catheters and, less frequently, invasion starting from a local infective focus. In the absence of candida blood stream infection primary invasive candidiasis of the lung may occur, however, its incidence is ill-defined and probably low (Masur *et al.*, 1977; Kontoyiannis *et al.*, 2002; Haron *et al.*, 1993).

Clinical presentation

The clinical manifestations of invasive candidiasis are often unspecific. In the neutropenic patient, fever or progressive sepsis, refractory to broad spectrum antibiotics, as well as multiple organ failure, are clinical clues. In acute disseminated candidiasis, indicative organ specific symptoms include maculopapular rash (Bodey and Luna, 1974) and endophthalmitis (Bouza *et al.*, 2000). Chronic disseminated candidiasis is usually confined to the liver and spleen, presenting as hepatomegaly accompanied by abdominal pain, nausea and vomiting. In general, pulmonary invasion during candidiasis remains asymptomatic. Nevertheless, cough, pleuritic chest pain, tachypnea and hemoptysis have been observed in probable cases of primary *Candida* pneumonia (Masur *et al.*, 1977; Haron *et al.*, 1993).

Diagnosis

Radiographic signs of pulmonary candidiasis are nonspecific and overlap with the findings in other opportunistic infections. Mixed bilateral alveolar-interstitial infiltrates (Figure 6.6) is the most common presentation (Buff *et al.*, 1982; Haron *et al.*, 1993; Masur *et al.*, 1977) but exsudative pleural effusions as well as unilateral lobar or segmental disease have also been reported (Buff *et al.*, 1982). Only one case of cavitation is known (Watanakunakorn, 1983) and this sign might rather be used as an exclusion criteria. Lucencies in the liver and spleen on ultrasound, magnetic resonance imaging, or CT scan are typical signs of chronic disseminated candidiasis.

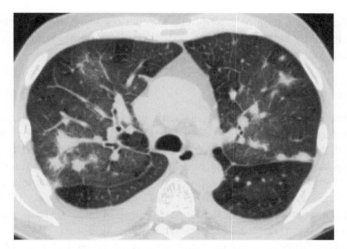

Figure 6.6 Mixed interstitial and patchy infiltrates caused by *Candida* sp. infection in a neutropenic patient.

The definite laboratory diagnosis of invasive candidiasis can be made by culture of usually sterile body fluids or tissues and/or cyto- or histopathological examination of biopsy specimens (Ascioglu *et al.*, 2002). However, it should be noted that in leukemia patients, only 25% disseminated candida infections can be identified by a positive blood culture (Pagano *et al.*, 2002). For a serologic result to be considered significant, a fourfold increase in paired serologies is required, representing a rarity in the immuno-compromised host. Molecular diagnostic methods are still in the investigatory phase. Chronic invasive candidiasis is frequently accompanied by elevation of the serum alkaline phosphatase.

Treatment

Fluconazole, voriconazole, liposomal amphotericin B and the three echinocandins, caspofungin, anidulafungin and micafungin are gradually replacing the former gold standard amphotericin B deoxycholate. While the azoles may be administered orally, the echinocandins may be valued due to their favourable interaction and toxicity profiles.

Outcome

With promptly administered therapy, mortality in invasive candidiasis is 10–17% (Kuse *et al.*, 2007; Reboli *et al.*, 2007).

Cryctococcal pneumonia

Patients with lymphoproliferative disorders and haematological malignancies are at risk of reactivation of latent *Cryptococcus neoformans* infection. Clinical disease may remain confined to the lung or disseminate to other organs, particularly the CNS. The diagnosis is made by culture, histology and – most importantly – antigen assay. First-line treatment: amphotericin B plus flucytosine. Survival rate: 95%.

Etiology and epidemiology

C. neoformans is an encapsulated yeast with a worldwide geographical distribution pattern. Its natural habitat has been associated with soil contaminated by bird droppings as well as with the presence of certain trees. The infection is contracted by inhalation of the basidiospore form of the fungus. Immunocompromised individuals, including patients with lymphoproliferative disorders or certain hematologic malignancies, such as chronic lymphocytic leukemia (Collins *et al.*, 1951; Kaplan *et al.*, 1977; Huter and Collins, 1962) are at an increased risk of reactivation of latent disease. Additional risk factors include organ failure, diabetes, rheumatic diseases, HIV, treatment with corticosteroids or tumour necrosis factor antagonist (Arend *et al.*, 2004; Cameron *et al.*, 1991; Kerkering *et al.*, 1981; Pappas *et al.*, 2001).

Pathogenesis

Once the inhaled basidiospores reach the alveoli, macrophages are activated, inducing Th1 response and granulomatous inflammation. Consequently, a primary complex similar to that seen in tuberculosis may develop (Baker, 1976). Therein, the pathogens remain dormant until future deterioration of the host's immune status. In the immuno-compromised individual, prompt proliferation and dissemination of the pathogen may ensue, resulting in clinical disease.

Clinical presentation

Patients with pulmonary cryptococcosis are usually symptomatic, presenting with fever, chest pain, dyspnea, haemoptysis, weight loss and night sweats. Progression may be rapid (Henson and Hill, 1984) leading to adult respiratory distress syndrome and dissemination to other organs, particularly the CNS (Kerkering *et al.*, 1981; Pappas *et al.*, 2001).

Diagnosis

Radiological signs vary widely and often mimic malignant disease. At the initial stage of disease, the primary complex often appears as a well defined, non-calcified node. Sometimes multiple nodes may be observed. Other radiological findings include lobar infiltrates, hilar adenopathy, cavitation and pleural effusion (Hunt *et al.*, 1976; Feigin, 1983).

The diagnosis of pulmonary cryptococcosis is made by positive culture of respiratory specimens or by histology of infected tissue. Serum cryptococcal antigen testing is far less reliable for non–HIV-infected patients than for HIV-positive patients (Jensen *et al.*,

1985; Pappas *et al.*, 2001) but a positive result suggests deep tissue invasion with a high likelihood of disseminated disease. CNS involvement should always be ruled out using India ink examination, culture and cryptococcal antigen assay of CSF specimens.

Treatment

Induction therapy with a combination of amphotericin B and flucytosine is recommended during the first 14–21 days of treatment (Pappas *et al.*, 2001), followed by 8–10 weeks of oral fluconazole (400–800 mg qd). Afterwards, low dose fluconazole (200 mg qd) should be maintained over 6–12 months (Saag *et al.*, 2000).

Outcome

A 12 month survival rate of 95% in non-HIV immunocompromised patients with pulmonary cryptococcosis has been reported. Age over 60 years and concomitant organ failure significantly influenced the outcome (Pappas *et al.*, 2001).

Viral pneumonia

Cytomegalovirus (CMV) and the community acquired respiratory viruses (CRV) are common causative agents of viral pneumonia in the neutropenic patient, associated with significant morbidity and mortality rates. Viral pneumonia in the neutropenic patients is marked by its severity and its great variability of clinical and radiological signs. Viral culture, detection of viral antigen or nucleic acid, and to a lesser extent, serologic analysis, can be used for diagnosis. Ganciclovir is the gold standard in the prophylaxis and treatment of CMV pneumonia after allogeneic hematopoietic stem cell transplantation (HSCT). Few options exist for the prophylaxis and treatment of the CRV.

Etiology and epidemiology

Traditionally, bacteria, fungi and CMV were considered to be the main infectious etiologies of lower respiratory disease in the neutropenic patient. Recent diagnostic advances have, however, revealed that the community acquired respiratory viruses (CRV), including respiratory syncytical virus (RSV), parainfluenza, adenovirus and influenza A and B, also play a significant role in this setting. In rare cases, pulmonary infection may be caused by Herpes simplex virus (HSV), Varizella zoster virus (VZV) and Epstein Barr virus (EBV).

Patients undergoing allogeneic HSCT are particularly prone to viral pulmonary infections. T-cell depletion, unrelated or HLA-mismatched transplants and severe graft versus host disease represent additional risk factors (Shenoy *et al.*, 1999; Holler, 2002; Cornely *et al.*, 2004), while the duration and severity of neutropenia are of less importance. In this setting, CMV pneumonia is the most common life-threatening disease (Meyers *et al.*, 1986) with mortality rates of up to 84%, usually occurring during the first 30 to 100 days after transplantation (Meyers *et al.*, 1986). With the availability of prophylactic strategies, the risk of CMV infection after HSCT is of 1–3% (Boeckh *et al.*, 1996b). Pulmonary CRV infection usually occurs during pre- and early post-engraftment and is associated with significant morbidity and mortality rates (Kim *et al.*, 2007). HSV predominates in the pre-engraftment phase, while VZV and EBV are more common three to six months after engraftment.

Pathogenesis

In the neutropenic patient, CMV, HSV, VZV, EBV and adenovirus infections are mostly reactivations of latent asymptomatic infections and thus occur throughout the year. RSV, influenza and parainfluenza are exogenous infections transmitted by contact with infectious secretions or inhalation of aerosols. They obey a seasonal pattern, even in the immunocompromised patient.

Clinical presentation

Viral pneumonia in the neutropenic patient is characterized by its particular severity, prolonged duration and variability of symptoms. After an incubation period of about two to five days, initial infection often presents with mild to moderate symptoms of an upper respiratory tract infection, such as rhinorrea, sinus congestion, sore throat and otitis media. Instead of resolution after two to four days, aggravation of symptoms, including cough, dyspnea and wheezing, indicates progression to the lower respiratory tract. Respiratory failure requiring assisted ventilation often ensues. Auscultation reveals focal chest signs such as rales, rhonchi and expiratory wheezing. Superinfection of viral pneumonia with microbial and fungal pathogens is common.

In CMV, HSV, VZV and adenovirus infections, additional symptoms of disseminated disease may be observed. In influenza A and B infections are characterized by a short incubation time of only one or two days. Thereafter, systemic symptoms, such as rapidly rising, persisting high fevers, myalgias, headache, chills and anorexia predominate.

Diagnosis

Compared to the immunocompetent patient with viral pneumonia whose chest radiographs and CT are characterized by interstitial infiltration, the neutropenic patient often displays an increased variety of radiological signs. Findings may include focal interstitial infiltrates (see Figure 6.7), lobar consolidation and diffuse alveolar-interstitial infiltrates (Hall, 2001).

A wide spectrum of techniques for the diagnosis of viral diseases is available. In CMV infection, serology is mainly used to determine the serostatus of patients in high risk situations. Active CMV infection can be identified in culture, but some molecular approaches have the advantage of yielding both, qualitative and quantitative results. The detection of CMV matrix protein pp65 (van der Bij *et al.*, 1988), CMV DNA PCR assays (Schulenburg *et al.*, 2001; Boivin *et al.*, 2000; Masaoka *et al.*, 2001; Sia *et al.*, 2000) and Hybrid Capture CMV DNA assay (Ho *et al.*, 2000; Mazzulli *et al.*, 1999) have been adapted by clinical laboratories.

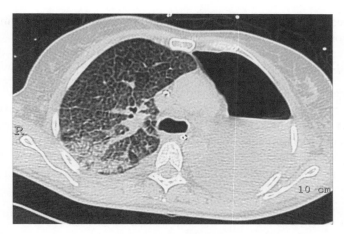

Figure 6.7 CMV pneumonitis with typical interstitial infiltrates in a pneumectomized neutropenic patient.

Similar approaches based on viral culture, detection of viral antigen or nucleic acid, and to a lesser extent, serologic analysis, are used for diagnosis of the other viral infections mentioned above.

Prophylaxis and treatment

Since allogeneic HSCT is the most common underlying immunosuppressive factor in viral pneumonia in the haemato-oncological patient, discussion of prophylaxis and treatment will be limited to this setting.

Cytomegalovirus (CMV)

The gold standard in the treatment of CMV pneumonia during allogeneic HSCT is a combination of ganciclovir and high-titer CMV immune globulin (Reed *et al.*, 1988; Schmidt *et al.*, 1988). Preventive strategies rely on two approaches, antiviral CMV prophylaxis and pre-emptive treatment. Owing to toxicity and the development of late-onset CMV disease after prolonged ganciclovir treatment, prophylaxis with ganciclovir cannot be generally recommended. Only in specific settings, such as T-cell depletion, severe chronic GvHD and intensive use of glucocorticoids can its use be justified (Zaia, 2002). Pre-emptive therapy depends on the results of weekly monitoring of CMV replication (Boeckh *et al.*, 1996b; Einsele *et al.*, 1995). Therapy with ganciclovir should be initiated after a single positive pp65 antigen test or after two consecutive positive CMV PCR assays. Continuation of weekly monitoring is recommended until at least 100 days after HSCT (Guidelines, 2000a) but should be extended up to one year in patients with chronic GvHD, prolonged immunosuppression or T-cell depletion. Even though official approval is still lacking, pre-emptive therapy of CMV infection with foscarnet shows similar efficacy as with ganciclovir, while bearing a lower incidence of neutropenia (Reusser *et al.*, 2002). Valganciclovir, an oral antiviral drug, allowing for outpatient treatment, has already been approved for CMV prophylaxis in solid organ transplantation but not in HSCT.

Herpes simplex virus (HSV) and varizella zoster virus (VZV)

During allogeneic HSCT, acyclovir should be administered to all HSV seropositive patients (Saral *et al.*, 1983). VZV seronegative patients should be protected from persons with active chickenpox or zoster, and if exposure occurs, passive VZV immunization is recommended if concomitant risk factors, such as chronic GvHD, immunosuppressive medication or a period of over two years after HSCT are present (Sandherr *et al.*, 2006). Active HSV or VZV disease may be treated with acyclovir as well.

Esptein Barr virus (EBV)

EBV seronegative patients with additional risk factors, including T-cell depletion, antithymocyte globulin therapy, anti-CD3 antibody therapy and unrelated or HLA-mismatch transplantation should be submitted to biweekly monitoring. In the presence of ≥ 1000 genome equivalents/ml or a steeply rising titer, a single dose of rituximab should be considered (van Esser *et al.*, 2002).

Community acquired respiratory viruses (CRV)

Prevention of CRV infection relies mainly on taking standard and contact precautions. FDA (Food and Drug Administration) approved prevention and treatment regimen of CRV infections in the neutropenic patient are limited. In paediatric patients, palivizumab has been approved for prevention of RSV infection in patients at high risk. The preventive and therapeutical use of aerosolized ribavirin (Boeckh *et al.*, 2007; Harrington *et al.*, 1992) and of RSV immune globulins (Schmidt *et al.*, 1988; DeVincenzo *et al.*, 2000; Ghosh *et al.*, 2000) has been discussed controversially.

Influenzaviruses

The medical staff caring for patients undergoing HSCT as well as close relatives should receive regular influenza vaccinations. The neuraminidase inhibitors oseltamivir or zanamivir can be considered in endemic regions and seasons (Smith *et al.*, 2006). They are also indicated in the treatment of active influenza disease (Hayden *et al.*, 1997; Hayden *et al.*, 1999; Treanor *et al.*, 2000). The use of amantadine and rimantadine has been abandoned due to emerging resistances.

Outcome

Complete recovery of viral pulmonary infection takes at least four to eight weeks, but may be impeded in patients with significant pulmonary fibrosis or an immunocompromising condition such as GvHD or prolonged use of glucocorticosteroids (Whimbey and Ghosh, 2000).

Tuberculosis

Since neutropenia is not per se a risk factor for tuberculosis, the incidence of tuberculosis largely depends on the risk factors originating from endemic countries and possible recent infection. Since the incidence is low also in endemic countries, and since presenting disease patterns may be altered, the diagnosis must rely on a high index of suspicion. Culture and susceptibility testing remains the mainstay for the design of adequate antituberculous treatment. Treatment regimen and the management of complications or drug resistance as well as preventive measures should follow the general national or international recommendations for the management of tuberculosis. The outcome is usually favourable.

Epidemiology

Tuberculosis as an infectious complication of neutropenia is only rarely found in Western countries. In a large recent survey of the M. D. Anderson Cancer Center of patients with tuberculosis from January 2001 until April 2005, 18 patients with active tuberculosis and cancer were identified. The overall rate of active tuberculosis during this period was 0.2 in 1000 new cancer diagnoses. There were 18 men (69%), the median age was 54 years (range, 3–84 years), and 16 patients (62%) were born in the US. Only five patients had a hematologic malignancy (three of those non-Hodgkin lymphoma). No patient had a recent history (within the past four weeks) of chemotherapy; only four patients had neutropenia (Aisenberg et al.,).

In fact, the incidence of tuberculosis strongly depends on the rate of latent tuberculosis infection (LTBI) in a given population and the risk of acquiring a new tuberculous infection; neutropenia itself does not contribute significantly to the risk of manifest tuberculosis. Also treatment with monoclonal antibodies in neutropenic patients has as yet not been associated with significant increased rates of tuberculosis (Wendtner et al., 2004).

Having said this, it is understandable that most reports of tuberculosis in neutropenia come from endemic areas. For example in a series over a two-year period of 130 consecutive patients with acute leukemia from India, nine cases (6.9%) had active tuberculosis. Interestingly, patients with AML were more likely to develop TB as compared to patients with acute lymphoblastic leukemia (ALL) despite the wider use of steroids and radiotherapy in ALL protocols (Mishra et al., 2006). In another series over a two-year period of 91 consecutive patients with acute leukemia from India, tuberculosis was found in only two of the 162 febrile episodes during neutropenia (Jagarlamudi et al., 2000). In one review of tuberculosis in blood and bone marrow transplant patients, the overall frequency was 52 cases among 13 881 BMT recipients (0.4%). Risk factors associated with tuberculosis were endemic countries, allogeneic transplantation, graft-versus-host disease, and total body irradiation. However, among the 48 cases in whom the time of manifestation was reported, only one case manifested during the neutropenic period (day 11) (Yuen and Woo, 2002). In one recent series from India covering a 15-year period and including 297 patients undergoing 304 allogenic transplants, only 2.3% of patients developed tuberculosis (George et al., 2004).

Pathogenesis

Antimycobacterial immune response mainly involves T lymphocytes activating the macrophages and their microbicidal functions through the release of interferon-gamma (IFN-gamma). After the priming in lymph nodes, memory CD4 and CD8-cells become central components of immunity. Humoural immunity plays little part in protection against tuberculosis. Numerous host genes have been identified favouring *M. tuberculosis* infections. Individuals with defective cellular immunity such as HIV-infection or after solid organ transplantation are much more susceptible to disease from *M. tuberculosis* and are more likely to have a disseminated form of tuberculosis. Patients with neutropenia are not per se at increased risk to develop active tuberculosis.

Clinical presentation

Descriptions of the clinical presentation of tuberculosis in neutropenic patients are scarce. In the M. D. Anderson Cancer Center survey addressed above, 15 patients (58%) had extrapulmonary infection, including five patients with concurrent pulmonary involvement; seven noncancer patients (88%) and eight cancer patients (44%, $p = 0.22$) had extrapulmonary disease. In 11 patients (42%), the lungs were the only site of active tuberculosis. Cavitary tuberculosis was present only in three of 16 patients (19%) (Aisenberg *et al.*,). In fact, it seems at least in patients with BMT, clinical patterns usually mimic other more common infectious and non-infectious complications after BMT. Thus, beyond classical clinical signs and radiographic patterns, a high index of suspicion, particularly in patients from endemic countries is mandatory to make the appropriate diagnosis.

Diagnosis

The diagnosis of tuberculosis is made by smear and culture from respiratory and other clinical samples such as sputum, bronchoalveolar lavage fluid, pleural fluid, and urine. Rapid diagnosis may be established by PCR for Mycobacterium tuberculosis. Pathogen isolation and susceptibility testing is mandatory in every case.

The Infectious Disease Society of Taiwan has published guidelines for use of antimicrobial agents in patients with febrile neutropenia and included special considerations for the diagnosis of tuberculosis due to its high prevalence in Taiwan (although a relatively uncommon pathogen of febrile neutropenia even there) (Infectious Diseases Society of Taiwan, 2005). According to this guideline, febrile neutropenic patients with a normal chest radiography and persistent fever after more than two weeks and patients with old TB or nonspecific changes in chest radiography should be evaluated for tuberculosis. This algorithm may be useful also for patients from endemic regions in Western countries.

Treatment

Patients born in non-endemic areas can safely be treated with standard regimen including four drugs (H, R, Z, E) during two months and two drugs (H, R) for the following seven months. In patients born and/or living in endemic countries with high incidence of multiresistance, it may be prudent to start with a five drug regimen (H, R, Z, E, S) and continue according to susceptibility testing. The management of patients intolerant to antituberculous medications or drug resistance should follow general national or international recommendations as provided, for example, by the ATS/CDC/ IDSA (Blumberg *et al.*, 2003).

Prophylaxis

Chemoprophylaxis and preventive treatment should also follow general national or international recommendations as provided, for example, by the ATS/CDC/IDSA (American Thoracic Society, 2005). There are no specific considerations for patients expected to undergo neutropenia.

Outcome

The outcome is usually favourable, provided that the treatment regimen was adequate and the patient was compliant. There are no data about the outcome of neutropenic patients with multidrug resistant tuberculosis.

Toxoplasmosis

Toxoplasma gondii is a worldwide protozoon. Recipients of allogeneic haemato-poietic stem cell (HSCT) transplantation may experience recrudescence of latent infection in the post-engraftment phase. Pulmonary involvement occurs within the clinical picture of disseminated toxoplasmosis and is associated with high mortality rates. First-line prophylaxis and treatment for allogeneic HSCT recipients: trimethoprim-sulfamethoxazole (TMZ-SMZ).

Etiology and epidemiology

T. gondii is an intracellular protozoon with worldwide geographic distribution, belonging to the subphylum *Apicomplexa*. Felines, the definite hosts, shed infectious oocysts in their faeces. Active disease in the immunocompromised individual usually occurs through reactivation of latent infection. Apart from HIV patients, this may also be observed among individuals with complex immune deficiencies, for example, allogeneic HSCT recipients (Martino *et al.*, 2000). In this subpopulation, the incidence of toxoplasmosis ranges from 0.3 to 5%. Risk factors include the presence of pre-transplant antibodies and concomitant Graft-versus-host-disease (GvHD) (Mele *et al.*, 2002). Primary infection of sero-negative HSCT recipients is an infrequent event that may occur via ingestion of contaminated water, food or undercooked meat or reception of blood products or transplants (Dubey *et al.*, 1998).

Pathogenesis

Following ingestion, bradyzoites released from tissue cysts or sporozoites released from oocytes invade the epithelium of the gastrointestinal tract. After intracellular multiplication, spread to distant organs, particularly the CNS, lung and muscles, occurs via mesenteric lymph nodes.

Clinical presentation

In allogeneic HSCT recipients, clinical signs and symptoms may be limited. Clinical disease is generally confined to the CNS. Isolated infection of the lung is rare (Chandrasekar and Momin, 1997) and pulmonary symptons, such as dyspnoea, hypoxemia, tachypnea, cough and/or fever usually suggest dissemination, particularly if presented between 30 and 100 days after HSCT (Mele *et al.*, 2002). In this case, progression to adult respiratory distress syndrome often ensues (Sing *et al.*, 1999).

Diagnosis

Radiological signs of pulmonary toxoplasmosis are highly variable. Interstitial infiltrates are the most common presentation, but alveolar infiltrates, consolidation and pleural effusion may also be observed (Mariuz *et al.*, 1997).

Pre-transplantation serum IgG titers should be obtained from all allogeneic HSCT recipients, allowing for the identification of seropositive patients. Post-engraftment titers are not reliable. In pulmonary toxoplasmosis, the microscopic examination of bronchoalveolar lavage (BAL) fluid may reveal the presence of tachyzoites within alveolocytes and alveolar macrophages, and *T. gondii* DNA may be detected using PCR.

Treatment and prophylaxis

Seronegative allogeneic HSCT recipients should be informed of the risks for contracting toxoplasmosis. Additionally, TMP-SMZ prophylaxis is administered to seropositive patients with concomitant risk factors, such as active GvHD or a prior history of toxoplasma chorioretinitis (Peacock *et al.*, 1995; Foot *et al.*, 1994). The optimum dosage for this indication is still unknown. The rare occurrence of primary infection in seronegative individuals undergoing HSCT (Chandrasekar and Momin, 1997) has raised the question whether the indication for prophylaxis should be extended. TMP-SMZ is also used in the treatment of active toxoplasmosis. A combination of clindamycin, pyrimethamine and leucovorin is a valuable second line option (Koplan *et al.*, 2000). Subsequent secondary prophylaxis is recommended.

Outcome

Pulmonary toxoplasmosis in the immunocompromised patient has been associated with mortality rates higher than 90% (Sing *et al.*, 1999).

References

Abernathy-Carver, K.J., Fan, L.L., Boguniewicz, M., Larsen, G.L. and Leung, D.Y. (1994) Legionella and Pneumocystis pneumonias in asthmatic children on high doses of systemic steroids. *Pediatric Pulmonology*, **18**, 135–138.

Afessa, B., Peters, S.G. (2006) Major complications following hematopoietic stem cell transplantation. *Seminar in Respiratory and Critical Care Medicine*, **27**(3), 297–309.

Aisenberg, G.M., Jacobson, K., Chemaly, R.F., Rolston, K.V., Raad, I.I. and Safdar, A. (2005) Extrapulmonary tuberculosis active infection misdiagnosed as cancer: Mycobacterium tuberculosis disease in patients at a Comprehensive Cancer Center (2001–2005). *Cancer*, **104**, 2882–2887.

American Thoracic Society; Centers for Disease Control and Prevention; Infectious Diseases Society of America (2005) American Thoracic Society/Centers for Disease Control and Prevention/Infectious Diseases Society of America: controlling tuberculosis in the United States. *American Journal of Respiratory and Critical Care Medicine*, **172**, 1169–1227.

Ammari, L.K., Puck, J.M. and Mcgowan, K.L. (1993) Catheter-related Fusarium solani fungemia and pulmonary infection in a patient with leukemia in remission. *Clinical Infectious Diseases*, **16**, 148–150.

Arend, S.M., Kuijper, E.J., Allaart, C.F., Muller, W.H. and van Dissel, J.T. (2004) Cavitating pneumonia after treatment with infliximab and prednisone. *European Journal of Clinical Microbiology & Infectious Diseases*, **23**, 638–641.

Ascioglu, S., Rex, J.H., de Pauw, B., DBennett, J.E., Bille, J., Crokaert, F., Denning, D.W., Donnelly, J.P., Edwards, J.E., Erjavec, Z., Fiere, D., Lortholary, O., Maertens, J., Meis, J.F., Patterson, T.F., Ritter, J., Selleslag, D., Shah, P.M., Stevens, D.A. and Walsh, T.J. (2002) Defining opportunistic invasive fungal infections in immunocompromised patients with cancer and hematopoietic stem cell transplants: an international consensus. *Clinical Infectious Diseases*, **34**, 7–14.

Baker, R.D. (1976) The primary pulmonary lymph node complex of cryptococcosis. *American Journal of Clinical Pathology*, **65**, 83–92.

Bergmann, L., Fenchel, K., Jahn, B., Mitrou, P.S. and Hoelzer, D. (1993) Immunosuppressive effects and clinical response of fludarabine in refractory chronic lymphocytic leukemia. *Annals of Oncology*, **4**, 371–375.

Blumberg, H.M., Burman, W.J., Chaisson, R.E., Daley, C.L., Etkinf, S.C., Friedman, L.N., Fujiwara, P., Gremzska, M., Hopewell, P.C., Iseman, M.D., Jasmer, R.M., Koppaka, V., Menzies, R.I., O'Brien, R.J., Reves, R.R., Reichman, L.B., Simone, P.M., Starke, J.R. and Vernon, A.A. (2003) American Thoracic Society, Centers for Disease Control, Prevention, the Infectious Disease Society. *American Journal of Respiratory and Critical Care Medicine*, **167**, 603–662.

Bodey, G., Bueltmann, B., Duguid, W., Gibbs, D., Hanak, H., Hotchi, M., Mall, G., Martino, P., Meunier, F., Milliken, S. *et al.* (1992) Fungal infections in cancer patients: an international autopsy survey. *European Journal of Clinical Microbiology & Infectious Diseases*, **11**, 99–109.

Bodey, G.P., Buckley, M., Sathe, Y.S. and Freireich, E.J. (1966) Quantitative relationships between circulating leukocytes and infection in patients with acute leukemia. *Annals of Internal Medicine*, **64**, 328–340.

Bodey, G.P. and Luna, M. (1974) Skin lesions associated with disseminated candidiasis. *The Journal of the American Medical Association*, **229**, 1466–1468.

Bodey, G.P. and Luna, M.A. (1998) Disseminated candidiasis in patients with acute leukemia: two diseases? *Clinical Infectious Diseases*, **27**, 238.

Boeckh, M., Englund, J., Li, Y., Miller, C., Cross, A., Fernandez, H., Kuypers, J., Kim, H., Gnann, J. and Whitley, R. (2007) Randomized controlled multicenter trial of aerosolized ribavirin for respiratory syncytial virus upper respiratory tract infection in hematopoietic cell transplant recipients. *Clinical Infectious Diseases*, **44**, 245–249.

Boeckh, M., Gooley, T.A., Myerson, D., Cunningham, T., Schoch, G. and Bowden, R.A. (1996a) Cytomegalovirus pp65 antigenemia-guided early treatment with ganciclovir versus ganciclovir at engraftment after allogeneic marrow transplantation: a randomized double-blind study. *Blood*, **88**, 4063–4071.

Boeckh, M., Gooley, T.A., Myerson, D., Cunningham, T., Schoch, G. and Bowden, R.A., (1996b) Cytomegalovirus pp65 antigenemia-guided early treatment with ganciclovir versus ganciclovir at engraftment after allogeneic marrow transplantation: a randomized double-blind study. *Blood*, **88**, 4063–4071.

Boersma, W.G., Erjavec, Z., van der Werf, T.S., de Vries-Hosper, H.G., Gouw, A.S. and Manson, W.L. (2007) Bronchoscopic diagnosis of pulmonary infiltrates in granulocytopenic patients with hematologic malignancies: BAL versus PSB and PBAL. *Respiratory Medicine*, **101**(2), 317–325.

Boivin, G., Belanger, R., Delage, R., Beliveau, C., Demers, C., Goyette, N. and Roy, J. (2000) Quantitative analysis of cytomegalovirus (CMV) viremia using the pp65 antigenemia assay and the COBAS AMPLICOR CMV MONITOR PCR test after blood and marrow allogeneic transplantation. *Journal of Clinical Microbiology*, **38**, 4356–4360.

Boutati, E.I. and Anaissie, E.J. (1997) Fusarium, a significant emerging pathogen in patients with hematologic malignancy: ten years' experience at a cancer center and implications for management. *Blood*, **90**, 999–1008.

Bouza, E., Cobo-Soriano, R., Rodriguez-Creixems, M., Munoz, P., Suarez-Leoz, M. and Cortes, C. (2000) A prospective search for ocular lesions in hospitalized patients with significant bacteremia. *Clinical Infectious Diseases*, **30**, 306–312.

Bretagne, S., Costa, J.M., Foulet, F., Jabot-Lestang, L., Baud-Camus, F. and Cordonnier, C. (2000) Prospective study of toxoplasma reactivation by polymerase chain reaction in allogeneic stem-cell transplant recipients. *Transplant Infectious Disease*, **2**, 127–132.

Buff, S.J., McLelland, R., Gallis, H.A., Matthay, R. and Putman, C.E. (1982) Candida albicans pneumonia: radiographic appearance. *American Journal of Roentgenology*, **138**, 645–648.

Caillot, D., Couaillier, J.F., Bernard, A., Casasnovas, O., Denning, D.W., Mannone, L., Lopez, J., Couillault, G., Piard, F., Vagner, O. and Guy, H. (2001) Increasing volume and changing characteristics of invasive pulmonary aspergillosis on sequential thoracic computed tomography scans in patients with neutropenia. *Journal of Clinical Oncology*, **19**, 253–259.

Cameron, M.L., Bartlett, J.A., Gallis, H.A. and Waskin, H.A. (1991) Manifestations of pulmonary cryptococcosis in patients with acquired immunodeficiency syndrome. *Reviews of Infectious Diseases*, **13**, 64–67.

Canadian Clinical Trials Group (2006) A randomized trial of diagnostic techniques for ventilator-associated pneumonia. *The New England Journal of Medicine*, **355**, 2619–2630.

Chandrasekar, P.H. and Momin, F. (1997) Disseminated toxoplasmosis in marrow recipients: a report of three cases and a review of the literature. Bone Marrow Transplant Team. *Bone Marrow Transplantation*, **19**, 685–689.

Chayakulkeeree, M., Ghannoum, M.A. and Perfect, J.R. (2006) Zygomycosis: the re-emerging fungal infection. *European Journal of Clinical Microbiology & Infectious Diseases*, **25**, 215–229.

Chen, S., Slavin, M., Nguyen, Q., Marriott, D., Playford, E.G., Ellis, D. and Sorrell, T. (2006) Active surveillance for candidemia, Australia. *Emerging Infectious Diseases*, **12**, 1508–1516.

Chong, S., Lee, K.S., Kim, T.S., Chung, M.J., Chung, M.P. and Han, J. (2006) Adenovirus pneumonia in adults: radiographic and high-resolution CT findings in five patients. *American Journal of Roentgenology*, **186**, 1288–1293.

Cohen, M.L., Murphy, M.T., Counts, G.W., Buckner, C.D., Clift, R.A. and Meyers, J.D. (1983) Prediction by surveillance cultures of bacteremia among neutropenic patients treated in a protective environment. *The Journal of Infectious Diseases*, **147**, 789–793.

Collins, V.P., Gellhorn, A. and Trimble, J.R. (1951) The coincidence of cryptococcosis and disease of the reticulo-endothelial and lymphatic systems. *Cancer*, **4**, 883–889.

Cornely, O.A., Maertens, J., Bresnik, M., Ebrahimi, R., Ullmann, A.J., Bouza, E., Heussel, C.P., Lortholary, O., Rieger, C., Boehme, A., Aoun, M., Horst, H.A., Thiebaut, A., Ruhnke, M., Reichert, D., Vianelli, N., Krause, S.W., Olavarria, E. and Herbrecht, R. (2007a) Liposomal amphotericin B as initial therapy for invasive mold infection: a randomized trial comparing a high-loading dose regimen with standard dosing (AmBiLoad trial). *Clinical Infectious Diseases*, **44**, 1289–1297.

Cornely, O.A., Maertens, J., Winston, D.J., Perfect, J., Ullmann, A.J., Walsh, T.J., Helfgott, D., Holowiecki, J., Stockelberg, D., Goh, Y.T., Petrini, M., Hardalo, C., Suresh, R. and Angulo-Gonzalez, D. (2007b) Posaconazole vs. fluconazole or itraconazole prophylaxis in patients with neutropenia. *The New England Journal of Medicine*, **356**, 348–359.

Cornely, O.A., Ullmann, A.J. and Karthaus, M. (2003) Evidence-based assessment of primary antifungal prophylaxis in patients with hematologic malignancies. *Blood*, **101**, 3365–3372.

Cornely, O.A., Ullmann, A.J. and Karthaus, M. (2004) Opportunistic infections after treatment with monoclonal antibodies. *Wien Med Wochenschr*, **154**, 209–217.

Daw, M.A., Munnelly, P., Mccann, S.R., Daly, P.A., Falkiner, F.R. and Keane, C.T. (1988) Value of surveillance cultures in the management of neutropenic patients. *European Journal of Clinical Microbiology & Infectious Diseases*, **7**, 742–747.

Daxboeck, F., Rabitsch, W., Blacky, A., Stadler, M., Kyrle, P.A., Hirschl, A.M. and Koller, W. (2004) Influence of selective bowel decontamination on the organisms recovered during bacteremia in neutropenic patients. *Infection Control and Hospital Epidemiology*, **25**, 685–689.

Delorenzo, L.J., Huang, C.T., Maguire, G.P. and Stone, D.J. (1987) Roentgenographic patterns of Pneumocystis carinii pneumonia in 104 patients with AIDS. *Chest*, **91**, 323–327.

Denning, D.W. (1998) Invasive aspergillosis. *Clinical Infectious Diseases*, **26**, 781–803; quiz 804–805.

Devincenzo, J.P., Hirsch, R.L., Fuentes, R.J. and Top, F.H.J. (2000) Respiratory syncytial virus immune globulin treatment of lower respiratory tract infection in pediatric patients undergoing bone marrow transplantation – a compassionate use experience. *Bone Marrow Transplantation*, **25**, 161–165.

Dornbusch, H.J., Strenger, V., Kerbl, R., Lackner, H., Schwinger, W., Sovinz, P. and Urban, C. (2005) Procalcitonin–a marker of invasive fungal infection? *Support Care Cancer*, **13**, 343–346.

Dubey, J.P., Lindsay, D.S. and Speer, C.A. (1998) Structures of toxoplasma gondii tachyzoites, bradyzoites, and sporozoites and biology and development of tissue cysts. *Clinical Microbiology Reviews*, **11**, 267–299.

Eckmanns, T., Ruden, H. and Gastmeier, P. (2006) The influence of high-efficiency particulate air filtration on mortality and fungal infection among highly immunosuppressed patients: a systematic review. *The Journal of Infectious Diseases*, **193**, 1408–1418.

Einsele, H., Ehninger, G., Hebart, H., Wittkowski, K.M., Schuler, U., Jahn, G., Mackes, P., Herter, M., Klingebiel, T. and Loffler, J., (1995) Polymerase chain reaction monitoring reduces the incidence of cytomegalovirus disease and the duration and side effects of antiviral therapy after bone marrow transplantation. *Blood*, **86**, 2815–2820.

Einsele, H., Hebart, H., Kauffmann-Schneider, C., Sinzger, C., Jahn, G., Bader, P., Klingebiel, T., Dietz, K., Loffler, J., Bokemeyer, C., Muller, C.A. and Kanz, L. (2000) Risk factors for treatment failures in patients receiving PCR-based preemptive therapy for CMV infection. *Bone Marrow Transplantation*, **25**, 757–763.

El-Sadr, W.M., Murphy, R.L., Yurik, T.M., Luskin-Hawk, R., Cheung, T.W., Balfour, H.H., Jr, Eng, R., Hooton, T.M., Kerkering, T.M., Schutz, M., van der Horst, C. and Hafner, R. (1998) Atovaquone compared with dapsone for the prevention of Pneumocystis carinii pneumonia in patients with HIV infection who cannot tolerate trimethoprim, sulfonamides, or both. Community Program for Clinical Research on AIDS and the AIDS Clinical Trials Group. *The New England Journal of Medicine*, **339**, 1889–1895.

Elting, L.S., Rubenstein, E.B., Rolston, K.V. and Bodey, G.P. (1997) Outcomes of bacteremia in patients with cancer and neutropenia: observations from two decades of epidemiological and clinical trials. *Clinical Infectious Diseases*, **25**, 247–259.

Fauci, A.S., Dale, D.C. and Balow, J.E. (1976) Glucocorticosteroid therapy: mechanisms of action and clinical considerations. *Annals of Internal Medicine*, **84**, 304–315.

Feigin, D.S. (1983) Pulmonary cryptococcosis: radiologic-pathologic correlates of its three forms. *American Journal of Roentgenology*, **141**, 1262–1272.

Ferns, R.B. (2006) Evaluation of the role of real-time PCR in the diagnosis of invasive aspergillosis. *Leukemia & Lymphoma*, **47**, 15–20.

Florent, M., Katsahian, S., Vekhoff, A., Levy, V., Rio, B., Marie, J.P., Bouvet, A. and Cornet, M. (2006) Prospective evaluation of a polymerase chain reaction-ELISA targeted to Aspergillus fumigatus and Aspergillus flavus for the early diagnosis of invasive aspergillosis in patients with hematological malignancies. *The Journal of Infectious Diseases*, **193**, 741–747.

Foot, A.B., Garin, Y.J., Ribaud, P., Devergie, A., Derouin, F. and Gluckman, E. (1994) Prophylaxis of toxoplasmosis infection with pyrimethamine/sulfadoxine (Fansidar) in bone marrow transplant recipients. *Bone Marrow Transplantation*, **14**, 241–245.

Frampton, J.E. and Wagstaff, A.J. (2003) *Alemtuzumab Drugs*, **63**, 1229–1243; discussion 1245–1246.

Gafter-Gvili, A., Fraser, A., Paul, M., van de Wetering, M., Kremer, L. and Leibovici, L. (2005) Antibiotic prophylaxis for bacterial infections in afebrile neutropenic patients following chemotherapy. *Cochrane Database of Systematic Reviews*, CD004386.

Gasparetto, E.L., Escuissato, D.L., Marchiori, E., Ono, S., Frare, E., Silva, R.L. and Muller, N.L. (2004) High-resolution CT findings of respiratory syncytial virus pneumonia after bone marrow transplantation. *American Journal of Roentgenology*, **182**, 1133–1137.

George, B., Mathews, V., Srivastava, A. and Chandy, M. (2004) Infections among allogenic bone marrow transplant recipients in India. *Bone Marrow Transplantation*, **33**, 311–315.

Gerson, S.L., Talbot, G.H., Hurwitz, S., Strom, B.L., Lusk, E.J. and Cassileth, P.A. (1984) Prolonged granulocytopenia: the major risk factor for invasive pulmonary aspergillosis in patients with acute leukemia. *Annals of Internal Medicine*, **100**, 345–351.

Ghosh, S., Champlin, R.E., Englund, J., Giralt, S.A., Rolston, K., Raad, I., Jacobson, K., Neumann, J., Ippoliti, C., Mallik, S. and Whimbey, E. (2000) Respiratory syncytial virus upper respiratory tract illnesses in adult blood and marrow transplant recipients: combination therapy with aerosolized ribavirin and intravenous immunoglobulin. *Bone Marrow Transplantation*, **25**, 751–755.

Ginzler, E., Diamond, H., Kaplan, D., Weiner, M., Schlesinger, M. and Seleznick, M. (1978) Computer analysis of factors influencing frequency of infection in systemic lupus erythematosus. *Arthritis and Rheumatism*, **21**, 37–44.

Gonzalez, C.E., Rinaldi, M.G. and Sugar, A.M. (2002) Zygomycosis. *Infectious Disease Clinics of North America*, **16**, 895–914, vi.

Goodman, J.L., Winston, D.J., Greenfield, R.A., Chandrasekar, P.H., Fox, B., Kaizer, H., Shadduck, R. K., Shea, T.C., Stiff, P., Friedman, D.J. *et al.* (1992) A controlled trial of fluconazole to prevent fungal infections in patients undergoing bone marrow transplantation. *The New England Journal of Medicine*, **326**, 845–851.

Goodman, L.S., Wintrobe, M.M., Dameshek, W., Goodman, M.J., Gilman, A. and Mclennan, M.T. (1984) Landmark article Sept. 21, 1946: Nitrogen mustard therapy. Use of methyl-bis(beta-chloroethyl)amine hydrochloride and tris(beta-chloroethyl)amine hydrochloride for Hodgkin's disease, lymphosarcoma, leukemia and certain allied and miscellaneous disorders. By Louis S. Goodman, Maxwell M. Wintrobe, William Dameshek, Morton J. Goodman, Alfred Gilman and Margaret T. McLennan. *The Journal of the American Medical Association*, **251**, 2255–2261.

Gratwohl, A., Baldomero, H., Frauendorfer, K., Urbano-Ispizua, A. and Niederwieser, D. (2007) Results of the EBMT activity survey 2005 on haematopoietic stem cell transplantation: focus on increasing use of unrelated donors. *Bone Marrow Transplantation*, **39**, 71–87.

Greene, R.E., Schlamm, H.T., Stark, P. *et al.* (2003) Radiological findings in acute invasive pulmonary aspergillosis: Utility and reliability of halo sign and air-crescent sign for diagnosis and treatment of IPA in high-risk patients (Abstract O397), 13th European Congress of Clinical Microbiology and Infectious Diseases. glasgow.

Guidelines (2000a) Guidelines for preventing opportunistic infections among hematopoietic stem cell transplant recipients. *Biology of Blood and Marrow Transplantation*, **6**, 659–713; 715; 717–727.

Guidelines (2000b) Targeted Tuberculin Testing and Treatment of Latent Tuberculosis Infection. This Official Statement of the American Thoracic Society was adopted by the ATS Board of Directors, July 1999. This is a Joint Statement of the American Thoracic Society (ATS) and the Centers for Disease Control and Prevention (CDC). This Statement was endorsed by the Council of the Infectious Diseases Society of America (IDSA), September 1999, and the sections of this Statement as it relates to infants and children were endorsed by the American Academy of Pediatrics (AAP), August 1999. *American Journal of Respiratory and Critical Care Medicine*, **161**, 221S–247S.

Gruson, D., Hilbert, G., Valentino, R., Vargas, F., Chene, G., Bebear, C., Allery, A., Pigneux, A., Gbikpi-Benissan, G. and Cardinaud, J.P. (2000) Utility of fiberoptic bronchoscopy in neutropenic patients admitted to the intensive care unit with pulmonary infiltrates. *Critical Care Medicine*, **28** (7), 2224–2230.

Guarro, J. and Gene, J. (1995) Opportunistic fusarial infections in humans. *European Journal of Clinical Microbiology & Infectious Diseases*, **14**, 741–754.

Hajjeh, R.A., Sofair, A.N., Harrison, L.H., Lyon, G.M., Arthington-Skaggs, B.A., Mirza, S.A., Phelan, M., Morgan, J., Lee-Yang, W., Ciblak, M.A., Benjamin, L.E., Thomson Sanza, L., Huie, S., Yeo, S. F., Brandt, M.E. and Warnock, D.W. (2004) Incidence of bloodstream infections due to candida species and In vitro susceptibilities of isolates collected from 1998 to 2000 in a population-based active surveillance program. *Journal of Clinical Microbiology*, **42**, 1519–1527.

Hall, C.B. (2001) Respiratory syncytial virus and parainfluenza virus. *The New England Journal of Medicine*, **344**, 1917–1928.

Haron, E., Vartivarian, S., Anaissie, E., Dekmezian, R. and Bodey, G.P. (1993) Primary Candida pneumonia. Experience at a large cancer center and review of the literature. *Medicine (Baltimore)*, **72**, 137–142.

Harrington, R.D., Hooton, T.M., Hackman, R.C., Storch, G.A., Osborne, B., Gleaves, C.A., Benson, A. and Meyers, J.D. (1992) An outbreak of respiratory syncytial virus in a bone marrow transplant center. *The Journal of Infectious Diseases*, **165**, 987–993.

Hayden, F.G., Osterhaus, A.D., Treanor, J.J., Fleming, D.M., Aoki, F.Y., Nicholson, K.G., Bohnen, A.M., Hirst, H.M., Keene, O. and Wightman, K. (1997) Efficacy and safety of the neuraminidase inhibitor zanamivir in the treatment of influenzavirus infections. GG167 Influenza Study Group. *The New England Journal of Medicine*, **337**, 874–880.

Hayden, F.G., Treanor, J.J., Fritz, R.S., Lobo, M., Betts, R.F., Miller, M., Kinnersley, N., Mills, R.G., Ward, P. and Straus, S.E. (1999) Use of the oral neuraminidase inhibitor oseltamivir in experimental human influenza: randomized controlled trials for prevention and treatment. *The Journal of the American Medical Association*, **282**, 1240–1246.

Henson, D.J. and Hill, A.R. (1984) Cryptococcal pneumonia: a fulminant presentation. *The American Journal of the Medical Sciences*, **288**, 221–222.

Herbrecht, R., Denning, D.W., Patterson, T.F., Bennett, J.E., Greene, R.E., Oestmann, J.W., Kern, W.V., Marr, K.A., Ribaud, P., Lortholary, O., Sylvester, R., Rubin, R.H., Wingard, J.R., Stark, P., Durand, C., Caillot, D., Thiel, E., Chandrasekar, P.H., Hodges, M.R., Schlamm, H.T., Troke, P.F. and de Pauw, B. (2002) Voriconazole versus amphotericin B for primary therapy of invasive aspergillosis. *The New England Journal of Medicine*, **347**, 408–415.

Heussel, C.P., Kauczor, H.U., Heussel, G.E., Fischer, B., Begrich, M., Mildenberger, P. and Thelen, M. (1999) Pneumonia in febrile neutropenic patients and in bone marrow and blood stem-cell transplant recipients: use of high-resolution computed tomography. *Journal of Clinical Oncology*, **17**, 796–805.

Hidalgo, A., Falco, V., Mauleon, S., Andreu, J., Crespo, M., Ribera, E., Pahissa, A. and Caceres, J. (2003) Accuracy of high-resolution CT in distinguishing between Pneumocystis carinii pneumonia and non- Pneumocystis carinii pneumonia in AIDS patients. *European Radiology*, **13**, 1179–1184.

Hilbert, G., Gruson, D., Vargas, F., Valentino, R., Gbikpi-Benissan, G., Dupon, M., Reiffers, J. and Cardinaud, J.P. (2001) Noninvasive ventilation in immunosuppressed patients with pulmonary infiltrates, fever, and acute respiratory failure. *The New England Journal of Medicine*, **344**(7), 481–487.

Ho, S.K., Li, F.K., Lai, K.N. and Chan, T.M. (2000) Comparison of the CMV brite turbo assay and the digene hybrid capture CMV DNA (Version 2.0) assay for quantitation of cytomegalovirus in renal transplant recipients. *Journal of Clinical Microbiology*, **38**, 3743–3745.

Hof, H. (2006) A new, broad-spectrum azole antifungal: posaconazole–mechanisms of action and resistance, spectrum of activity. *Mycoses*, **49** (Suppl 1), 2–6.

Hohenadel, I.A., Kiworr, M., Genitsariotis, R., Zeidler, D. and Lorenz, J. (2001) Role of bronchoalveolar lavage in immunocompromised patients with pneumonia treated with a broad spectrum antibiotic and antifugal regimen. *Thorax*, **56** (2), 115–120.

Holler, E. (2002) Cytokines, viruses, and graft-versus-host disease. *Current Opinion in Hematology*, **9**, 479–484.

Holmberg, L.A., Boeckh, M., Hooper, H., Leisenring, W., Rowley, S., Heimfeld, S., Press, O., Maloney, D.G., Mcsweeney, P., Corey, L., Maziarz, R.T., Appelbaum, F.R. and Bensinger, W. (1999) Increased incidence of cytomegalovirus disease after autologous CD34-selected peripheral blood stem cell transplantation. *Blood*, **94**, 4029–4035.

Hughes, W.T. (1982) Systemic candidiasis: a study of 109 fatal cases. *Pediatric Infectious Disease Journal*, **1**, 11–18.

Hughes, W.T., Armstrong, D., Bodey, G.P., Bow, E.J., Brown, A.E., Calandra, T., Feld, R., Pizzo, P.A., Rolston, K.V., Shenep, J.L. and Young, L.S. (2002) 2002 guidelines for the use of antimicrobial agents in neutropenic patients with cancer. *Clinical Infectious Diseases*, **34**, 730–751.

Hughes, W.T., Feldman, S., Chaudhary, S.C., Ossi, M.J., Cox, F. and Sanyal, S.K. (1978) Comparison of pentamidine isethionate and trimethoprim-sulfamethoxazole in the treatment of Pneumocystis carinii pneumonia. *The Journal of Pediatrics*, **92**, 285–291.

Hughes, W.T., Rivera, G.K., Schell, M.J., Thornton, D. and Lott, L. (1987) Successful intermittent chemoprophylaxis for Pneumocystis carinii pneumonitis. *The New England Journal of Medicine*, **316**, 1627–1632.

Hunt, K.K., Enquist, R.W. and Bowen, T.E. (1976) Multiple pulmonary nodules with central cavitation. *Chest*, **69**, 529–530.

Huter, R.V. and Collins, H.S. (1962) The occurrence of opportunistic fungus infections in a cancer hospital. *Laboratory Investigation; A Journal of Technical Methods and Pathology*, **11**, 1035–1045.

Infectious Diseases Society of Taiwan (2005) Guidelines for the use of antimicrobial agents in patients with febrile neutropenia in Taiwan. *Journal of Microbiology, Immunology and Infection*, **38**, 455–457.

Jagarlamudi, R., Kumar, L., Kochupillai, V., Kapil, A., Banerjee, U. and Thulkar, S. (2000) Infections in acute leukemia: an analysis of 240 febrile episodes. *Medical Oncology (Northwood, London, England)*, **17**, 111–116.

Jain, P., Sandur, S., Meli, Y., Arroliga, A.C., Stoller, J.K. and Mehta, A.C. (2004) Role of flexible bronchoscopy in immunocompromised patients with lung infiltrates. *Chest*, **125**(2):712–722.

Jensen, W.A., Rose, R.M., Hammer, S.M. and Karchmer, A.W. (1985) Serologic diagnosis of focal pneumonia caused by Cryptococcus neoformans. *The American Review of Respiratory Disease*, **132**, 189–191.

Kaplan, M.H., Rosen, P.P. and Armstrong, D. (1977) Cryptococcosis in a cancer hospital: clinical and pathological correlates in forty-six patients. *Cancer*, **39**, 2265–2274.

Karnak, D., Kayacan, O. and Beder, S. (2002) Reactivation of pulmonary tuberculosis in malignancy. *Tumori*, **88**, 251–254.

Kerkering, T.M., Duma, R.J. and Shadomy, S. (1981) The evolution of pulmonary cryptococcosis: clinical implications from a study of 41 patients with and without compromising host factors. *Annals of Internal Medicine*, **94**, 611–616.

Kern, W.V., Beyer, J., Bohme, A., Buchheidt, D., Cornely, O., Einsele, H., Kisro, J., Kruger, W., Maschmeyer, G., Ruhnke, M., Schmidt, C.A., Schwartz, S. and Szelenyi, H. (2000) Prophylaxis of infection in neutropenic patients. Guidelines of the Working Party on Infections in Hematology and Oncology. *Deutsche Medizinische Wochenschrift (1946)*, **125**, 1582–1588.

Kim, Y.J., Boeckh, M. and Englund, J.A. (2007) Community respiratory virus infections in immunocompromised patients: hematopoietic stem cell and solid organ transplant recipients, and individuals with human immunodeficiency virus infection. *Seminars in Respiratory and Critical Care Medicine*, **28**, 222–242.

Klastersky, J., Ameye, L., Maertens, J., Georgala, A., Muanza, F., Aoun, M., Ferrant, A., Rapoport, B., Rolston, K. and Paesmans, M. (2007) Bacteraemia in febrile neutropenic cancer patients. *International Journal of Antimicrobial Agents*, Epub ahead of print.

Klein, N.C., Duncanson, F.P., Lenox, T.H., Forszpaniak, C., Sherer, C.B., Quentzel, H., Nunez, M., Suarez, M., Kawwaff, O., Pitta-Alvarez, A. *et al.* (1992) Trimethoprim-sulfamethoxazole versus pentamidine for Pneumocystis carinii pneumonia in AIDS patients: results of a large prospective randomized treatment trial. *AIDS (London, England)*, **6**, 301–305.

Klimowski, L.L., Rotstein, C. and Cummings, K.M. (1989) Incidence of nosocomial aspergillosis in patients with leukemia over a twenty-year period. *Infection Control and Hospital Epidemiology*, **10**, 299–305.

Klont, R.R., Mennink-Kersten, M.A., Ruegebrink, D., Rijs, A.J., Blijlevens, N.M., Donnelly, J.P. and Verweij, P.E. (2006) Paradoxical increase in circulating Aspergillus antigen during treatment with caspofungin in a patient with pulmonary aspergillosis. *Clinical Infectious Diseases*, **43**, e23–e25.

Kontoyiannis, D.P. (2002) Why prior fluconazole use is associated with an increased risk of invasive mold infections in immunosuppressed hosts: an alternative hypothesis. *Clinical Infectious Diseases*, **34**, 1281–1283; author reply 1283.

Kontoyiannis, D.P., Lionakis, M.S., Lewis, R.E., Chamilos, G., Healy, M., Perego, C., Safdar, A., Kantarjian, H., Champlin, R., Walsh, T.J. and Raad, I.I. (2005) Zygomycosis in a tertiary-care cancer center in the era of Aspergillus-active antifungal therapy: a case-control observational study of 27 recent cases. *The Journal of Infectious Diseases*, **191**, 1350–1360.

Kontoyiannis, D.P., Reddy, B.T., Torres, H.A., Luna, M., Lewis, R.E., Tarrand, J., Bodey, G.P. and Raad, I.I. (2002) Pulmonary candidiasis in patients with cancer: an autopsy study. *Clinical Infectious Diseases*, **34**, 400–403.

Koplan, J.P., Hughes, J.M., Jaffe, H.W., Holloway, B.R., Ward, J.W., Hewitt, S.M., Smith-Akin, C.K., Cupell, L.G., Higgins, M., Renshaw, M.D. and Shaver, E.R. (2000) IDSA/CDC guidelines for preventing opportunistic infections among HSCT recipients. *Centers for Disease Control and Prevention Morbidity and Mortality, Weekly Report*, **49**, 1.

Krause, R., Auner, H.W., Gorkiewicz, G., Wolfler, A., Daxboeck, F., Linkesch, W., Krejs, G.J., Wenisch, C. and Reisinger, E.C. (2004) Detection of catheter-related bloodstream infections by the differential-time-to-positivity method and gram stain-acridine orange leukocyte cytospin test in neutropenic patients after hematopoietic stem cell transplantation. *Journal of Clinical Microbiology*, **42**, 4835–4837.

Kruger, W.H., Zollner, B., Kaulfers, P.M. and Zander, A.R. (2003) Effective protection of allogeneic stem cell recipients against Aspergillosis by HEPA air filtration during a period of construction–a prospective survey. *Journal of Hematotherapy & Stem Cell Research*, **12**, 301–307.

Kuse, E.R., Chetchotisakd, P., da Cunha, C.A., Ruhnke, M., Barrios, C., Raghunadharao, D., Sekhon, J.S., Freire, A., Ramasubramanian, V., Demeyer, I., Nucci, M., Leelarasamee, A., Jacobs, F., Decruyenaere, J., Pittet, D., Ullmann, A.J., Ostrosky-Zeichner, L., Lortholary, O., Koblinger, S., Diekmann-Berndt, H. and Cornely, O.A. (2007) Micafungin versus liposomal amphotericin B for candidaemia and invasive candidosis: a phase III randomised double-blind trial. *Lancet*, **369**, 1519-1527.

Leal, F.E., Cavazzana, C.L., de Andrade, H.F., Jr, Galisteo, A.J., Jr, de Mendonca, J.S. and Kallas, E.G. (2007) Toxoplasma gondii pneumonia in immunocompetent subjects: case report and review. *Clinical Infectious Diseases*, **44**, e62-e66.

Lee, D.G., Choi, S.M., Choi, J.H., Yoo, J.H., Park, Y.H., Kim, Y.J., Lee, S., Min, C.K., Kim, H.J., Kim, D.W., Lee, J.W., Min, W.S., Shin, W.S. and Kim, C.C. (2002) Selective bowel decontamination for the prevention of infection in acute myelogenous leukemia: a prospective randomized trial. *The Korean Journal of Internal Medicine*, **17**, 38-44.

Lionakis, M.S. and Kontoyiannis, D.P. (2004) Fusarium infections in critically ill patients. *Seminars in Respiratory and Critical Care Medicine*, **25**, 159-169.

Lorente, L., Henry, C., Martin, M.M., Jimenez, A. and Mora, M.L. (2005) Central venous catheter-related infection in a prospective and observational study of 2,595 catheters. *Critical Care (London, England)*, **9**, R631-R635.

Maertens, J., Raad, I., Petrikkos, G., Boogaerts, M., Selleslag, D., Petersen, F.B., Sable, C.A., Kartsonis, N.A., Ngai, A., Taylor, A., Patterson, T.F., Denning, D.W. and Walsh, T.J. (2004) Efficacy and safety of caspofungin for treatment of invasive aspergillosis in patients refractory to or intolerant of conventional antifungal therapy. *Clinical Infectious Diseases*, **39**, 1563-1571.

Mansharamani, N.G., Garland, R., Delaney, D. and Koziel, H. (2000) Management and outcome patterns for adult Pneumocystis carinii pneumonia, 1985 to 1995: comparison of HIV-associated cases to other immunocompromised states. *Chest*, **118**, 704-711.

Mariuz, P., Bosler, E.M. and Luft, B.J. (1997) Toxoplasma pneumonia. *Seminars in Respiratory Infections*, **12**, 40-43.

Marr, K.A., Carter, R.A., Crippa, F., Wald, A. and Corey, L. (2002) Epidemiology and outcome of mould infections in hematopoietic stem cell transplant recipients. *Clinical Infectious Diseases*, **34**, 909-917.

Marr, K.A., Seidel, K., White, T.C. and Bowden, R.A. (2000) Candidemia in allogeneic blood and marrow transplant recipients: evolution of risk factors after the adoption of prophylactic fluconazole. *The Journal of Infectious Diseases*, **181**, 309-316.

Marron, A., Carratala, J., Gonzalez-Barca, E., Fernandez-Sevilla, A., Alcaide, F. and Gudiol, F. (2000) Serious complications of bacteremia caused by Viridans streptococci in neutropenic patients with cancer. *Clinical Infectious Diseases*, **31**, 1126-1130.

Martino, R., Bretagne, S., Rovira, M., Ullmann, A.J., Maertens, J., Held, T., Deconinck, E. and Cordonnier, C. (2000) Toxoplasmosis after hematopoietic stem transplantation. Report of a 5-year survey from the Infectious Diseases Working Party of the European Group for Blood and Marrow Transplantation. *Bone Marrow Transplantation*, **25**, 1111-1114.

Martino, R., Parody, R., Fukuda, T., Maertens, J., Theunissen, K., Ho, A., Mufti, G.J., Kroger, N., Zander, A.R., Heim, D., Paluszewska, M., Selleslag, D., Steinerova, K., Ljungman, P., Cesaro, S., Nihtinen, A., Cordonnier, C., Vazquez, L., Lopez-Duarte, M., Lopez, J., Cabrera, R., Rovira, M., Neuburger, S., Cornely, O., Hunter, A.E., Marr, K.A., Dornbusch, H.J. and Einsele, H. (2006) Impact of the intensity of the pretransplantation conditioning regimen in patients with prior invasive aspergillosis undergoing allogeneic hematopoietic stem cell transplantation: A retrospective survey of the Infectious Diseases Working Party of the European Group for Blood and Marrow Transplantation. *Blood*, **108**, 2928-2936.

Masaoka, T., Hiraoka, A., Ohta, K., Tatsumi, N., Watanabe, S., Hotta, T., Yabe, H., Kato, S., Aikawa, A., Ohara, T., Hasegawa, A., Tanabe, K., Toma, H., Yasuoka, A. and Oka, S. (2001) Evaluation of the

AMPLICOR CMV, COBAS AMPLICOR CMV monitor and antigenemia assay for cytomegalovirus disease. *Japanese Journal of Infectious Diseases*, **54**, 12–16.

Maschmeyer, G., Beinert, T., Buchheidt, D., Einsele, H., Heussel, C.P., Kiehl, M. and Lorenz, J. (2003) Diagnosis and antimicrobial therapy of pulmonary infiltrates in febrile neutropenic patients–guidelines of the Infectious Diseases Working Party (AGIHO) of the German Society of Hematology and Oncology (DGHO). *Annals of Hematology*, **82** (Suppl 2), S118–S126.

Maschmeyer, G., Haas, A. and Cornely, O.A., (2007) Aspergillosis. *Drugs*.

Masur, H., Rosen, P.P. and Armstrong, D. (1977) Pulmonary disease caused by Candida species. *The American Journal of Medicine*, **63**, 914–925.

Mazzulli, T., Drew, L.W., Yen-Lieberman, B., Jekic-Mcmullen, D., Kohn, D.J., Isada, C., Moussa, G., Chua, R. and Walmsley, S. (1999) Multicenter comparison of the digene hybrid capture CMV DNA assay (version 2.0), the pp65 antigenemia assay, and cell culture for detection of cytomegalovirus viremia. *Journal of Clinical Microbiology*, **37**, 958–963.

Mele, A., Paterson, P.J., Prentice, H.G., Leoni, P. and Kibbler, C.C. (2002) Toxoplasmosis in bone marrow transplantation: a report of two cases and systematic review of the literature. *Bone Marrow Transplantation*, **29**, 691–698.

Meyers, J.D., Flournoy, N. and Thomas, E.D. (1986) Risk factors for cytomegalovirus infection after human marrow transplantation. *The Journal of Infectious Diseases*, **153**, 478–488.

Mishra, P., Kumar, R., Mahapatra, M., Sharma, S., Dixit, A., Chaterjee, T., Choudhry, D.R., Saxena, R. and Choudry, V.P. (2006) Tuberculosis in acute leukemia: a clinico-hematological profile. *Hematology (Amsterdam, Netherlands)*, **11**, 335–340.

Moody, K., Charlson, M.E. and Finlay, J. (2002) The neutropenic diet: what's the evidence? *Journal of Pediatric Hematology and Oncology*, **24**, 717–721.

Moody, K., Finlay, J., Mancuso, C. and Charlson, M. (2006) Feasibility and safety of a pilot randomized trial of infection rate: neutropenic diet versus standard food safety guidelines. *Journal of Pediatric Hematology/Oncology*, **28**, 126–133.

Morris, A., Lundgren, J.D., Masur, H., Walzer, P.D., Hanson, D.L., Frederick, T., Huang, L., Beard, C.B. and Kaplan, J.E. (2004) Current epidemiology of Pneumocystis pneumonia. *Emerging Infectious Diseases*, **10**, 1713–1720.

Muhlemann, K., Wenger, C., Zenhausern, R. and Tauber, M.G. (2005) Risk factors for invasive aspergillosis in neutropenic patients with hematologic malignancies. *Leukemia*, **19**, 545–550.

Nucci, M., Marr, K.A., Queiroz-Telles, F., Martins, C.A., Trabasso, P., Costa, S., Voltarelli, J.C., Colombo, A.L., Imhof, A., Pasquini, R., Maiolino, A., Souza, C.A. and Anaissie, E. (2004) Fusarium infection in hematopoietic stem cell transplant recipients. *Clinical Infectious Diseases*, **38**, 1237–1242.

Obayashi, T., Yoshida, M., Mori, T., Goto, H., Yasuoka, A., Iwasaki, H., Teshima, H., Kohno, S., Horiuchi, A., Ito, A. et al. (1995) Plasma $(1 \rightarrow 3)$-beta-D-glucan measurement in diagnosis of invasive deep mycosis and fungal febrile episodes. *Lancet*, **345**, 17–20.

Odabasi, Z., Mattiuzzi, G., Estey, E., Kantarjian, H., Saeki, F., Ridge, R.J., Ketchum, P.A., Finkelman, M.A., Rex, J.H. and Ostrosky-Zeichner, L. (2004) Beta-D-glucan as a diagnostic adjunct for invasive fungal infections: validation, cutoff development, and performance in patients with acute myelogenous leukemia and myelodysplastic syndrome. *Clinical Infectious Diseases*, **39**, 199–205.

Onishi, Y., Mori, S., Higuchi, A., Kim, S.W., Fukuda, T., Heike, Y., Tanosaki, R., Minematsu, T., Takaue, Y., Sasaki, T. and Furuta, K. (2006) Early detection of plasma cytomegalovirus DNA by real-time PCR after allogeneic hematopoietic stem cell transplantation. *The Tohoku Journal of Experimental Medicine*, **210**, 125–135.

Ostrosky-Zeichner, L., Alexander, B.D., Kett, D.H., Vazquez, J., Pappas, P.G., Saeki, F., Ketchum, P.A., Wingard, J., Schiff, R., Tamura, H., Finkelman, M.A. and Rex, J.H. (2005) Multicenter clinical evaluation of the $(1 \rightarrow 3)$ beta-D-glucan assay as an aid to diagnosis of fungal infections in humans. *Clinical Infectious Diseases*, **41**, 654–659.

Pagano, L., Mele, L., Fianchi, L., Melillo, L., Martino, B., D'Antonio, D., Tosti, M.E., Posteraro, B., Sanguinetti, M., Trape, G., Equitani, F., Carotenuto, M. and Leone, G. (2002) Chronic disseminated candidiasis in patients with hematologic malignancies. Clinical features and outcome of 29 episodes. *Haematologica*, **87**, 535–541.

Paphitou, N.I., Ostrosky-Zeichner, L., Paetznick, V.L., Rodriguez, J.R., Chen, E. and Rex, J.H. (2002) In vitro activities of investigational triazoles against Fusarium species: effects of inoculum size and incubation time on broth microdilution susceptibility test results. *Antimicrobial Agents and Chemotherapy*, **46**, 3298–3300.

Pappas, P.G., Perfect, J.R., Cloud, G.A., Larsen, R.A., Pankey, G.A., Lancaster, D.J., Henderson, H., Kauffman, C.A., Haas, D.W., Saccente, M., Hamill, R.J., Holloway, M.S., Warren, R.M. and Dismukes, W.E. (2001) Cryptococcosis in human immunodeficiency virus-negative patients in the era of effective azole therapy. *Clinical Infectious Diseases*, **33**, 690–699.

Pareja, J.G., Garland, R. and Koziel, H. (1998) Use of adjunctive corticosteroids in severe adult non-HIV Pneumocystis carinii pneumonia. *Chest*, **113**, 1215–1224.

Pascoe, J. and Cullen, M. (2006) The prevention of febrile neutropenia. *Current Opinion in Oncology*, **18**, 325–329.

Patel, N.R., Lee, P.S., Kim, J.H., Weinhouse, G.L. and Koziel, H. (2005) The influence of diagnostic bronchoscopy on clinical outcomes comparing adult autologous and allogeneic bone marrow transplant patients. *Chest*, **127**(4), 1388–1396.

Patterson, T.F., Kirkpatrick, W.R., White, M., Hiemenz, J.W., Wingard, J.R., Dupont, B., Rinaldi, M.G., Stevens, D.A. and Graybill, J.R. (2000) Invasive aspergillosis. Disease spectrum, treatment practices, and outcomes. I3 Aspergillus Study Group. *Medicine (Baltimore)*, **79**, 250–260.

Pazos, C., Ponton, J. and del Palacio, A. (2005) Contribution of $(1 \rightarrow 3)$-beta-D-glucan chromogenic assay to diagnosis and therapeutic monitoring of invasive aspergillosis in neutropenic adult patients: a comparison with serial screening for circulating galactomannan. *Journal of Clinical Microbiology*, **43**, 299–305.

Peacock, J.E., Jr, Greven, C.M., Cruz, J.M. and Hurd, D.D. (1995) Reactivation toxoplasmic retinochoroiditis in patients undergoing bone marrow transplantation: is there a role for chemoprophylaxis? *Bone Marrow Transplantation*, **15**, 983–987.

Peikert, T., Rana, S. and Edell, E.S. (2005) Safety, diagnostic yield, and therapeutic implications of flexible bronchoscopy in patients with febrile neutropenia and pulmonary infiltrates. *Mayo Clinical Proceeding*, **80**(11),1414–1420.

Penack, O., Keilholz, U., Thiel, E. and Blau, I.W. (2005) Value of surveillance blood cultures in neutropenic patients–a pilot study. *Japanese Journal of Infectious Diseases*, **58**, 171–173.

Perfect, J.R. (2005) Treatment of non-Aspergillus moulds in immunocompromised patients, with amphotericin B lipid complex. *Clinical Infectious Diseases*, **40** (Suppl 6), S401–S408.

Perfect, J.R., Marr, K.A., Walsh, T.J., Greenberg, R.N., Dupont, B., de la Torre-Cisneros, J., Just-Nubling, G., Schlamm, H.T., Lutsar, I., Espinel-Ingroff, A. and Johnson, E. (2003) Voriconazole treatment for less-common, emerging, or refractory fungal infections. *Clinical Infectious Diseases*, **36**, 1122–1131.

Petrikkos, G.L., Christofilopoulou, S.A., Tentolouris, N.K., Charvalos, E.A., Kosmidis, C.J. and Daikos, G.L. (2005) Value of measuring serum procalcitonin, C-reactive protein, and mannan antigens to distinguish fungal from bacterial infections. *European Journal of Clinical Microbiology & Infectious Diseases*, **24**, 272–275.

Pfaller, M.A., Diekema, D.J., Gibbs, D.L., Newell, V.A., Meis, J.F., Gould, I.M., Fu, W., Colombo, A.L. and Rodriguez-Noriega, E. (2007) Results from the ARTEMIS DISK Global Antifungal Surveillance study, 1997 to 2005: an 8.5-year analysis of susceptibilities of Candida species and other yeast species to fluconazole and voriconazole determined by CLSI standardized disk diffusion testing. *Journal of Clinical Microbiology*, **45**, 1735–1745.

Pfaller, M.A., Jones, R.N., Messer, S.A., Edmond, M.B. and Wenzel, R.P. (1998a) National surveillance of nosocomial blood stream infection due to Candida albicans: frequency of occurrence and antifungal susceptibility in the SCOPE Program. *Diagnostic Microbiology and Infectious Disease*, **31**, 327–332.

Pfaller, M.A., Jones, R.N., Messer, S.A., Edmond, M.B. and Wenzel, R.P. (1998b) National surveillance of nosocomial blood stream infection due to species of Candida other than Candida albicans: frequency of occurrence and antifungal susceptibility in the SCOPE Program. SCOPE Participant Group. Surveillance and Control of Pathogens of Epidemiologic. *Diagnostic Microbiology and Infectious Disease*, **30**, 121–129.

Pfeiffer, C.D., Fine, J.P. and Safdar, N. (2006a) Diagnosis of invasive aspergillosis using a galactomannan assay: a meta-analysis. *Clinical Infectious Diseases*, **42**, 1417–1427.

Pfeiffer, C.D., Fine, J.P. and Safdar, N. (2006b) Diagnosis of invasive aspergillosis using a galactomannan assay: a meta-analysis. *Clinical Infectious Diseases*, **42**, 1417–1727.

Principi, T., Pantanetti, S., Catani, F., Elisei, D., Gabbanelli, V., Pelaia, P. and Leoni, P. (2004) Noninvasive continuous positive airway pressure delivered by helmet in hematological malignancy patients with hypoxemic acute respiratory failure. *Intensive Care Medicine*, **30**, 147–150.

Quist, J. and Hill, A.R. (1995) Serum lactate dehydrogenase (LDH) in Pneumocystis carinii pneumonia, tuberculosis, and bacterial pneumonia. *Chest*, **108**, 415–418.

Ramphal, R. (2004) Changes in the etiology of bacteremia in febrile neutropenic patients and the susceptibilities of the currently isolated pathogens. *Clinical Infectious Diseases*, **39** (Suppl 1), S25–S31.

Rañó, A., Agustí, C., Jimenez, P., Angrill, J., Benito, N., Danés, C., González, J., Rovira M., Pumarola, T., Moreno, A. and Torres, A. (2001) Pulmonary infiltrates in non-HIV immunocompromised patients: a diagnostic approach using non-invasive and bronchoscopic procedures. *Thorax*, **56**(5), 379–387.

Reboli, A.C., Rotstein, C., Pappas, P.G., Chapman, S.W., Kett, D.H., Kumar, D., Betts, R., Wible, M., Goldstein, B.P., Schranz, J., Krause, D.S. and Walsh, T.J. (2007) Anidulafungin versus fluconazole for invasive candidiasis. *The New England Journal of Medicine*, **356**, 2472–2482.

Reed, E.C., Bowden, R.A., Dandliker, P.S., Lilleby, K.E. and Meyers, J.D. (1988) Treatment of cytomegalovirus pneumonia with ganciclovir and intravenous cytomegalovirus immunoglobulin in patients with bone marrow transplants. *Annals of Internal Medicine*, **109**, 783–788.

Regazzi, M.B., Iacona, I., Avanzini, M.A., Arcaini, L., Merlini, G., Perfetti, V., Zaja, F., Montagna, M., Morra, E. and Lazzarino, M. (2005) Pharmacokinetic behavior of rituximab: a study of different schedules of administration for heterogeneous clinical settings. *Therapeutic Drug Monitoring*, **27**, 785–792.

Reich, G., Mapara, M.Y., Reichardt, P., Dorken, B. and Maschmeyer, G. (2001) Infectious complications after high-dose chemotherapy and autologous stem cell transplantation: comparison between patients with lymphoma or multiple myeloma and patients with solid tumors. *Bone Marrow Transplantation*, **27**, 525–529.

Reusser, P., Einsele, H., Lee, J., Volin, L., Rovira, M., Engelhard, D., Finke, J., Cordonnier, C., Link, H. and Ljungman, P., (2002) Randomized multicenter trial of foscarnet versus ganciclovir for preemptive therapy of cytomegalovirus infection after allogeneic stem cell transplantation. *Blood*, **99**, 1159–1164.

Rocco, M., Dellùtri, D., Morelli, A., Spadetta, G., Conti, G., Antonelli, M. and Pietropaoli, P. (2004) Nonivasive ventilation by helmet of face mask in immunocompromised patients: a case-control study. *Chest*, **126**, 1508–1515.

Roden, M.M., Zaoutis, T.E., Buchanan, W.L., Knudsen, T.A., Sarkisova, T.A., Schaufele, R.L., Sein, M., Sein, T., Chiou, C.C., Chu, J.H., Kontoyiannis, D.P. and Walsh, T.J. (2005) Epidemiology and outcome of zygomycosis: a review of 929 reported cases. *Clinical Infectious Diseases*, **41**, 634–653.

Rotstein, C., Bow, E.J., Laverdiere, M., Ioannou, S., Carr, D. and Moghaddam, N. (1999) Randomized placebo-controlled trial of fluconazole prophylaxis for neutropenic cancer patients: benefit based on purpose and intensity of cytotoxic therapy. The Canadian Fluconazole Prophylaxis Study Group. *Clinical Infectious Diseases*, **28**, 331–340.

Saag, M.S., Graybill, R.J., Larsen, R.A., Pappas, P.G., Perfect, J.R., Powderly, W.G., Sobel, J.D. and Dismukes, W.E. (2000) Practice guidelines for the management of cryptococcal disease. Infectious Diseases Society of America. *Clinical Infectious Diseases*, **30**, 710–718.

Sandherr, M., Einsele, H., Hebart, H., Kahl, C., Kern, W., Kiehl, M., Massenkeil, G., Penack, O., Schiel, X., Schuettrumpf, S., Ullmann, A.J. and Cornely, O.A. (2006) Antiviral prophylaxis in patients with haematological malignancies and solid tumours: Guidelines of the Infectious Diseases Working Party (AGIHO) of the German Society for Hematology and Oncology (DGHO). *Annals of Oncology*, **17**, 1051–1059.

Saral, R., Ambinder, R.F., Burns, W.H., Angelopulos, C.M., Griffin, D.E., Burke, P.J. and Lietman, P.S. (1983) Acyclovir prophylaxis against herpes simplex virus infection in patients with leukemia. A randomized, double-blind, placebo-controlled study. *Annals of Internal Medicine*, **99**, 773–776.

Schmidt, G.M., Kovacs, A., Zaia, J.A., Horak, D.A., Blume, K.G., Nademanee, A.P., O'Donnell, M.R., Snyder, D.S. and Forman, S.J. (1988) Ganciclovir/immunoglobulin combination therapy for the treatment of human cytomegalovirus-associated interstitial pneumonia in bone marrow allograft recipients. *Transplantation*, **46**, 905–907.

Schulenburg, A., Watkins-Riedel, T., Greinix, H.T., Rabitsch, W., Loidolt, H., Keil, F., Mitterbauer, M. and Kalhs, P. (2001) CMV monitoring after peripheral blood stem cell and bone marrow transplantation by pp65 antigen and quantitative PCR. *Bone Marrow Transplantation*, **28**, 765–768.

Shenoy, S., Mohanakumar, T., Todd, G., Westhoff, W., Dunnigan, K., Adkins, D.R., Brown, R.A. and Dipersio, J.F. (1999) Immune reconstitution following allogeneic peripheral blood stem cell transplants. *Bone Marrow Transplantation*, **23**, 335–346.

Sia, I.G., Wilson, J.A., Espy, M.J., Paya, C.V. and Smith, T.F. (2000) Evaluation of the COBAS AMPLICOR CMV MONITOR test for detection of viral DNA in specimens taken from patients after liver transplantation. *Journal of Clinical Microbiology*, **38**, 600–606.

Siegel, S.E., Wolff, L.J., Baehner, R.L. and Hammond, D. (1984) Treatment of Pneumocystis carinii pneumonitis. A comparative trial of sulfamethoxazole-trimethoprim v pentamidine in pediatric patients with cancer: report from the Children's Cancer Study Group. *American Journal of Diseases of Children*, **138**, 1051–1054.

Simon, L., Gauvin, F., Amre, D.K., Saint-Louis, P. and Lacroix, J. (2004) Serum procalcitonin and C-reactive protein levels as markers of bacterial infection: a systematic review and meta-analysis. *Clinical Infectious Diseases*, **39**, 206–217.

Sing, A., Leitritz, L., Roggenkamp, A., Kolb, H.J., Szabados, A., Fingerle, V., Autenrieth, I.B. and Heesemann, J. (1999) Pulmonary toxoplasmosis in bone marrow transplant recipients: report of two cases and review. *Clinical Infectious Diseases*, **29**, 429–433.

Singh, N., Avery, R.K., Munoz, P., Pruett, T.L., Alexander, B., Jacobs, R., Tollemar, J.G., Dominguez, E.A., Yu, C.M., Paterson, D.L., Husain, S., Kusne, S. and Linden, P. (2003) Trends in risk profiles for and mortality associated with invasive aspergillosis among liver transplant recipients. *Clinical Infectious Diseases*, **36**, 46–52.

Siwek, G.T., Dodgson, K.J., de Magalhaes-Silverman, M., Bartelt, L.A., Kilborn, S.B., Hoth, P.L., Diekema, D.J. and Pfaller, M.A. (2004) Invasive zygomycosis in hematopoietic stem cell transplant recipients receiving voriconazole prophylaxis. *Clinical Infectious Diseases*, **39**, 584–587.

Skapova, D., Racil, Z., Dvorakova, D., Minarikova, D. and Mayer, J. (2005) Significance of qualitative PCR detection method for preemptive therapy of cytomegalovirus infection in patients after allogeneic hematopoietic stem cell transplantation – single-centre experience. *Neoplasma*, **52**, 137–142.

Slavin, M.A., Osborne, B., Adams, R., Levenstein, M.J., Schoch, H.G., Feldman, A.R., Meyers, J.D. and Bowden, R.A. (1995) Efficacy and safety of fluconazole prophylaxis for fungal infections after marrow transplantation–a prospective, randomized, double-blind study. *The Journal of Infectious Diseases*, **171**, 1545–1552.

Smith, N.M., Bresee, J.S., Shay, D.K., Uyeki, T.M., Cox, N.J. and Strikas, R.A. (2006) Prevention and control of influenza: recommendations of the Advisory Committee on Immunization Practices (ACIP). *MMWR Recommendations Reports*, **55**, 1–42.

Sparrelid, E., Hagglund, H., Remberger, M., Ringden, O., Lonnqvist, B., Ljungman, P. and Andersson, J. (1998) Bacteraemia during the aplastic phase after allogeneic bone marrow transplantation is associated with early death from invasive fungal infection. *Bone Marrow Transplantation*, **22**, 795–800.

Spellberg, B., Edwards, J. Jr. and Ibrahim, A. (2005) Novel perspectives on mucormycosis: pathophysiology, presentation, and management. *Clinical Microbiology Reviews*, **18**, 556–569.

Stuck, A.E., Minder, C.E. and Frey, F.J. (1989) Risk of infectious complications in patients taking glucocorticosteroids. *Reviews of Infectious Diseases*, **11**, 954–963.

Sutton, D.A., Fothergill, A.W. and Rinaldi, M.G. (2004) Aspergillus in vitro antifungal susceptibility data: new millennium trends, in Advances Against Aspergillosis, San Francisco.

Toikka, P., Irjala, K., Juven, T., Virkki, R., Mertsola, J., Leinonen, M. and Ruuskanen, O. (2000) Serum procalcitonin, C-reactive protein and interleukin-6 for distinguishing bacterial and viral pneumonia in children. *The Pediatric Infectious Disease Journal*, **19**, 598–602.

Torres, H.A., Chemaly, R.F., Storey, R., Aguilera, E.A., Nogueras, G.M., Safdar, A., Rolston, K.V., Raad, I.I. and Kontoyiannis, D.P. (2006) Influence of type of cancer and hematopoietic stem cell transplantation on clinical presentation of Pneumocystis jiroveci pneumonia in cancer patients. *European Journal of Clinical Microbiology & Infectious Diseases*, **25**, 382–388.

Torres, H.A., Raad, I.I. and Kontoyiannis, D.P. (2003) Infections caused by Fusarium species. *J Chemother*, **15** (Suppl 2), 28–35.

Treanor, J.J., Hayden, F.G., Vrooman, P.S., Barbarash, R., Bettis, R., Riff, D., Singh, S., Kinnersley, N., Ward, P. and Mills, R.G. (2000) Efficacy and safety of the oral neuraminidase inhibitor oseltamivir in treating acute influenza: a randomized controlled trial. US Oral Neuraminidase Study Group. *The Journal of the American Medical Association*, **283**, 1016–1024.

Ullmann, A.J., Lipton, J.H., Vesole, D.H., Chandrasekar, P., Langston, A., Tarantolo, S.R., Greinix, H., Morais de Azevedo, W., Reddy, V., Boparai, N., Pedicone, L., Patino, H. and Durrant, S. (2007) Posaconazole or fluconazole for prophylaxis in severe graft-versus-host disease. *The New England Journal of Medicine*, **356**, 335–347.

van Burik, J.H., Leisenring, W., Myerson, D., Hackman, R.C., Shulman, H.M., Sale, G.E., Bowden, R.A. and Mcdonald, G.B. (1998) The effect of prophylactic fluconazole on the clinical spectrum of fungal diseases in bone marrow transplant recipients with special attention to hepatic candidiasis. An autopsy study of 355 patients. *Medicine (Baltimore)*, **77**, 246–254.

van der Bij, W., Schirm, J., Torensma, R., van Son, W.J., Tegzess, A.M. and The, T.H., (1988) Comparison between viremia and antigenemia for detection of cytomegalovirus in blood. *Journal of Clinical Microbiology*, **26**, 2531–2535.

van Esser, J.W.J., Niesters, H.G.M., van der Holt, B., Meijer, E., Osterhaus, A.D.M.E., Gratama, J.W., Verdonck, L.F., Lowenberg, B. and Cornelissen, J.J. (2002) Prevention of Epstein-Barr virus-lymphoproliferative disease by molecular monitoring and preemptive rituximab in high-risk patients after allogeneic stem cell transplantation. *Blood*, **99**, 4364–4369.

Vardakas, K.Z., Michalopoulos, A. and Falagas, M.E. (2005) Fluconazole versus itraconazole for antifungal prophylaxis in neutropenic patients with haematological malignancies: a meta-analysis of randomised-controlled trials. *British Journal of Haematology*, **131**, 22–28.

Vasconcelles, M.J., Bernardo, M.V., King, C., Weller, E.A. and Antin, J.H. (2000) Aerosolized pentamidine as pneumocystis prophylaxis after bone marrow transplantation is inferior to other regimens and is associated with decreased survival and an increased risk of other infections. *Biology of Blood and Marrow Transplantation*, **6**, 35–43.

Verhoef, J., Verhage, E.A. and Visser, M.R. (1993) A decade of experience with selective decontamination of the digestive tract as prophylaxis for infections in patients in the intensive care unit: what have we learned? *Clinical Infectious Diseases*, **17**, 1047–1054.

Viscoli, C., Girmenia, C., Marinus, A., Collette, L., Martino, P., Vandercam, B., Doyen, C., Lebeau, B., Spence, D., Krcmery, V., de Pauw, B. and Meunier, F. (1999) Candidemia in cancer patients: a prospective, multicenter surveillance study by the Invasive Fungal Infection Group (IFIG) of the European Organization for Research and Treatment of Cancer (EORTC). *Clinical Infectious Diseases*, **28**, 1071–1079.

Walsh, T.J., Raad, I., Patterson, T.F., Chandrasekar, P., Donowitz, G.R., Graybill, R., Greene, R.E., Hachem, R., Hadley, S., Herbrecht, R., Langston, A., Louie, A., Ribaud, P., Segal, B.H., Stevens, D. A., van Burik, J.A., White, C.S., Corcoran, G., Gogate, J., Krishna, G., Pedicone, L., Hardalo, C. and Perfect, J.R. (2007) Treatment of invasive aspergillosis with posaconazole in patients who are refractory to or intolerant of conventional therapy: an externally controlled trial. *Clinical Infectious Diseases*, **44**, 2–12.

Warren, E., George, S., You, J. and Kazanjian, P. (1997) Advances in the treatment and prophylaxis of Pneumocystis carinii pneumonia. *Pharmacotherapy*, **17**, 900–916.

Watanakunakorn, C. (1983) Acute pulmonary mycetoma due to Candida albicans with complete resolution. *The Journal of Infectious Diseases*, **148**, 1131.

Wendtner, C.M., Ritgen, M., Schweighofer, C.D., Fingerle-Rowson, G., Campe, H., Jäger, G., Eichhorst, B., Busch, R., Diem, H., Engert, A., Stilgenbauer, S., Döhner, H., Kneba, M., Emmerich, B. and Hallek, M., Germann CLL Study Group (GCLLSG) (2004) Consolidation with alemtuzumab in patients with chronic lymphocytic leukemia (CLL) in first remission–experience on safety and efficacy within a randomized multicenter phase III trial of the German CLL Study Group (GCLLSG). *Leukemia*, **18**, 1093–1101.

Whimbey, E. and Ghosh, S. (2000) Respiratory syncytial virus infections in immunocompromised adults. *Current Clinical Topics in Infectious Diseases*, **20**, 232–255.

Willocks, L., Burns, S., Cossar, R. and Brettle, R. (1993) Diagnosis of Pneumocystis carinii pneumonia in a population of HIV-positive drug users, with particular reference to sputum induction and fluorescent antibody techniques. *The Journal of Infection*, **26**, 257–264.

Winston, D.J., Chandrasekar, P.H., Lazarus, H.M., Goodman, J.L., Silber, J.L., Horowitz, H., Shadduck, R.K., Rosenfeld, C.S., Ho, W.G., Islam, M.Z. and Buell, D.N. (1993) Fluconazole prophylaxis of fungal infections in patients with acute leukemia. Results of a randomized placebo-controlled, double-blind, multicenter trial. *Annals of Internal Medicine*, **118**, 495–503.

Yen, K.T., Lee, A.S., Krowka, M.J. and Burger, C.D. (2004) Pulmonary complications in bone marrow transplantation: a practical approach to diagnosis and treatment. *Clinical Chest Medicine*, **25**(1), 189–201

Yuen, K.Y. and Woo, P.C. (2002) Tuberculosis in blood and marrow transplant recipients. *Hematological Oncology*, **20**, 51–62.

Zaia, J.A. (2002) Prevention of cytomegalovirus disease in hematopoietic stem cell transplantation. *Clinical Infectious Diseases*, **35**, 999–1004.

7

General management of suspected pneumonia in the solid organ transplant patient

Andrew F. Shorr

Pulmonary and Critical Care Medicine Section, Washington Hospital Center, Washington DC

7.1 Introduction

Over 40 000 solid organ transplants (SOTs) are performed annually in the United States (www.unos.org). Often these operations are undertaken for persons with advanced, end-organ cardiopulmonary or liver disease. As such, these procedures represent the only means available to forestall mortality. Additionally, for others, such as individuals with end-stage renal disease, SOT enhances quality of life. With improvements in surgical techniques and different strategies for immunosuppression, SOT recipients are living longer post-transplant then they had previously. Hence, there is a large and growing population of SOT patients.

Frequently SOT patients develop pulmonary disease. Generally the lungs represent a major site for injury because they are constantly exposed to the environment. The lungs may be injured directly through an infectious or toxic insult. Conversely lung disease may result as a secondary event. Pulmonary complications may also develop acutely or arise more gradually. The management of these pulmonary issues following transplant necessitates an appreciation of: the epidemiology of post-transplant pulmonary complications, the differential diagnoses for these processes, the diagnostic approach to the SOT patient with radiographic infiltrates, and the characteristics and treatments for the unique organisms that can cause pneumonia in this population.

7.2 Epidemiology

Little literature exists describing the general frequency of either pulmonary complications or pneumonia following SOT. Pulmonary complications appear to vary in frequency based on the type of organ transplant. For example, pneumonia is relatively

Pulmonary Infection in the Immunocompromised Patient, Edited by Carlos Agustí and Antoni Torres
© 2009 John Wiley & Sons, Ltd.

rare following kidney transplant while pulmonary complications occur more often in heart, lung and liver transplant patients (Kotloff, Ahya and Crawford, 2004). In lung and heart transplant patients, the lung is the most common site for post-transplant infection while it is the second most common source of infection in those receiving abdominal transplants. The fact that pneumonia remains rare following kidney transplant reflects that this is a comparatively less rigorous surgical procedure than other forms of transplantation and because these subjects often require less intense immunosuppression (Kotloff, Ahya and Crawford, 2004).

The list of potential pathogens causing pneumonia in SOT patients is extensive and diverse. However, several epidemiologic themes emerge. Initially, early following transplant, traditional bacterial pathogens predominate. This reflects the fact that immediately following surgery many SOT patients require monitoring in the intensive care unit (ICU) and may undergo somewhat prolonged courses of mechanical ventilation. Moreover, the immunosuppression used to prevent rejection often has not reached its peak activity until several weeks following organ placement. Pneumonia during this phase may also be caused by pathogens which previously colonized either the recipient, or in the case of the pulmonary transplant, the donor lung(s). Recent surveys suggest that bacterial pneumonia occurs in fewer than 10% of non-pulmonary SOT patients, while in lung transplant patients, approximately 15% of patients suffer from acute pneumonia (Duncan and Wilkes, 2005). The increased risk for pneumonia after lung transplant is due to an unpredictable interaction of factors. For example, intra-operative surgical issues and anastamotic complications may contribute to pneumonia during the early post-transplant period. Ischemia of the bronchial mucosa, an important component of innate pulmonary immunity, can additionally increase the risk for early pneumonia in these patients, as can the loss of the cough reflex which may follow implantation of a devenerated donor lung (Gasink and Blumberg, 2005).

Later, usually following hospital discharge, opportunistic organisms become more of a concern (Fishman and Rubin, 1998). As a result, these patients routinely receive prophylaxis for multiple potential infectious agents. Both the type of prophylaxis and compliance with it alters the range of organisms which may cause pneumonia during this time frame. Agents used for induction of immunosuppression earlier may also now exert their effect on the risk and form of pneumonia. Recently, Peleg and colleagues explored the link between use of alemtuzumab, an anti-CD-52 monoclonal antibody that results in sustained lymphocyte depletion, and infection in persons receiving SOTs (Peleg et al., 2007). They noted that persons given this during immunosuppression tended to suffer infection approximately 120 days following its administration (Peleg et al., 2007). This observation underscores that management decisions made early post-SOT have implications during later phases of recovery and highlights that clinicians must take a detailed immunosuppression history when evaluating SOT recipients for pneumonia.

During long-term follow-up, the risk for pneumonia and the types of pathogens causing it often are a function of the underlying state of immunosuppression and other host factors. The central host factor is the development of rejection. Acute rejection itself may be a risk factor for pneumonia with certain types of pathogens (for example, invasive mould). Additionally, acute rejection routinely necessitates augmentation of immunosuppression. This, too, affects the probability of pneumonia and must be considered when evaluating SOT patients with pulmonary infiltrates. Furthermore, traditional community-acquired organisms become more evident in this period. These three phases of risk for pneumonia are divided roughly into distinct time periods ranging from the transplant to the first month post-transplant, then the first to sixth month after SOT, and finally thereafter beyond the sixth month (Fishman and Rubin, 1998).

7.3 Differential diagnosis and non-infectious complications

The differential diagnosis for radiographic infiltrates in the SOT remains broad and is summarized in Table 7.1. It is important to note that both infectious and non-infectious processes may lead to pulmonary symptoms and abnormal findings on thoracic imaging. Additionally, the signs and symptoms of a pulmonary process in a SOT patient may be subtle. Because of their immunosuppression, for instance, they may not be able to mount a fever in response to infection (Shorr, Susla and O'Grady, 2004). Infectious causes of pulmonary disease in SOT patients are described in detail in the section addressing the organisms which cause pneumonia after SOT.

Fortunately, compared to persons either receiving high-dose chemotherapy for haematologic malignancies or undergoing haematologic stem cell transplantation (HSCT), the differential diagnosis for pulmonary disease is more limited in the SOT subject. For example, engraftment syndrome and diffuse alveolar haemorrhage which may complicate HSCT are not an issue in the SOT recipient (Kotloff, Ahya and Crawford, 2004). Similarly, the physician need not consider leukemic infiltrates or idiopathic pneumonia syndrome. Additionally, many of the chemotherapeutic agents given for HSCT may cause direct pulmonary toxicity.

Despite the more limited differential diagnosis compared to the HSCT subject, a variety of non-infectious causes may account for radiographic infiltrates mimicking pneumonia. Both cardiogenic and non-cardiogenic pulmonary edema can lead to diffuse

Table 7.1 Differential diagnosis of pulmonary infiltrates in solid organ transplant patients.

Infectious Causes
- Bacteria (*Pseudomonas aeruginosa, Methicillin-resistant Staphylococcus aureus, Streptococcus pneumonia, Legionella spp.*)
- Fungi (Aspergillus, Pneumocystis jeroviici)
- Viruses (CMV, HSV, RSV, parainlfuenza, influenza)
- Mycobateria (Mycobacterium tuberculosis, non-tuberculosis mycobacteria)

Non-infectious causes
- Pulmonary oedema
- Acute lung injury
- Transfusion-related acute lung injury
- Drug reaction (e.g. sirolimus)
- Malignancy (Post-transplant lymphoproliferative disorder)

Abbreviations: CMV – cytomegalovirus, HSV – herpes simplex virus, RSV – respiratory syncytial virus.

infiltrates and hypoxemia. With fluid shifts and transfusions intraoperatively, fluid overload is frequent following SOT. Transfusion may also cause acute lung injury (TRALI). The true incidence of TRALI is unknown but it is likely underappreciated; and transplant patients, because of immunosuppression, may be at higher risk for it (Swanson *et al.*, 2006).

Among pulmonary transplant patients, reperfusion injury will also lead to diffuse infiltrates and a clinical scenario consistent with acute lung injury. Currently this condition is termed 'primary graft dysfunction' and represents a diagnosis of exclusion (Ahya and Kawut, 2005). This syndrome usually arises in the immediate post-transplant period and is usually the result of multiple insults to the allograft which alter pulmonary microvascular permeability. Alternatively, acute pulmonary rejection usually presents as new infiltrates arising three to five days after graft insertion.

More focal or scattered infiltrates may arise as a result of drug reactions. Multiple agents used for immunosuppression lead to pulmonary toxicity. Three agents of particular concern are: sirolimus, OKT3 and basilizimab. Sirolimus is a potent immunosuppressive that binds to a kinase which prevents mRNA translation and thus affects many aspects of cell cycle regulation. Reliance on sirolimus has increased because this agent causes significantly less nephrotoxicity than calcineurin inhibitors. Sirolimus, though, has been reported to cause an interstitial pneumonitis (Pham *et al.*, 2004; Buhaescu, Izzedine and Covic, 2006). Initially, investigators believed that this arose in association with excess blood levels of sirolimus. Recent case reports, however, describe this syndrome in persons whose blood concentrations were normal (Pham *et al.*, 2004). These reports also note lung injury related to sirolimus arising several months after the initiation of therapy. Hence, sirolimus pulmonary toxicity may either present as a fulminant condition with rapidly progressive respiratory failure or, more commonly, as an indolent process. Often patients complain of dyspnea and cough, and more than half of affected subjects report fever. Radiographically, sirolimus toxicity appears as either diffuse or bilateral infiltrates. CT scanning may reveal ground glass opacifications (Pham *et al.*, 2004; Buhaescu, Izzedine and Covic, 2006). On the other hand, sirolimus pulmonary disease may take the form of small bilateral nodules. The findings on lung biopsy have been mixed with descriptions of sirolimus associated with cryptogenic organizing pneumonia (COP), lymphocytic alveolar aggregates, and non-necrotizing granulomas. Irrespective of the histopathologic appearance, infection must be excluded as a consideration. With discontinuation of the drug pulmonary function improves. The role for corticosteroids is unclear.

OKT-3 is a murine anti-IgG antibody directed against T cells. Use of OKT-3 has diminished substantially. Because of its mechanism of action which requires initial T cell activation, OKT-3 may cause a cytokine release syndrome. With respect to lung injury, OKT-3 has been implicated as a risk factor for ARDS following renal transplantation. In an analysis of over 40 000 kidney transplants, OKT-3 increased the risk for ARDS more than threefold (Shorr, Abbott and Agadoa, 2003).

Basilizimab, another monoclonal antibody, is an interlukein-2 receptor antagonist. Because it is well tolerated, this agent is increasingly employed for immunosuppression induction. With broader utilization, several cases of acute lung injury associated with basilizimab administration have been reported. The reason for this reaction remains undefined (Bamgbola *et al.*, 2003).

In addition to drug toxicity and various types of pulmonary oedema, physicians must include post-transplant lymphoproliferative disease (PTLD) in the initial differential diagnosis of SOT patients with abnormal chest radiographs. PTLD represents a heterogeneous collection of abnormal lymphoid proliferations, often of B cell origin. The vast majority of cases are associated with Epstein-Barr virus (EBV) infection. PTLD affects up to 15% of SOT recipients (Loren and Tsai, 2005). Lung transplant and heart-lung transplant patients are at highest risk for this condition. Although usually diagnosed approximately six months following SOT, PTLD can occur at any point. Patients often present with a non-specific syndrome and specific pulmonary complaints such as dyspnea, cough and haemoptysis are not major features. The key factors suggesting PTLD relate to its radiographic appearance. PTLD usually appears as multiple discrete nodules in the lung (Loren and Tsai, 2005). The edges of the nodules may be either smooth or irregular and thus PTLD can mimic fungal infections, septic emboli, or pulmonary metastases. Unlike most invasive mould infections, nodules caused by PTLD rarely cavitate. Factors associated with a better prognosis include limitation of the PTLD to the allograft and EBV positivity. Reduction of immunosuppression remains the cornerstone of therapy. Chemotherapy and other alternatives are reserved for patients who fail despite a reduction in immunosuppression.

7.4 Diagnostic approach

Central to efforts to diagnose pneumonia following SOT is a low threshold to evaluate patients for non-specific pulmonary complaints. In certain instances, the symptoms may be obvious and alert the clinician to the likelihood of pneumonia. However, because of immunosuppression, the presentation of pneumonia may be more subtle. For example, fever may be absent and cough may be minimal.

When taking the patient's history as part of the evaluation for pneumonia in the SOT recipient, one must remember to inquire about the agents used for infection prophylaxis and compliance with these medications. The broad utilization of prophylaxis for Pneumocytisi jirovecii (PJP) and CMV disease makes these less likely in persons who have been compliant with their preventive regimens. Similarly, knowing if acute rejection has occurred and how it was treated may help direct the evaluation, particularly since acute rejection is a risk factor for invasive mould infection. Investigating the subject's CMV status and that of the donor further aids in prioritizing the possible infectious causes of pneumonia. The presence of non-pulmonary symptoms, particularly gastrointestinal ones, may suggest CMV infection. Finally, a history of recent travel or occupational exposures can prove helpful in identifying potential pathogens.

Radiology

Radiographic imaging provides important information beyond the history. First, a normal chest radiograph (CXR) does not preclude the diagnosis of pneumonia.

Approximately, 10% of immunosuppressed patients with pneumonia present with initially normal CXRs (Franquet, Gimenez and Hidalgo, 2004). Because immunosuppression may blunt the inflammatory response the CXR can be relatively insensitive. In other words, evidence of pulmonary disease may only be present on CT imaging. Confirming this supposition, Heussel *et al.* performed CT scans in neutropenic patients with fever but normal CXRs (Heussel *et al.*, 1999). In 60% of subjects, the CT identified a pneumonic process up to five days before the CXR became abnormal (Heussel *et al.*, 1999). Thus, in SOT subjects with pulmonary complaints or unexplained fever, early CT is warranted to facilitate the evaluation. Moreover, a CT scan tends to reveal information that may not be readily noted on a CXR. Adenopathy, an important diagnostic clue as to the cause of a pulmonary process, is often missed on plain radiographs. The pattern of infiltrates noted on a CT can also be helpful in forming a differential diagnosis while at the same time help guide decision as to where to perform invasive sampling. No pattern on CT, however, is pathognomic for a particular process.

Typical patterns noted on CT scanning in SOT patients with pneumonia are shown in Table 7.2. Generally, CT scans tend to reveal either diffuse or focal processes. Diffuse infiltrates may be caused by either cardiogenic or non-cardiogenic oedema. These diffuse infiltrates also tend to be bilateral. In the pulmonary transplant subject, a patchy infiltrate seen only in the allograft may suggest reperfusion injury or acute rejection, depending on the infiltrates' onset relative to the timing of the transplant (Ahya and Kawut, 2005). Usually, the infiltrates associated with reperfusion injury are mild and

Table 7.2   Patterns seen on CT scans in SOT patients with pneumonia.

Diffuse, Bilateral Infiltrates
- Pulmonary oedema
- Acute lung injury
- Transfusion-related acute lung injury
- Reperfusion injury (seen in the allograft in lung transplant recipients, may be unilateral if single lung

Focal Infiltrates (may be unilateral or bilateral)

Alveolar consolidation
- Bacterial pneumonia
- Non-bacterial infections (e.g. Mycobacterial and fungal disease)
- Malignancy

Ground glass opacities
- Opportunistic infections (e.g. Pnuemocystis, viruses)
- Drug toxicity
- Acute rejection (e.g. lung transplant)

Peripheral Nodules (single or multiple)
- Infection (e.g. Aspergillosis, Nocardia)
- Malignancy (e.g. post-transplant lymphoproliferative disease)

Centrilobular Nodules
- Infections
- Bronchiolitis obliterans syndrome

clear shortly after day five following organ insertion. Drug toxicity also can manifest as diffuse infiltrates (Ahya and Kawut, 2005).

Focal consolidation takes many forms. Acute airspace disease in a classic lobar pattern suggests a bacterial pneumonia. Some pathogens, such as actinomycoses, though, do not always respect anatomical borders. Additionally, infections may cause patchy disease rather than dense consolidations. A chemical pneumonitis following aspiration can mimic an infectious pneumonia as well. The sensitivity and specificity of particular findings on CT for bacterial infection are generally thought to be poor and therefore the results of the CT ought not to be used to narrow the initial antibiotic prescription in the absence of specific clinical and microbiologic data (Shah and Miller, 2005). Illustrating the non-specific nature of airspace consolidation, tuberculosis (TB) often presents atypically in those infected following SOT with cavitary disease being noted in fewer then 5% of subjects (Singh and Paterson, 1998). A dense consolidation represents one of the more common radiographic presentations of TB infection following SOT.

Ground glass opacities represent another pattern often noted on CT scans in immunocompromised patients. The differential diagnosis for ground glass attenuation is diverse. Both infectious and non-infectious diseases can lead to ground glass changes on CT. Two major infections tend to manifest as ground glass opacities: Pneumocystis jerovecii (PJP) and CMV. PJP causes bilateral disease but there may be asymmetry with respect to the apparent lung involvement. Infiltrates due to PJP may be either homogeneous or may be associated with a reticular-nodular pattern. Adenopathy is rarely noted in PJP.

CMV is the most common viral cause of pneumonia in SOT recipients. Up to 9% of SOT patients with CMV pneumonia present with normal CXRs (Franquet, Lee and Muller, 2003). On CT, ground glass is commonly noted with CMV. However, CMV, unlike PJP, often has a significant nodular component. Infiltrates secondary to CMV infection may be patchy or diffuse depending on the extent of the infection. Effusions are more commonly seen with CMV than PJP, occurring in approximately 20% of CT scans of patients eventually diagnosed with CMV (Leung et al., 1999). Readers should note that most other respiratory viruses, such as respiratory syncytical virus and varciella, radiographically appear similar to CMV. Hence, in persons demonstrating ground glass on a CT scan and in whom the diagnosis of CMV is unlikely because of either donor serostatus or because of the use of prophylaxis, one must consider these other viruses.

Just as ground glass may be due to either infectious or non-infectious complications of SOT, nodules too may be caused by both infectious and non-infectious insults. Nodules related to mould infection may be either single or multiple. The nodules are often less than 5 mm in size. Depending on the time course of the infection, the nodules arising due to invasive mould may be either cavitary or solid. In fact, cavitation is often a late finding and the absence of cavitation does not preclude a diagnosis of either *Aspergillus* or *Mucormycosis* (Segal and Walsh, 2006). Often peripheral, these nodules can occasionally coalesce to form a large mass which may be mistaken for a primary lung neoplasm. Because it is angioinvasive, *Aspergillus* infection can lead to peripheral, wedge shaped opacities, which resemble those seen after pulmonary infarction from a pulmonary embolism. In some cases, necrosis results in local haemorrhage causing an area of ground glass near the nodules. The air-crescent sign is a late finding in invasive mould disease and is caused by contraction of infracted tissue surrounding the site of infection (Lee *et al.*, 2005). Conversely, the halo sign, an area of low attenuation near the primary lesion is an early finding that often is transient. These two signs are somewhat specific for invasive *Aspergillosis* but lack sensitivity. Therefore the diagnosis of *Aspergillus* requires a high index of suspicion. If cavities do form following *Aspergillus* infection often they are thick walled. Other fungi, such as *Coccidiomycoses* and Fusarium spp., result in thin walled cavities. Nocardia, now a rare complication of SOT given the broad use of prophylaxis, should be considered in persons being evaluated for invasive *Aspergillosis*. Nocardia pneumonia too may appear as either single or multiple nodules with or without cavitation (Husain *et al.*, 2002). PTLD and primary lung cancer should also be considered in the differential of peripheral nodules in the SOT subject.

Physicians may observe more central nodules in traditional bacterial infections (for example, the round pneumonia). Alternatively, when associated with evidence of bronchiolar inflammation potential etiologies include community-acquired respiratory viruses such as influenza, parainfluenza and RSV. If nodules display clustering with extension into the adjoining airway, this is referred to as 'tree in bud' appearance. The tree-in-bud pattern is classically described in infections due to non-tuberculus mycobacteria. In persons with underlying bronchiestasis (for example, due to either cystic fibrosis of idiopathic pulmonary fibrosis) the tree in bud appearance may also be seen in association with bacterial infection.

Non-invasive testing

Before moving to invasive testing in suspected pneumonia in the SOT recipient, non-invasive testing plays an important role in the diagnostic evaluation. Components of the non-invasive evaluation include blood cultures, use of the urinary antigens for *Steptococus pneumoniae* and *Legionealla*, and serologic testing for CMV, and sputum culture and gram stain. The primary purpose of these non-invasive tests is to obviate the need for more invasive testing and the risks associated with those techniques.

In prior reports describing the epidemiology of pneumonia following SOT, the yield for blood cultures is variable. In a review of 83 cases of pneumonia in organ transplant patients, Cervera *et al.* noted that blood cultures result in a diagnosis in approximately 3% of subjects (Cervera *et al.*, 2006). Rano and colleagues focusing on mixed population of non-HIV immunocompromised hosts observed that blood cultures aided in pathogen identification more often (15% of cases) (Rano *et al.*, 2001). It appears that the utility of blood cultures varies based on the probability that the individual's clinical syndrome is a bacterial infection. Therefore, the value of blood cultures is often higher during the early post-transplant period when persons are at high risk for infection with traditional nosocomial pathogens and during the late post transplant time frame when the likelihood of CAP increases.

Sputum cultures also appear to have a variable value. However, for Tuberculosis, sputum culture with appropriate staining remains an important tool. Urinary antigens for S. pneumoniae and Legionella have excellent specificity but somewhat limited sensitivity (Bartlett, 2004). This is particularly true for Legionella given that the current antigen testing methodology only identifies infection with serotype 1 (Bartlett, 2004). Nonetheless, several case series suggest that urinary antigen testing may identify the cause of infiltrates in 3–5% of patients (Cervera et al., 2006; Rano et al., 2001).

Bronchoscopy

Many conditions potentially responsible for infiltrates and pneumonia following organ transplant cannot reliably be detected without bronchoscopy. For example, bronchoscopy represents an accurate tool for diagnosing both PJP and CMV infection. Empiric therapy for both of these conditions may be warranted in many transplant patients with infiltrates. However, the therapies for CMV and PJP can be toxic so extended empiric treatment based solely on clinical grounds would expose the majority of patients to unacceptable and unnecessary risks. Moreover, diagnosis of non-infectious causes of infiltrates in this setting routinely requires the exclusion of alternative, infectious processes. Again, this can usually only be accomplished with bronchoscopy. Finally, these non-infectious conditions may require treatment with corticosteroids. Since corticosteroids (1) have side-effects and (2) can exacerbate underlying infection, one needs to be certain as to the likelihood of a non-infectious injury and should strive to exclude infection as a significant issue.

The sensitivity of bronchoscopy at identifying the etiology of pneumonia in immunocompromised transplant patients varies based on the population studied, the offending pathogen, and the techniques used. Bronchoscopy has a high sensitivity for CMV and certain other opportunistic pathogens. Review of cytology specimens from bronchoscopy can reveal viral inclusions consistent with CMV. Additionally, bronchoalveolar lavage (BAL) fluid can be tested for the presence of anti-CMV antibodies and be sent for direct shell viral culture. Overall the reported sensitivity and specificity of BAL for CMV are approximately 90 and 98% respectively (Tamm et al., 2001; Tiroke, Bewig and Haverich, 1999).

In contrast, bronchoscopy is less reliable in suspected mould infections. By their nature, Aspergillus and other invasive moulds tend to cause patchy involvement in the lung and also can be angioinvasive. This probably explains why BAL is only positive half the time in either known or probable invasive Aspergillosis (Paterson and Singh, 1999). The role for transbronchial biopsy (TBB) to increase the yield of bronchoscopy for suspected invasive Aspergillus is controversial. First, many patients with this condition are coagulopathic or thrombocytopenic which may preclude TBB. Second, because it is patchy by nature, the bronchoscopist may simply fail to biopsy a site of involvement. A newer area of research to enhance the value of bronchoscopy in Aspergillus infection addresses the use of the current assay for Galacomannan (GM) (Verdaguer et al., 2007). GM is a component of the Aspergillus that is released in areas of tissue invasion. As a serologic test, GM has proved less useful than was hoped. However, one can measure GM concentrations in BAL fluid. Efforts to enhance the yield of the GM assays have explored its use on BAL fluid. One recent study in over 100 patients indicates that this approach has significant promise (Husain *et al.*, 2007). Although the recovery of *Aspergillosis* from the airways almost always suggests infection and not colonization, negative stains and cultures for mould should not preclude treatment if this is highly suspected by the physician.

Several recent studies, summarized in Table 7.3 have examined the potential role and yield of bronchoscopy in the immunosuppressed transplant host. These case series have confirmed the importance of bronchoscopy. These reports have described outcomes either in homogenous cohorts of persons who have undergone a specific type of SOT or in heterogeneous populations of immunocompromised hosts. Chang *et al.* reviewed the records of 92 renal transplant patients with suspected pneumonia (Chang *et al.*, 2004). In 71 instances, the investigators confirmed a final etiologic diagnosis. The most common pathogens identified included *S. aureus*, *P. aeruginosa*, and *Klebsiella pneumoniae*. Of the 64 subjects who underwent bronchoscopy, the diagnostic yield approached 60% (Chang *et al.*, 2004).

In a similar review of bronchoscopy in heart transplant recipients, Lehto *et al.* observed that bronchoscopy resulted in a diagnosis of pneumonia in 41% of cases (Lehto *et al.*, 2004). Common pathogens identified with the aid of invasive testing were *P. aeruginosa*, PJP and CMV. More importantly, bronchoscopy altered management (for example, addition or discontinuation of therapies) in 14 of 44 patients (Lehto *et al.*, 2004). Confirming the report of Chang and co-workers, SOT recipients tolerated bronchoscopy well, and major complications were rare. These same investigators also described their experience with bronchoscopy for infection in lung and heart-lung transplant patients. Bronchoscopy in those who have received a lung allograft is somewhat unique since it represents a means for identifying rejection and therefore is often performed on a routine, surveillance basis. In this description of over 600 bronchoscopies, 60% were performed for suspected infection with the remainder done as part of a surveillance protocol (Lehto *et al.*, 2005). In half of the clinically indicated bronchoscopies, this procedure identified an offending pathogen. Again, bacterial pathogens and CMV predominated (Lehto *et al.*, 2005). Bronchoscopy, though, also led to the diagnosis of invasive mould, mycobacteria and community respiratory viruses. Despite having undergone lung transplant, the procedure was remarkably safe with only two small pneumothoracies reported.

Unique because of its prospective design, Torres *et al.* studied pneumonia in liver transplant recipients (Torres *et al.*, 2000). The authors diagnosed pneumonia in half the cohort and 30% were classified as 'probable pneumonia'. With the aid of bronchoscopy, 32 distinct pathogens were identified (Torres *et al.*, 2000). Highlighting the importance of invasive testing, findings from bronchoscopy led to treatment alterations in 35% of patients. These researchers performed both BAL and protected specimen brush. In comparing the two, the correlation was moderate (kappa = 0.52) (Torres *et al.*, 2000). Among the study population, the mortality rate was high with 16 subjects dying.

Table 7.3 Recent studies describing the yield of bronchoscopy in solid organ transplant patients.

References	Population	Sample size	Yield of bronchoscopy	Complications from bronchoscopy	Overall mortality
Torres *et al.*, 2000	Liver Transplant	50	53%	NR	32%
Chang *et al.*, 2004	Renal Transplant	92	59%	NR	29%
Lehto *et al.*, 2004	Heart Transplant	44	41%	8% (none fatal)	23%
Lehto *et al.*, 2005	Thoracic Transplant	190 (clinically suspected infection)	51%	2% (none fatal)	NR
Rano *et al.*, 2001	Non-HIV Immunocompromised	200	59%	NR	35%
Danes *et al.*, 2002	Mixed Immunocompromised	241	52%	NR	NR
Jain *et al.*, 2004	Non-HIV Immunocompromised	104	51%	21% overall, but 1 major bleed; 4 PTX, none fatal	NR
Cervera *et al.*, 2006	Mixed Solid Organ Transplant	83	66%	NR	36%

Abbreviations: NR – not reported, PTX – pneumothorax.

Systemic utilization of bronchoscopy along with non-invasive testing in mixed groups of immunosuppressed transplant patients substantiates the findings seen in evaluations of this approach in cohorts of selected SOT subjects. Rano *et al.* applied a systematic diagnostic algorithm including serologic testing, blood antigen testing, and blood and sputum cultures (Rano *et al.*, 2001). If these tests proved unrevealing, individuals underwent bronchoscopy. These investigators employed their protocol in 200 cases of suspected pneumonia, one quarter of whom had received organ transplants. In approximately 80% of cases a diagnosis was made, and in three-quarters of persons with a final diagnosis, the researchers identified an infectious process (Rano *et al.*, 2001). In patients undergoing bronchoscopy, the reported yield was similar to that seen in other trials. The procedure itself directly facilitated diagnosis in 50% of persons undergoing bronchoscopy. (Rano *et al.*, 2001). More strikingly, half of patients had a change in their treatment paradigm based on utilization of this systematic protocol.

Extending their work in this area, these investigators continued to rely on a systematic protocol for evaluation of infiltrates in immunocompromised patients. Among an additional 241 immunosuppressed persons, bacterial infections predominated followed by fungal and viral pathogens (Agusti *et al.*, 2003). Again, bronchoscopy proved pivotal in making a diagnosis in nearly half of patients. In exploring the value of cell counts on BAL fluid, they observed that the proportion of inflammatory cells may help in the diagnostic process. Specifically, as one might expect, in bacterial pneumonia, most patients had a BAL cell count with greater than 50% neturophils and lymphocytes (Agusti *et al.*, 2003). Conversely, in fungal and viral infections, neutrophilia was less extensive and there was a greater proportion of lymphocytes.

The most recent prospective analysis of diagnostic testing including bronchoscopy in mixed SOT recipients included 80 cases of suspected pneumonia in 83 patients (Cervera *et al.*, 2006). Forty of the subjects had undergone renal transplant and the median time from transplantation to pneumonia in the entire population was 112 days. (Cervera *et al.*, 2006). Nearly 40% of pneumonias presented during the first three months following organ implantation. Although the yield for bronchoscopy was high (66%), the value of the procedure varied based on the timing of the onset of pneumonia. (Cervera *et al.*, 2006). In persons with relatively early post-transplant pneumonia, bronchoscopy was more often performed and had a higher diagnostic yield. In those presenting with pneumonia after the first three months post-transplant, bronchoscopy was only diagnostic in 45% of cases. This difference probably arises because bacterial pathogens predominate early following transplant, and bronchoscopy has a high sensitivity for these types of infections. Overall the mortality of pneumonia in SOT recipients remained elevated (36%) (Cervera *et al.*, 2006). Significant factors associated with mortality included the need for mechanical ventilation and early onset pneumonia. Although the presence of *Aspergillus* infection correlated with death in univariate analysis, it was not an independent predictor of mortality in logistic regression.

In summary, bronchoscopy is safe, easy to perform, and aids in the diagnosis of pneumonia in SOT patients. Often, the findings from bronchoscopy alter management. Even when non-diagnostic, use of this procedure to exclude certain diagnoses for which presumptive therapy can be toxic (e.g. PJP) can benefit the patient. Additionally,

information for BAL cell count can help narrow the differential diagnosis while awaiting final cultures and biopsy reports.

Recommended diagnostic strategy

Based on these reports, we propose clinicians employ a systematic, protocolized
approach in evaluation of SOT patients with suspected pneumonia. First, and concurrent
with diagnostic testing, it is prudent to begin broad-spectrum anti-infective therapy.
Multiple analyses in both immunocompetent and immunosuppressed persons document that delay in initiation of therapy is an important independent risk factor for death
(Iregui *et al.*, 2002; Morrell, Fraser and Kollef, 2005). For SOT recipients, since the list
of potential pathogens is so broad, it becomes important to rapidly eliminate certain
possibilities and to tailor therapy to the needs and condition of the individual patient.

Initial antibiotic therapy should be based on the suspected bacterial epidemiology and
resistance patterns and be modified in light of agents the patient might have received in
the past. Prior exposure to one antibiotic increases the potential for subsequent infection
with a new pathogen which is resistant to what the patient has been given previously
(Fishman, 2006). In general it is crucial to cover non-lactose fermenting gram negative
rods, MRSA, *S. pneumoniae* and *Legionella*. Added therapy for PJP, CMV and fungi
should be considered depending on the patient's severity of illness, underlying immune
status, and prophylaxis used. Findings on CT scanning may also help physicians
determine whether or not to treat PJP, CMV and fungi while awaiting further testing.
Sputum, blood and urine cultures along with urine antigen testing and serologic studies
should be performed soon after pneumonia is suspected. As noted earlier, given that
CT scanning can help either limit or expand the differential diagnosis in SOT subjects,
this should be completed expeditiously.

Bronchoscopy should follow if either the non-invasive testing is inconclusive or if the
patient is too unstable to undergo the procedure. The exact timing of bronchoscopy
remains controversial. Given that processing of BAL specimens requires special
techniques, the bronchoscopist must coordinate with colleagues to ensure pathology
and lab support is readily available. There is little reason to expose the patient to the
limited risks associated with bronchoscopy if the specimens and cultures will not be
processed for several days.

Is there a role for surgical lung biopsy (SLB) if all other testing is non-diagnostic?
SLB represents the 'gold standard' and provides the pathologist with a large piece
of tissue to evaluate histologically. SLB, though, is very invasive. More significantly, it
is unclear how SLB alters management in SOT patients. Immunosuppressed persons
undergoing SOT already face a high risk for death because their condition has remained
undiagnosed for an extended period of time. Moreover, most infectious conditions will
be diagnosed with less invasive testing and bronchoscopy. (Ahya and Kawut, 2005).
Likely diagnoses in SOT patients found only on SLB include cryptogenic organizing
pneumonia, malignancy and drug reactions. Unfortunately, there is little descriptive
literature exploring SLB in persons who have undergone SOT. In haematologic
transplant patients, SLB has been utilized somewhat more frequently and been found

to alter management in some patients. (White, Wong and Downey, 2000). It seems, though, that findings from HSCT patients are not directly applicable to SOT subjects. HSCT patients are more significantly immunosuppressed than SOT recipients, and the differential diagnosis for pneumonia following HSCT is more extensive than the differential diagnosis in SOT subjects. In light of these considerations, the decision to pursue SLB must be undertaken carefully.

7.5   Conclusion

Pneumonia in the SOT patient remains a challenge. Although the differential diagnosis remains exceedingly broad, the physician must recall that both infectious and non-infectious processes may cause pulmonary infiltrates following SOT. Both the appearance of the infiltrates and their pattern along with the timing of onset of the syndrome provide important clues as to possible etiology. Despite using a traditional approach and structuring the list of possible conditions as to their likelihood, it is important to note that no constellation of signs and symptoms ever provides sufficient diagnostic certainty as to the cause of pneumonia in a SOT recipient. As such, invasive and aggressive diagnostic interventions are not only warranted but are crucial. Precision as to the diagnosis allows one: (1) to ensure that the patient is receiving anti-infective appropriate for his/her syndrome and; (2) to withdraw treatments that are not indicated and which may, in fact, be harmful. In selected cases, OLB may be necessary.

Irrespective of the type of SOT or the patient's presentation, the prompt and timely administration of anti-infective therapy remains central to improving outcomes. Delay in therapy increases the potential for poor outcome and for mortality. With both aggressive diagnostic and treatment strategies, clinics can strive to improve outcomes for SOT patients who develop pneumonia.

References

Agusti, C., Rano, A., Sibila, O. and Torres, A. (2003) Nosocomial pneumonia in immunosuppressed patients. *Infectious Disease Clinics of North America*, **17** (4), 785–800.

Ahya, V.N. and Kawut, S.M. (2005) Noninfectious pulmonary complications after lung transplantation. *Clinics in Chest Medicine*, **26** (4), 613–622.

United Network for Organ Sharing website (2007) www.unos.org. Accessed.

Bamgbola, F.O., Del Rio, M., Kaskel, F.J. and Flynn, J.T. (2003) Non-cardiogenic pulmonary edema during basiliximab induction in three adolescent renal transplant patients. *Pediatric Transplantation*, **7** (4), 315–320.

Bartlett, J.G. (2004) Diagnostic test for etiologic agents of community-acquired pneumonia. *Infectious Disease Clinics of North America*, **18** (4), 809–827.

Buhaescu, I., Izzedine, H. and Covic, A. (2006) Sirolimus–challenging current perspectives. *Therapeutic Drug Monitoring*, **28** (5), 577–584.

Cervera, C., Agusti, C., Angeles Marcos, M., Pumarola, T., Cofan, F., Navasa, M., Perez-Villa, F., Torres, A. and Moreno, A. (2006) Microbiologic features and outcome of pneumonia in transplanted patients. *Diagnostic Microbiology and Infectious Disease*, **55** (1), 47–54.

Chang, G.C., Wu, C.L., Pan, S.H., Yang, T.Y., Chin, C.S., Yang, Y.C. and Chiang, C.D. (2004) The diagnosis of pneumonia in renal transplant recipients using invasive and noninvasive procedures. *Chest*, **125** (2), 541–547.

Danés, C., González-Martín, J., Pumarola, T., Rañó, A., Benito, N., Torres, A., Moreno, A., Rovira, M. and Puig de la Bellacasa, J. (2002) Pulmonary infiltrates in immunosuppressed patients: analysis of a diagnostic protocol. *Journal of Clinical Microbiology*, **40** (6), 2134–2140.

Duncan, M.D. and Wilkes, D.S. (2005) Transplant-related immunosuppression: a review of immuno-suppression and pulmonary infections. *Proceedings of the American Thoracic Society*, **2** (5), 449–455.

Fishman, N. (2006) Antimicrobial stewardship. *The American Journal of Medicine*, **119** (6 Suppl 1), S53–S61.

Fishman, J.A. and Rubin, R.H. (1998) Infection in organ-transplant recipients. *The New England Journal of Medicine*, **338** (24), 1741–1751.

Franquet, T., Lee, K.S. and Muller, N.L. (2003) Thin-section CT findings in 32 immunocompromised patients with cytomegalovirus pneumonia who do not have AIDS. *AJR American Journal of Roentgenology*, **181** (4), 1059–1063.

Franquet, T., Gimenez, A. and Hidalgo, A. (2004) Imaging of opportunistic fungal infections in immunocompromised patient. *European Journal of Radiology*, **51** (2), 130–138.

Gasink, L.B. and Blumberg, E.A. (2005) Bacterial and mycobacterial pneumonia in transplant recipients. *Clinics in Chest Medicine*, **26** (4), 647–659.

Heussel, C.P., Kauczor, H.U., Heussel, G.E., Fischer, B., Begrich, M., Mildenberger, P. and Thelen, M. (1999) Pneumonia in febrile neutropenic patients and in bone ma rrow and blood stem-cell transplant recipients: use of high-resolution computed tomography. *Journal of Clinical Oncology*, **17** (3), 796–805.

Husain, S., McCurry, K., Dauber, J., Singh, N. and Kusne, S. (2002) Nocardia infection in lung transplant recipients. *The Journal of Heart and Lung Transplantation*, **21** (3), 354–359.

Husain, S., Paterson, D.L., Studer, S.M., Crespo, M., Pilewski, J., Durkin, M., Wheat, J.L., Johnson, B., McLaughlin, L., Bentsen, C., McCurry, K.R. and Singh, N. (2007) Aspergillus Galactomannan Antigen in the Bronchoalveolar Lavage Fluid for the Diagnosis of Invasive Aspergillosis in Lung Transplant Recipients. *Transplantation*, **83** (10), 1330–1336.

Iregui, M., Ward, S., Sherman, G., Fraser, V.J. and Kollef, M.H. (2002) Clinical importance of delays in the initiation of appropriate antibiotic treatment for ventilator-associated pneumonia. *Chest*, **122** (1), 262–268.

Jain, P., Sandur, S., Meli, Y., Arroliga, A.C., Stoller, J.K. and Mehta, A.C. (2004) Role of flexible bronchoscopy in immunocompromised patients with lung infiltrates. *Chest*, **125** (2), 712–722.

Kotloff, R.M., Ahya, V.N. and Crawford, S.W. (2004) Pulmonary complications of solid organ and hematopoietic stem cell transplantation. *American Journal of Respiratory and Critical Care Medicine*, **170** (1), 22–48.

Lee, Y.R., Choi, Y.W., Lee, K.J., Jeon, S.C., Park, C.K. and Heo, J.N. (2005) CT halo sign: the spectrum of pulmonary diseases. *British Journal of Radiology*, **78** (933), 862–865.

Lehto, J.T., Anttila, V.J., Lommi, J., Nieminen, M.S., Harjula, A., Taskinen, E., Tukiainen, P. and Halme, M. (2004) Clinical usefulness of bronchoalveolar lavage in heart transplant recipients with suspected lower respiratory tract infection. *The Journal of Heart and Lung Transplantation*, **23** (5), 570–576.

Lehto, J.T., Koskinen, P.K., Anttila, V.J., Lautenschlager, I., Lemstrom, K., Sipponen, J., Tukiainen, P. and Halme, M. (2005) Bronchoscopy in the diagnosis and surveillance of respiratory infections in lung and heart-lung transplant recipients. *Transplant International*, **18** (5), 562–571.

Leung, A.N., Gosselin, M.V., Napper, C.H., Braun, S.G., Hu, W.W., Wong, R.M. and Gasman, J. (1999) Pulmonary infections after bone marrow transplantation: clinical and radiographic findings. *Radiology*, **210** (3), 699–710.

Loren, A.W. and Tsai, D.E. (2005) Post-transplant lymphoproliferative disorder. *Clinics in Chest Medicine*, **26** (4), 631–645.

Morrell, M., Fraser, V.J. and Kollef, M.H. (2005) Delaying the empiric treatment of candida bloodstream infection until positive blood culture results are obtained: a potential risk factor for hospital mortality. *Antimicrobial Agents and Chemotherapy*, **49** (9), 3640–3645.

Paterson, D.L. and Singh, N. (1999) Invasive aspergillosis in transplant recipients. *Medicine (Baltimore)*, **78** (2), 123–138.

Peleg, A.Y., Husain, S., Kwak, E.J., Silveira, F.P., Ndirangu, M., Tran, J., Shutt, K.A., Shapiro, R., Thai, N., Abu-Elmagd, K., McCurry, K.R., Marcos, A. and Paterson, D.L. (2007) Opportunistic infections in 547 organ transplant recipients receiving alemtuzumab, a humanized monoclonal CD-52 antibody. *Clinical Infectious Diseases*, **44** (2), 204–212.

Pham, P.T., Pham, P.C., Danovitch, G.M., Ross, D.J., Gritsch, H.A., Kendrick, E.A., Singer, J., Shah, T. and Wilkinson, A.H. (2004) Sirolimus-associated pulmonary toxicity. *Transplantation*, **77** (8), 1215–1220.

Rano, A., Agusti, C., Jimenez, P., Angrill, J., Benito, N., Danes, C., Gonzalez, J., Rovira, M., Pumarola, T., Moreno, A. and Torres, A. (2001) Pulmonary infiltrates in non-HIV immunocompromised patients: a diagnostic approach using non-invasive and bronchoscopic procedures. *Thorax*, **56** (5), 379–387.

Segal, B.H. and Walsh, T.J. (2006) Current approaches to diagnosis and treatment of invasive aspergillosis. *American Journal of Respiratory and Critical Care Medicine*, **173** (7), 707–717.

Shah, R.M. and Miller, W. Jr, (2005) Pulmonary complications of transplantation: radiographic considerations. *Clinics in Chest Medicine*, **26** (4), 545–560.

Shorr, A.F., Abbott, K.C. and Agadoa, L.Y. (2003) Acute respiratory distress syndrome after kidney transplantation: epidemiology, risk factors, and outcomes. *Critical Care Medicine*, **31** (5), 1325–1330.

Shorr, A.F., Susla, G.M. and O'Grady, N.P. (2004) Pulmonary infiltrates in the non-HIV-infected immunocompromised patient: etiologies, diagnostic strategies, and outcomes. *Chest*, **125** (1), 260–271.

Singh, N. and Paterson, D.L. (1998) Mycobacterium tuberculosis infection in solid-organ transplant recipients: impact and implications for management. *Clinical Infectious Diseases*, **27** (5), 1266–1277.

Swanson, K., Dwyre, D.M., Krochmal, J. and Raife, T.J. (2006) Transfusion-related acute lung injury (TRALI): current clinical and pathophysiologic considerations. *Lung*, **184** (3), 177–185.

Tamm, M., Traenkle, P., Grilli, B., Soler, M., Bolliger, C.T., Dalquen, P. and Cathomas, G. (2001) Pulmonary cytomegalovirus infection in immunocompromised patients. *Chest*, **119** (3), 838–843.

Tiroke, A.H., Bewig, B. and Haverich, A. (1999) Bronchoalveolar lavage in lung transplantation. State of the art. *Clinical Transplantation*, **13** (2), 131–157.

Torres, A., Ewig, S., Insausti, J., Guergue, J.M., Xaubet, A., Mas, A. and Salmeron, J.M. (2000) Etiology and microbial patterns of pulmonary infiltrates in patients with orthotopic liver transplantation. *Chest*, **117** (2), 494–502.

Verdaguer, V., Walsh, T.J., Hope, W. and Cortez, K.J. (2007) Galactomannan antigen detection in the diagnosis of invasive aspergillosis. *Expert Review of Molecular Diagnostics*, **7** (1), 21–32.

White, D.A., Wong, P.W. and Downey, R. (2000) The utility of open lung biopsy in patients with hematologic malignancies. *American Journal of Respiratory and Critical Care Medicine*, **161** (3 Pt 1), 723–729.

8

Respiratory infections following haematopoietic stem cell transplantation

Ayman O. Soubani

Division of Pulmonary, Allergy, Critical Care and Sleep Medicine, Karmanos Cancer Center and Wayne State University School of Medicine, Detroit, Michigan, USA

Haematopoietic stem cell transplantation (HSCT) is an important treatment for a variety of neoplastic diseases, haematologic disorders, immunodeficiency syndromes, congenital enzyme deficiencies, and autoimmune disorders (for example, systemic lupus erythematosus or multiple sclerosis). During the last few decades, there has been significant progress in the procedure and care of patients after transplantation. Annually, there are more than 30 000 cases of autologous HSCT and 15 000 cases of allogeneic HSCT performed worldwide (www.ibmtr.org). Haematopoietic stem cells may be obtained from bone marrow, peripheral blood, or umbilical cord blood. Depending on the source of these stem cells, HSCT is classified as autologous if the cells are taken from an individual patient and stored for reinfusion after high-dose chemotherapy, and it is classified as allogeneic if the stem cells are donated from another individual (who may or may not be related). In the case of allogeneic HSCT, the conditioning regimen before transplantation may be myeloablative, in which supra-lethal doses of chemotherapy and irradiation are given, leading to significant toxicity and immunosuppression. More recently, nonmyeloablative regimens have been used to minimize the toxicity related to the conditioning regimen and allow for immuno-logically mediated killing of tumour cells (graft vs. tumour effect).

Despite the advances in HSCT, the procedure remains limited by the high rate of severe complications that are generally related to toxicity of conditioning regimen, immunosuppression, and graft-vs.-host disease (GVHD). GVHD is a condition in which the donated cells recognize the recipient's cells as nonself and attack them. Efforts to prevent or treat GVHD include harvesting haematopoietic stem cells from an HLA matched donor and use of immunosuppressive and immunomodulatory therapy

Pulmonary Infection in the Immunocompromised Patient, Edited by Carlos Agustí and Antoni Torres
© 2009 John Wiley & Sons, Ltd.

Table 8.1 Spectrum and frequency of respiratory infectious and noninfectious complication following HSCT.[a]

Disease	Autologous	Allogeneic
Infectious		
- Bacteria	++	++
- Mycobacteria	±	+
- *Nocardia*	±	+
- *Aspergillus*	+	++
- Non-aspergillus fungal	±	+
- *P. jiroveci*	±	+
- CMV	+	++
- Community respiratory viruses	±	+
Non-infectious		
- Pulmonary oedema	++	++
- Engraftment syndrome	++	+
- Diffuse alveolar haemorrhage	+	++
- Idiopathic pneumonia syndrome	+	++
- Delayed pulmonary toxicity syndrome	++	+
- Bronchiolitis obliterans organizing pneumonia	+	+
- Bronchiolitis obliterans	±	++

[a] ++ = high incidence (>10%), + = low incidence (<10%), ± = very rare (<1%).

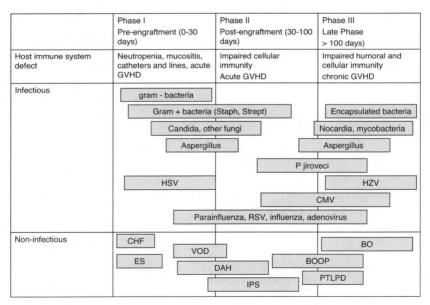

Figure 8.1 The time line of pulmonary complications following HSCT. Abbreviations: HSV = herpes simplex virus, HZV = herpes zoster virus, CMV = cytomegalovirus, RSV = respiratory syncytial virus, CHF = congestive heart failure, BO = bronchiolitis obliterans, VOD = veno-occlusive disease, ES = engraftment syndrome, DAH = diffuse alveolar hemorrhage, BOOP = bronchiolitis obliterans organizing pneumonia, IPS = idiopathic pneumonia syndrome, PTLPD = post transplant lymphoproliferative disorder.

Table 8.2 Factors that predispose to respiratory infections following HSCT.

Pre-transplantation
   - older age
   - pre-transplant immune status
   - underlying pulmonary disease
   - CMV status of the donor and recipient
   - residence in endemic areas
Transplantation
   - allogeneic
   - type and intensity of conditioning regimen
   - total body irradiation
   - delayed engraftment
Post-transplantation
   - mucositis
   - severity and duration of neutropenia
   - acute GVHD and its treatment
   - chronic GVHD and its treatment
   - T-cell depleting strategies
   - hospital environment (construction, type of air filtration,
     transmission of infection by healthcare providers)

such as corticosteroids, cyclosporine or tacrolimus (FK506) or TNF-α blocking agents (Lazarus, Vogelsang and Rowe, 1997). The use of these agents entails further hazards for infectious complications and relapse of the underlying neoplastic disease for which the transplant was performed. Pulmonary complications following HSCT, both infectious and noninfectious, develop in up to 60% of patients and are a significant cause of morbidity and mortality (Soubani, Miller and Hassoun, 1996) (Table 8.1). These complications tend to follow a characteristic sequence, and are more common following allogeneic HSCT especially in the setting of GVHD (Figure 8.1). Table 8.2 summarizes the general factors that predispose to respiratory infections following HSCT. Despite the advances in prophylaxis and treatment of these infectious processes, they remain a cause of death in more than 40% of HSCT recipients (Soubani, Miller and Hassoun, 1996). This chapter details the spectrum of respiratory infections following HSCT and describes the incidence, risk factors, clinical presentation and recent advances in the diagnosis and management of these infections.

8.1 Immune system recovery after HSCT

During the first year after an HSCT, recipients typically follow a predictable pattern of immune system deficiency and recovery, which begins with the conditioning regimen. In addition to destruction of the malignant cells, high dose chemotherapy (with or without total body irradiation) also destroys normal haematopoiesis for neutrophils, monocytes and macrophages and damages mucosal cells, causing a temporary loss of mucosal barrier integrity. In addition, HSCT recipients rapidly lose all T- and

B-lymphocytes after conditioning, losing immune memory accumulated through a lifetime of exposure to infectious agents, environmental antigens and vaccines.

Phase 1 (pre-engraftment): During the first month after HSCT, the major host-defence deficits include neutropenia and damaged mucocutaneous barriers that may lead to the translocation of gastrointestinal and cutaneous bacteria to the bloodstream. Additionally, indwelling intravenous catheters are frequently placed and left *in situ* for weeks to administer parenteral medications, blood products and nutritional supplements. These catheters serve as another portal of entry for opportunistic pathogens from organisms colonizing the skin. The organisms that commonly cause infection during this period include gram-negative bacilli such as *Klebsiella*, *Escherichia* and *Pseudomonas*, gram-positive cocci such coagulase negative and coagulase positive Staphylococci, *Enterococcus*, *Candida* species, and Herpes simplex virus. *Aspergillus* spp. may lead to infection if neutropenia persists. During preengraftment, the risks for infection are the same for autologous or allogeneic patients, and infection may present as febrile neutropenia. Although a recipient's first fever during preengraftment is probably caused by a bacterial pathogen, rarely is an organism or site of infection identified. Instead, such infections are usually treated preemptively or empirically until the neutropenia resolves. Growth factors can be administered during phase I to decrease neutropenia duration and complications.

These risks persist until the engraftment of the stem cells which is defined as sustained absolute neutrophil count of $>500/\mathrm{mm}^3$ and sustained platelet count of $>20\,000$, lasting more than 3 consecutive days without transfusions. Among unrelated allogeneic recipients, engraftment occurs at a median of 22 days after HSCT (range 6–84 days).

Phase II (30–100 days): Following engraftment and in the absence of corticosteroid therapy, neutrophil function is restored which results in a decreased risk for bacterial and fungal infections. However, all HSCT recipients and particularly allogeneic recipients, experience an immune system dysfunction for months after engraftment. They may have abnormal CD4/CD8 T-cell ratios, reflecting their decreased CD4 and increased CD8 T-cell counts (Lazarus, Vogelsang and Rowe, 1997). They might also have immunoglobulin G and immunoglobulin A deficiencies for months after HSCT and have difficulty switching from immunoglobulin M to immunoglobulin G production after antigen exposure. Immune system recovery might be delayed further by Cytomegalovirus (CMV) infection (Paulin, Ringden and Lonnqvist, 1985).

During this phase, allogeneic HSCT recipients usually develop acute GVHD that manifests as skin, gastrointestinal and liver injury. GVHD is associated with increased risk of infection due to delayed immunologic recovery. Furthermore, the immunosuppressive therapy used for GVHD prophylaxis and therapy makes HSCT recipients at an increased risk for opportunistic viral and fungal infections. The usual infectious agents during this phase include CMV, *Aspergillus* and *P. jiroveci*.

Phase III: (>100 days): Some patients with allogeneic HSCT develop chronic GVHD that is similar to connective tissue disorders (for example, scleroderma and sicca syndromes). This phase may be associated with cellular and humoural immuno-deficiencies, including macrophage deficiency, impaired neutrophil chemotaxis and poor response to vaccination. Also patients may experience long-lasting IgA and IgG deficiencies, poor opsonization and impaired reticuloendothelial function (Witherspoon *et al.*, 1981; Aucouturier *et al.*, 1987). After chronic GVHD resolves, which might take years, cell-mediated and humoural immunity function are gradually restored. Patients in this phase are at greater risk for infections caused by encapsulated organisms such as *S. pneumoniae, H. influenzae,* or *N. meningitidis.* They may also develop infections due to CMV, herpes zoster virus, community respiratory viral infections and *Aspergillus.*

8.2 Bacterial pneumonia

Bacterial pneumonia caused by gram-positive or gram-negative organisms is a significant problem following HSCT. These bacteria may lead to community or hospital acquired pneumonia. They account for 15% of all respiratory infections in HSCT recipients (Kotloff, Ahya and Crawford, 2004). Based on open lung biopsy, bacterial pneumonia is estimated to be in 2%, but increases to more than 25% when documented by autopsy (Sloane *et al.*, 1983). The mortality associated with bacterial pneumonia in HSCT recipients is 22% (Lossos *et al.*, 1995). One of the main challenges in the diagnosis of bacterial pneumonia following HSCT is the inability to identify the organism in the majority of these patients, which may underestimate the incidence of these infections. This is related to the contamination of respiratory samples by upper airways organisms, the fact that most of these patients are on prophylactic antibiotics, and the limitations in performing invasive procedures such as bronchoscopy to confirm the cause of infection.

Factors that generally increase the risk of bacterial pneumonia following HSCT include pre-transplantation immune status, type of conditioning regimen, degree and duration of neutropenia (Soubani, Miller and Hassoun, 1996; Wingard, 1999). Allogeneic HSCT and the presence of GVHD significantly increase the risk of bacterial pneumonia due to slower reconstitution of the immune system, impairment of the reticuloendothelial system and opsonization. Furthermore, the immunosuppressive therapy to treat GVHD increases the risk of bacterial pneumonia in these patients (Wingard, 1999).

HSCT recipients are at highest risk for bacterial pneumonia in the pre-engraftment phase within the first 30 days following transplantation. The factors that increase the risk of bacterial pneumonia in this phase are neutropenia, mucositis that increases the risk of aspiration especially with the use of narcotic analgesics. Indwelling catheters increase the risk of bacteremia and septic embolization to the lungs (Poutsiaka *et al.*, 2007). The presentation of bacterial pneumonia during this phase may be subtle, as the patient may present with neutropenic fever with no localizing symptoms and signs due to blunted inflammatory response (Rolston, 2001). Radiological signs may also be scarce. The chest radiograph usually shows focal consolidation, however this may be normal. The infiltrates may progress quickly to multifocal or diffuse changes that are compatible with ARDS. HRCT of the chest is recommended in febrile neutropenic patients, which may show pulmonary infiltrates in up to 50% of patients with negative chest radiograph (Heussel *et al.*, 1997; Anon, 2000).

Documentation of the microorganism causing the pneumonia may be difficult especially during the pre-engraftment period due to colonization of respiratory airways, or contamination of respiratory specimens by upper airways organisms. Coagulopathy and poor general health, may also hinder the routine performance of invasive procedures to document the cause of pneumonia. In addition, there is controversy on the value of such invasive procedures in these circumstances (Hofmeister *et al.*, 2006).

The main organisms identified as cause of bacterial pneumonia in the pre-engraftment phase are usually gram negative bacteria such as *Pseudomonas*, *Klebsiella* and *Enterobacter*. In a recent report of the utility of bronchoscopy following HSCT, the most commonly isolated bacteria following HSCT was *Pseudomonas* that was resistant to the current antibiotics (Hofmeister *et al.*, 2006). There is also increasing incidence of gram positive bacteria such as *S. aureus*, *E. faecium*, and α-haemolytic *Streptococcus*, which may be associated with septic shock and ARDS. Anaerobic organisms may be causative agents in the case of aspiration (Poutsiaka *et al.*, 2007; Laws *et al.*, 2006; Narreddy *et al.*, 2007). Broad spectrum antibiotics with activity against *Pseudomonas* and gram-positive cocci should be started immediately in all patients suspected to have bacterial pneumonia during this phase (Anon, 2000). Institutional resistance pattern needs to be considered when determining the choice of antibiotics (Anon, 2000).

Bacterial pneumonia is less common in the post-engraftment period (30–100 days). Allogeneic HSCT with acute GVHD increase the risk of bacterial pneumonia during this period. The clinical and radiological picture is usually classical for bacterial pneumonia. Antibiotics therapy during this period should be based on the organisms suspected or identified. A retrospective report on invasive *Pseudomonas* infection following HSCT revealed the incidence to be 1.65% a median of 63 days post HSCT. Attributable mortality was 36%. The risk factors for poor outcome were the presence of co pathogens and high dose corticosteroid therapy. Sixteen per cent had recurrence of *Pseudomonas* infection (Hakki *et al.*, 2007). Outbreaks of *Legionella* pneumonia have been described in HSCT recipients during this phase. Allogeneic HSCT recipients with GVHD seem to be at highest risk of this infection (Rolston, 2001; Oren *et al.*, 2002).

After the first 100 days, the risk of bacterial pneumonia is generally low except in patients with chronic GHVD. These patients continue to have defects in the immune system that result in infection with encapsulated organisms such as *S. pneumoniae* and *H. influenzae*. However, gram-negative organisms may be the etiology in up to 25% of patients (Kotloff, Ahya and Crawford, 2004; Lossos *et al.*, 1995; Wingard, 1999; Chen *et al.*, 2003). In a report of 1359 HSCT recipients, 25% of the patients developed at least one episode of pneumonia. Bacterial pneumonia was documented in 9% of all patients and was the most common etiology in those in whom an organism was identified. The most frequent isolate was *S. pneumoniae*, and gram-negative organisms were isolated in 23% of those patients. Late bacterial pneumonia was usually associated with chronic

GVHD. The one year survival of patients after bacterial pneumonia was 71% (Chen *et al.*, 2003). In another report, *S. pneumoniae* pneumonia was documented in 0.7% of HSCT recipients. The majority of these patients underwent allogeneic HSCT and had chronic GVHD. Infection was more common in patients with a history of lymphoma and in those on high dose corticosteroids therapy. Pneumococcal vaccine breakthrough developed in 11% of the cases. The infection occurred a mean of 433 ± 669 days post transplantation, and 76% of the patients had bacteremia. Mortality due to pneumococcal infection was 13%. Admission to critical care unit and higher APACHE II score were associated with worse outcome (Youssef *et al.*, 2007).

Empiric broad spectrum antibiotics should be started immediately when bacterial pneumonia is suspected following HSCT. The American Thoracic Society guidelines for the treatment of healthcare associated pneumonia in patients with risk factors such as HSCT or neutropenia recommend a regimen that includes antipseudomonal cephalosporin or carbepenem, or β lactam plus antipseudomonal fluroquinolone or aminoglycoside, plus linezolid or vancomycin if methacillin resistant *S. aureus* is suspected. In patients who develop bacterial pneumonia late following HSCT, coverage of encapsulated organisms with a flouroquinolone is recommended. The antibiotics regimen should be narrowed if the etiologic agent is identified (Niederman *et al.*, 2001; Anon, 2005).

Prophylactic measures against bacterial pneumonia include intravenous immunoglobulins in allogeneic HSCT recipients with low IgG level (Sullivan *et al.*, 2001) (Table 8.3). Antibiotics with activity against encapsulated organisms are recommended during the treatment of chronic GVHD. However, it should be noted that the routine use of prophylactic fluoroquinolones in the early post transplant phase may be associated with increased infections due to coagulase negative staphylococci and gram-negative rods resistant to fluorquinolones (Bonadio *et al.*, 2005).

Nocardia pneumonia

Nocardia infection has been rarely reported in HSCT recipients with an incidence ranging between 0.3 to 1.7% (Daly, McGeer and Lipton, 2003; van Burik *et al.*, 1997). Almost all cases reported were in allogeneic HSCT recipients on treatment for severe GVHD. In a study of 6759 HSCT recipients, 22 cases of proven or probable *Nocardia* infection were reported (van Burik *et al.*, 1997). The infection was diagnosed a median of 210 days following transplantation. The main predisposing factors for developing nocardiosis were neutropenia, active acute or chronic GVHD, and lack of prophylaxis with trimethoprim-Sulfamethoxezole (TMP-SMZ). In all except one patient *N. astroides* was the causative agent. Pulmonary involvement occurs in 56% of patients, and the most common radiological findings were nodules with or without infiltrates. The diagnosis of *Nocardia* pneumonia is usually made by Bronchoalveolar lavage (BAL), although occasionally the organism is detected by culture of sputum or tracheal secretions. If these methods are nondiagnostic then the diagnosis could be confirmed by CT guided aspirate of a pulmonary nodule or open lung biopsy. In 36% of patients there is co-infection with other organisms such as CMV and *Aspergillus*.

Table 8.3 Suggested prophylactic options against respiratory infections following HSCT.

Infection	First choice	Alternate choice	Comments
Bacteria (general)	- intravenous immunoglobulins		Intravenous immunoglobulins only if IgG level <400 mg/dl
- pneumococcus - H. influenzae	- Pneumococcal vaccine at 12, 24 mo - H. influenzae B vaccine at 12, 14, 24 mo		
Mycobacteria	Isoniazid 300 mg/day		9 mo therapy Add pyridoxine 25–50 mg daily
Aspergillus	Posaconazole 200 mg three times daily	- voriconazole - itraconazole - echinocandins	Until engraftment and during neutropenia
Candida	Fluconazole 400 mg/day orally or IV	- echinocandins	Until engraftment and during neutropenia
P. jiroveci	TMP/SMZ double strength 1 tablet/day or 3 times/wk	- Dapsone - aerosolized pentamidine	From engraftment for 6 mo and during immunosuppressive therapy for GVHD
CMV	Gancyclovir 5 mg/kg/dose bid for 7–14 d, followed by 5 mg/kg/day for 5 d/wk	- Foscarnet - valgancyclovir	Until day 100 or for a minimum of 3 wks. Monitor CMV antigen for duration of treatment
RSV	RSV immunoglobulins 750 mg/kg/month	Aerosolized ribavirin	Based on paediatric HSCT during the high season months
Influenza	Lifelong annual seasonal Influenza vaccine before HSCT, and restarting 6 mo after HSCT	- Rimantadine - amantadine	
Herpes	Acyclovir 200 mg orally 3 times/day or 250 mg/m2/dose bid intravenously	Valacyclovir	Until engraftment or day 30
Herpes Zoster Virus	Herpes zoster immunoglobulin 625 U IM		

Treatment of *Nocardia* infection is by prolonged administration of TMP-SMZ. Second line agents are available if there is allergy or side effects associated with sulfa preparations. These second line agents include amikacin, minocycline, cephalosporin or imipenem. Response to treatment is generally good, and long term survival in patients with nocardiosis is not significantly different from controls (van Burik *et al.*, 1997). Prophylaxis against *P. jiroveci* using low dose TMP-SMZ has an added benefit of reducing the incidence of *Nocardia* infection in HSCT recipients.

Mycobacterial infection

M. tuberculosis is reported in 0.4–5.5% of HSCT recipients (Roy and Weisdorf, 1997; de la Camara *et al.*, 2000; Cordonnier *et al.*, 2004; Ip *et al.*, 1998; Ku *et al.*, 2001; Yuen and Woo, 2002), and is a concern in endemic areas, or in patients who lived in an endemic area prior to HSCT. The prevalence of *M. tuberculosis* in autologous HSCT is similar to the general population, while in allogeneic HSCT recipients, the *M. tuberculosis* infection increased by threefold (de la Camara *et al.*, 2000).

A recent review of the literature reported the overall frequency of *M. tuberculosis* infection to be 0.4%, with only 2% of infections developing during neutropenia, 23% were during the first 100 days post-transplantation, and 75% were after the first 100 days (Yuen and Woo, 2002). In another review of 2241 patients who underwent HSCT, only 11 patients (0.49%) had mycobacterial infection; two patients had *M. tuberculosis*, two *M. avium intracellulare*, and the rest had rapidly growing mycobacteria organisms. All patients responded well to antimycobacterial treatment (Roy and Weisdorf, 1997).

The main risk factors for *M. tuberculosis* in HSCT are allogeneic transplantation, total body irradiation, chronic GVHD, corticosteroid therapy and residence in endemic areas (de la Camara *et al.*, 2000; Cordonnier *et al.*, 2004; Ip *et al.*, 1998; Ku *et al.*, 2001; Yuen and Woo, 2002). The median time for *M. tuberculosis* infection was 324 days in one study (de la Camara *et al.*, 2000). The clinical and radiological picture of *M. tuberculosis* infection in HSCT recipients is generally similar to non-transplant patients. However, atypical presentations including rapidly progressive disease have been described in HSCT recipients (Keung *et al.*, 1999).

Treatment of *M. tuberculosis* infection is similar to non-transplant patients; however rifampin should be avoided because of potential interaction with commonly used medications in this patient population such as fluconazole and calcineurin inhibitors (Anon, 2000; Anon, 2004a). Some studies suggested a full one year of treatment (Yuen and Woo, 2002). It is important to mention in this context that the diagnosis of latent *M. tuberculosis* may be difficult in HSCT recipients given the degree of immuno-suppression. Tuberculin skin test with 5 mm or more induration is an indication for treatment for latent *M. tuberculosis* infection, as well as patients with significant exposure to patients with active *M. tuberculosis* infection even with a negative tuberculin skin test (Anon, 2000). Treatment in these circumstances is by isoniazid for nine months (Anon, 2000).

Nontuberculous mycobacterial infections (such as *M. avium* complex, *M. kansasii*, *M. chelonae*) are rare in HSCT recipients, and are generally reported in less than 1% of all patients (Doucette and Fishman, 2004). However in one report from Memorial Sloan

Kettering Hospital the incidence of Nontuberculous mycobacterial infection was 2.8% of HSCT recipients (Weinstock *et al.*, 2003). This higher incidence was felt to be related to environmental and historical factors. In a review of 93 cases of Nontuberculous mycobacterial infection in HSCT recipients reported in the literature, the median time to diagnosis was four months, and 46% of patients had GVHD. Sixty-two per cent of patients had resolution of infection with medical therapy. The attributed mortality to Nontuberculous mycobacteria was 7.5% (Doucette and Fishman, 2004).

It is known that Nontuberculous mycobacteria colonize the airways of patients with chronic lung disease such as bronchiectasis, which may create a challenge in determining the significance of isolating Nontuberculous mycobacteria from lower respiratory tract samples of HSCT recipients. The diagnostic criteria of pulmonary Nontuberculous mycobacteria infection were detailed in published guidelines and should include signs and symptoms compatible with the diagnosis and isolation of Nontuberculous mycobacteria from respiratory tract specimen or other body tissues (Anon, 2004b; Griffith *et al.*, 2007). In the case of *M. avium intracellulare*, first line agents include clarithromycin, azithormycin, ethambutol, rifampin and rifabutin for 18 months that include 12 months of negative culture.

8.3   Invasive pulmonary aspergillosis

Aspergillus is a filamentous fungus that is ubiquitous in the environment. The *Aspergillus spp.* are present in the environment as small conidia that are regularly inhaled into the lungs. In the lungs, they change into hyphae that are short and septate, with acute angle branching. Alveolar macorphages and peripheral blood neutrophils are the primary defence mechanism against this fungus. T helper cells and their cytokines (such as TNF-α, interferon-γ, IL-12, and IL-15) augment the activity of macrophages and neutrophils against *Aspergillus*. Neutropenia and defects in T-helper cell function following HSCT make these patients especially vulnerable to invasive disease by *Aspergillus*.

Invasive pulmonary aspergillosis (IPA) is a major problem following HSCT, with steady rise in the documented cases of IPA post-transplantation. The risk for IPA is much higher following allogeneic HSCT when compared to autologous transplantation (incidence is 0.5–4% in autologous HSCT compared to 2.3–15% in allogeneic HSCT (Morgan *et al.*, 2005; Wald *et al.*, 1997; Marr *et al.*, 2002; Fukuda *et al.*, 2003; Marr *et al.*, 2002)). After autologous HSCT, IPA is mainly seen during the neutropenic phase. In allogeneic HSCT, the highest risk is in patients with severe GVHD (grade III-IV). In a study by Marr *et al.*, the probability of IPA following allogeneic HSCT reached approximately 5% at two months, 9% at six months, and 10% at one year following allogeneic HSCT. By the third year after transplantation, the probability of IPA increased minimally, to 11.1% (Marr *et al.*, 2002). In these patients, the timeline for IPA infection follows a bimodal distribution, with a peak in the first month following HSCT, which is associated with neutropenia. The second peak is during the treatment for GVHD (median 78–112 days post transplantation) (Wald *et al.*, 1997; Fukuda *et al.*, 2003; Baddley *et al.*, 2001). The first peak is currently less significant due to the routine use of stem cell instead of bone marrow for transplantation, non-myeloablative regimens, the use of colony stimulating factors during neutropenia, and the widespread use of antifungal agents have significantly decreased the incidence of IPA during this period (Wald *et al.*, 1997; Junghanss *et al.*, 2002). On the other hand, the incidence of IPA during the treatment of GVHD has become more significant, especially with higher incidence of GVHD associated with unrelated allogeneic transplantation and non-myeloablative HSCT. Cord blood HSCT is also associated with increased risk of IPA. In one study of patients who received low intensity cord blood transplantation, the three-year accumulative incidence of IPA was 10% with mortality of 86%. All of these patients developed IPA in the first 100 days post transplantation (median 20 days) (Miyakoshi *et al.*, 2007).

Also, the risk of IPA increases with the use of Alemutuzumab, which is an anti-DC52 monoclonal antibody used to deplete peripheral B and T lymphocytes (Wald *et al.*, 1997; Marr *et al.*, 2002; Marr *et al.*, 2002). Treatment of GVHD with intensive immunosuppressive therapy including corticosteroids, cyclosporine A, and anti-TNF-α agents further increases the risk of IPA (Wald *et al.*, 1997; Marr *et al.*, 2002; Warris, Bjorneklett and Gaustad, 2001; Cordonnier *et al.*, 2006; Ribaud *et al.*, 1999). There is evidence that CMV infection in these patients increases the risk of IPA (Marr *et al.*, 2002; Nichols *et al.*, 2002). The hazards ratio for IPA in the setting of CMV disease increases by 13.3 fold (95% CI 4.7–37.7) (Fukuda *et al.*, 2003).

Aspergillus is most often introduced to the lower respiratory tract by inhalation of the infectious spores. Less commonly, IPA may start in locations other than the lungs, like sinuses, the gastrointestinal tract, or the skin (intravenous catheters or prolonged skin contact with adhesive tapes) (Iwen *et al.*, 1998; Young *et al.*, 1970; Prystowsky *et al.*, 1976; Allo *et al.*, 1987). Patients present with symptoms that are usually non-specific, and consistent with bronchopneumonia, with fever unresponsive to antibiotics, cough, sputum production and dyspnea. Patients may also present with pleuritic chest pain (due to vascular invasion leading to small pulmonary infarcts) and haemoptysis which is usually mild, but could be massive. IPA is one of the most common causes of haemoptysis in neutropenic patients, and has been reported to be associated with cavitation that occurs with neutrophil recovery (Albelda *et al.*, 1985). *Aspergillus* infection may also disseminate and spread haematogenously to other organs, most commonly the brain (leading to seizures, ring-enhancing lesions, cerebral infarctions, intracranial haemorrhage, meningitis and epidural abscess), and less frequently other organs such as skin, kidneys, pleura, heart, oesophagus and liver may be involved (Denning, 1998).

The diagnosis of IPA is challenging. Early diagnosis of IPA in HSCT recipients remains difficult, and high index of suspicion is necessary in patients with risk factors for invasive disease. Histopathological diagnosis by examining lung tissue obtained by thoracoscopic or open lung biopsy remains the 'gold standard' in the diagnosis of IPA (Ruhnke *et al.*, 2003). The presence of septate, acute, branching hyphae invading the lung tissue samples along with a culture that is positive for *Aspergillus* from the same site are diagnostic of IPA. Histopathological examination also allows for the exclusion of other diagnoses, such as malignancy or nonfungal infectious diseases. The histopathological findings associated with IPA have been recently shown to differ according to the underlying host. In patients with allogeneic HSCT and GVHD there is intense inflammation with neutrophilic infiltration, minimal coagulation necrosis, and low fungal burden. On the other hand, IPA in neutropenic patients is characterized by scant inflammation, extensive coagulation necrosis associated with hyphal angio-invasion, and high fungal burden. Dissemination to other organs is equally high in both groups (Chamilos *et al.*, 2006).

The chest radiograph has a small role in the early stages of the disease because the incidence of non-specific changes is high. Usual findings include rounded densities, pleural-based infiltrates that are suggestive of pulmonary infarctions and cavitations. Pleural effusions are uncommon (Libshitz and Pagani, 1981; Kuhlman, Fishman and Siegelman, 1985). Chest CT scan, especially when combined with high resolution images (HRCT), is a much more helpful tool in the diagnosis of IPA. The routine use of HRCT of the chest early in the course of IPA has been shown to lead to earlier diagnosis and improved outcome of these patients (Caillot *et al.*, 1997; Caillot *et al.*, 2001). It also aids further diagnostic studies such as bronchoscopy and open lung biopsy (Kuhlman, Fishman and Siegelman, 1987). The typical chest CT scan findings in patients suspected to have IPA include: multiple nodules and the halo sign, which is mainly seen in neutropenic patients early in the course of infection (usually in the first week), and appears as a zone of low attenuation due to haemorrhage surrounding the pulmonary nodule. Another late radiological sign is the air crescent sign, which represents crescent-shaped lucency in the region of the original nodule secondary to necrosis (Kuhlman, Fishman and Siegelman, 1985; Curtis, Smith and Ravin, 1979). Both the halo and the air crescent signs are neither sensitive nor pathognomic of IPA. The halo sign may be found as a result of metastasis, bronchiolitis obliterans organizing pneumonia, or other fungal infection (Gaeta *et al.*, 1999). Greene *et al.* found that 94% of 235 patients with a confirmed diagnosis of IPA had at least one nodular region (Greene, 2005). Another recent report of 27 patients with IPA following allogeneic HSCT, the most common radiological findings were ill defined consolidation (48%), nodules with halo sign (44%), centrilobular nodules (44%), ground glass attenuation (22%), and pleural effusion (26%) (Kojima *et al.*, 2005). In a retrospective study done on 45 patients, Horger *et al.* found that none of the early HRCT signs (nodule, consolidation, peribronchial infiltrates) seems to predict patient outcome or the development of pulmonary haemorrhage (Horger *et al.*, 2005). However, pulmonary haemorrhage is expected to occur in the presence of large cavitating nodules or consolidations located close to larger pulmonary vessels.

The significance of isolating *Aspergillus* spp. in sputum samples depends on the immune status of the host. In HSCT recipients, isolation of an *Aspergillus* species from sputum is highly predictive of invasive disease. Studies have shown that sputum samples that are positive for *Aspergillus* in these patients have a positive predictive value of 80–90% (Soubani and Qureshi, 2002; Horvath and Dummer, 1996; Yu, Muder and Poorsattar, 1986). However, sputum samples that are negative couldn't role out IPA; since negative sputum studies have been noted in 70% of patients with confirmed IPA (Yu, Muder and Poorsattar, 1986; Tang and Cohen, 1992). Blood cultures are rarely positive in patients with confirmed IPA (Duthie and Denning, 1995).

Bronchoscopy with BAL is generally helpful in the diagnosis of IPA, especially in patients with diffuse lung involvement. The sensitivity and specificity of a positive result of BAL fluid is around 50 and 97% respectively. This yield of BAL in the diagnosis of IPA is not consistent, and there are reports of much lower diagnostic yield (Soubani and Qureshi, 2002; Horvath and Dummer, 1996; Albelda *et al.*, 1984; Kahn, Jones and England, 1986; Levy *et al.*, 1992; Reichenberger *et al.*, 1999; Maschmeyer *et al.*, 2003). BAL is generally a safe and useful tool in HSCT recipients suspected to have IPA. In addition to obtaining samples for fungal stain and culture, it may be useful in detecting *Aspergillus* antigens in the BAL fluid, and excluding other infections. Transbronchial biopsies usually do not add much to the diagnosis of IPA, and are associated with increased risk of bleeding, so they are usually not performed (Soubani and Qureshi, 2002).

In the setting of diagnostic work up for IPA, it is important to send samples such as sputum, BAL fluid, or lung tissue for culture as well as for histological examination. This is because other fungal species, such as *Scedosporium, Pseudallescheria* and *Fusarium*, may have similar histological appearance as *Aspergillus* (Panackal and Marr, 2004). Furthermore, there are different species of *Aspergillus* that may lead to IPA. While *A. fumigatus* is the most common cause of IPA, there are increasing reports of IPA in cancer patients due to other species such as *A. niger, A. terreus* and *A. flavus* (Walsh and Groll, 2001; Lass-Florl *et al.*, 2005; Steinbach *et al.*, 2004; Hachem *et al.*, 2004; Kontoyiannis *et al.*, 2002). Some of these species (such as *A. terreus* and *A. nidulans*) are resistant to amphotericin B (Lass-Florl *et al.*, 2005; Kontoyiannis *et al.*, 2002). In a review of 300 cases (40% were HSCT recipients) with proven IPA, *A. terreus* was the second most common species isolated with a frequency of 23%. The risk factors and outcome for *A. terrues* infection were similar to those for *A. fumigatus* infection, however the former was significantly more likely to be nosocomial in origin, and more likely to be resistant to amphotericin B (Hachem *et al.*, 2004). The new triazole antifungal agents such as voriconazole and posaconazole have significantly better efficacy against *A. terreus* (Lass-Florl *et al.*, 2005; Steinbach *et al.*, 2004; Walsh *et al.*, 2007).

The most recent advances in the diagnosis of IPA are related to detecting *Aspergillus* antigens in body fluids. Galactomannan (GM) is a polysaccharide cell-wall component that is released by *Aspergillus* during growth. A double sandwich ELISA for the detection of GM in serum was recently approved by the Food and Drug Administration for the diagnosis of IPA, with a threshold of 0.5 ng/ml. It is reported that serum GM can be detected several days before the presence of clinical signs, an abnormal chest radiograph, or positive culture. Thus, GM detection may allow earlier confirmation of the diagnosis and serial determination of serum GM values may be useful in assessing the evolution of infection during treatment (Boutboul *et al.*, 2002; Marr *et al.*, 2004).

A meta-analysis study was undertaken by Pfeiffer *et al.* to assess the accuracy of a GM assay for diagnosing IPA. Twenty-seven studies from 1996 to 2005 were included and cases were diagnosed to have IPA according to the European Organization for Research on Treatment of Cancer/Mycoses Study Group (EORTC/MSG) criteria. Overall, the GM assay had a sensitivity of 71% and specificity of 89% for proven cases of invasive aspergillosis. The negative predictive value was 92–98% and the positive predictive value was between 25 to 62% (Pfeiffer, Fine and Safdar, 2006). Pfeiffer and colleagues concluded that GM assay is more useful in patients who have haematological malignancy or who have undergone allogeneic HSCT than in solid-organ transplant recipients or nonneutropenic patients.

GM is found in food and may be absorbed by the digestive tract, especially in patients with postchemotherapy mucositis, resulting in false positive reaction. Also medications such as β-lactam antibiotics (for example, piperacillin/tazobactam) may be associated with false positive GM assay, while antifungal agents with activity against *Aspergillus* may lead to a false negative test (Herbrecht *et al.*, 2002; Singh *et al.*, 2004; Marr *et al.*, 2005; Ansorg, van den Boom and Rath, 1997).

One of the major limitations of the GM test is the species-specificity of the assay. Consequently, it is not possible to exclude the involvement of other moulds such as *Fusarium*, Zygomycetes and dematiaceous fungi (Busca *et al.*, 2006). As a result, it is worthwhile recalling that GM detection doesn't replace careful microbiological and clinical evaluations.

There is evidence that GM is detected in other body fluids such as BAL, urine and cerebrospinal fluid, and that these tests may become positive prior to clinical and radiological findings suggestive of IPA (Busca *et al.*, 2006; Musher *et al.*, 2004; Klont, Mennink-Kersten and Verweij, 2004; Salonen *et al.*, 2000). Prospective studies are needed to study and compare the performance of *Aspergillus* antigen detection in samples other than serum. A retrospective study done by Musher *et al.* showed that incorporating GM assay and quantitative PCR assay into standard BAL fluid analysis may enhance bronchoscopic identification of *Aspergillus* species as the cause of pulmonary disease in HSCT recipients (Musher *et al.*, 2004).

Polymerase chain reaction (PCR) is another way to diagnose IPA by the detection of *Aspergillus* DNA in BAL fluid and serum. A positive *Aspergillus* PCR in BAL fluid has an estimated sensitivity of 67–100% and specificity between 55 and 95% (Hizel *et al.*, 2004). PCR sensitivity and specificity have also been reported as 100% and 65–92%, respectively in serum samples (Hizel *et al.*, 2004; Buchheidt *et al.*, 2001; Loeffler *et al.*, 2002; Halliday *et al.*, 2006). However, this test is often associated with false positive results because it doesn't discriminate between colonization and infection. PCR for *Aspergillus* nucleic acid detection remains restricted to highly specialized laboratories and can not be considered as a routine test.

Detection of serum $(1 \rightarrow 3)$-β-D-glucan, a fungal cell wall constituent has recently received Food and Drug Administration approval. Determination of plasma $(1 \rightarrow 3)$-β-D-glucan has been reported to be a highly sensitive and specific test for invasive deep mycosis, including candidiasis, fusariosis and aspergillosis, and could be useful in the immunocompromised patients (Obayashi *et al.*, 1995). However, the utility of this assay in allogeneic HSCT recipients at high risk for IPA is not yet defined.

The role of GM and other serological studies in the diagnosis of IPA is evolving. Furthermore, their role in different hosts, as surveillance tools, and their impact on the outcome of patients are not clear. There are ongoing prospective studies to address these issues. Until solid data are available, these tests should be considered as adjunct

Table 8.4 The diagnostic criteria for IPA.

Diagnosis	Criteria
Proven IPA	Histopathologic or cytopathologic examination of lung tissue showing hyphae from needle aspiration or biopsy specimen with evidence of associated tissue damage; *OR*
	Positive culture result for *Aspergillus* from a sample obtained by sterile procedure from the lung and clinically or radiologically abnormal site consistent with infection
Probable IPA	Host risk factor; *AND*
	Microbiological criteria (positive *Aspergillus* microscopy or culture from the sputum or BAL, or positive GM assay); *AND*
	Clinical criteria consistent with the infection (1 major or 2 minor)[a]
Possible IPA	Host risk factor; *AND*
	Microbiological criteria (positive *Aspergillus* microscopy or culture from the sputum or BAL, or positive GM assay); *OR*
	Clinical criteria consistent with the infection (1 major or 2 minor)[a]

[a]Major clinical criteria are: new characteristic infiltrates on CT imaging (halo sign, air-crescent sign, or cavity within area of consolidation). Minor Clinical criteria are: Symptoms of LRTI (cough, chest pain, hemoptysis, or dyspnea); physical finding of pleural rub; any new infiltrate not fulfilling major criterion; pleural effusion.

diagnostic studies, and should not replace appropriate clinical and radiological evaluation, and in selected cases, invasive procedures to confirm the diagnosis of IPA.

The EORTC/MSG has proposed several criteria for the diagnosis of invasive fungal infections (Ascioglu *et al.*, 2002). These criteria consist of host factors, microbiologic, minor and major clinical criteria (Table 8.4). Two consecutive positive serum GM, with the appropriate host and clinical factors can be considered as 'probable' IPA (Ascioglu *et al.*, 2002). The EORTC/MSG criteria are not evidence-based, and are not prospectively validated. Instead, they are meant to serve as a guide for clinical and epidemiological research, and need not be present in every patient to treat for IPA.

The treatment of IPA is difficult and mortality rate is still high despite the introduction of several new antifungal agents. Therapy should be considered as soon as there is a clinical suspicion of IPA, and while a workup is underway. For many years, amphotericin B has been the first line of therapy for IPA. The recommended dose is 1 to 1.5 mg/kg/day. Amphotericin B is known, however, to cause serious side effects including nephrotoxicity, electrolyte disturbances, and hypersensitivity. For these reasons, this agent nowadays has little role to play in the treatment of IPA, and newer lipid-based preparations of amphotericin B (for example, liposomal amphotericin B and lipid complex amphotericin B) have been introduced to minimize these side effects. Higher doses of the lipid formulations are needed for equivalent antifungal efficacy to amphotericin B.

Voriconazole is a new broad-spectrum triazole which is approved as the initial treatment of invasive aspergillosis, and is currently considered the treatment of choice in many patients with IPA (Johnson and Kauffman, 2003; Sambatakou *et al.*, 2006; Ghannoum and Kuhn, 2002). In a large prospective, randomized, multicentre trial, voriconazole was compared to amphotericin B as the primary therapy for IPA (Herbrecht *et al.*, 2002). Patients receiving voriconazole had a higher favourable response rate at week 12 (53% compared with 32% in patients receiving amphotericin B), and a higher 12-week survival (71% compared with 58%). Voriconazole is available in both intravenous and oral formulations. The recommended dose is 6 mg/kg twice daily intravenously on day one followed by 4 mg/kg/d. After seven days, switching to 200 mg PO twice daily may be considered. Voriconazole has a milder side effect profile, and is much better tolerated than amphotericin B. The most frequent adverse effect is visual disturbances described as blurred vision, photophobia and altered colour perception. Liver function test abnormalities and skin reactions are less common side effects associated with voriconazole treatment. It is important to note that voriconazole is associated with a significant number of drug-drug interactions such as cyclosporine, warfarin, terfenadine, carbamazepine, quinidine, rifampin, statins and sulfonylureas (Johnson and Kauffman, 2003).

Posaconazole is another broad-spectrum triazole that has been shown to be effective and safe as salvage therapy in patients with invasive aspergillosis refractory to standard antifungal therapy (Walsh *et al.*, 2007; Segal *et al.*, 2005; Pitisuttithum *et al.*, 2005).

Echinocandin derivatives such as caspofungin, micafungin and anidulafungin are effective agents in the treatment of IPA refractory to standard treatment, or if the patient could not tolerate first line agents (Spanakis, Aperis and Mylonakis, 2006; Cohen-Wolkowiez *et al.*, 2006). Since echinocandins inhibit the $(1 \rightarrow 3)$-β-D-glucan constituent of the fungal cell wall, unlike polyenes and azoles which target the fungal cell membrane, combination antifungal therapy could be a strategy to treat refractory IPA (Aliff *et al.*, 2003; Kontoyiannis *et al.*, 2003). There are no prospective randomized studies that show superior efficacy of combination therapy over single agent in the management of primary IPA. There are *in vitro* and limited clinical studies in the form of case reports and retrospective case series that show a benefit from combining antifungal agents as salvage therapy in refractory IPA (Kontoyiannis *et al.*, 2003; Graybill *et al.*, 2003; Marr *et al.*, 2004; Perea *et al.*, 2002). The combination of caspofungin and liposomal amphotericin B as a salvage therapy showed an overall response rate of 42%, however in patients with progressive documented IPA, the response rate was only 18% (Kontoyiannis *et al.*, 2003). A survival advantage of voriconazole plus caspofungin compared with voriconazole alone was reported by Marr *et al.* in a retrospective analysis of salvage therapy for IPA (Marr *et al.*, 2004). On the other hand, the report by Denning *et al.*, showed no difference in the response rate between patients who received micafungin alone or in combination with other antifungal agents as primary or salvage therapy for acute IPA (Denning *et al.*, 2006). Combination therapy of an echinocandin with either a lipid formulation of amphotericin B or triazole agent appear to be promising, however cannot be recommended for the routine treatment of primary IPA. Controlled randomized prospective studies are needed to document the value of this approach. Because GM is covalently bound to $(1 \rightarrow 3)$-β-D-glucan in the fungal cell wall, an initial increase in circulating GM might be expected in patients treated with echinocandins (Klont *et al.*, 2006).

Surgical resection has a limited role in the management of patients with IPA; however it should be considered in cases of massive haemoptysis, or pulmonary lesions close to the great blood vessels or pericardium, or the resection of residual localized pulmonary lesions in patients with continuing immunosuppression. Several reports have shown the relative efficacy and safety of surgical intervention – in addition to antifungal therapy – in these situations (Caillot *et al.*, 2001; Moreau *et al.*, 1993; Reichenberger *et al.*, 1998; Habicht *et al.*, 1999; Pidhorecky, Urschel and Anderson, 2000; Matt *et al.*, 2004; Baron *et al.*, 1998).

Immunomodulatory therapy such as using colony stimulating factors (for example, granulocyte-colony stimulating factors, granulocyte macrophage-colony stimulating therapy) or interferon-γ could be used to decrease the degree of immunosuppression, and as an adjunct to antifungal therapy for the treatment of IPA. Colony stimulating factors stimulate the bone marrow to produce more neutrophils, and have been shown to augment the phagocytic activity of neutrophils against fungi, including *Aspergillus* spp. (Giles, 1998; Roilides *et al.*, 1994; Roilides *et al.*, 1995). There is a theoretical advantage from adding these agents to the treatment of neutropenic patients suspected to have IPA. In one randomized study in patients receiving chemotherapy for acute myelogenous leukemia, prophylaxis with granulocyte macrophage-colony stimulating factor led to a lower frequency of fatal fungal infections compared with placebo (1.9 vs. 19% respectively) and reduced overall mortality (Rowe *et al.*, 1995). It is recommended to consider colony stimulating factors in neutropenic patients with serious infections, however there are no definitive studies that show benefit in patients with IPA (Ozer *et al.*, 2000). Interferon-γ is another cytokine that has been shown *in vitro* and in animal models to augment immunity by increasing neutrophil and monocyte activity against *Aspergillus* (Roilides *et al.*, 1994; Roilides *et al.*, 1993; Nagai *et al.*, 1995). The value of adding interferon-γ as an adjunct treatment of IPA is limited to case reports and small reports, and there are no guidelines on its role in the treatment of IPA (Safdar, 2006). There was a concern about the use of interferon-γ in allogeneic HSCT recipients, since it may worsen GVHD, however a recent trial showed that GVHD may actually improve during this therapy (Safdar *et al.*, 2005). Granulocyte transfusion is another potential supportive therapy for patients with prolonged neutropenia and life-threatening infections refractory to conventional therapy. It has been shown that it is safe for potential donors to donate neutrophils by granulocytophoresis, however there are no randomized studies that prove the benefit of adjuvant granulocyte transfusion in the treatment of IPA (Price *et al.*, 2000). It is also important in patients with IPA, whenever possible, to decrease the dose of systemic corticosteroids and immunosuppressive agents.

The management of IPA is difficult and an important approach to this problem is prophylaxis for those patients who are at increased risk for IPA. Avoiding the hospitalization of patients in areas where there are construction and the use of high-efficiency particulate air (HEPA) filtration with or without laminar air flow ventilation have proven to be efficient (Sherertz *et al.*, 1987). A meta-analysis suggested that itraconazole was effective in preventing fungal infections in neutropenic patients (Mattiuzzi, Kantarjian and O'Brien, 2004). Recent data also suggest the efficacy of posaconazole in the prophylaxis against IPA in patients with severe GVHD and other haematological malignancies (Ullmann and Cornely, 2006; Ullmann *et al.*, 2007).

Currently, chemoprophylaxis trials using other antifungal agents (such as voriconazole, caspofungin, micafungin) are underway in high risk patients.

Other fungal infections

HSCT predisposes to other invasive fungal infections (other than *Aspergillus*) that primarily involve the lungs but may disseminate to other organs. These invasive fungal infections are mainly seen in patients with neutropenia, allogeneic HSCT and GVHD (Marr *et al.*, 2002; Nucci, Marr and Queiroz-Telles, 2004; Boutati and Anaissie, 1997; Gaziev *et al.*, 1996; Maertens *et al.*, 1999).

The main invasive fungal infections that are reported in HSCT include hyaline hyphomycetes such as *Fusarium, Scedosporium, Zygomycetes* and endemic fungi. In a Centers for Disease Control sponsored surveillance programme for invasive fungal infections, there were 886 patients with invasive fungal infections out of 20 000 HSCT and solid organ transplant recipients (Costa and Alexander, 2005). Non-*Apsergillus* mould were responsible for 14% of infections, Cryptococcus in 4%, endemic fungi in 3% and *P. jiroveci* in 2%.

Hyaline hyphomycetes such as Fusarium and Scedosporium are the main non-*Aspergillus* moulds that are reported following HSCT. These organisms resemble *Aspergillus* histologically with septate hyphae that invade blood vessels (Marr *et al.*, 2002; Groll and Walsh, 2001; Jahagirdar and Morrison, 2002). Culture is the only means to distinguish these organisms from *Aspergillus*. The lungs are the primary site of infection, however these organisms have the tendency to disseminate. In one study, fusarium infection involved the lungs in 81% of the cases, and was disseminated in 74% of the patients (Marr *et al.*, 2002). Fungemia due to *Fusarium* is reported in 20–70% of patients (Sampathkumar and Paya, 2001). These infections usually occur early (in the first two months) following allogeneic HSCT. *Scedosporium* has been isolated from the air in hospitals (Jahagirdar and Morrison, 2002). In the lungs, these organisms usually present with thin wall cavities or nodules with or without air-crescent sign that are refractory to antibiotics and antifungal therapy (Castiglioni *et al.*, 2002). The diagnosis is usually confirmed by isolating the organisms by culture of BAL fluid or lung tissue obtained by open lung biopsy. Occasionally the diagnosis is obtained by fungal blood cultures.

These fungal agents are resistant to amphotericin B, however respond to voriconazole in 40–60% of cases (Costa and Alexander, 2005). In the case of *S. prolificans*, this organism is resistant to all available antifungal agents including the newer azoles (Berenguer *et al.*, 1997; Espinel-Ingroff, 2001). Mortality associated with these fungal infections remains very high, in the range of 70–100% (Sampathkumar and Paya, 2001; Husain *et al.*, 2005).

Zygomycetes such as Rhizopus and *Mucor* are characterized by sparsely septate, broad hyphae with irregular branching. They have the tendency to invade blood vessels with thrombosis and tissue necrosis. They usually involve the sinopulmonary tree; however dissemination to other organs is rare. The incidence of Zygomycetes infections in HSCT recipients is rare (0.5–1.9%) (Marr *et al.*, 2002; Gaziev *et al.*, 1996; Maertens *et al.*, 1999). The best approach to treatment is the combination of high dose amphtericin B preparation and surgical debridement. It is important to note that these organisms may be resistant to voriconazole (Trifilio *et al.*, 2007). Recent reports suggest good response to posaconazole (Page *et al.*, 2007). Mortality associated with Zygomycetes infection in HSCT recipient is 75–80% (Marr *et al.*, 2002; Gaziev *et al.*, 1996; Maertens *et al.*, 1999).

Endemic mycoses such as histoplasmosis, blastomycosis and coccidiomycosis are rare after HSCT (Glenn, Blair and Adams, 2005). These infections tend to have geographical distribution, and are usually caused by endogenous reactivation of a latent infection. The infection usually presents with progressive pulmonary disease that disseminates to other organs. Treatment is with high dose amphotericin B preparation (Groll and Walsh, 2001). After controlling the infection, an azole such as itraconazole (or fluconazole in the case of coccidiomycosis) can be used as a continuing treatment (Costa and Alexander, 2005).

Invasive Candida infection develops in 11–16% of HSCT recipients and pulmonary involvement is usually secondary to disseminated candidiasis or candidemia. Autopsy studies suggest that 50% of infected patients have pulmonary involvement (Goodrich *et al.*, 1991). Primary *Candida* pneumonia is extremely rare. The universal prophylaxis with fluconazole has significantly decreased the incidence of *Candida* infections. However, there is a shift in the *Candida* species from *C. albicans* to more resistant species such as *C. glabarata* and *C. krusei*.

Pneumocystosis: Pneumocystis pneumonia is caused by *P. jiroveci* which is a fungal agent (Stringer *et al.*, 2002). Infection is caused by inhalation of aerosolized organisms. The incidence of *Pneumocystis* pneumonia following HSCT was historically 5–15%, usually in the second to the sixth month following HSCT (Soubani, Miller and Hassoun, 1996). However, the routine prophylaxis with TMX/SMZ during this period has significantly decreased the incidence of this infection to negligible values. Breakthrough infection in patients on TMP/SMZ prophylaxis is extremely rare, however, is possible in patients on other prophylactic agents such as low dose atevaquone, or aerosolized pentamidine (Rodriguez, Sifri and Fishman, 2004; Torre-Cisneros *et al.*, 1999; Marras *et al.*, 2002). In a recent report, *P. jiroveci* infection was documented in 13 out of 519 patients undergoing allogeneic HSCT (2.5%). The majority of cases occurred late in the course following HSCT (median 14.5 months). The CD4 + T cell count was low, and 70% of patients were on immunosuppressive therapy for chronic GVHD. In all these patients, prophylaxis against *P. jiroveci* had been discontinued due to suspected bone marrow toxicity of the prophylactic regimen (De Castro *et al.*, 2005).

The patient usually presents with progressive dyspnea, nonproductive cough, fever and hypoxemia, a median of 60 days following HSCT. Radiologically, there are perihilar interstitial or alveolar infiltrates. Ground glass opacification may be the prominent finding on HRCT of the chest. LDH may be elevated. The diagnosis is usually made by bronchoscopy with BAL, however, the sensitivity of this procedure is lower than that reported in patients with AIDS due to the lower burden of the organism (Soubani, Miller and Hassoun, 1996).

TMP/SMZ with or without systemic corticosteroids is the agent of choice in the treatment of *P. jiroveci* pneumonia following HSCT. Alternative agents in the case of allergy or side effects (gastrointestinal and marrow suppression) associated with TMP/ SMZ are less effective and include intravenous pentamidine, dapsone and trimethoprim, atevaqoune, or clindamycin and primaqine (Anon, 2000). Mortality has been recently reported to be 34%, and the only predictor of poor outcome based on multivariate analysis was the use of mechanical ventilation (Torres *et al.*, 2006). Prophylaxis against *P. jiroveci* pneumonia is initiated by starting TMP/SMZ following engraftment for 120 days, however, if the patient has chronic GVHD, prophylactic treatment is recommended as long as they are on treatment for chronic GVHD.

8.4   Cytomegalovirus

It is important at the outset to define the different manifestations of CMV infection following HSCT. CMV infection is defined as isolation of the CMV virus or its proteins or nucleic acid from body fluids or tissue specimens. CMV viremia is isolation of CMV from blood by culture. CMV antigenemia is detection of CMV pp65 in circulating leukocytes or CMV nucleic acid by PCR techniques. CMV disease is the presence of signs and symptoms related to CMV infection, and may manifest as hepatitis, gastroenteritis, encephalitis, or a systemic syndrome. CMV pneumonitis is one of the most frequent and severe manifestations of CMV disease in HSCT recipient. It is defined as pulmonary signs and symptoms combined with detection of CMV in pulmonary samples (sputum, BAL, or lung tissue). It is important to note that some patients may shed CMV in sputum or BAL fluid in the absence of invasive disease. It is also important to note that CMV affects the immune system and promotes other infections. Co-infection with other organisms such as *P. jiroveci*, *Aspergillus*, or other viruses is reported in up to one third of cases (Ison and Fishman, 2005).

Traditionally, CMV pneumonia was a relatively frequent infection in HSCT recipients. It was diagnosed in 20–35% of patients, and 60–80% of those with diffuse pneumonitis following HSCT (Sullivan *et al.*, 2001; Meyers, Flournoy and Thomas, 1982; Crawford *et al.*, 1988). CMV pneumonia usually presented in the first two months post-transplantation (median 44 days), and was associated with high mortality ranging between 80 to 100% (Meyers, Flournoy and Thomas, 1982). However, antiviral prophylaxis for high risk patients and preemptive therapy have changed the epidemiology of CMV pneumonia in HSCT recipients. Currently in allogeneic HSCT recipients, the incidence of CMV pneumonia is 10–30%, while in autologous recipients, CMV pneumonia is extremely rare (1–9%) (Blacklock *et al.*, 1985; Taplitz and Jordan, 2002; Konoplev *et al.*, 2001; Shepp *et al.*, 1985).

Prophylactic and preemptive antiviral therapy have also shifted the onset of CMV pneumonia in allogeneic HSCT to after the first 100 days (median 169 days), especially in patients with non-myeloablative HSCT and during the treatment of chronic GVHD (Boeckh *et al.*, 2003; Junghanss *et al.*, 2002).

CMV pneumonia is mainly seen after allogeneic HSCT, and the highest risk is in seropositive recipients. CMV disease is reported in 14% of seropostive recipients who received a seropositive graft and in 12% of seropositive recipients and seronegative grafts. On the other hand, the risk of CMV disease is lower in seronegative recipients who had HSCT from seropositive donors (incidence is less than 5%) (Ljungman *et al.*, 1998). Additional risk factors for CMV pneumonia include older age, total body irradiation, myeloablative chemotherapy, the presence and acuity of acute GVHD, and the use of T-cell depletion strategies (Meyers, Flournoy and Thomas, 1982; Reusser, 1991; Enright *et al.*, 1993).

In autologous HSCT, the main risk factors for CMV pneumonia are the presence of CMV infection prior to transplantation, CD-34 enriched stem cells, probably due to lower number of T cells and delayed immunologic reconstitution (Holmberg *et al.*, 1999).

CMV pneumonia presents clinically with rapid onset of fever, nonproductive cough, dyspnea and hypoxemia. Pleurisy may be present. The respiratory symptoms usually progress to acute respiratory failure within two weeks. Radiologically, the most common findings are an interstitial pattern with tiny pulmonary nodules and patchy areas of consolidation. Rarely CMV pneumonia may present with focal infiltrate (Leung *et al.*, 1999; Franquet, Lee and Muller, 2003). HRCT of the chest is more sensitive in detecting the findings related to CMV pneumonia including diffuse or patchy ground glass opacification, thickened interlobular septa, tree on bud nodular changes. Pleural effusion may be present in around a quarter of patients (Franquet, Lee and Muller, 2003). The differential diagnosis of these clinical and radiological findings includes *P. jiroveci*, other viral infections, pulmonary haemorrhage, drug induced lung injury, pulmonary oedema, or tumour recurrence. Some of these conditions may co-exist with CMV pneumonia.

The hallmark of the histopathological findings of CMV pneumonia is demonstrating the intracytoplasmic inclusion bodies within areas of inflammation on lung biopsy. These eosinophilic bodies may be absent early in the process. There are also areas of mononuclear interstitial pneumonitis with or without alveolar epithelial desquamation and hyaline membrane formation. These findings can be rarely demonstrated by bronchoscopic biopsy, however, usually open lung biopsy by video-assisted thoraco-scopy is necessary.

Cytological examination of the BAL fluid to detect the inclusion bodies within the lower respiratory tract epithelial cells is highly specific (98%) for CMV pneumonia, but has low sensitivity (90%), with positive predicted value of 73%, and a negative predictive value of 99.5% (Tamm *et al.*, 2001). On the other hand, rapid culture of the BAL fluid using shell viral technique is highly sensitive (99%) in detecting the virus, but lacks the specificity (67–83%), since it cannot differentiate between viral shedding and invasive disease (Tamm *et al.*, 2001; Sakamaki *et al.*, 1997).

The value of detecting CMV antigens in the diagnosis of CMV pneumonia is controversial. CMV pp65 antigen assay is based on staining blood neutrophil for the pp65 antigen. The test requires an adequate number of neutrophils (>1000 cells/mm^3), so it is not useful in the presence of neutropenia (Michaelides *et al.*, 2001). Another way to quantitatively measure CMV viral load is by detecting the viral DNA by PCR which could be done on whole blood, plasma, leukocytes, BAL, urine and cerebrospinal fluid. Detection of CMV viral DNA in the BAL fluid is suggestive of CMV pneumonia, however false positive results are frequent (Westall *et al.*, 2004). Detecting blood CMV antigens – by either method – correlates well with the CMV pneumonia (Humar *et al.*, 2001; Leruez-Ville *et al.*, 2003). However, it is possible for CMV pneumonia to develop without antigenemia (Reinke *et al.*, 1999). CMV antigens in blood samples may precede clinical features of CMV pneumonia by up to three weeks (Bordon *et al.*, 2007). These tests are also useful in monitoring response to antiviral therapy. Persistence of CMV antigenemia after two weeks of therapy, should raise suspicion of antiviral resistance.

Gancyclovir as a single agent or in combination with CMV immunoglobulins has been shown to be effective in uncontrolled trials in the treatment of CMV pneumonia and is currently the standard of care in the management of this condition following HSCT (Blacklock *et al.*, 1985; Shepp *et al.*, 1985). With this approach, mortality has decreased to 0–47% provided treatment is started prior to the onset of acute respiratory failure. Survival of patients with respiratory failure at the time of initiation of therapy remains infrequent.

Gancyclovir is a nucleotide analogue of ghanosine which is an inhibitor of CMV DNA polymerase. The main side effect associated with this treatment is neutropenia, which is reported in 25–50% of treated patients and usually occurs after the first two weeks of treatment. Valgancyclovir is an oral agent that has 60% bioavailability, and a daily dose of 900mg is equivalent to 5 mg/kg/day of intravenous gancyclovir (Ison and Fishman, 2005). CMV IgG is prepared from a pooled adult human plasma that contain CMV antibodies. It is not useful as the sole treatment for CMV pneumonia (Blacklock *et al.*, 1985). Second line agents include foscarnet and cidofivir. The main problem with these agents is nephrotoxicity, especially if the patient is already receiving other nephrotoxic agents. CMV resistance to gancyclovir should be suspected when there is lack of clinical response or failure of decline in the viral load after the second week of therapy. In these cases, second line agents may be effective. There is also evidence that the combination of gancyclovir and foscarnet provides synergy (Bacigalupo *et al.*, 1996).

Prevention of CMV infection is the best approach to avoid disease. Use of CMV negative stem cells and seronegative or leukocyte-filtered blood products for CMV seronegative recipients decreases the risk of infection to 2–4% (Bowden *et al.*, 1995; Nichols *et al.*, 2003). Antiviral prophylaxis and viral monitoring with pre-emptive therapy are at present the two main antiviral strategies used in the prevention of CMV infection and disease. Gancyclovir prophylaxis administered in seropositive patients or in seronegative subjects receiving graft from a seropositive donor, from five days before engraftment to 100 days after transplant reduces the risk of CMV infection and invasive disease, as well as mortality (Zaia, 1993). However, this approach did not change the overall survival owing to increased sepsis associated with gancyclovir induced neutro-penia, and shift in the onset of the CMV disease later in the course following HSCT when the prophylactic treatment is discontinued (Goodrich *et al.*, 1993). Valgancyclovir showed promise as an alternative antiviral agent for preemptive treatment of CMV reactivation following allogeneic HSCT (Busca *et al.*, 2007). The use of a cut-off of the number of CMV DNA copies in whole blood samples (10 000 DNA copies/ml) may be useful in avoiding unnecessary antiviral treatment (Lilleri *et al.*, 2007). Other inter-ventions that are under evaluation include infusion of donor derived CMV specific cytotoxic T lymphocyte infusion and CMV vaccine (Walter *et al.*, 1995).

8.5 Community respiratory viruses

There are four main community respiratory viral agents that lead to infection following HSCT. These are respiratory syncytial virus (RSV), parainfluenza, influenza and adenovirus. The information on the significance of community respiratory viral infections following HSCT is limited for several reasons including reports based on small case series, the seasonal nature of the infection that may change the frequency of these infections depending on the time and location of the study, and the fact that many of the patients with community respiratory viral infections may be asymptomatic. Nevertheless, there have been recent large trials that have been helpful in better understanding the role of community respiratory viral infections in HSCT recipients. Overall, it appears that the incidence of these viral infections following HSCT ranges between 11 to 65% (Lujan-Zilbermann et al., 2001; Roghmann et al., 2003; van Kraaij et al., 2005; Chemaly et al., 2006). In one study of community respiratory viral infections following HSCT, the main viruses were RSV (35%), parainfluenza (30%), rhinovirus (25%) and influenza virus (11%). Of these, pneumonia occurred in 49% of patients with RSV infection, 22% of those with parainfluenza virus, and 3% of rhinovirus infection (Bowden, 1997). In another recent review of 343 cases of community respiratory viral infections in 306 adult HSCT recipients, parainfluenza (mainly type 3) accounted for 27% of infections, influenza (mainly type A) in 33% of infections and RSV in 31% of infections. Community respiratory viral infections progressed to pneumonia in 35% of patients with equal frequency among the three viruses. The patients at high risk for community respiratory viral infections included allogeneic HSCT, leukemia, age older than 65 years, and presence of severe neutropenia or lymphopenia. The overall mortality for community respiratory viral pneumonia was 15%. The only independent predictor of fatal outcome was absolute lymphopenia in patients with influenza pneumonia (Chemaly et al., 2006).

The diagnosis of lower respiratory tract community respiratory viral infection is usually suspected in patients with preceding upper respiratory tract infection. The HRCT of the chest usually shows patchy or extensive ground glass opacities, or a mixture of patterns including ground glass attenuation, thickening of the bronchial walls, and multiple small nodules that may have centrilobular or random distribution. Consolidation and pleural effusions are less common (Franquet et al., 2006). The diagnosis is usually made using the combination of direct fluorescent antibody (DFA) and indirect fluorescent antibody (IFA) testing, and viral cultures of clinical specimens. The results of the former tests are usually available within 24 hours, while cultures usually take 7–14 days. The clinical specimens are best obtained by nasopharyngeal wash or swabs. The sensitivity of direct DFA and IFA in detecting infection in HSCT recipients ranges between 20 to 52% (Whimbey, Englund and Couch, 1997; Raboni et al., 2003; Bredius et al., 2004). BAL fluid may also be helpful when lower respiratory tract infection is suspected with a sensitivity of around 70% (van Kraaij et al., 2005). It is important to note in this context that community respiratory viruses are often co-pathogens with other organisms including bacteria, fungi (such as *Aspergillus* and *P. jiroveci*) or other viruses (such as CMV) (Nichols et al., 2001). In one study of community respiratory viral pneumonia, 119 patients had BAL specimen, and in 14% had other pathogens cultured (Chemaly *et al.*, 2006). This may create a challenge to clinicians, and every effort should be made to exclude such infections in which community respiratory viruses are isolated.

Community respiratory viruses associated with upper respiratory tract infections in HSCT recipients are usually self-limiting, and are not associated with increased mortality. However, it is common for these patients to develop lower respiratory tract infection that is associated with high mortality (Chemaly *et al.*, 2006). Another potential risk associated with community respiratory viral infections is the development of bronchiolitis obliterans following allogeneic HSCT. In the large series of new onset airflow obstruction following allogeneic HSCT, one of the main risk factors was respiratory viral infections within the first 100 days following transplantation (Soubani and Uberti, 2007). Lower respiratory tract parainfluenza (OR 17.9 (95% CI, 2.0–160) and RSV (OR 3.6, 95% CI, 1.0–13) infections were independent risk factors for development of airflow decline one year after allogeneic HSCT (Erard *et al.*, 2006).

Given the high mortality associated with community respiratory viral lower respiratory tract infections in HSCT recipients, preventive measures play an important role in avoiding infection in these patients. Simple measures such as hand washing are very effective against infection (except for influenza which is transmitted by aerosolized droplets). In addition, isolating patients suspected to have community respiratory viral infection, even before the infection is confirmed, has been shown to be effective (Anon, 2000). Symptomatic healthcare providers should be restricted from contact with HSCT recipients (Garcia *et al.*, 1997). It is also advisable to limit visitors to HSCT recipients during the winter months (Anon, 2000).

Respiratory syncytial virus (RSV)

RSV is the most common community respiratory virus infection in HSCT recipients. It has seasonal variation with the highest incidence in late autumn and winter. Children are more affected than adults, and outbreaks of RSV infections have been described in HSCT units (Hall, 2000; Ghosh *et al.*, 2001; Abdallah *et al.*, 2003). There are several reasons to explain these outbreaks including community based outbreaks, transmission from other infected HSCT recipients who may shed the virus for a long time, or asymptomatic healthcare providers. The reported incidence of RSV infection ranges between 3.5 to 6.3% following allogeneic HSCT and 0.4–1.5% following autologous HSCT (Small *et al.*, 2002; Ljungman, 1997).

RSV infection usually starts with upper respiratory tract symptoms including cough, rhinorrhea and sinus congestion. Wheezing may develop in 30%, however fever may not be present even with lower respiratory tract infection (Falsey and Walsh, 2000). The most serious complication of RSV infection in this patient population is the development of lower respiratory tract infection which happens in 30–50% of patients and is associated with high mortality (19%) (Chemaly *et al.*, 2006; Barton and Blumberg, 2005). Lack of RSV directed antiviral therapy and older age are associated with increased risk of progression to pneumonia (Chemaly *et al.*, 2006). Lower respiratory tract infection is characterized by progressive dyspnea and hypoxemia. Fever may be absent. The radiological findings of RSV pneumonia include multiple small nodules, bud on tree pattern, diffuse ground glass infiltrates, and bronchial thickening (Escuissato *et al.*, 2005).

The diagnosis of RSV lower respiratory tract infection could be made by DFA or IFA of nasopharyngeal specimens which have a sensitivity of 15%. However, DFA on BAL samples has a much higher sensitivity (67–90%) (Englund *et al.*, 1996). PCR test on BAL fluid may have a higher sensitivity (90%) (Falsey and Walsh, 2000).

The role of pharmacological therapy in RSV infection following HSCT remains controversial. Several studies have suggested benefit from ribavirin (intravenously, orally or aerosolized) with or without RSV specific intravenous immunoglobulins (Englund, Piedra and Whimbey, 1997; Anon, 2004c). Delivery of aerosolized ribavirin requires a special machine that is not widely available. Care should be taken during aerosolization of this medication since those who are exposed to it may develop headache, skin rash and conjunctivitis. Furthermore, ribavirin has teratogenic effects and pregnant women should not enter the patient's room during treatment (Anon, 2004c). Other therapeutic modalities, such as high titer monoclonal antibody against RSV are under investigation (Ottolini *et al.*, 2002). Treatment of upper respiratory tract RSV infection to avoid progression to lower respiratory tract infection which is associated with high mortality has been suggested by some studies with good results (Small *et al.*, 2002). However, this approach is not widely adopted. A recent randomized trial of HSCT recipients with upper respiratory tract RSV infection were randomized to preemptive aerosolized ribavirin or supportive therapy to prevent progression to lower respiratory tract infection. The intervention was safe and was associated with reduced viral load, however the study could not prove the efficacy of aerosolized ribavirin in preventing progression to lower respiratory tract RSV infection (Boeckh *et al.*, 2007). On the other hand, starting antiviral therapy once the patient develops acute respiratory failure requiring mechanical ventilation is usually not effective, with high mortality that reaches 90% (Englund, Piedra and Whimbey, 1997).

Parainfluenza virus

Parainfluenza is another important cause of community respiratory viral infections following HSCT. It accounts for 5–50% of community respiratory viral infections, with equal incidence following autologous and allogeneic HSCT (Bowden, 1997; Whimbey *et al.*, 1993; Elizaga *et al.*, 2001). Parainfluenza has four serotypes, and serotypes 1 and 3 are reportedly the most common causes of infection in HSCT recipients. Parainfluenza infection is variable throughout the year, with outbreaks reported in winter, and sometimes in spring and summer.

Parainfluenza infection usually presents with a cough, however, rhinorrhea and fever are uncommon. Lower respiratory tract infection is the most serious complication of parainfluenza infection, and is reported in 18–100% (mean 33%) of patients, with mortality ranging between 15 to 73% (mean 50%) (Barton and Blumberg, 2005). It is estimated that up to 50% of patients with parainfluenza lower respiratory tract infection have co-infection with bacteria or fungi (Elizaga *et al.*, 2001). The diagnosis of parainfluenza infection is usually made by IFA or DFA and culture of respiratory samples. Real time PCR is under development and is not available for clinical practice.

Treatment of parainfluenza infection is supportive. Ribavirin has activity against parainfluenza, and has been shown to be helpful in small studies (Anon, 2004c; McCurdy, Milstone and Dummer, 2003), however large studies failed to demonstrate benefit from this therapy (Elizaga *et al.*, 2001). It is recommended to consider aerosolized ribavirin in the treatment of parainfluenza lower respiratory tract infection, although experience to date provides little evidence of efficacy (Anon, 2004c).

Influenza

Influenza infection has been described in HSCT recipients as a community or nosocomial infection. It usually develops in the winter months, and the clinical picture is similar to normal hosts with fever, rhinorrhea, coryza, mayalgia and headache. The frequency of influenza infection is similar in autologous and allogeneic HSCT recipients. Lower respiratory tract infections are rare, and co-infection with bacteria has been reported. The overall mortality with influenza lower respiratory tract infection following HSCT is low, however the prognosis is worse if the patient develops the infection early post transplantation (Nichols *et al.*, 2004). Lower respiratory tract influenza infection is more in those who develop infection early post-transplantation (median 36 days vs. 61 days), and those with lymphopenia (Chemaly *et al.*, 2006; Nichols *et al.*, 2004). The diagnosis of influenza infection is made by DFA or IFA or viral cultures on upper respiratory tract samples obtained by nasopharyngeal wash or swab. BAL is adequate if lower respiratory tract infection is suspected.

The treatment of influenza infection is supportive. Antiviral agents such as amantadine, rimantadine, oseltamir, zanamivir may be considered in HSCT patients with severe infection (Vu *et al.*, 2007). In one report, early treatment with oseltamivir was associated with a trend for less progression to lower respiratory tract infection, and decrease viral shedding (Nichols *et al.*, 2004). Vaccination against influenza is effective, however live attenuated preparations should be avoided in these patients, and it is necessary to take into consideration that HSCT recipients may respond poorly to vaccination in the first two years following transplantation (Anon, 2004c).

Adenovirus

Adenovirus infection accounts for 0–21% of community respiratory viral infections following HSCT, and is more common in children (Barton and Blumberg, 2005; Symeonidis *et al.*, 2007). While infection may be acquired by person to person transmission, most of the cases are due to reactivation of latent infection. Patients with allogeneic HSCT may have delayed adenovirus specific T cell immune recovery, which correlates with increased risk of adenovirus associated morbidity and mortality (Myers *et al.*, 2007).

Adenovirus infection may be asymptomatic, or lead to pneumonia or to a disseminated disease with gastroenteritis, hepatitis and hemorrhagic cystitis, with or without respiratory involvement. Approximately 20% of HSCT recipients with adenovirus infection develop pneumonia (Shields *et al.*, 1985). The diagnosis of adenovirus lower respiratory tract infection is made by IFA or DFA or viral cultures of BAL fluid or lung biopsy. Histologically, the diagnosis is suggested by the presence of the characteristic smudge cells (Shields *et al.*, 1985).

Morality associated with adenovirus infection ranges between 38 to 100%, with accumulative mortality of 56% (Raboni *et al.*, 2003; Bredius *et al.*, 2004; Ljungman, 1997). Prognosis is usually dependent on the degree of dissemination. Given this high mortality, early and aggressive treatment is warranted. There are limited antiviral agents with activity against adenovirus. Ribavirin and gancyclovir have no significant activity against this virus (Anon, 2004d). Cidofivir has been shown to improve outcome in small studies (Anon, 2004d). However, this agent is associated with significant nephrotoxicity.

Other viral infections

Rhinovirus is an important cause of the common cold. Its significance in HSCT recipients is not well known. In prospective studies on HSCT recipients, 25% of patients with viral infections were documented to have rhinovirus, and in 3–17% of these patients the infection progressed to the lower respiratory tract with mortality up to 33% (Bowden, 1997; Hassan *et al.*, 2003). There is no specific treatment for rhinovirus infection.

Herpes viruses have been reported as a cause of lower respiratory tract infection following HSCT. Herpes simplex virus-1 reactivates in 80% of HSCT recipients and occasionally may be associated with pneumonia. Pneumonia generally develops due to contiguous spread from the oropharynx and trachea, although it may be due to generalized viremia. Universal prophylaxis with acyclovir and gancyclovir have significantly reduced the incidence of herpes simplex virus serious infections, including pneumonia, following HSCT (Taplitz and Jordan, 2002). Herpes zoster virus may also lead to lower respiratory tract infection following HSCT, and is usually preceded by the characteristic skin rash. Human herpes virus (HHV-6) has been suggested to have a role in the pathogenesis of idiopathic pneumonia syndrome following HSCT (Buchbinder *et al.*, 2000). It may act as a co-pathogen with CMV or act as an isolated cause of pneumonia (Buchbinder *et al.*, 2000). In a recent report HHV-6 was isolated from 56.6% of peripheral blood or other specimen tested following HSCT, however it was associated with interstitial/alveolar pneumonia in only 2% of patients. HHV-6 reactivation was significantly associated with GVHD, *Epstein Barr* viral co infection, and unrelated donor transplantation (Hentrich *et al.*, 2005).

8.6 Non-infectious pulmonary complications

In addition to the wide variety of pulmonary infectious complications following HSCT, these patients are prone to several noninfectious pulmonary conditions that are a major cause of morbidity and mortality following HSCT. The advances in the diagnosis, prophylaxis and management of the infectious complications following HSCT, has increased the significance of these noninfectious complications on the outcome of HSCT. The other significant point is that several of these complications such as diffuse alveolar haemorrhage, idiopathic pneumonia syndrome and bronchiolitis obliterans organizing pneumonia have similar presentation to infectious processes with dyspnea, cough, fever and pulmonary infiltrates, which makes the differentiation between these two categories difficult. Commonly these patients require invasive procedures to differentiate between the two and in those patients in whom the diagnosis is not clear, broad spectrum antibiotics should be started until infection is excluded.

The noninfectious pulmonary complications also tend to follow a predictable time line following HSCT (Figure 8.1). Cardiogenic pulmonary oedema may develop in the peri-transplant period due to fluid overload and cardiac toxicity secondary to high dose chemotherapy. This is usually a reversible process and management is supportive and may include diuretics.

HSCT recipients may also develop generalized capillary leak that develops within 96 hr of engraftment. The engraftment syndrome is seen more commonly following autologous HSCT and is due to the recovery of neutrophils and is felt to be due to overproduction of inflammatory cytokines such as TNF-α, IL-1B and IL-8. These patients have fever, diffuse erthymatous rash and diffuse pulmonary infiltrates with hypoxemia (Gorak et al., 2005). The patients may also have other organ involvement including the liver, kidneys and central nervous system. The management of engraftment syndrome is supportive and the prognosis is generally good. Some reports suggest discontinuing granulocyte-colony stimulating factor which has been implicated in the pathogenesis of engraftment syndrome. Patients with severe manifestations including acute respiratory failure respond very well to high dose corticosteroid therapy (Spitzer, 2001).

Diffuse alveolar haemorrhage is another cause of acute lung injury following HSCT. It is reported in 1–21% (average 5%) of HSCT recipients with equal incidence following autologous and allogeneic HSCT (Afessa et al., 2002). The patients usually present a median of 24 days following HSCT with dyspnea, fever and cough and hypoxemia. Haemoptysis is reported in a minority of patients. The chest radiography shows bilateral interstitial and alveolar infiltrates that tend to be perihilar and in the middle and lower lobes (Afessa et al., 2002). Characteristically, BAL reveals a progressively bloodier return from at least three separate subsegmental bronchi. Diffuse alveolar haemorrhage is not due to an infectious process and does not correlate with coagulopathy or thrombocytopenia. It is probably related to recovery of neutrophils following HSCT. There are no prospective trials in the management of diffuse alveolar haemorrhage. These patients require supportive treatment with mechanical ventilation, excluding infection and may benefit from high dose systemic corticosteroid therapy. Prognosis is poor with mortality reported to reach 70%, however recent reports suggest a better outcome, with mortality of 48% (Afessa et al., 2002). Death is usually due to multiorgan system failure and sepsis. Allogeneic HSCT, late onset (after the first 30 days), and mechanical ventilation are associated with a worse outcome.

Idiopathic pneumonia syndrome develops later following HSCT, usually in the second and third month following HSCT. It is reported in around 10% of patients and is more common following allogeneic HSCT (Afessa, Litzow and Tefferi, 2001). The syndrome is diagnosed by the presence of widespread alveolar injury manifested by multilobar infiltrates, symptoms and signs of pneumonia that does not respond to antibiotics with negative cultures on BAL. Idiopathic pneumonia syndrome is probably related to high dose chemotherapy and is more commonly reported following myeloablative regimen and total body irradiation as compared to nonmyeloablative HSCT. There is also some evidence that it may be a manifestation of acute GVHD. The management of idiopathic pneumonia syndrome is supportive with oxygen supplementation and corticosteroids therapy. There is anecdotal evidence that anti-TNF-α antibodies may be helpful. The prognosis of idiopathic pneumonia syndrome is poor and mortality reaches a mean of 74% (Afessa, Litzow and Tefferi, 2001). Mortality is primarily related to progressive respiratory failure.

The main late noninfectious pulmonary complication following allogeneic HSCT is bronchiolitis obliterans which is characterized by new onset of airflow obstruction that usually develops after the first 100 days post transplantation. The incidence of bronchiolitis obliterans is reported to be 6–20%, however a recent report of large cohort of allogeneic HSCT recipients report the incidence of new airflow obstruction to be 26% and in 32% of those patients with chronic GVHD. The main risk factors for bronchiolitis obliterans are older age, the presence of airflow obstruction prior to transplantation, the presence of chronic GVHD and a history of respiratory viral infection (especially parainfluenza and RSV) in the first 100 days post transplantation (Soubani and Uberti, 2007). The patients have insidious onset of dyspnea with cough and wheezing. Pulmonary functions show progressive airflow obstruction and high resolution chest CT scan with inspiratory and expiratory views showing evidence of air trapping and later may have bronchiectatic changes. Bronchiolitis obliterans is not associated with infection, however, at a later stage the airways become colonized with bacteria including *Staphylococci* and *Pseudomonas* that lead to recurrent bronchopneumonia. There are no prospective randomized trials on the management of bronchiolitis obliterans, however several reports suggest augmenting immunosuppressive therapy and systemic corticosteroids therapy. This may increase the risk of opportunistic infections and these patients should be put on the appropriate prophylactic therapy. There are few reports that suggest some patients with bronchiolitis obliterans may benefit from maintenance therapy with macrolides, however there are no randomized trials to suggest benefit from this treatment (Soubani and Uberti, 2007). Bronchiolitis obliterans increases the late mortality due to allogeneic HSCT (HR 2.3, range 1.6–3.3), with attributable mortality of 9% at three years (Chien *et al.*, 2003).

8.7 Conclusion

HSCT is an established treatment for a variety of malignancies and may see further indications in the future. The procedure remains limited by a range of infectious and noninfectious complications that are related to the conditioning regimen, immunosuppressive therapy and GVHD. Pulmonary conditions are a major component of these post transplantation complications. However, there have been significant advances in the diagnosis and management of respiratory infections following HSCT. *P. jiroveci* and CMV infections are very rare. The treatment of bacterial pneumonia has improved with the availability of broad spectrum antibiotics. The management of fungal infections, including IPA, is enhanced by the introduction of noninvasive diagnostic methods such as galactomannan assay and better tolerated antifungal agents.

Future directions in the management of respiratory infections following HSCT need to focus on more robust and validated noninvasive diagnostic assays that allow for earlier detection and preemptive therapy of fungal and viral infections. Also more emphasis is needed on prevention of respiratory infections and the management of the acute lung injury and systemic response secondary to infections in HSCT recipients. More effective and safer antiviral agents should be another area of research and development as well as the role of combination antimicrobial agents in the management of severe viral and fungal infections.

Respiratory infections following HSCT can also be minimized by improved transplantation techniques that are associated with better engraftment and less GVHD. Also more target-specific immunosuppressive agents and better management of GVHD decrease the risk of opportunistic infection following HSCT. Enhanced understanding, diagnosis and management of the noninfectious pulmonary complications of HSCT such as diffuse alveolar haemorrhage, idiopathic pneumonia syndrome and bronchiolitis obliterans, will in turn decrease the risk of respiratory infections in this patient population.

References

Abdallah, A., Rowland, K.E., Schepetiuk, S.K., To, L.B. and Bardy, P. (2003) An outbreak of respiratory syncytial virus infection in a bone marrow transplant unit: effect on engraftment and outcome of pneumonia without specific antiviral treatment. *Bone Marrow Transplantation*, **32** (2), 195–203.

Afessa, B., Litzow, M.R. and Tefferi, A. (2001) Bronchiolitis obliterans and other late onset noninfectious pulmonary complications in hematopoietic stem cell transplantation. *Bone Marrow Transplantation*, **28** (5), 425–434.

Afessa, B., Tefferi, A., Litzow, M.R., Krowka, M.J., Wylam, M.E. and Peters, S.G. (2002) Diffuse alveolar hemorrhage in hematopoietic stem cell transplant recipients. *American Journal of Respiratory and Critical Care Medicine*, **166** (5), 641–645.

Afessa, B., Tefferi, A., Litzow, M.R. and Peters, S.G. (2002) Outcome of diffuse alveolar hemorrhage in hematopoietic stem cell transplant recipients. *American Journal of Respiratory and Critical Care Medicine*, **166** (10), 1364–1368.

Albelda, S.M., Talbot, G.H., Gerson, S.L., Miller, W.T. and Cassileth, P.A. (1984) Role of fiberoptic bronchoscopy in the diagnosis of invasive pulmonary aspergillosis in patients with acute leukemia. *The American Journal of Medicine*, **76** (6), 1027–1034.

Albelda, S.M., Talbot, G.H., Gerson, S.L., Miller, W.T. and Cassileth, P.A. (1985) Pulmonary cavitation and massive hemoptysis in invasive pulmonary aspergillosis. Influence of bone marrow recovery in patients with acute leukemia. *The American Review of Respiratory Disease*, **131** (1), 115–120.

Aliff, T.B., Maslak, P.G., Jurcic, J.G. *et al.* (2003) Refractory Aspergillus pneumonia in patients with acute leukemia: successful therapy with combination caspofungin and liposomal amphotericin. *Cancer*, **97** (4), 1025–1032.

Allo, M.D., Miller, J., Townsend, T. and Tan, C. (1987) Primary cutaneous aspergillosis associated with Hickman intravenous catheters. *The New England Journal of Medicine*, **317** (18), 1105–1108.

Anon (2000) Guidelines for preventing opportunistic infections among hematopoietic stem cell transplant recipients. MMWR Recommendations Reports, 49, (RR-10), 1–125. CE1-7.

Anon (2004a) Mycobacterium tuberculosis. *American Journal of Transplantation*, **4** (Suppl 10), 37–41.

Anon (2004b) Nontuberculous mycobacteria. *American Journal of Transplantation*, **4** (Suppl 10), 42–46.

Anon (2004c) Community-acquired respiratory viruses. *American Journal of Transplantation*, **4** (Suppl 10) 105–109.

Anon (2004d) Adenovirus. *American Journal of Transplantation*, **4** (Suppl 10), 101–104.

Anon (2005) Guidelines for the management of adults with hospital-acquired, ventilator-associated, and healthcare-associated, pneumonia. *American Journal of Respiratory and Critical Care Medicine*, **171**, 4, 388–416.

Anon (2007) www.ibmtr.org. Accessed.

Ansorg, R., van den Boom, R. and Rath, P.M. (1997) Detection of Aspergillus galactomannan antigen in foods and antibiotics. *Mycoses*, **40** (9–10), 353–357.

Ascioglu, S., Rex, J.H., de Pauw, B. *et al.* (2002) Defining opportunistic invasive fungal infections in immunocompromised patients with cancer and hematopoietic stem cell transplants: an international consensus. *Clinical Infectious Diseases: An Official Publication of the Infectious Diseases Society of America*, **34** (1), 7–14.

Aucouturier, P., Barra, A., Intrator, L. *et al.* (1987) Long lasting IgG subclass and antibacterial polysaccharide antibody deficiency after allogeneic bone marrow transplantation. *Blood*, **70** (3), 779–785.

Bacigalupo, A., Bregante, S., Tedone, E. *et al.* (1996) Combined foscarnet -ganciclovir treatment for cytomegalovirus infections after allogeneic hemopoietic stem cell transplantation (Hsct). *Bone Marrow Transplantation*, **18** (Suppl 2), 110–114.

Baddley, J.W., Stroud, T.P., Salzman, D. and Pappas, P.G. (2001) Invasive mold infections in allogeneic bone marrow transplant recipients. *Clinical Infectious Diseases: An Official Publication of the Infectious Diseases Society of America*, **32** (9), 1319–1324.

Baron, O., Guillaume, B., Moreau, P. *et al.* (1998) Aggressive surgical management in localized pulmonary mycotic and nonmycotic infections for neutropenic patients with acute leukemia: report of eighteen cases. *The Journal of Thoracic and Cardiovascular Surgery*, **115** (1) 63–68 discussion 8–9.

Barton, T.D. and Blumberg, E.A. (2005) Viral pneumonias other than cytomegalovirus in transplant recipients. *Clinics in Chest Medicine*, **26** (4), 707–720, viii.

Berenguer, J., Rodriguez-Tudela, J.L., Richard, C. *et al.* (1997) Deep infections caused by Scedosporium prolificans. A report on 16 cases in Spain and a review of the literature. Scedosporium Prolificans Spanish Study Group. *Medicine (Baltimore)*, **76** (4), 256–265.

Blacklock, H.A., Griffiths, P., Stirk, P. and Prentice, H.G. (1985) Specific hyperimmune globulin for cytomegalovirus pneumonitis. *Lancet*, **2** (8447), 152–153.

Boeckh, M., Leisenring, W., Riddell, S.R. *et al.* (2003) Late cytomegalovirus disease and mortality in recipients of allogeneic hematopoietic stem cell transplants: importance of viral load and T-cell immunity. *Blood*, **101** (2), 407–414.

Boeckh, M., Englund, J., Li, Y. *et al.* (2007) Randomized controlled multicenter trial of aerosolized ribavirin for respiratory syncytial virus upper respiratory tract infection in hematopoietic cell transplant recipients. *Clinical Infectious Diseases: An Official Publication of the Infectious Diseases Society of America*, **44** (2), 245–249.

Bonadio, M., Morelli, G., Mori, S., Riccioni, R., Papineschi, F. and Petrini, M. (2005) Fluoroquinolone resistance in hematopoietic stem cell transplant recipients with infectious complications. *Biomedicine & Pharmacotherapy = Biomedecine & Pharmacotherapie*, **59** (9), 511–516.

Bordon, V., Bravo, S., Van Rentergem, L. *et al.* (2007) Surveillance of cytomegalovirus (CMV) DNAemia in pediatric allogeneic stem cell transplantation: incidence and outcome of CMV infection and disease. *Transplant Infectious Disease: An Official Journal of the Transplantation Society.*

Boutati, E.I. and Anaissie, E.J. (1997) Fusarium, a significant emerging pathogen in patients with hematologic malignancy: ten years' experience at a cancer center and implications for management. *Blood*, **90** (3), 999–1008.

Boutboul, F., Alberti, C., Leblanc, T. *et al.* (2002) Invasive aspergillosis in allogeneic stem cell transplant recipients: increasing antigenemia is associated with progressive disease. *Clinical Infectious Diseases: An Official Publication of the Infectious Diseases Society of America*, **34** (7), 939–943.

Bowden, R.A. (1997) Respiratory virus infections after marrow transplant: the Fred Hutchinson Cancer Research Center experience. *The American Journal of Medicine*, **102** (3A) 27–30 discussion 42–43.

Bowden, R.A., Slichter, S.J., Sayers, M. *et al.* (1995) A comparison of filtered leukocyte-reduced and cytomegalovirus (CMV) seronegative blood products for the prevention of transfusion-associated CMV infection after marrow transplant. *Blood*, **86** (9), 3598–3603.

Bredius, R.G., Templeton, K.E., Scheltinga, S.A., Claas, E.C., Kroes, A.C. and Vossen, J.M. (2004) Prospective study of respiratory viral infections in pediatric, hemopoietic stem cell transplantation patients. *The Pediatric Infectious Disease Journal*, **23** (6), 518–522.

Buchbinder, S., Elmaagacli, A.H., Schaefer, U.W. and Roggendorf, M. (2000) Human herpesvirus 6 is an important pathogen in infectious lung disease after allogeneic bone marrow transplantation. *Bone Marrow Transplantation*, **26** (6), 639–644.

Buchheidt, D., Baust, C., Skladny, H. *et al.* (2001) Detection of Aspergillus species in blood and bronchoalveolar lavage samples from immunocompromised patients by means of 2-step polymerase chain reaction: clinical results. *Clinical Infectious Diseases: An Official Publication of the Infectious Diseases Society of America*, **33** (4), 428–435.

Busca, A., Locatelli, F., Barbui, A. *et al.* (2006) Usefulness of sequential Aspergillus galactomannan antigen detection combined with early radiologic evaluation for diagnosis of invasive pulmonary aspergillosis in patients undergoing allogeneic stem cell transplantation. *Transplantation Proceedings*, **38** (5), 1610–1613.

Busca, A., de Fabritiis, P., Ghisetti, V. *et al.* (2007) Oral valganciclovir as preemptive therapy for cytomegalovirus infection post allogeneic stem cell transplantation. *Transplant Infectious Disease: An Official Journal of the Transplantation Society*, **9** (2), 102–107.

Caillot, D., Casasnovas, O., Bernard, A. *et al.* (1997) Improved management of invasive pulmonary aspergillosis in neutropenic patients using early thoracic computed tomographic scan and surgery. *Journal of Clinical Oncology: Official Journal of the American Society of Clinical Oncology*, **15** (1), 139–147.

Caillot, D., Mannone, L., Cuisenier, B. and Couaillier, J.F. (2001) Role of early diagnosis and aggressive surgery in the management of invasive pulmonary aspergillosis in neutropenic patients. *Clinical Microbiology and Infection: The Official Publication of the European Society of Clinical Microbiology and Infectious Diseases*, **7** (Suppl 2), 54–61.

Castiglioni, B., Sutton, D.A., Rinaldi, M.G., Fung, J. and Kusne, S. (2002) Pseudallescheria boydii (Anamorph Scedosporium apiospermum). Infection in solid organ transplant recipients in a tertiary medical, center and review of the literature. *Medicine (Baltimore)* **81** (5), 333–348.

Chamilos, G., Luna, M., Lewis, R.E. *et al.* (2006) Invasive fungal infections in patients with hematologic malignancies in a tertiary care cancer center: an autopsy study over a 15-year period (1989–2003). *Haematologica*, **91** (7), 986–989.

Chemaly, R.F., Ghosh, S., Bodey, G.P. *et al.* (2006) Respiratory viral infections in adults with hematologic malignancies and human stem cell transplantation recipients: a retrospective study at a major cancer center. *Medicine (Baltimore)*, **85** (5), 278–287.

Chen, C.S., Boeckh, M., Seidel, K. *et al.* (2003) Incidence, risk factors, and mortality from pneumonia developing late after hematopoietic stem cell transplantation. *Bone Marrow Transplantation*, **32** (5), 515–522.

Chien, J.W., Martin, P.J., Gooley, T.A. *et al.* (2003) Airflow obstruction after myeloablative allogeneic hematopoietic stem cell transplantation. *American Journal of Respiratory and Critical Care Medicine*, **168** (2), 208–214.

Cohen-Wolkowiez, M., Benjamin, D.K., Jr, Steinbach, W.J. and Smith, P.B. (2006) Anidulafungin: a new echinocandin for the treatment of fungal, infections. *Drugs of Today (Barcelona, Spain: 1998)*, **42** (8), 533–544.

Cordonnier, C., Martino, R., Trabasso, P. *et al.* (2004) Mycobacterial infection: a difficult and late diagnosis in stem cell transplant recipients. *Clinical Infectious Diseases: An Official Publication of the Infectious Diseases Society of America*, **38** (9), 1229–1236.

Cordonnier, C., Ribaud, P., Herbrecht, R. *et al.* (2006) Prognostic factors for death due to invasive aspergillosis after hematopoietic stem cell transplantation: a 1-year retrospective study of consecutive patients at French transplantation centers. *Clinical Infectious Diseases: An Official Publication of the Infectious Diseases Society of America*, **42** (7), 955–963.

Costa, S.F. and Alexander, B.D. (2005) Non-Aspergillus fungal pneumonia in transplant recipients. *Clinics in Chest Medicine*, **26** (4) 675–690 vii.

Crawford, S.W., Bowden, R.A., Hackman, R.C., Gleaves, C.A., Meyers, J.D. and Clark, J.G. (1988) Rapid detection of cytomegalovirus pulmonary infection by bronchoalveolar lavage and centrifugation culture. *Annals of Internal Medicine*, **108** (2), 180–185.

Curtis, A.M., Smith, G.J. and Ravin, C.E. (1979) Air crescent sign of invasive aspergillosis. *Radiology*, **133** (1), 17–21.

Daly, A.S., McGeer, A. and Lipton, J.H. (2003) Systemic nocardiosis following allogeneic bone marrow transplantation. *Transplant Infectious Disease: An Official Journal of the Transplantation Society*, **5** (1), 16–20.

De Castro, N., Neuville, S. Sarfati, C. *et al.* (2005) Occurrence of Pneumocystis jiroveci pneumonia after allogeneic stem cell transplantation: a 6-year retrospective study. *Bone Marrow Transplantation*, **36** (10), 879–883.

de la Camara, R., Martino, R., Granados, E. *et al.* (2000) Tuberculosis after hematopoietic stem cell transplantation: incidence, clinical characteristics and outcome. Spanish group on infectious complications in hematopoietic transplantation. *Bone Marrow Transplantation*, **26** (3), 291–298.

Denning, D.W. (1998) Invasive aspergillosis. *Clinical Infectious Diseases: An Official Publication of the Infectious Diseases Society of America*, **26** (4) 781–803 quiz 4–5.

Denning, D.W., Marr, K.A., Lau, W.M. *et al.* (2006) Micafungin (FK463), alone or in combination with other systemic antifungal agents, for the treatment of acute invasive aspergillosis. *The Journal of Infection*, **53** (5), 337–349.

Doucette, K. and Fishman, J.A. (2004) Nontuberculous mycobacterial infection in hematopoietic stem cell and solid organ transplant recipients. *Clinical Infectious Diseases: An Official Publication of the Infectious Diseases Society of America*, **38** (10), 1428–1439.

Duthie, R. and Denning, D.W. (1995) Aspergillus fungemia: report of two cases and review. *Clinical Infectious Diseases: An Official Publication of the Infectious Diseases Society of America*, **20** (3), 598–605.

Elizaga, J., Olavarria, E., Apperley, J., Goldman, J. and Ward, K. (2001) Parainfluenza virus 3 infection after stem cell transplant: relevance to outcome of rapid diagnosis and ribavirin treatment. *Clinical*

Infectious Diseases: An Official Publication of the Infectious Diseases Society of America, **32** (3), 413–418.

Englund, J.A., Piedra, P.A., Jewell, A., Patel, K., Baxter, B.B. and Whimbey, E. (1996) Rapid diagnosis of respiratory syncytial virus infections in immunocompromised adults. *Journal of Clinical Microbiology*, **34** (7), 1649–1653.

Englund, J.A., Piedra, P.A. and Whimbey, E. (1997) Prevention and treatment of respiratory syncytial virus and parainfluenza viruses in immunocompromised patients. *The American Journal of Medicine*, **102** (3A), 61–70. discussion 5–6.

Enright, H., Haake, R., Weisdorf, D. *et al.* (1993) Cytomegalovirus pneumonia after bone marrow transplantation. Risk factors and response to therapy. *Transplantation*, **55** (6), 1339–1346.

Erard, V., Chien, J.W., Kim, H.W. *et al.* (2006) Airflow decline after myeloablative allogeneic hematopoietic cell transplantation: the role of community respiratory viruses. *The Journal of Infectious Diseases*, **193** (12), 1619–1625.

Escuissato, D.L., Gasparetto, E.L., Marchiori, E. *et al.* (2005) Pulmonary infections after bone marrow transplantation: high-resolution CT findings in 111 patients. *AJR American Journal of Roentgenology*, **185** (3), 608–615.

Espinel-Ingroff, A. (2001) In vitro fungicidal activities of voriconazole, itraconazole, and amphotericin B against opportunistic moniliaceous and dematiaceous fungi. *Journal of Clinical Microbiology*, **39** (3), 954–958.

Falsey, A.R. and Walsh, E.E. (2000) Respiratory syncytial virus infection in adults. *Clinical Microbiology Reviews*, **13** (3), 371–384.

Franquet, T., Lee, K.S. and Muller, N.L. (2003) Thin-section CT findings in 32 immunocompromised patients with cytomegalovirus pneumonia who do not have AIDS. *AJR American Journal of Roentgenology*, **181** (4), 1059–1063.

Franquet, T., Rodriguez, S., Martino, R., Gimenez, A., Salinas, T. and Hidalgo, A. (2006) Thin-section CT findings in hematopoietic stem cell transplantation recipients with respiratory virus pneumonia. *AJR American Journal of Roentgenology*, **187** (4), 1085–1090.

Fukuda, T., Boeckh, M., Carter, R.A. *et al.* (2003) Risks and outcomes of invasive fungal infections in recipients of allogeneic hematopoietic stem cell transplants after nonmyeloablative conditioning. *Blood*, **102** (3), 827–833.

Gaeta, M., Blandino, A., Scribano, E., Minutoli, F., Volta, S. and Pandolfo, I. (1999) Computed tomography halo sign in pulmonary nodules: frequency and diagnostic value. *Journal of Thoracic Imaging*, **14** (2), 109–113.

Garcia, R., Raad, I., Abi-Said, D. *et al.* (1997) Nosocomial respiratory syncytial virus infections: prevention and control in bone marrow transplant patients. *Infection Control and Hospital Epidemiology*, **18** (6), 412–416.

Gaziev, D., Baronciani, D., Galimberti, M. *et al.* (1996) Mucormycosis after bone marrow transplantation: report of four cases in thalassemia and review of the literature. *Bone Marrow Transplantation*, **17** (3), 409–414.

Ghannoum, M.A. and Kuhn, D.M. (2002) Voriconazole – better chances for patients with invasive mycoses. *European Journal of Medical Research*, **7** (5), 242–256.

Ghosh, S., Champlin, R.E., Ueno, N.T. *et al.* (2001) Respiratory syncytial virus infections in autologous blood and marrow transplant recipients with breast cancer: combination therapy with aerosolized ribavirin and parenteral immunoglobulins. *Bone Marrow Transplantation*, **28** (3), 271–275.

Giles, F.J. (1998) Monocyte-macrophages, granulocyte-macrophage colony-stimulating factor, and prolonged survival among patients with acute myeloid leukemia and stem cell transplants. *Clinical Infectious Diseases: An Official Publication of the Infectious Diseases Society of America*, **26** (6), 1282–1289.

Glenn, T.J., Blair, J.E. and Adams, R.H. (2005) Coccidioidomycosis in hematopoietic stem cell transplant recipients. *Medical Mycology: Official Publication of the International Society for Human and Animal Mycology*, **43** (8), 705–710.

Goodrich, J.M., Reed, E.C., Mori, M. *et al.* (1991) Clinical features and analysis of risk factors for invasive candidal infection after marrow transplantation. *The Journal of Infectious Diseases*, **164** (4), 731–740.

Goodrich, J.M., Bowden, R.A., Fisher, L., Keller, C., Schoch, G. and Meyers, J.D. (1993) Ganciclovir prophylaxis to prevent cytomegalovirus disease after allogeneic marrow transplant. *Annals of Internal Medicine*, **118** (3), 173–178.

Gorak, E., Geller, N., Srinivasan, R. *et al.* (2005) Engraftment syndrome after nonmyeloablative allogeneic hematopoietic stem cell transplantation: incidence and effects on survival. *Biology of Blood and Marrow Transplantation: Journal of the American Society for Blood and Marrow Transplantation*, **11** (7), 542–550.

Graybill, J.R., Bocanegra, R., Gonzalez, G.M. and Najvar, L.K. (2003) Combination antifungal therapy of murine aspergillosis: liposomal amphotericin B and micafungin. *The Journal of Antimicrobial Chemotherapy*, **52** (4), 656–662.

Greene, R. (2005) The radiological spectrum of pulmonary aspergillosis. *Medical Mycology: Official Publication of the International Society for Human and Animal Mycology*, **43** (Suppl 1), S147–S154.

Griffith, D.E., Aksamit, T., Brown-Elliott, B.A. *et al.* (2007) An official ATS/IDSA statement: diagnosis, treatment, and prevention of nontuberculous mycobacterial diseases. *American Journal of Respiratory and Critical Care Medicine*, **175** (4), 367–416.

Groll, A.H. and Walsh, T.J. (2001) Uncommon opportunistic fungi: new nosocomial threats. *Clinical Microbiology and Infection: The Official Publication of the European Society of Clinical Microbiology and Infectious Diseases*, **7** (Suppl 2), 8–24.

Habicht, J.M., Reichenberger, F., Gratwohl, A., Zerkowski, H.R. and Tamm, M. (1999) Surgical aspects of resection for suspected invasive pulmonary fungal infection in neutropenic patients. *The Annals of Thoracic Surgery*, **68** (2), 321–325.

Hachem, R.Y., Kontoyiannis, D.P., Boktour, M.R. *et al.* (2004) Aspergillus terreus: an emerging amphotericin B-resistant opportunistic mold in patients with hematologic malignancies. *Cancer*, **101** (7), 1594–1600.

Hakki, M., Limaye, A.P., Kim, H.W., Kirby, K.A., Corey, L. and Boeckh, M. (2007) Invasive Pseudomonas aeruginosa infections: high rate of recurrence and mortality after hematopoietic cell transplantation. *Bone Marrow Transplantation*, **39** (11), 687–693.

Hall, C.B. (2000) Nosocomial respiratory syncytial virus infections: the 'Cold War' has not ended. *Clinical Infectious Diseases: An Official Publication of the Infectious Diseases Society of America*, **31** (2), 590–596.

Halliday, C., Hoile, R., Sorrell, T. *et al.* (2006) Role of prospective screening of blood for invasive aspergillosis by polymerase chain reaction in febrile neutropenic recipients of haematopoietic stem cell transplants and patients with acute leukaemia. *British Journal of Haematology*, **132** (4), 478–486.

Hassan, I.A., Chopra, R., Swindell, R. and Mutton, K.J. (2003) Respiratory viral infections after bone marrow/peripheral stem-cell transplantation: the Christie hospital experience. *Bone Marrow Transplantation*, **32** (1), 73–77.

Hentrich, M., Oruzio, D., Jager, G. *et al.* (2005) Impact of human herpesvirus-6 after haematopoietic stem cell transplantation. *British Journal of Haematology*, **128** (1), 66–72.

Herbrecht, R., Letscher-Bru, V., Oprea, C. *et al.* (2002) Aspergillus galactomannan detection in the diagnosis of invasive aspergillosis in cancer patients. *Journal of Clinical Oncology: Official Journal of the American Society of Clinical Oncology*, **20** (7), 1898–1906.

Herbrecht, R., Denning, D.W., Patterson, T.F. *et al.* (2002) Voriconazole versus amphotericin B for primary therapy of invasive aspergillosis. *The New England Journal of Medicine*, **347** (6), 408–415.

Heussel, C.P., Kauczor, H.U., Heussel, G., Fischer, B., Mildenberger, P. and Thelen, M. (1997) Early detection of pneumonia in febrile neutropenic patients: use of thin-section CT. *AJR American Journal of Roentgenology*, **169** (5), 1347–1353.

Hizel, K., Kokturk, N., Kalkanci, A., Ozturk, C., Kustimur, S. and Tufan, M. (2004) Polymerase chain reaction in the diagnosis of invasive aspergillosis. *Mycoses*, **47** (7), 338–342.

Hofmeister, C.C., Czerlanis, C., Forsythe, S. and Stiff, P.J. (2006) Retrospective utility of bronchoscopy after hematopoietic stem cell transplant. *Bone Marrow Transplantation*, **38** (10), 693–698.

Holmberg, L.A., Boeckh, M., Hooper, H. *et al.* (1999) Increased incidence of cytomegalovirus disease after autologous CD34-selected peripheral blood stem cell transplantation. *Blood*, **94** (12), 4029–4035.

Horger, M., Hebart, H., Einsele, H. *et al.* (2005) Initial CT manifestations of invasive pulmonary aspergillosis in 45, non-HIV immunocompromised patients: association with patient outcome? *European Journal of Radiology*, **55** (3), 437–444.

Horvath, J.A. and Dummer, S. (1996) The use of respiratory-tract cultures in the diagnosis of invasive pulmonary aspergillosis. *The American Journal of Medicine*, **100** (2), 171–178.

Humar, A., Lipton, J., Welsh, S., Moussa, G., Messner, H. and Mazzulli, T. (2001) A randomised trial comparing cytomegalovirus antigenemia assay vs screening bronchoscopy for the early detection and prevention of disease in allogeneic bone marrow and peripheral blood stem cell transplant recipients. *Bone Marrow Transplantation*, **28** (5), 485–490.

Husain, S., Munoz, P., Forrest, G. *et al.* (2005) Infections due to Scedosporium apiospermum and Scedosporium prolificans in transplant recipients: clinical characteristics and impact of antifungal agent therapy on outcome. *Clinical Infectious Diseases: An Official Publication of the Infectious Diseases Society of America*, **40** (1), 89–99.

Ip, M.S., Yuen, K.Y., Woo, P.C. *et al.* (1998) Risk factors for pulmonary tuberculosis in bone marrow transplant recipients. *American Journal of Respiratory and Critical Care Medicine*, **158** (4), 1173–1177.

Ison, M.G. and Fishman, J.A. (2005) Cytomegalovirus pneumonia in transplant recipients. *Clinics in Chest Medicine*, **26** (4), 691–705. viii.

Iwen, P.C., Rupp, M.E., Langnas, A.N., Reed, E.C. and Hinrichs, S.H. (1998) Invasive pulmonary aspergillosis due to Aspergillus terreus: 12-year experience and review of the literature. *Clinical Infectious Diseases: An Official Publication of the Infectious Diseases Society of America*, **26** (5), 1092–1097.

Jahagirdar, B.N. and Morrison, V.A. (2002) Emerging fungal pathogens in patients with hematologic malignancies and marrow/stem-cell transplant recipients. *Seminars in Respiratory Infections*, **17** (2), 113–120.

Johnson, L.B. and Kauffman, C.A. (2003) Voriconazole: a new triazole antifungal agent. *Clinical Infectious Diseases: An Official Publication of the Infectious Diseases Society of America*, **36** (5), 630–637.

Junghanss, C., Marr, K.A., Carter, R.A. *et al.* (2002) Incidence and outcome of bacterial and fungal infections following nonmyeloablative compared with myeloablative allogeneic hematopoietic stem cell transplantation: a matched control study. *Biology of Blood and Marrow Transplantation: Journal of the American Society for Blood and Marrow Transplantation*, **8** (9), 512–520.

Junghanss, C., Boeckh, M., Carter, R.A. *et al.* (2002) Incidence and outcome of cytomegalovirus infections following nonmyeloablative compared with myeloablative allogeneic stem cell transplantation, a matched control study. *Blood*, **99** (6), 1978–1985.

Kahn, F.W., Jones, J.M. and England, D.M. (1986) The role of bronchoalveolar lavage in the diagnosis of invasive pulmonary aspergillosis. *American Journal of Clinical Pathology*, **86** (4), 518–523.

Keung, Y.K., Nugent, K., Jumper, C. and Cobos, E. (1999) Mycobacterium tuberculosis infection masquerading as diffuse alveolar hemorrhage after autologous stem cell transplant. *Bone Marrow Transplantation*, **23** (7), 737–738.

Klont, R.R., Mennink-Kersten, M.A. and Verweij, P.E. (2004) Utility of Aspergillus antigen detection in specimens other than serum specimens. *Clinical Infectious Diseases: An Official Publication of the Infectious Diseases Society of America*, **39** (10), 1467–1474.

Klont, R.R., Mennink-Kersten, M.A., Ruegebrink, D. *et al.* (2006) Paradoxical increase in circulating Aspergillus antigen during treatment with caspofungin in a patient with pulmonary aspergillosis. *Clinical Infectious Diseases: An Official Publication of the Infectious Diseases Society of America*, **43** (3), e23–e25.

Kojima, R., Tateishi, U., Kami, M. *et al.* (2005) Chest computed tomography of late invasive aspergillosis after allogeneic hematopoietic stem cell transplantation. *Biology of Blood and Marrow Transplantation: Journal of the American Society for Blood and Marrow Transplantation*, **11** (7), 506–511.

Konoplev, S., Champlin, R.E., Giralt, S. *et al.* (2001) Cytomegalovirus pneumonia in adult autologous blood and marrow transplant recipients. *Bone Marrow Transplantation*, **27** (8), 877–881.

Kontoyiannis, D.P., Lewis, R.E., May, G.S., Osherov, N. and Rinaldi, M.G. (2002) Aspergillus nidulans is frequently resistant to amphotericin B. *Mycoses*, **45** (9–10), 406–407.

Kontoyiannis, D.P., Hachem, R., Lewis, R.E. *et al.* (2003) Efficacy and toxicity of caspofungin in combination with liposomal amphotericin B as primary or salvage treatment of invasive aspergillosis in patients with hematologic malignancies. *Cancer*, **98** (2), 292–299.

Kotloff, R.M., Ahya, V.N. and Crawford, S.W. (2004) Pulmonary complications of solid organ and hematopoietic stem cell transplantation. *American Journal of Respiratory and Critical Care Medicine*, **170** (1), 22–48.

Ku, S.C., Tang, J.L., Hsueh, P.R., Luh, K.T., Yu, C.J. and Yang, P.C. (2001) Pulmonary tuberculosis in allogeneic hematopoietic stem cell transplantation. *Bone Marrow Transplantation*, **27** (12), 1293–1297.

Kuhlman, J.E., Fishman, E.K. and Siegelman, S.S. (1985) Invasive pulmonary aspergillosis in acute leukemia: characteristic findings on CT, the CT halo sign, and the role of CT in early diagnosis. *Radiology*, **157** (3), 611–614.

Kuhlman, J.E., Fishman, E.K., Burch, P.A., Karp, J.E., Zerhouni, E.A. and Siegelman, S.S. (1987) Invasive pulmonary aspergillosis in acute leukemia. The contribution of CT to early diagnosis and aggressive management. *Chest*, **92** (1), 95–99.

Lass-Florl, C., Griff, K., Mayr, A. *et al.* (2005) Epidemiology and outcome of infections due to Aspergillus terreus: 10-year single centre experience. *British Journal of Haematology*, **131** (2), 201–207.

Laws, H.J., Kobbe, G., Dilloo, D. *et al.* (2006) Surveillance of nosocomial infections in paediatric recipients of bone marrow or peripheral blood stem cell transplantation during neutropenia, compared with adult recipients. *The Journal of Hospital Infection*, **62** (1), 80–88.

Lazarus, H.M., Vogelsang, G.B. and Rowe, J.M. (1997) Prevention and treatment of acute graft-versus-host disease: the old and the new. A report from the Eastern Cooperative Oncology Group (ECOG). *Bone Marrow Transplantation*, **19** (6), 577–600.

Leruez-Ville, M., Ouachee, M., Delarue, R. *et al.* (2003) Monitoring cytomegalovirus infection in adult and pediatric bone marrow transplant recipients by a real-time PCR assay performed with blood plasma. *Journal of Clinical Microbiology*, **41** (5), 2040–2046.

Leung, A.N., Gosselin, M.V., Napper, C.H. *et al.* (1999) Pulmonary infections after bone marrow transplantation: clinical and radiographic findings. *Radiology*, **210** (3), 699–710.

Levy, H., Horak, D.A., Tegtmeier, B.R., Yokota, S.B. and Forman, S.J. (1992) The value of bronchoalveolar lavage and bronchial washings in the diagnosis of invasive pulmonary aspergillosis. *Respiratory Medicine*, **86** (3), 243–248.

Libshitz, H.I. and Pagani, J.J. (1981) Aspergillosis and mucormycosis: two types of opportunistic fungal pneumonia. *Radiology*, **140** (2), 301–306.

Lilleri, D., Gerna, G., Furione, M. *et al.* (2007) Use of a DNAemia cut-off for monitoring human cytomegalovirus infection reduces the number of pre-emptively treated children and young adults receiving haematopoietic stem cell transplantation as compared to qualitative pp65-antigenemia. *Blood*.

Ljungman, P. (1997) Respiratory virus infections in bone marrow transplant recipients: the European perspective. *The American Journal of Medicine*, **102** (3A), 44–47.

Ljungman, P., Aschan, J., Lewensohn-Fuchs, I. *et al.* (1998) Results of different strategies for reducing cytomegalovirus-associated mortality in allogeneic stem cell transplant recipients. *Transplantation*, **66** (10), 1330–1334.

Loeffler, J., Kloepfer, K., Hebart, H. *et al.* (2002) Polymerase chain reaction detection of aspergillus DNA in experimental models of invasive aspergillosis. *The Journal of Infectious Diseases*, **185** (8), 1203–1206.

Lossos, I.S., Breuer, R., Or, R. *et al.* (1995) Bacterial pneumonia in recipients of bone marrow transplantation. A five-year prospective study. *Transplantation*, **60** (7), 672–678.

Lujan-Zilbermann, J., Benaim, E., Tong, X., Srivastava, D.K., Patrick, C.C. and DeVincenzo, J.P. (2001) Respiratory virus infections in pediatric hematopoietic stem cell transplantation. *Clinical Infectious Diseases: An Official Publication of the Infectious Diseases Society of America*, **33** (7), 962–968.

Maertens, J., Demuynck, H., Verbeken, E.K. *et al.* (1999) Mucormycosis in allogeneic bone marrow transplant recipients: report of five cases and review of the role of iron overload in the pathogenesis. *Bone Marrow Transplantation*, **24** (3), 307–312.

Marr, K.A., Carter, R.A., Boeckh, M., Martin, P. and Corey, L. (2002) Invasive aspergillosis in allogeneic stem cell transplant recipients: changes in epidemiology and risk factors. *Blood*, **100** (13), 4358–4366.

Marr, K.A., Carter, R.A., Crippa, F., Wald, A. and Corey, L. (2002) Epidemiology and outcome of mould infections in hematopoietic stem cell transplant recipients. *Clinical Infectious Diseases: An Official Publication of the Infectious Diseases Society of America*, **34** (7), 909–917.

Marr, K.A., Balajee, S.A., McLaughlin, L., Tabouret, M., Bentsen, C. and Walsh, T.J. (2004) Detection of galactomannan antigenemia by enzyme immunoassay for the diagnosis of invasive aspergillosis: variables that affect performance. *The Journal of Infectious Diseases*, **190** (3), 641–649.

Marr, K.A., Boeckh, M., Carter, R.A., Kim, H.W. and Corey, L. (2004) Combination antifungal therapy for invasive aspergillosis. *Clinical Infectious Diseases: An Official Publication of the Infectious Diseases Society of America*, **39** (6), 797–802.

Marr, K.A., Laverdiere, M., Gugel, A. and Leisenring, W. (2005) Antifungal therapy decreases sensitivity of the Aspergillus galactomannan enzyme immunoassay. *Clinical Infectious Diseases: An Official Publication of the Infectious Diseases Society of America*, **40** (12), 1762–1769.

Marras, T.K., Sanders, K., Lipton, J.H., Messner, H.A., Conly, J. and Chan, C.K. (2002) Aerosolized pentamidine prophylaxis for Pneumocystis carinii pneumonia after allogeneic marrow transplantation. *Transplant Infectious Disease: An Official Journal of the Transplantation Society*, **4** (2), 66–74.

Maschmeyer, G., Beinert, T., Buchheidt, D. *et al.* (2003) Diagnosis and antimicrobial therapy of pulmonary infiltrates in febrile neutropenic patients–guidelines of the infectious diseases working party (AGIHO) of the German society of hematology and oncology (DGHO). *Annals of Hematology*, **82** (Suppl 2), S118–S126.

Matt, P., Bernet, F., Habicht, J. *et al.* (2004) Predicting outcome after lung resection for invasive pulmonary aspergillosis in patients with neutropenia. *Chest*, **126** (6), 1783–1788.

Mattiuzzi, G.N., Kantarjian, H., O'Brien, S. *et al.* (2004) Intravenous itraconazole for prophylaxis of systemic fungal infections in patients with acute myelogenous leukemia and high-risk myelodysplastic syndrome undergoing induction chemotherapy. *Cancer*, **100** (3), 568–573.

McCurdy, L.H., Milstone, A. and Dummer, S. (2003) Clinical features and outcomes of paramyxoviral infection in lung transplant recipients treated with ribavirin. *The Journal of Heart and Lung Transplantation: The Official Publication of the International Society for Heart Transplantation*, **22** (7), 745–753.

Meyers, J.D., Flournoy, N. and Thomas, E.D. (1982) Nonbacterial pneumonia after allogeneic marrow transplantation: a review of ten years' experience. *Reviews of Infectious Diseases*, **4** (6), 1119–1132.

Michaelides, A., Liolios, L., Glare, E.M. *et al.* (2001) Increased human cytomegalovirus (HCMV) DNA load in peripheral blood leukocytes after lung transplantation correlates with HCMV pneumonitis. *Transplantation*, **72** (1), 141–147.

Miyakoshi, S., Kusumi, E., Matsumura, T. *et al.* (2007) Invasive fungal infection following reduced-intensity cord blood transplantation for adult patients with hematologic diseases. *Biology of Blood and Marrow Transplantation: Journal of the American Society for Blood and Marrow Transplantation*, **13** (7), 771–777.

Moreau, P., Zahar, J.R., Milpied, N. *et al.* (1993) Localized invasive pulmonary aspergillosis in patients with neutropenia. Effectiveness of surgical resection. *Cancer*, **72** (11), 3223–3226.

Morgan, J., Wannemuehler, K.A., Marr, K.A. *et al.* (2005) Incidence of invasive aspergillosis following hematopoietic stem cell and solid organ transplantation: interim results of a prospective multicenter surveillance program. *Medical Mycology: Official Publication of the International Society for Human and Animal Mycology*, **43** (Suppl 1), S49–S58.

Musher, B., Fredricks, D., Leisenring, W., Balajee, S.A., Smith, C. and Marr, K.A. (2004) Aspergillus galactomannan enzyme immunoassay and quantitative PCR for diagnosis of invasive aspergillosis with bronchoalveolar lavage fluid. *Journal of Clinical Microbiology*, **42** (12), 5517–5522.

Myers, G.D., Bollard, C.M., Wu, M.F. *et al.* (2007) Reconstitution of adenovirus-specific cell-mediated immunity in pediatric patients after hematopoietic stem cell transplantation. *Bone Marrow Transplantation*, **39** (11), 677–686.

Nagai, H., Guo, J., Choi, H. and Kurup, V. (1995) Interferon-gamma and tumor necrosis factor-alpha protect mice from invasive aspergillosis. *The Journal of Infectious Diseases*, **172** (6), 1554–1560.

Narreddy, S., Mellon-Reppen, S., Abidi, M.H. *et al.* (2007) Non-bacterial infections in allogeneic non-myeloablative stem cell transplant recipients. *Transplant Infectious Disease: An Official Journal of the Transplantation Society*, **9** (1), 3–10.

Nichols, W.G., Corey, L., Gooley, T., Davis, C. and Boeckh, M. (2001) Parainfluenza virus infections after hematopoietic stem cell transplantation: risk factors, response to antiviral therapy, and effect on transplant outcome. *Blood*, **98** (3), 573–578.

Nichols, W.G., Corey, L., Gooley, T., Davis, C. and Boeckh, M. (2002) High risk of death due to bacterial and fungal infection among cytomegalovirus (CMV)-seronegative recipients of stem cell transplants from seropositive donors: evidence for indirect effects of primary CMV infection. *The Journal of Infectious Diseases*, **185** (3), 273–282.

Nichols, W.G., Price, T.H., Gooley, T., Corey, L. and Boeckh, M. (2003) Transfusion-transmitted cytomegalovirus infection after receipt of leukoreduced blood products. *Blood*, **101** (10), 4195–4200.

Nichols, W.G., Guthrie, K.A., Corey, L. and Boeckh, M. (2004) Influenza infections after hematopoietic stem cell transplantation: risk factors, mortality, and the effect of antiviral therapy. *Clinical Infectious Diseases: An Official Publication of the Infectious Diseases Society of America*, **39** (9), 1300–1306.

Niederman, M.S., Mandell, L.A., Anzueto, A. *et al.* (2001) Guidelines for the management of adults with community-acquired pneumonia. Diagnosis, assessment of severity, antimicrobial therapy, and, prevention. *American Journal of Respiratory and Critical Care Medicine*, **163** (7), 1730–1754.

Nucci, M., Marr, K.A., Queiroz-Telles, F. *et al.* (2004) Fusarium infection in hematopoietic stem cell transplant recipients. *Clinical Infectious Diseases: An Official Publication of the Infectious Diseases Society of America*, **38** (9), 1237–1242.

Obayashi, T., Yoshida, M., Mori, T. *et al.* (1995) Plasma $(1 \rightarrow 3)$-beta-D-glucan measurement in diagnosis of invasive deep mycosis and fungal febrile episodes. *Lancet*, **345** (8941), 17–20.

Oren, I., Zuckerman, T., Avivi, I., Finkelstein, R., Yigla, M. and Rowe, J.M. (2002) Nosocomial outbreak of Legionella pneumophila serogroup 3 pneumonia in a new bone marrow transplant unit: evaluation, treatment and control. *Bone Marrow Transplantation*, **30** (3), 175–179.

Ottolini, M.G., Curtis, S.R., Mathews, A., Ottolini, S.R. and Prince, G.A. (2002) Palivizumab is highly effective in suppressing respiratory syncytial virus in an immunosuppressed animal model. *Bone Marrow Transplantation*, **29** (2), 117–120.

Ozer, H., Armitage, J.O., Bennett, C.L. *et al.* (2000) 2000 update of recommendations for the use of hematopoietic colony-stimulating factors: evidence-based, clinical practice guidelines. American Society of Clinical Oncology Growth Factors Expert Panel. *Journal of Clinical Oncology: Official Journal of the American Society of Clinical Oncology*, **18** (20), 3558–3585.

Page, R.L., 2nd, Schwiesow, J. and Hilts, A. (2007) Posaconazole as salvage therapy in a patient with disseminated zygomycosis: case report and review of the literature. *Pharmacotherapy*, **27** (2), 290–298.

Panackal, A.A. and Marr, K.A. (2004) Scedosporium/Pseudallescheria infections. *Seminars in Respiratory and Critical Care Medicine*, **25** (2), 171–181.

Paulin, T., Ringden, O. and Lonnqvist, B. (1985) Faster immunological recovery after bone marrow transplantation in patients without cytomegalovirus infection. *Transplantation*, **39** (4), 377–384.

Perea, S., Gonzalez, G., Fothergill, A.W., Kirkpatrick, W.R., Rinaldi, M.G. and Patterson, T.F. (2002) In vitro interaction of caspofungin acetate with voriconazole against clinical isolates of Aspergillus spp. *Antimicrobial Agents and Chemotherapy*, **46** (9), 3039–3041.

Pfeiffer, C.D., Fine, J.P. and Safdar, N. (2006) Diagnosis of invasive aspergillosis using a galacto-mannan assay: a meta-analysis. *Clinical Infectious Diseases: An Official Publication of the Infectious Diseases Society of America*, **42** (10), 1417–1727.

Pidhorecky, I., Urschel, J. and Anderson, T. (2000) Resection of invasive pulmonary aspergillosis in immunocompromised patients. *Annals of Surgical Oncology: The Official Journal of the Society of Surgical Oncology*, **7** (4), 312–317.

Pitisuttithum, P., Negroni, R., Graybill, J.R. *et al.* (2005) Activity of posaconazole in the treatment of central nervous system fungal infections. *The Journal of Antimicrobial Chemotherapy*, **56** (4), 745–755.

Poutsiaka, D.D., Price, L.L., Ucuzian, A., Chan, G.W., Miller, K.B. and Snydman, D.R. (2007) Blood stream infection after hematopoietic stem cell transplantation is associated with increased mortality. *Bone Marrow Transplantation*, **40** (1), 63–70.

Price, T.H., Bowden, R.A., Boeckh, M. *et al.* (2000) Phase I/II trial of neutrophil transfusions from donors stimulated with G-CSF and dexamethasone for treatment of patients with infections in hematopoietic stem cell transplantation. *Blood*, **95** (11), 3302–3309.

Prystowsky, S.D., Vogelstein, B., Ettinger, D.S. *et al.* (1976) Invasive aspergillosis. *The New England Journal of Medicine*, **295** (12), 655–658.

Raboni, S.M., Nogueira, M.B., Tsuchiya, L.R. *et al.* (2003) Respiratory tract viral infections in bone marrow transplant patients. *Transplantation*, **76** (1), 142–146.

Reichenberger, F., Habicht, J., Kaim, A. *et al.* (1998) Lung resection for invasive pulmonary aspergillosis in neutropenic patients with hematologic diseases. *American Journal of Respiratory and Critical Care Medicine*, **158** (3), 885–890.

Reichenberger, F., Habicht, J., Matt, P. *et al.* (1999) Diagnostic yield of bronchoscopy in histologically proven invasive pulmonary aspergillosis. *Bone Marrow Transplantation*, **24** (11), 1195–1199.

Reinke, P., Prosch, S., Kern, F. and Volk, H.D. (1999) Mechanisms of human cytomegalovirus (HCMV) (re)activation and its impact on organ transplant patients. *Transplant Infectious Disease: An Official Journal of the Transplantation Society*, **1** (3), 157–164.

Reusser, P. (1991) Cytomegalovirus infection and disease after bone marrow transplantation: epidemiology, prevention, and treatment. *Bone Marrow Transplantation*, **7** (Suppl 3), 52–56.

Ribaud, P., Chastang, C., Latge, J.P. *et al.* (1999) Survival and prognostic factors of invasive aspergillosis after allogeneic bone marrow transplantation. *Clinical Infectious Diseases: An Official Publication of the Infectious Diseases Society of America*, **28** (2), 322–330.

Rodriguez, M., Sifri, C.D. and Fishman, J.A. (2004) Failure of low-dose atovaquone prophylaxis against Pneumocystis jiroveci infection in transplant recipients. *Clinical Infectious Diseases: An Official Publication of the Infectious Diseases Society of America*, **38** (8), e76–e78.

Roghmann, M., Ball, K., Erdman, D., Lovchik, J., Anderson, L.J. and Edelman, R. (2003) Active surveillance for respiratory virus infections in adults who have undergone bone marrow and peripheral blood stem cell transplantation. *Bone Marrow Transplantation*, **32** (11), 1085–1088.

Roilides, E., Uhlig, K., Venzon, D., Pizzo, P.A. and Walsh, T.J. (1993) Prevention of corticosteroid-induced suppression of human polymorphonuclear leukocyte-induced damage of Aspergillus fumigatus hyphae by granulocyte colony-stimulating factor and gamma interferon. *Infection and Immunity*, **61** (11), 4870–4877.

Roilides, E., Holmes, A., Blake, C., Venzon, D., Pizzo, P.A. and Walsh, T.J. (1994) Antifungal activity of elutriated human monocytes against Aspergillus fumigatus hyphae: enhancement by granulocyte-macrophage colony-stimulating factor and interferon-gamma. *The Journal of Infectious Diseases*, **170** (4), 894–899.

Roilides, E., Sein, T., Holmes, A. *et al.* (1995) Effects of macrophage colony-stimulating factor on antifungal activity of mononuclear phagocytes against Aspergillus fumigatus. *The Journal of Infectious Diseases*, **172** (4), 1028–1034.

Rolston, K.V. (2001) The spectrum of pulmonary infections in cancer patients. *Current Opinion in Oncology*, **13** (4), 218–223.

Rowe, J.M., Andersen, J.W., Mazza, J.J. *et al.* (1995) A randomized placebo-controlled phase III study of granulocyte-macrophage colony-stimulating factor in adult patients (>55 to 70 years of age) with acute myelogenous leukemia: a study of the Eastern Cooperative Oncology Group (E1490). *Blood*, **86** (2), 457–462.

Roy, V. and Weisdorf, D. (1997) Mycobacterial infections following bone marrow transplantation: a 20 year retrospective review. *Bone Marrow Transplantation*, **19** (5), 467–470.

Ruhnke, M., Bohme, A., Buchheidt, D. *et al.* (2003) Diagnosis of invasive fungal infections in hematology and oncology–guidelines of the Infectious Diseases Working Party (AGIHO) of the German Society of Hematology and Oncology (DGHO). *Annals of Hematology*, **82** (Suppl 2), S141–S148.

Safdar, A. (2006) Strategies to enhance immune function in hematopoietic transplantation recipients who have fungal infections. *Bone Marrow Transplantation*, **38** (5), 327–337.

Safdar, A., Rodriguez, G., Ohmagari, N. *et al.* (2005) The safety of interferon-gamma-1b therapy for invasive fungal infections after hematopoietic stem cell transplantation. *Cancer*, **103** (4), 731–739.

Sakamaki, H., Yuasa, K., Goto, H. *et al.* (1997) Comparison of cytomegalovirus (CMV) antigenemia and CMV in bronchoalveolar lavage fluid for diagnosis of CMV pulmonary infection after bone marrow transplantation. *Bone Marrow Transplantation*, **20** (2), 143–147.

Salonen, J., Lehtonen, O.P., Terasjarvi, M.R. and Nikoskelainen, J. (2000) Aspergillus antigen in serum, urine and bronchoalveolar lavage specimens of neutropenic patients in relation to clinical outcome. *Scandinavian Journal of Infectious Diseases*, **32** (5), 485–490.

Sambatakou, H., Dupont, B., Lode, H. and Denning, D.W. (2006) Voriconazole treatment for subacute invasive and chronic pulmonary aspergillosis. *The American Journal of Medicine*, **119** (6) 527. e17–24.

Sampathkumar, P. and Paya, C.V. (2001) Fusarium infection after solid-organ transplantation. *Clinical Infectious Diseases: An Official Publication of the Infectious Diseases Society of America*, **32** (8), 1237–1240.

Segal, B.H., Barnhart, L.A., Anderson, V.L., Walsh, T.J., Malech, H.L. and Holland, S.M. (2005) Posaconazole as salvage therapy in patients with chronic granulomatous disease and invasive filamentous fungal infection. *Clinical Infectious Diseases: An Official Publication of the Infectious Diseases Society of America*, **40** (11), 1684–1688.

Shepp, D.H., Dandliker, P.S., de Miranda, P. *et al.* (1985) Activity of 9-[2-hydroxy-1-(hydroxymethyl) ethoxymethyl]guanine in the treatment of cytomegalovirus pneumonia. *Annals of Internal Medicine*, **103** (3), 368–373.

Sherertz, R.J., Belani, A., Kramer, B.S. *et al.* (1987) Impact of air filtration on nosocomial Aspergillus infections. Unique risk of bone marrow transplant recipients. *The American Journal of Medicine*, **83** (4), 709–718.

Shields, A.F., Hackman, R.C., Fife, K.H., Corey, L. and Meyers, J.D. (1985) Adenovirus infections in patients undergoing bone-marrow transplantation. *The New England Journal of Medicine*, **312** (9), 529–533.

Singh, N., Obman, A., Husain, S., Aspinall, S., Mietzner, S. and Stout, J.E. (2004) Reactivity of platelia Aspergillus galactomannan antigen with piperacillin-tazobactam: clinical implications based on achievable concentrations in serum. *Antimicrobial Agents and Chemotherapy*, **48** (6), 1989–1992.

Sloane, J.P., Depledge, M.H., Powles, R.L., Morgenstern, G.R., Trickey, B.S. and Dady, P.J. (1983) Histopathology of the lung after bone marrow transplantation. *Journal of Clinical Pathology*, **36** (5), 546–554.

Small, T.N., Casson, A., Malak, S.F. *et al.* (2002) Respiratory syncytial virus infection following hematopoietic stem cell transplantation. *Bone Marrow Transplantation*, **29** (4), 321–327.

Soubani, A.O. and Qureshi, M.A. (2002) Invasive pulmonary aspergillosis following bone marrow, transplantation: risk factors and diagnostic aspect. *Haematologia*, **32** (4), 427–437.

Soubani, A.O. and Uberti, J.P. (2007) Bronchiolitis obliterans following haematopoietic stem cell, transplantation. *The European Respiratory Journal: Official Journal of the European Society for Clinical Respiratory Physiology*, **29** (5), 1007–1019.

Soubani, A.O., Miller, K.B. and Hassoun, P.M. (1996) Pulmonary complications of bone marrow transplantation. *Chest*, **109** (4), 1066–1077.

Spanakis, E.K., Aperis, G. and Mylonakis, E. (2006) New agents for the treatment of fungal infections: clinical efficacy and gaps in coverage. *Clinical Infectious Diseases: An Official Publication of the Infectious Diseases Society of America*, **43** (8), 1060–1068.

Spitzer, T.R. (2001) Engraftment syndrome following hematopoietic stem cell transplantation. *Bone Marrow Transplantation*, **27** (9), 893–898.

Steinbach, W.J., Benjamin, D.K., Jr, Kontoyiannis, D.P. *et al.* (2004) Infections due to Aspergillus terreus: a multicenter retrospective analysis of 83 cases. *Clinical Infectious Diseases: An Official Publication of the Infectious Diseases Society of America*, **39** (2), 192–198.

Stringer, J.R., Beard, C.B., Miller, R.F. and Wakefield, A.E. (2002) A new name (Pneumocystis jiroveci) for Pneumocystis from humans. *Emerging Infectious Diseases*, **8** (9), 891–896.

Sullivan, K.M., Dykewicz, C.A. Longworth. D.L. *et al.* (2001) Preventing opportunistic infections after hematopoietic stem cell transplantation: the Centers for Disease Control and Prevention, Infectious Diseases Society of America, and American Society for Blood and Marrow Transplantation Practice Guidelines and beyond. *Hematology, the American Society of Hematology Education Program*, 392–421.

Symeonidis, N., Jakubowski, A., Pierre-Louis, S. *et al.* (2007) Invasive adenoviral infections in T-cell-depleted allogeneic hematopoietic stem cell transplantation: high mortality in the era of cidofovir. *Transplant Infectious Disease: An Official Journal of the Transplantation Society*, **9** (2), 108–113.

Tamm, M., Traenkle, P., Grilli, B. *et al.* (2001) Pulmonary cytomegalovirus infection in immuno-compromised patients. *Chest*, **119** (3), 838–843.

Tang, C.M. and Cohen, J. (1992) Diagnosing fungal infections in immunocompromised hosts. *Journal of Clinical Pathology*, **45** (1), 1–5.

Taplitz, R.A. and Jordan, M.C. (2002) Pneumonia caused by herpesviruses in recipients of hematopoietic cell transplants. *Seminars in Respiratory Infections*, **17** (2), 121–129.

Torre-Cisneros, J., De la Mata, M., Pozo, J.C. *et al.* (1999) Randomized trial of weekly sulfadoxine/pyrimethamine vs. daily low-dose trimethoprim-sulfamethoxazole for the prophylaxis of Pneumocystis carinii pneumonia after liver transplantation. *Clinical Infectious Diseases: An Official Publication of the Infectious Diseases Society of America*, **29** (4), 771–774.

Torres, H.A., Chemaly, R.F., Storey, R. *et al.* (2006) Influence of type of cancer and hematopoietic stem cell transplantation on clinical presentation of Pneumocystis jiroveci pneumonia in cancer patients. *European Journal of Clinical Microbiology & Infectious Diseases: Official Publication of the European Society of Clinical Microbiology*, **25** (6), 382–388.

Trifilio, S., Singhal, S., Williams, S. *et al.* (2007) Breakthrough fungal infections after allogeneic hematopoietic stem cell transplantation in patients on prophylactic voriconazole. *Bone Marrow Transplantation*.

Ullmann, A.J. and Cornely, O.A. (2006) Antifungal prophylaxis for invasive mycoses in high risk patients. *Current Opinion in Infectious Diseases*, **19** (6), 571–576.

Ullmann, A.J., Lipton, J.H., Vesole, D.H. *et al.* (2007) Posaconazole or fluconazole for prophylaxis in severe graft-versus-host disease. *The New England Journal of Medicine*, **356** (4), 335–347.

van Burik, J.A., Hackman, R.C., Nadeem, S.Q. *et al.* (1997) Nocardiosis after bone marrow transplantation: a retrospective study. *Clinical Infectious Diseases: An Official Publication of the Infectious Diseases Society of America*, **24** (6), 1154–1160.

van Kraaij, M.G., van Elden, L.J., van Loon, A.M. *et al.* (2005) Frequent detection of respiratory viruses in adult recipients of stem cell transplants with the use of real-time polymerase chain reaction, compared with viral culture. *Clinical Infectious Diseases: An Official Publication of the Infectious Diseases Society of America*, **40** (5), 662–669.

Vu, D., Peck, A.J., Nichols, W.G. *et al.* (2007) Safety and tolerability of oseltamivir prophylaxis in hematopoietic stem cell transplant recipients: a retrospective case-control study. *Clinical Infectious Diseases: An Official Publication of the Infectious Diseases Society of America*, **45** (2), 187–193.

Wald, A., Leisenring, W., van Burik, J.A. and Bowden, R.A. (1997) Epidemiology of Aspergillus infections in a large cohort of patients undergoing bone marrow transplantation. *The Journal of Infectious Diseases*, **175** (6), 1459–1466.

Walsh, T.J. and Groll, A.H. (2001) Overview: non-fumigatus species of Aspergillus: perspectives on emerging pathogens in immunocompromised hosts. *Current Opinion in Investigational Drugs*, **2** (10), 1366–1367.

Walsh, T.J., Raad, I., Patterson, T.F. *et al.* (2007) Treatment of invasive aspergillosis with posaconazole in patients who are refractory to or intolerant of conventional therapy: an externally controlled trial. *Clinical Infectious Diseases: An Official Publication of the Infectious Diseases Society of America*, **44** (1), 2–12.

Walter, E.A., Greenberg, P.D., Gilbert, M.J. *et al.* (1995) Reconstitution of cellular immunity against cytomegalovirus in recipients of allogeneic bone marrow by transfer of T-cell clones from the donor. *The New England Journal of Medicine*, **333** (16), 1038–1044.

Warris, A., Bjorneklett, A. and Gaustad, P. (2001) Invasive pulmonary aspergillosis associated with infliximab therapy. *The New England Journal of Medicine*, **344** (14), 1099–1100.

Weinstock, D.M., Feinstein, M.B., Sepkowitz, K.A. and Jakubowski, A. (2003) High rates of infection and colonization by nontuberculous mycobacteria after allogeneic hematopoietic stem cell transplantation. *Bone Marrow Transplantation*, **31** (11), 1015–1021.

Westall, G.P., Michaelides, A., Williams, T.J., Snell, G.I. and Kotsimbos, T.C. (2004) Human cytomegalovirus load in plasma and bronchoalveolar lavage fluid: a longitudinal study of lung transplant recipients. *The Journal of Infectious Diseases*, **190** (6), 1076–1083.

Whimbey, E., Vartivarian, S.E., Champlin, R.E., Elting, L.S., Luna, M. and Bodey, G.P. (1993) Parainfluenza virus infection in adult bone marrow transplant recipients. *European Journal of Clinical Microbiology & Infectious Diseases: Official Publication of the European Society of Clinical Microbiology*, **12** (9), 699–701.

Whimbey, E., Englund, J.A. and Couch, R.B. (1997) Community respiratory virus infections in immunocompromised patients with cancer. *The American Journal of Medicine*, **102** (3A) 10–18 discussion 25–26.

Wingard, J.R. (1999) Opportunistic infections after blood and marrow transplantation. *Transplant Infectious Disease: An Official Journal of the Transplantation Society*, **1** (1), 3–20.

Witherspoon, R.P., Storb, R., Ochs, H.D. *et al.* (1981) Recovery of antibody production in human allogeneic marrow graft recipients: influence of time posttransplantation, the presence or absence of chronic graft-versus-host disease, and antithymocyte globulin treatment. *Blood*, **58** (2), 360–368.

Young, R.C., Bennett, J.E., Vogel, C.L., Carbone, P.P. and DeVita, V.T. (1970) Aspergillosis. The spectrum of the disease in 98 patients. *Medicine (Baltimore)*, **49** (2), 147–173.

Youssef, S., Rodriguez, G., Rolston, K.V., Champlin, R.E., Raad, I.I. and Safdar, A. (2007) Streptococcus pneumoniae infections in 47 hematopoietic stem cell transplantation recipients: clinical characteristics of infections and vaccine-breakthrough infections, 1989–2005. *Medicine (Baltimore)*, **86** (2), 69–77.

Yu, V.L., Muder, R.R. and Poorsattar, A. (1986) Significance of isolation of Aspergillus from the respiratory tract in diagnosis of invasive pulmonary aspergillosis. Results from a three-year prospective study. *The American Journal of Medicine*, **81** (2), 249–254.

Yuen, K.Y. and Woo, P.C. (2002) Tuberculosis in blood and marrow transplant recipients. *Hematological Oncology*, **20** (2), 51–62.

Zaia, J.A. (1993) Prevention and treatment of cytomegalovirus pneumonia in transplant recipients. *Clinical Infectious Diseases: An Official Publication of the Infectious Diseases Society of America*, **17** (Suppl 2), S392–S399.

9

Chronic non-infectious pulmonary complications in haematopoietic stem cell transplantation

Bekele Afessa and Steve G. Peters

Division of Pulmonary and Critical Care Medicine, Department of Medicine, Mayo Clinic College of Medicine, Rochester MN, USA

9.1 Introduction

Tens of thousands of patients undergo haematopoietic stem cell transplantation (HSCT) annually, primarily for haematologic and lymphoid cancers, but also for other disorders (Copelan, 2006). HSCT entails the intravenous infusion of haematopoietic progenitor (stem) cells to replace the malignant or ablated bone marrow cells. The pre-transplant conditioning regimen virtually eliminates all pre-existing innate and acquired immunity (Matulis and High, 2002). The post-transplant period is divided into three phases: pre-engraftment, early post-transplant, and late post-transplant (Gosselin and Adams, 2002). Pulmonary complications develop in 30–60% of HSCT recipients (Afessa and Peters, 2005). They are the immediate cause of death in approximately 61% (Roychowdhury *et al.*, 2005; Sharma *et al.*, 2005). Risk factors for the development of pulmonary complications include pre-transplant radiation and chemotherapy, total body irradiation, allogeneic stem cell source and graft-versus-host disease (GVHD) (Afessa and Peters, 2005; Afessa and Peters, 2006). Pulmonary complications are less common in T-cell depleted HSCT recipients (Huisman *et al.*, 2006).

There are several non-infectious pulmonary complications that develop in HSCT recipients, and some follow characteristic temporal patterns (Table 9.1) (Figure 9.1) (Afessa and Peters, 2005; Afessa and Peters, 2006; Peters and Afessa, 2005). The characteristics of the main non-infectious pulmonary complications are listed in Table 9.2. This chapter describes the chronic non-infectious pulmonary complications that develop in HSCT recipients.

When HSCT recipients present with pulmonary symptoms and signs, they are usually treated with antibiotics empirically. When initial evaluation reveals no infectious

Pulmonary Infection in the Immunocompromised Patient, Edited by Carlos Agustí and Antoni Torres
© 2009 John Wiley & Sons, Ltd.

Table 9.1   Non-infectious pulmonary complications in haematopoietic stem cell transplant recipients.

Isolated abnormality in pulmonary function
Asthma
Acute pulmonary oedema
Diffuse alveolar haemorrhage
Periengraftment respiratory distress syndrome
Bronchiolitis obliterans
Bronchiolitis obliterans organizing pneumonia
Idiopathic pneumonia syndrome
Delayed pulmonary toxicity syndrome
Pulmonary cytolytic thrombi
Pulmonary veno-occlusive disease
Progressive pulmonary fibrosis
Pulmonary hypertension
Hepatopulmonary syndrome
Pulmonary alveolar proteinosis
Eosinophilic pneumonia

etiology, and empiric therapy fails, a systemic diagnostic approach is required. The diagnostic tools include high resolution computed tomography (HRCT), pulmonary function testing (PFT), bronchoalveolar lavage (BAL) with transbronchial lung biopsy if tolerated, and if needed, video-assisted thoracoscopic lung biopsy (Figure 9.2) (Afessa and Peters, 2006). For peripherally located nodules and masses, fluoroscopy

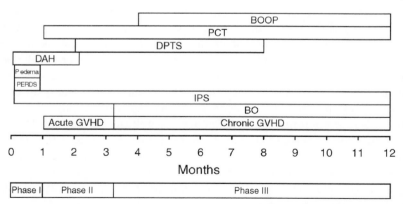

Figure 9.1   Timing of the major non-infectious pulmonary complications following haematopoietic stem cell transplantation. BO = Bronchiolitis obliterans; BOOP = Bronchiolitis obliterans organizing pneumonia; DAH = Diffuse alveolar haemorrhage; DPTS = Delayed pulmonary toxicity syndrome; GVHD = Graft-versus-host-disease; IPS = Idiopathic pneumonia syndrome; P edema = Pulmonary oedema; PCT = Pulmonary cytolytic thrombi; PERDS = Peri-engraftment respiratory distress syndrome; Phase I = Pre-engraftment period; Phase II = Early post-engraftment period; Phase III = Late post-engraftment period.

Table 9.2 The characteristics of the main non-infectious pulmonary complications in haematopoietic stem cell transplant recipients.

Pulmonary complications	Distinguishing features
Bronchiolitis obliterans	No sign of pulmonary infection and presence of airway obstruction
Bronchiolitis obliterans organizing pneumonia	Fever, patchy pulmonary airspace consolidation, and typical lung histology
Idiopathic pneumonia syndrome	Findings of acute lung injury and exclusion of infectious pneumonia and other causes
Diffuse alveolar haemorrhage	Diffuse pulmonary infiltrates and bronchoalveolar lavage with progressively bloodier return and/or ≥20% haemosiderin-laden macrophages
Peri-engraftment respiratory distress syndrome	Acute lung injury onset within 5 d of neutrophil engraftment and exclusion of cardiac and infectious causes
Delayed pulmonary toxicity syndrome	In autologous haematopoietic stem cell recipients with breast cancer, and following high dose pre-transplant chemotherapy; good prognosis
Pulmonary cytolytic thrombi	Fever and pulmonary nodules in children with graft-versus-host disease, and typical lung histology

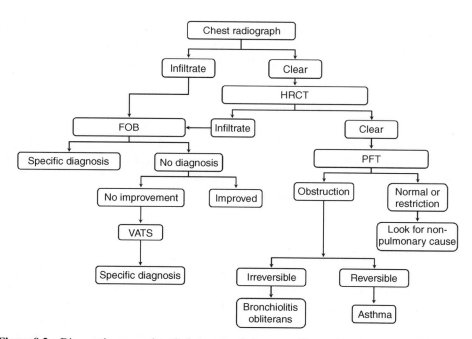

Figure 9.2 Diagnostic approach to the haematopoietic stem cell transplant recipient with pulmonary complication. FOB = Fibreoptic bronchoscopy; HRCT = High-resolution computed tomography of the chest; PFT = Pulmonary function test; VATS = Video-assisted thoracoscopic surgery.

or computed tomography (CT) guided transthoracic fine needle aspiration may be helpful (Afessa and Peters, 2006).

9.2 Bronchiolitis obliterans (BO)

The histologic pulmonary manifestations of GVHD include diffuse alveolar damage, lymphocytic bronchitis/bronchiolitis with interstitial pneumonitis, bronchiolitis obliterans organizing pneumonia (BOOP), and BO (Yousem, 1995). BO is a severe manifestation of chronic GVHD, characterized by airflow limitation. The pathogenesis of BO in HSCT recipients is not well understood. GVHD, recurrent aspiration, abnormal local immunoglobulin secretory function in the lungs, and unrecognized infections are implicated (Afessa, Litzow and Tefferi, 2001; Afessa and Peters, 2005). About 45% of long-term survivor allogeneic HSCT recipients develop chronic GVHD (Carlens et al., 1998).

Incidence

With the exception of rare case reports in autologous recipients (Paz et al., 1992), BO almost exclusively affects allogeneic HSCT recipients with GVHD. Because of the heterogeneity of the patient populations and diagnostic criteria, the reported incidence of BO has varied from study to study. Although some studies have included pathologic findings, most of the reported cases of BO in HSCT recipients are defined by the presence of airflow limitation in the appropriate clinical setting. BO may develop in up to 35% of long-term survivors with GVHD. However, the overall frequency in allogeneic HSCT recipients is about 3.9% (Afessa, Litzow and Tefferi, 2001; Afessa and Peters, 2005).

Risk factors

Risk factors for BO include GVHD, advanced donor and recipient age, myeloablative conditioning, methotrexate use, antecedent respiratory infection and serum immunoglobulin deficiency (Afessa, Litzow and Tefferi, 2001; Afessa and Peters, 2005). T-cell depletion may prevent BO in allogeneic HSCT recipients (Ditschkowski et al., 2007; Huisman et al., 2006).

Clinical findings and diagnostic evaluation

Airway obstruction usually develops between 80 and 700 days following HSCT in patients with BO (Afessa, Litzow and Tefferi, 2001; Afessa and Peters, 2005). The clinical presentation includes dry cough and dyspnea in most, wheezing in about 40%, and antecedent cold symptoms in 20% (Afessa, Litzow and Tefferi, 2001). Twenty per cent of the patients with BO have no respiratory symptoms at the time of the abnormal PFT (Clark et al., 1989). Since the presenting respiratory symptoms are non-specific, the diagnostic work-up should focus on multiple organs likely to be affected by GVHD

Table 9.3 Stages of BO severity (Estenne *et al.*, 2002).

Stage	FEV1 (% of baseline)
Mild	66–80
Moderate	51–65
Severe	≤50

(Afessa, Litzow and Tefferi, 2001). Microbiological evaluation should be undertaken to exclude infection. Complete blood count with differential, blood urea nitrogen, creatinine, total bilirubin, hepatic transaminases, gammaglobulin levels and subclasses, and urinalysis are recommended (Crawford and Clark, 1993).

Although normal airflow has been reported in HSCT recipients with histologically proven BO (Paz *et al.*, 1992), irreversible airflow obstruction, with decrease in forced expiratory volume in one second (FEV1) and FEV1 to force vital capacity (FVC) ratio, is the hallmark of BO. Based on spirometric measurements, BO can be classified into three severity stages (Table 9.3) (Estenne *et al.*, 2002).

Chest radiograph is usually normal or may show hyperinflation (Afessa, Litzow and Tefferi, 2001; Afessa and Peters, 2005). Decreased lung attenuation, bronchial dilatation, centrilobular nodules and non-homogeneous air trapping are seen on HRCT of the chest (Figure 9.3) (Afessa, Litzow and Tefferi, 2001; Afessa and Peters, 2005; Jung *et al.*, 2004). Since there is a high prevalence of sinusitis in these patients, radiographic assessment of the paranasal sinuses is recommended (Crawford and Clark, 1993;

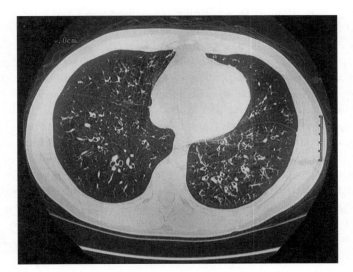

Figure 9.3 Computed tomography of the chest in a patient with bronchiolitis obliterans showing diffuse areas of parenchymal hypoattenuation, proximal bronchiectasis and subsegmental bronchial dilatation (Reprinted by permission from Bone Marrow Transplantation, Afessa *et al.* 2001; 28(5): 425–434.).

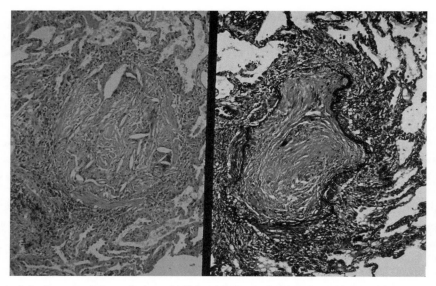

Figure 9.4 Lung pathology in bronchiolitis obliterans showing bronchiolar inflammation and luminal obliteration associated with excess fibrous connective tissue. Alveoli and their ducts are spared. (Haematoxylin and eosin and Verhoeff-Van Gieson elastic tissue stain) (Reprinted by permission from Bone Marrow Transplantation, Afessa *et al.* 2001; 28(5):425–434.).

Thompson *et al.*, 2002). If gastrointestinal GVHD or aspiration is a consideration, oesophageal studies should be performed (Crawford and Clark, 1993; McDonald, Sullivan and Plumley, 1984).

BAL may show neutrophilic and/or lymphocytic inflammation (St. John *et al.*, 1990; Trisolini *et al.*, 2001). Transbronchial lung biopsy is usually non-diagnostic. Video-assisted thoracoscopic lung biopsy, showing fibrinous obliteration of the small airway lumen, is required to make a definitive histologic diagnosis of BO (Figure 9.4) (Afessa, Litzow and Tefferi, 2001; Afessa and Peters, 2005). However, surgical biopsies are rarely indicated, since the diagnosis can usually be made clinically. The clinical criteria for the diagnosis of BO include the presence of obstructive airways disease with suspected bronchiolitis due to chronic GVHD, or the demonstration of new onset airflow obstruction on PFT in a HSCT recipient without pulmonary symptoms (Crawford and Clark, 1993). The presence of bronchiolitis is suspected by the presence of cough, wheezing, dyspnea or hypoxemia in a HSCT recipient with a normal chest radiograph (Crawford and Clark, 1993).

Treatment

The treatment of BO consists of corticosteroids and augmented immunosuppression, targeting chronic GVHD. However, only a minority of the patients show clinical improvement (Afessa, Litzow and Tefferi, 2001). There is a report of eight HSCT patients with BO whose pulmonary function improved after treatment with Azithromycin at an initial dose of 500 mg daily for three days followed by 250 mg three times weekly for 12 weeks (Khalid *et al.*, 2005). A randomized clinical trial is warranted to define the role of macrolide therapy for the treatment of BO in HSCT recipients. Although not confirmed by prospective clinical trials, inhaled Budesonide/Formoterol, a combination of an inhaled steroid and long-acting bronchodilatator, has been shown to improve the lung function of HSCT recipients with mild to moderately severe BO (Bergeron *et al.*, 2007). The role of blocking TNF-α awaits further trial (Fullmer *et al.*, 2005). In a recent pilot study of 19 patients with chronic GVHD, the addition of monteleukast to the standard immunosuppressant regimen improved the PFT of three of the five patients with lung involvement and no lung involvement occurred in the other 14 (Or *et al.*, 2007). One study reported improvement of lung function in one of the three patients with chronic GVHD using extracorporeal photochemotherapy (Bisaccia *et al.*, 2006).

In addition to immunosuppression and anti-inflammatory therapy, prophylaxis against *Pneumocystis jiroveci* and *Streptococcus pneumoniae* should be provided. In selected HSCT recipients with respiratory failure secondary to BO, lung transplantation is an option (Afessa, Litzow and Tefferi, 2001; Afessa and Peters, 2005; Favaloro *et al.*, 2004; Heath *et al.*, 2001; Pechet *et al.*, 2003; Rabitsch *et al.*, 2001; Redel-Montero *et al.*, 2006; Sano *et al.*, 2005).

Clinical course and prognosis

Serial PFTs in allogeneic HSCT recipients with BO have shown that the rates of decline in the FEV1 are widely variable (Clark *et al.*, 1989). Those who have rapid deterioration in FEV1 have a higher mortality rate than those with slow deterioration (Clark *et al.*, 1989). The airflow limitation in HSCT recipients with BO improves in only 8–20% (Afessa, Litzow and Tefferi, 2001; Afessa and Peters, 2005). The reported overall case fatality rate is 59%, range 14–100% (Afessa, Litzow and Tefferi, 2001; Afessa and Peters, 2005). In a recent study, the five-year survival rate of 47 HSCT recipients with BO was 10% compared to 40% for those without BO (Dudek *et al.*, 2003).

9.3 Bronchiolitis obliterans organizing pneumonia (BOOP)

BOOP is characterized by the presence of granulation tissue within the alveolar ducts and alveoli. It has clinical features more similar to pneumonia than airways disease. The first cases of BOOP in HSCT recipients were reported in the early 1990s (Mathew *et al.*, 1994; Thirman *et al.*, 1992). The published medical literature on BOOP in HSCT recipients is mostly limited to case reports (Afessa, Litzow and Tefferi, 2001; Afessa and Peters, 2005; Ditschkowski *et al.*, 2007). The occurrence of BOOP predominantly in allogeneic HSCT recipients with GVHD suggests that it may represent a form of alloimmune injury by the transplanted stem cell (Alasaly *et al.*, 1995). However, it has also been reported in autologous HSCT recipients, suggesting additional mechanisms (Hayes-Jordan *et al.*, 2002). Unrecognized infections may also play a role. Human leukocyte antigen (HLA) B35 may be a risk factor for the development of BOOP after HSCT (Yotsumoto *et al.*, 2007). T-cell depletion may prevent BOOP in allogeneic HSCT recipients (Ditschkowski *et al.*, 2007).

Clinical findings and evaluation

The onset of BOOP is typically one month to two years after transplant (Afessa, Litzow and Tefferi, 2001). Presenting symptoms include dry cough, dyspnea and fever. PFT shows a restrictive defect, decreased diffusing capacity for carbon monoxide (DLCO), normal airflow and hypoxemia (Afessa, Litzow and Tefferi, 2001; Afessa and Peters, 2005). Chest radiographs and CT show patchy air space consolidation, ground glass attenuation, and nodular opacities (Wah *et al.*, 2003). Although usually bilateral, the radiographic abnormalities can also be unilateral (Hayes-Jordan *et al.*, 2002). Exhaled nitric oxide concentration may be increased in HSCT recipients with BOOP and may decline in response to treatment (Kanamori *et al.*, 2002).

The definitive diagnosis of BOOP requires transbronchial, or, more commonly, surgical lung biopsy (Alasaly *et al.*, 1995). Typical findings include patchy intraluminal fibrosis, with polypoid plugs of immature fibroblasts resembling granulation tissue obliterating the distal airways, alveolar ducts and peribronchial alveolar space (Figure 9.5) (Myers and Colby, 1993).

Treatment and prognosis

About 80% of HSCT recipients with BOOP respond favourably to treatment with corticosteroids (Afessa, Litzow and Tefferi, 2001; Afessa and Peters, 2005). The duration and dosage of corticosteroid therapy have not been clearly defined. Radiographic

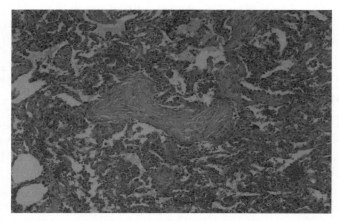

Figure 9.5   Lung pathology in bronchiolitis obliterans organizing pneumonia showing the presence of intraluminal granulation tissue in bronchioli alveolar ducts and alveoli. There is also interstitial infiltration with mononuclear cells and foamy macrophages (Haematoxylin and eosin stains) (Reprinted by permission from Bone Marrow Transplantation, Afessa *et al.* 2001; 28(5):425–434.).

abnormalities usually clear within one to three months of initiating corticosteroid therapy. Erythromycin has been used in conjunction with corticosteroid in one allogeneic HSCT recipient with BOOP with favourable outcome (Ishii *et al.*, 2000). The case fatality rate of BOOP in HSCT recipients is about 19% (Afessa, Litzow and Tefferi, 2001; Afessa and Peters, 2005).

9.4 Idiopathic pneumonia syndrome (IPS)

Despite aggressive diagnostic evaluation, no infectious etiology is identified in many HSCT recipients with suspected pneumonia. The term *idiopathic pneumonia* has been used for many years to describe pneumonia without infectious etiology in HSCT recipients. In a 1985 review of pulmonary complications in 4500 HSCT recipients, Krowka *et al.* reported a 35% incidence rate of idiopathic pneumonia (Krowka, Rosenow, III and Hoagland, 1985). There have been wide variations in the reported incidence of IPS due to the lack of uniform definition and diagnostic criteria. However, the problems of definitions and diagnostic criteria were addressed in 1993 by a workshop sponsored by the National Heart, Lung and Blood Institute (NHLBI) (Clark *et al.*, 1993). This workshop defined IPS as the presence of widespread alveolar injury in the absence of lower respiratory tract infection, characterized by acute, bilateral pulmonary infiltrates, associated symptoms of cough and dyspnea, hypoxemia and restrictive physiology, in the absence of infection or heart failure (Table 9.4). Absence of infection is typically established by negative BAL and by the lack of clinical response to antimicrobial therapy. Although diffuse alveolar haemorrhage (DAH) and peri-engraftment respiratory distress syndrome (PERDS) also fulfill the diagnostic criteria of IPS, their response to treatment and clinical course are different (Afessa *et al.*, 2002a; Capizzi *et al.*, 2001).

Incidence

The overall incidence of IPS is 10%, with a reported range 2–17% (Afessa, Litzow and Tefferi, 2001; Chen *et al.*, 2003; Wong *et al.*, 2003). The median time of onset of IPS is

Table 9.4 Criteria for the diagnosis of idiopathic pneumonia syndrome in haematopoietic stem cell transplant recipients (Clark *et al.*, 1993).

I. Evidence of widespread alveolar injury
   a. Multilobar infiltrate
   b. Symptoms and signs of pneumonia
   c. Abnormal pulmonary physiology with increased alveolar to arterial oxygen gradient and increased restrictive defect
II. Absence of lower respiratory tract infection after appropriate evaluation with
   a. Bronchoalveolar lavage negative for bacterial and nonbacterial pathogens
   b. Lack of improvement with broad spectrum antibiotics
   c. Transbronchial lung biopsy if tolerated
   d. A second confirmatory test for infection within 2–14 d

between 21 and 87 days, with a range 0–1653 days after transplant. Compared to patients with GVHD, IPS may present earlier in patients without GVHD (Kantrow *et al.*, 1997).

Risk factors

Risk factors for the development of IPS include old age, transplant for malignancy other than leukemia, pre-transplant chemotherapy, total body irradiation, GVHD and positive donor cytomegalovirus serology (Afessa, Litzow and Tefferi, 2001; Cooke and Yanik, 2004).

Pathogenesis

The pathogenesis of IPS is not well defined (Hauber *et al.*, 2002; Schots *et al.*, 2003; Yanik *et al.*, 2002). Lung tissue injury, inflammation and cytokine release are implicated. Pre-transplant radiation and chemotherapy, and undocumented infections may be responsible for the initial injury. The increased levels of interleukin-6, interleukin-8 and tumour necrosis factor (TNF)-alpha in the serum and BAL of HSCT recipients with IPS, and the clinical improvement following the administration of etanercept, suggest the role of these cytokines in the pathogenesis (Hauber *et al.*, 2002; Hildebrandt *et al.*, 2004; Schots *et al.*, 2003; Uberti *et al.*, 2005; Yanik *et al.*, 2002).

Clinical findings

The clinical presentation of IPS includes dyspnea, dry cough, hypoxemia and non-lobar radiographic infiltrates (Clark *et al.*, 1993). The clinical spectrum is broad, ranging from acute respiratory failure to incidental radiographic abnormalities (Clark *et al.*, 1993). The median time of onset of IPS is 21 to 65 days and the range 0–1653 days after transplant (Crawford and Hackman, 1993; Kantrow *et al.*, 1997; Wingard *et al.*, 1988a; Wingard *et al.*, 1988b). Despite this wide range, the time of onset of IPS is within the first 120 days following transplant in the majority. Compared to patients with grade 4 acute GVHD, IPS presents earlier in patients without GVHD (Kantrow *et al.*, 1997).

Diagnostic evaluation

The clinical presentation and radiographic findings in HSCT recipients cannot be used to differentiate between infectious and idiopathic pneumonia. PFT and CT of the chest are also nonspecific (Kantrow *et al.*, 1997). More than 90% of patients with IPS have diffuse infiltrate on chest radiograph (Crawford and Hackman, 1993). The NHLBI criteria require BAL or lung biopsy to exclude infectious etiology before entertaining the diagnosis of IPS (Clark *et al.*, 1993). BAL provides limited information about histopathological structure, interstitial fungus and neoplasms, vascular damage and other abnormalities of potential therapeutic or prognostic importance. In our diagnostic approach to patients with suspected IPS, we perform BAL and, if there are no contraindications, transbronchial lung biopsy. We resort to video assisted thoracoscopic lung biopsy if transbronchial lung biopsy is contraindicated or the transbronchial lung biopsy specimen is inadequate. Lung biopsies of patients with IPS may show diffuse alveolar damage, organizing or acute pneumonia, and interstitial lymphocytic inflammation (Griese *et al.*, 2000; Kantrow *et al.*, 1997).

Treatment

Despite case reports of patients with IPS responding to treatment with corticosteroids, larger studies have not shown any outcome benefit (Crawford, Longton and Storb, 1993; Griese *et al.*, 2000; Kantrow *et al.*, 1997). Currently, the only accepted treatment regimens are supportive care, and prevention and treatment of infection. There is a report of three cases of HSCT recipients with IPS whose lung function improved following the administration of etanercept (Yanik *et al.*, 2002). Lung transplantation may play a role in selected patients (Heath *et al.*, 2001).

Clinical course and prognosis

The pneumonitis resolves in about 31% of patients with IPS (Crawford, Longton and Storb, 1993; Kantrow *et al.*, 1997). However, the clinical course may often be complicated by viral and fungal infections, pneumothorax, pneumomediastinum, subcutaneous emphysema, pulmonary fibrosis and auto-immune polyserositis (Afessa, Litzow and Tefferi, 2001; Keates-Baleeiro *et al.*, 2006). The case fatality of IPS is about 74%, with a range between 60 and 86% (Afessa, Litzow and Tefferi, 2001). The reported one-year survival rate of IPS is less than 15% (Crawford and Hackman, 1993; Kantrow *et al.*, 1997). For those who require mechanical ventilation, the hospital mortality exceeds 95% (Kantrow *et al.*, 1997). However, more recent studies show a higher survival rate (Chen *et al.*, 2003; Wong *et al.*, 2003). Infectious complications and non-pulmonary organ failure contribute to the high mortality rate (Crawford and Hackman, 1993; Kantrow *et al.*, 1997).

9.5   Diffuse alveolar haemorrhage (DAH)

DAH occurs in approximately 5% of autologous and allogeneic HSCT recipients, with a range of approximately 2–21% (Afessa *et al.*, 2002a). The reported frequency is higher in patients identified in the intensive care unit or at autopsy (Agusti *et al.*, 1995; Bojko *et al.*, 1995; Huaringa *et al.*, 2000; Sloane *et al.*, 1983; Wojno *et al.*, 1994). The etiology and pathogenesis of DAH in the HSCT recipient have not been clearly established. Lung tissue injury, inflammation and cytokine release are implicated in the pathogenesis of DAH (Afessa *et al.*, 2002a).

Risk factors

Risk factors for DAH include age greater than 40 years, intensive chemotherapy and total body irradiation, and the presence of inflammatory cells in BAL fluid (Afessa *et al.*, 2002a). Following transplant, the development of high fever and severe mucositis, and acute GVHD are also risk factors for DAH. There are no associations between DAH and prolonged prothrombin or partial thromboplastin time or low platelets (Afessa *et al.*, 2002a). Although most patients with DAH have thrombocytopenia, DAH is not corrected with platelet transfusion (Robbins *et al.*, 1989). Pre-transplant pulmonary function is not predictive of DAH following HSCT, but evidence of airway inflammation, defined by BAL neutrophils higher than 20% and any eosinophils, has been associated with subsequent DAH (Sisson *et al.*, 1992).

Clinical findings and diagnostic evaluation

Symptoms of DAH typically include dyspnea, fever and cough (Robbins *et al.*, 1989). Haemoptysis is rare, reported in less than 20% (Afessa *et al.*, 2002a; Afessa *et al.*, 2002b). The onset of DAH is usually within the first 30 (median between 11 and 24) days following HSCT.

Measurements of spirometry, lung volume and DLCO are usually not available since HSCT recipients with DAH are too ill to perform PFT. Arterial blood gas studies show hypoxemia. Chest radiographs usually show alveolar and interstitial infiltrates involving middle and lower lung zones (Witte *et al.*, 1991). In its early phases, the radiographic changes may be subtle, unilateral or asymmetric (Witte *et al.*, 1991). Although CT of the chest may be helpful in patients in whom a focal abnormality is suspected, it has a limited role in DAH. The most common CT findings in DAH are bilateral areas of ground-glass attenuation or consolidation (Worthy, Flint and Muller, 1997).

The criteria for the diagnosis DAH are outlined in Table 9.5. The visual description of the BAL fluid and the presence of haemosiderin laden macrophages play a complementary role in the diagnosis of DAH (Afessa *et al.*, 2002b). Lung tissues in DAH show diffuse alveolar damage (Robbins *et al.*, 1989; Roychowdhury *et al.*, 2005).

Treatment

Based on retrospective studies, HSCT recipients with DAH are treated with systemic corticosteroids (Afessa *et al.*, 2002a; Afessa *et al.*, 2002b). We commonly use intravenous methylprednisolone approximately 1 g daily in four divided doses for five days, followed by 1 mg/kg for three days and tapering off over two to four weeks (Afessa *et al.*,

Table 9.5   Criteria for the diagnosis of diffuse alveolar haemorrhage {Afessa *et al.*, 2002a}.

1. Signs and symptoms of pneumonitis:
   a. Hypoxemia and/or restrictive ventilatory defects and
   b. Radiographic infiltrates involving multiple lobes;
2. No evidence of infection
3. Bronchoalveolar lavage showing
   a. Progressively bloodier return from separate subsegmental bronchi, OR
   b. ≥20% haemosiderin-laden alveolar macrophages

2002a). Although a retrospective study showed no outcome benefit (Gupta *et al.*, 2007), there are case reports of allogeneic HSCT recipients with DAH successfully treated with recombinant factor VIIa (Hicks, Peng and Gajewski, 2002; Pastores *et al.*, 2003).

Clinical course and prognosis

The majority of HSCT recipients with DAH require mechanical ventilator support for respiratory failure (Afessa *et al.*, 2002a; Afessa *et al.*, 2002b; Gupta *et al.*, 2007). HSCT recipients with DAH are at high risk for subsequent infectious complications (Mandanas *et al.*, 1996; Metcalf *et al.*, 1994). The reported mortality rate of DAH in HSCT recipients ranges between 48 and 100% (Afessa *et al.*, 2002a; Afessa *et al.*, 2002b; Gupta *et al.*, 2007). Although the initial presentation of DAH is usually respiratory failure, the two most common reported causes of death had been multiple organ failure and sepsis (Lewis, DeFor and Weisdorf, 2000; Metcalf *et al.*, 1994). However, in two recent studies, respiratory failure was the most common cause of death in HSCT recipients with DAH (Afessa *et al.*, 2002b; Gupta *et al.*, 2007).

9.6 Peri-engraftment respiratory distress syndrome (PERDS)

Engraftment syndrome is a poorly understood syndrome characterized by skin rash, non-infectious pulmonary infiltrates, fever, diarrhorea and capillary leak occurring in the peri-engraftment period. PERDS refers to the pulmonary component of the engraftment syndrome. It responds to treatment and has low case fatality rate (Capizzi *et al.*, 2001). There is overlap between PERDS and DAH, about one-third of DAH occurring during the peri-engraftment period and about one-third of patients with PERDS having DAH (Afessa *et al.*, 2002b; Capizzi *et al.*, 2001). The pathogenesis of PERDS is not well defined, but is believed to be complex interaction between the conditioning-related endothelial damage and the cytokine release associated with the neutrophil and lymphocyte recovery (Capizzi *et al.*, 2001).

Incidence

The engraftment syndrome, including non-pulmonary presentations, has been reported in up to 20% of autologous HSCT recipients (Akasheh, Eastwood and Vesole, 2003; Capizzi *et al.*, 2001; Maiolino *et al.*, 2003). Capizzi *et al.* reported the incidence of PERDS to be about 5% in autologous HSCT recipients (Capizzi *et al.*, 2001).

Clinical findings and diagnostic evaluation

The diagnostic criteria of PERDS include fever (greater than 38.3 °C) and pulmonary injury evidenced by hypoxia (arterial oxygen saturation less than 90%) and/or pulmonary infiltrates, in the absence of cardiac dysfunction and infection, within five days of neutrophil engraftment (Capizzi *et al.*, 2001). In the study by Capizzi *et al.*, the median time to onset of PERDS was 11 days (range, 4–25) after transplant (Capizzi *et al.*, 2001).

Dyspnea was the initial symptom in all the patients. Fever was present in 12 patients (63%) at the onset of symptoms. Bilateral pulmonary infiltrates may not be present on plain chest radiography at the onset of symptoms (Capizzi *et al.*, 2001).

BAL may show neutrophilic inflammation (Capizzi *et al.*, 2001). Transbronchial lung biopsy is usually contraindicated during the peri-engraftment period because of thrombocytopenia. Surgical lung biopsy may show diffuse alveolar damage but is rarely necessary.

Treatment/Prevention

HSCT recipients with PERDS are treated with high dose corticosteroids that usually lead to rapid clinical improvement (Capizzi *et al.*, 2001). A short course of corticosteroid therapy has been used effectively to reduce engraftment syndrome in autologous HSCT recipients (Mossad *et al.*, 2005).

Prognosis

Unlike DAH and IPS, only about one-third of HSCT recipients with PERDS require ICU admission and mechanical ventilation (Capizzi *et al.*, 2001). The reported mortality rate in PERDS is about 26%.

9.7   Delayed pulmonary toxicity syndrome (DPTS)

Chemotherapeutic agents and radiation therapy have been associated with pulmonary toxicities that manifest weeks to years later (Abratt *et al.*, 2004; Limper, 2004). In the 1990s, many patients with breast cancer were treated with a high dose chemotherapy regimen consisting of cyclophosphamide, cisplatin and bischloroethylinitrosurea (BCNU) followed by autologous HSCT (Pedrazzoli *et al.*, 2003). A significant number of these patients developed pulmonary complications, including DPTS (Afessa and Peters, 2005). The pathogenesis of DPTS is not known. The depletion of reduced glutathione and impaired antioxidant defences caused by cyclophosphamide and BCNU have been implicated (Todd *et al.*, 1993).

Incidence

DPTS develops in up to 72% of autologous HSCT recipients who have received high dose chemotherapy for breast cancer (Afessa and Peters, 2005). The relatively high frequency, low mortality and good response to corticosteroid treatment distinguish DPTS from IPS. Because recent studies have not shown a survival benefit, the use of autologous HSCT following high dose chemotherapy for breast cancer has declined.

Clinical findings and diagnostic evaluation

Patients with DPTS present with cough, dyspnea and fever (Afessa and Peters, 2005). The onset of symptoms ranges from two weeks to four months following transplantation.

In the context of prior breast cancer treated with high dose chemotherapy and autologous HSCT, DPTS is diagnosed by demonstrating a decline in DLCO and exclusion of infectious causes (Afessa and Peters, 2005). In patients with DPTS, the median absolute DLCO decrement is 26% (range, 10–73%) and a nadir is reached in 15–18 weeks following transplant. The most common findings on CT of the chest are ground glass opacities (Wilczynski *et al.*, 1998). Because of the typical clinical presentation and response to therapy, invasive procedures such as bronchoscopy are not required.

Prevention, treatment and prognosis

Corticosteroid therapy for DPTS usually results in resolution of symptoms and improvement in DLCO without long-term pulmonary sequelae (Afessa and Peters, 2005). One case of DPTS refractory to steroid was treated successfully with interferon-gamma (Suratt *et al.*, 2003). Prophylactic inhaled corticosteroids may reduce the frequency of DPTS (McGaughey *et al.*, 2001). No deaths attributable to DPTS have been reported (Afessa and Peters, 2005).

9.8 Pulmonary cytolytic thrombi (PCT)

PCT is a non-infectious pulmonary complication of unknown etiology. It occurs exclusively after allogeneic transplant, typically in the setting of GVHD. All but one of the 17 HSCT recipients with PCT reported in the medical literature are from a single institution (Gulbahce *et al.*, 2004; Morales *et al.*, 2003; Peters *et al.*, 2005). Sixteen of the 17 patients were under the age of 18 at the time of diagnosis. Despite the seemingly rare and previously unrecognized nature of PCT, it was found in 15 of 33 (45%) HSCT recipients who underwent surgical lung biopsy for diagnosis of pulmonary nodules at the University of Minnesota (Gulbahce *et al.*, 2004). The pathogenesis of PCT is not known. Although the haemorrhagic infarcts in PCT are similar to those seen in angioinvasive fungal infections, none of the lung biopsies in the reported PCT cases had evidence of infection (Gulbahce *et al.*, 2004; Morales *et al.*, 2003). The development of PCT exclusively in allogeneic HSCT recipients, chiefly in those with GVHD, suggests that it may be a manifestation of GVHD targeting the endothelium of the lungs (Gulbahce *et al.*, 2004).

Clinical findings and diagnostic evaluation

Most HSCT recipients with PCT have active GVHD at the time of presentation (Gulbahce, Manivel and Jessurun, 2000; Morales *et al.*, 2003; Woodard *et al.*, 2000). The onset of PCT is between 8 and 343 days (median 72) after transplantation (Gulbahce, Manivel and Jessurun, 2000; Morales *et al.*, 2003; Woodard *et al.*, 2000). All patients are febrile and some have a cough at presentation, but dyspnea has not been noted.

Chest radiographs may be normal in 25% of the patients with PCT (Woodard *et al.*, 2000). Abnormal chest radiographic findings include nodules, interstitial prominence and atelectasis. Chest CT shows multiple peripheral pulmonary nodules, ranging from a few mm to 4 cm in size.

Bronchoscopy with BAL is used to exclude infection. Because of the peripheral and intravascular location of the nodules in PCT, transbronchial lung biopsy is unlikely to yield a diagnosis. Histological demonstration of PCT requires surgical lung biopsy or necropsy (Morales *et al.*, 2003; Peters *et al.*, 2005; Woodard *et al.*, 2000). Features of PCT include occlusive vascular lesions and haemorrhagic infarcts due to thrombi that consist of intensely basophilic, amorphous material that may extend into the adjacent tissue through the vascular wall (Gulbahce *et al.*, 2004). The amorphous material suggests cellular breakdown products. Immunohistochemical studies show a discontinuous endothelial cell layer. The cells that make up PCT are exclusively monocytes (Peters *et al.*, 2005).

Treatment and prognosis

In one case report, treatment with corticosteroid and cyclosporin resulted in improvement (Morales *et al.*, 2003). Most of the patients with PCT improve clinically within one to two weeks and radiographically over weeks to months (Woodard *et al.*, 2000). There has been no reported death attributed to PCT (Gulbahce *et al.*, 2004; Morales *et al.*, 2003). Of the 15 HSCT recipients with PCT reported from the University of Minnesota, 10 were still alive at an average of 13 months after diagnosis and five died; one from GVHD and four from infectious complications (Gulbahce *et al.*, 2004).

9.9   Other non-infectious pulmonary complications

Pulmonary veno-occlusive disease (PVOD)

PVOD is a rare cause of pulmonary hypertension that has been associated with various conditions including HSCT. The incidence of PVOD in HSCT recipients is not known. Wingard *et al.* reported PVOD in 19 of 154 autopsies of allogeneic HSCT recipients (12%) (Wingard *et al.*, 1989). However, in a recent autopsy review of 71 adult HSCT recipients (39 allogeneic), no case of PVOD was identified (Sharma *et al.*, 2005). There are about 28 HSCT recipients with PVOD in the published literature (Afessa and Peters, 2005). There is no proven therapy for PVOD.

Pulmonary hypertension

Several cases of pulmonary arterial hypertension have been reported in HSCT recipients. Its pathogenesis is not clearly defined. Radiation and chemotherapy-associated endothelial damage may be the mechanism for the development of the pulmonary hypertension. Prostacyclin infusion and calcium channel antagonists have been used for the treatment of pulmonary hypertension in HSCT recipients (Bruckmann *et al.*, 1991; Shankar *et al.*, 2004; Vaksmann *et al.*, 2002).

Acute pulmonary oedema

Pulmonary oedema is quite common during the neutropenic phase and generally represents a combination of both cardiogenic and noncardiogenic (capillary leak) factors (Gosselin and Adams, 2002). It usually results from increased hydrostatic pressure due to large volumes of fluid, parenteral nutrition and blood products infused during conditioning and the immediate post-transplant period (Cahill, Spitzer and Mazumder, 1996; Dickout *et al.*, 1987). The heart may also be compromised by a number of chemotherapeutic drugs. Pulmonary oedema can be prevented by fluid restriction and diuretic therapy (Dickout *et al.*, 1987).

Pulmonary alveolar proteinosis (PAP)

PAP is characterized by excessive accumulation of surfactant lipoprotein in the alveoli, leading to abnormal gas exchange (Presneill *et al.*, 2004). In an autopsy study of 71 HSCT recipients, PAP was found in one (Sharma *et al.*, 2005). Cordonnier *et al.* described three allogeneic HSCT recipients with PAP (Cordonnier *et al.*, 1994). Chest radiographs showed diffuse infiltrates. Only one of the three survived. Because of the small number of cases reported in the literature, the roles of BAL and aerosolized granulocyte-macrophage colony-stimulating factor in HSCT recipients with pulmonary alveolar proteinosis are unknown.

Chronic eosinophilic pneumonia

Three cases of chronic eosinophilic pneumonia have been reported in HSCT recipients, one autologous and two allogeneic (Brunet, Muniz-Diaz and Baiget, 1994; Gross *et al.*, 1994; Richard *et al.*, 1994). Despite initial response to steroid therapy, one patient had a fatal outcome (Gross *et al.*, 1994).

Post-transplant lymphoproliferative disorder (PTLD)

PTLD is an uncommon complication of HSCT, occurring in less than 1% of patients (Gosselin and Adams, 2002). It is probably related to the Epstein–Barr virus stimulation of the B-cell lymphocytes and the ensuing imbalance between B cells and T cells. Radiographic abnormalities are often incidentally seen and usually manifest as multiple, well-defined nodules and occasionally as patchy consolidations (Au *et al.*, 2002; Monforte-Munoz, Kapoor and Saavedra, 2003; Shoji *et al.*, 2003; Tolar *et al.*, 2001). Mediastinal and hilar lymphadenopathy is relatively uncommon. There is one case report of PTLD in a HSCT recipient that presented as interstitial pneumonia and was successfully treated with rituximab (Kunitomi, Arima and Ishikawa, 2007). Initial treatment for PTLD usually involves discontinuation of immunosuppressants (Kang, Kirkpatrick and Halperin, 2003). Anti-CD20 monoclonal antibody and/or antivirals are employed for persistent disease. Chemotherapy is generally reserved as a final option.

Asthma

There are case reports of asthma developing after allogeneic HSCT (Afessa and Peters, 2005). Limited data suggest that the serum IgE of donor origin is elevated following transplantation. Allergen-specific IgE-mediated hypersensitivity can be transferred from donor to HSCT recipient by B cells with allergen-specific memory leading to atopic dermatitis, allergic rhinitis and asthma. The management of asthma in HSCT recipients is similar to the other population.

Transfusion-related acute lung injury (TRALI)

TRALI is a clinical syndrome characterized by bilateral pulmonary oedema in association with transfusion of blood products. There are few case reports of TRALI that developed following infusion of allogeneic stem cells (Knop *et al.*, 2004; Noji *et al.*, 2004; Urahama *et al.*, 2003).

Sarcoidosis

Sarcoidosis is uncommon in HSCT recipients (Gooneratne *et al.*, 2007; Padilla, Schilero and Teirstein, 2002). Until recently, the cases of the reported sarcoidosis were donor-acquired. Bhagat *et al.* reported four cases of de novo pulmonary sarcoidosis occurring post-HSCT (three autologous HSCT and one allogeneic HSCT) (Bhagat *et al.*, 2004).

Abnormal pulmonary function

Restrictive and obstructive ventilatory defects, and gas transfer abnormalities are frequent long-term sequelae following allogeneic transplantation. A systematic review of 20 publications published between 1996 and 2001 found decreased DLCO in 83%, restriction in 35% and obstruction in 23% of allogeneic HSCT recipients (Marras *et al.*, 2002). A more recent study of over 500 HSCT recipients documented somewhat lower frequencies: impaired diffusion in 35%, restriction in 12%, and obstruction in only 6% of long-term survivors (Marras *et al.*, 2004). The development of airflow obstruction increases the risk of mortality following transplantation (Chien *et al.*, 2003; Chien *et al.*, 2004; Marras *et al.*, 2004).

9.10   Summary

Non-infectious pulmonary complications develop in a large number of HSCT recipients, more commonly in the allogeneic. The main non-infectious pulmonary complications include BO, IPS, PERDS and DAH. BO occurs exclusively in allogeneic recipients and is characterized by the presence of irreversible airway obstruction in the absence of fever and pulmonary infiltrates. IPS, PERDS and DAH are characterized by diffuse pulmonary infiltrates on chest radiographs. BAL shows progressively bloodier return and/or more than 20% haemosiderin-laden macrophages in DAH. PERDS differs from IPS by its occurrence during the neutrophil peri-engraftment period and favourable response to corticosteroid therapy. DPTS occurs in autologous HSCT recipients with breast cancer, and following high dose pre-transplant chemotherapy. Since the use of HSCT for the treatment of metastatic breast cancer has declined, DPTS has become rare. The treatment of the non-infectious pulmonary complications is not based on randomized clinical trials.

References

Abratt, R.P., Morgan, G.W., Silvestri, G. and Willcox, P. (2004) Pulmonary complications of radiation therapy. *Clinics in Chest Medicine*, **25**, 167–177.

Afessa, B., Litzow, M.R. and Tefferi, A. (2001) Bronchiolitis obliterans and other late onset non-infectious pulmonary complications in hematopoietic stem cell transplantation. *Bone Marrow Transplantation*, **28**, 425–434.

Afessa, B. and Peters, S.G. (2005) Chronic lung disease after hematopoietic stem cell transplantation. *Clinics in Chest Medicine*, **26**, 571–586, vi.

Afessa, B. and Peters, S.G. (2006) Major complications following hematopoietic stem cell transplantation. *Seminars in Respiratory and Critical Care Medicine*, **27**, 297–309.

Afessa, B., Tefferi, A., Litzow, M.R. *et al.* (2002a) Diffuse alveolar hemorrhage in hematopoietic stem cell transplant recipients. *American Journal of Respiratory and Critical Care Medicine*, **166**, 641–645.

Afessa, B., Tefferi, A., Litzow, M.R. and Peters, S.G. (2002b) Outcome of diffuse alveolar hemorrhage in hematopoietic stem cell transplant recipients. *American Journal of Respiratory and Critical Care Medicine*, **166**, 1364–1368.

Agusti, C., Ramirez, J., Picado, C. *et al.* (1995) Diffuse alveolar hemorrhage in allogeneic bone marrow transplantation. A postmortem study. *American Journal of Respiratory and Critical Care Medicine*, **151**, 1006–1010.

Akasheh, M., Eastwood, D. and Vesole, D.H. (2003) Engraftment syndrome after autologous hematopoietic stem cell transplant supported by granulocyte-colony-stimulating factor (G-CSF) versus granulocyte-macrophage colony-stimulating factor (GM-CSF). *Bone Marrow Transplantation*, **31**, 113–116.

Alasaly, K., Muller, N., Ostrow, D.N. *et al.* (1995) Cryptogenic organizing pneumonia. A report of 25 cases and a review of the literature. *Medicine (Baltimore)*, **74**, 201–211.

Au, W.Y., Lie, A.K., Kwong, Y.L. *et al.* (2002) Post-transplantation lymphoproliferative disease in Chinese: the Queen Mary Hospital experience in Hong Kong. *Leukemia & Lymphoma*, **43**, 1403–1407.

Bergeron, A., Belle, A., Chevret, S. *et al.* (2007) Combined inhaled steroids and bronchodilatators in obstructive airway disease after allogeneic stem cell transplantation. *Bone Marrow Transplantation*, **39**, 547–553.

Bhagat, R., Rizzieri, D.A., Vredenburgh, J.J. *et al.* (2004) Pulmonary sarcoidosis following stem cell transplantation: is it more than a chance occurrence? *Chest*, **126**, 642–644.

Bisaccia, E., Palangio, M., Gonzalez, J. *et al.* (2006) Treatment of extensive chronic graft-versus-host disease with extracorporeal photochemotherapy. *Journal of Clinical Apheresis*, **21**, 181–187.

Bojko, T., Notterman, D.A., Greenwald, B.M. *et al.* (1995) Acute hypoxemic respiratory failure in children following bone marrow transplantation: an outcome and pathologic study. *Critical Care Medicine*, **23**, 755–759.

Bruckmann, C., Lindner, W., Roos, R. *et al.* (1991) Severe pulmonary vascular occlusive disease following bone marrow transplantation in Omenn syndrome. *European Journal of Pediatrics*, **150**, 242–245.

Brunet, S., Muniz-Diaz, E. and Baiget, M. (1994) Chronic eosinophilic pneumonia in a patient treated with allogeneic bone marrow transplantation. *Medicina Clinica (Barc)*, **103**, 677.

Cahill, R.A., Spitzer, T.R. and Mazumder, A. (1996) Marrow engraftment and clinical manifestations of capillary leak syndrome. *Bone Marrow Transplantation*, **18**, 177–184.

Capizzi, S.A., Kumar, S., Huneke, N.E. *et al.* (2001) Peri-engraftment respiratory distress syndrome during autologous hematopoietic stem cell transplantation. *Bone Marrow Transplantation*, **27**, 1299–1303.

Carlens, S., Ringden, O., Remberger, M. *et al.* (1998) Risk factors for chronic graft-versus-host disease after bone marrow transplantation: a retrospective single centre analysis. *Bone Marrow Transplantation*, **22**, 755–761.

Chen, C.S., Boeckh, M., Seidel, K. *et al.* (2003) Incidence, risk factors, and mortality from pneumonia developing late after hematopoietic stem cell transplantation. *Bone Marrow Transplantation*, **32**, 515–522.

Chien, J.W., Martin, P.J., Flowers, M.E. *et al.* (2004) Implications of early airflow decline after myeloablative allogeneic stem cell transplantation. *Bone Marrow Transplantation*, **33**, 759–764.

Chien, J.W., Martin, P.J., Gooley, T.A. *et al.* (2003) Airflow obstruction after myeloablative allogeneic hematopoietic stem cell transplantation. *American Journal of Respiratory and Critical Care Medicine*, **168**, 208–214.

Clark, J.G., Crawford, S.W., Madtes, D.K. and Sullivan, K.M. (1989) Obstructive lung disease after allogeneic marrow transplantation. Clinical presentation and course. *Annals of Internal Medicine*, **111**, 368–376.

Clark, J.G., Hansen, J.A., Hertz, M.I. *et al.* (1993) NHLBI workshop summary. Idiopathic pneumonia syndrome after bone marrow transplantation. *The American Review of Respiratory Disease*, **147**, 1601–1606.

Cooke, K.R. and Yanik, G. (2004) Acute lung injury after allogeneic stem cell transplantation: is the lung a target of acute graft-versus-host disease? *Bone Marrow Transplantation*, **34**, 753–765.

Copelan, E.A. (2006) Hematopoietic stem-cell transplantation. *The New England Journal of Medicine*, **354**, 1813–1826.

Cordonnier, C., Fleury-Feith, J., Escudier, E. *et al.* (1994) Secondary alveolar proteinosis is a reversible cause of respiratory failure in leukemic patients. *American Journal of Respiratory and Critical Care Medicine*, **149**, 788–794.

Crawford, S.W. and Clark, J.G. (1993) Bronchiolitis associated with bone marrow transplantation. *Clinics in Chest Medicine*, **14**, 741–749.

Crawford, S.W. and Hackman, R.C. (1993) Clinical course of idiopathic pneumonia after bone marrow transplantation. *The American Review of Respiratory Disease*, **147**, 1393–1400.

Crawford, S.W., Longton, G. and Storb, R. (1993) Acute graft-versus-host disease and the risks for idiopathic pneumonia after marrow transplantation for severe aplastic anemia. *Bone Marrow Transplantation*, **12**, 225–231.

Dickout, W.J., Chan, C.K., Hyland, R.H. *et al.* (1987) Prevention of acute pulmonary edema after bone marrow transplantation. *Chest*, **92**, 303–309.

Ditschkowski, M., Elmaagacli, A.H., Trenschel, R. *et al.* (2007) T-cell depletion prevents from bronchiolitis obliterans and bronchiolitis obliterans with organizing pneumonia after allogeneic hematopoietic stem cell transplantation with related donors. *Haematologica*, **92**, 558–561.

Dudek, A.Z., Mahaseth, H., DeFor, T.E. and Weisdorf, D.J. (2003) Bronchiolitis obliterans in chronic graft-versus-host disease: analysis of risk factors and treatment outcomes. *Biology of Blood and Marrow Transplantation*, **9**, 657–666.

Estenne, M., Maurer, J.R., Boehler, A. *et al.* (2002) Bronchiolitis obliterans syndrome 2001: an update of the diagnostic criteria. *The Journal of Heart and Lung Transplantation*, **21**, 297–310.

Favaloro, R., Bertolotti, A., Gomez, C. *et al.* (2004) Lung transplant at the Favaloro Foundation: a 13-year experience. *Transplantation Proceedings*, **36**, 1689–1691.

Fullmer, J.J., Fan, L.L., Dishop, M.K. *et al.* (2005) Successful treatment of bronchiolitis obliterans in a bone marrow transplant patient with tumor necrosis factor-alpha blockade. *Pediatrics*, **116**, 767–770.

Gooneratne, L., Lim, Z.Y., Vivier, A. *et al.* (2007) Sarcoidosis as an unusual cause of hepatic dysfunction following reduced intensity conditioned allogeneic stem cell transplantation. *Bone Marrow Transplantation*, **39**, 511–512.

Gosselin, M.V. and Adams, R.H. (2002) Pulmonary complications in bone marrow transplantation. *Journal of Thoracic Imaging*, **17**, 132–144.

Griese, M., Rampf, U., Hofmann, D. *et al.* (2000) Pulmonary complications after bone marrow transplantation in children: twenty-four years of experience in a single pediatric center. *Pediatric Pulmonology*, **30**, 393–401.

Gross, T.G., Hoge, F.J., Jackson, J.D. *et al.* (1994) Fatal eosinophilic disease following autologous bone marrow transplantation. *Bone Marrow Transplantation*, **14**, 333–337.

Gulbahce, H.E., Manivel, J.C. and Jessurun, J. (2000) Pulmonary cytolytic thrombi: a previously unrecognized complication of bone marrow transplantation. *The American Journal of Surgical Pathology*, **24**, 1147–1152.

Gulbahce, H.E., Pambuccian, S.E., Jessurun, J. *et al.* (2004) Pulmonary nodular lesions in bone marrow transplant recipients: impact of histologic diagnosis on patient management and prognosis. *American Journal of Clinical Pathology*, **121**, 205–210.

Gupta, S., Jain, A., Warneke, C.L. *et al.* (2007) Outcome of alveolar hemorrhage in hematopoietic stem cell transplant recipients. *Bone Marrow Transplantation*, **40**, 71–78.

Hauber, H.P., Mikkila, A., Erich, J.M. *et al.* (2002) TNFalpha, interleukin-10 and interleukin-18 expression in cells of the bronchoalveolar lavage in patients with pulmonary complications following bone marrow or peripheral stem cell transplantation: a preliminary study. *Bone Marrow Transplantation*, **30**, 485–490.

Hayes-Jordan, A., Benaim, E., Richardson, S. *et al.* (2002) Open lung biopsy in pediatric bone marrow transplant patients. *Journal of Pediatric Surgery*, **37**, 446–452.

Heath, J.A., Kurland, G., Spray, T.L. *et al.* (2001) Lung transplantation after allogeneic marrow transplantation in pediatric patients: the Memorial Sloan-Kettering experience. *Transplantation*, **72**, 1986–1990.

Hicks, K., Peng, D. and Gajewski, J.L. (2002) Treatment of diffuse alveolar hemorrhage after allogeneic bone marrow transplant with recombinant factor VIIa. *Bone Marrow Transplantation*, **30**, 975–978.

Hildebrandt, G.C., Olkiewicz, K.M., Corrion, L.A. *et al.* (2004) Donor-derived TNF-alpha regulates pulmonary chemokine expression and the development of idiopathic pneumonia syndrome after allogeneic bone marrow transplantation. *Blood*, **104**, 586–593.

Huaringa, A.J., Leyva, F.J., Giralt, S.A. *et al.* (2000) Outcome of bone marrow transplantation patients requiring mechanical ventilation [see comments]. *Critical Care Medicine*, **28**, 1014–1017.

Huisman, C., van der Straaten, H.M., Canninga-van Dijk, M.R. *et al.* (2006) Pulmonary complications after T-cell-depleted allogeneic stem cell transplantation: low incidence and strong association with acute graft-versus-host disease. *Bone Marrow Transplantation*, **38**, 561–566.

Ishii, T., Manabe, A., Ebihara, Y. *et al.* (2000) Improvement in bronchiolitis obliterans organizing pneumonia in a child after allogeneic bone marrow transplantation by a combination of oral prednisolone and low dose erythromycin [In Process Citation]. *Bone Marrow Transplantation*, **26**, 907–910.

Jung, J.I., Jung, W.S., Hahn, S.T. *et al.* (2004) Bronchiolitis obliterans after allogenic bone marrow transplantation: HRCT findings. *Korean Journal of Radiology*, **5**, 107–113.

Kanamori, H., Fujisawa, S., Tsuburai, T. *et al.* (2002) Increased exhaled nitric oxide in bronchiolitis obliterans organizing pneumonia after allogeneic bone marrow transplantation. *Transplantation*, **74**, 1356–1358.

Kang, S.K., Kirkpatrick, J.P. and Halperin, E.C. (2003) Low-dose radiation for posttransplant lymphoproliferative disorder. *American Journal of Clinical Oncology*, **26**, 210–214.

Kantrow, S.P., Hackman, R.C., Boeckh, M. *et al.* (1997) Idiopathic pneumonia syndrome: changing spectrum of lung injury after marrow transplantation. *Transplantation*, **63**, 1079–1086.

Keates-Baleeiro, J., Moore, P., Koyama, T. *et al.* (2006) Incidence and outcome of idiopathic pneumonia syndrome in pediatric stem cell transplant recipients. *Bone Marrow Transplantation*, **38**, 285–289.

Khalid, M., Al Saghir, A., Saleemi, S. *et al.* (2005) Azithromycin in bronchiolitis obliterans complicating bone marrow transplantation: a preliminary study. *The European Respiratory Journal*, **25**, 490–493.

Knop, S., Bux, J., Kroeber, S.M. *et al.* (2004) Fatal immune-mediated pancytopenia and a TRALI-like syndrome associated with high titers of recipient-type antibodies against donor-derived peripheral blood cells after allogeneic bone marrow transplantation following dose reduced conditioning. *Haematologica*, **89**, ECR12.

Krowka, M.J., Rosenow, E.C., III, Hoagland, H.C. (1985) Pulmonary complications of bone marrow transplantation. *Chest*, **87**, 237–246.

Kunitomi, A., Arima, N. and Ishikawa, T. (2007) Epstein-Barr virus-associated post-transplant lymphoproliferative disorders presented as interstitial pneumonia; successful recovery with rituximab. *Haematologica*, **92**, 92e049.

Lewis, I.D., DeFor, T. and Weisdorf, D.J. (2000) Increasing incidence of diffuse alveolar hemorrhage following allogeneic bone marrow transplantation: cryptic etiology and uncertain therapy. *Bone Marrow Transplantation*, **26**, 539–543.

Limper, A.H. (2004) Chemotherapy-induced lung disease. *Clinics in Chest Medicine*, **25**, 53–64.

Maiolino, A., Biasoli, I., Lima, J. *et al.* (2003) Engraftment syndrome following autologous hematopoietic stem cell transplantation: definition of diagnostic criteria. *Bone Marrow Transplantation*, **31**, 393–397.

Mandanas, R.A., Saez, R.A., Selby, G.B. and Confer, D.L. (1996) Cytomegalovirus surveillance and prevention in allogeneic bone marrow transplantation: examination of a preemptive plan of ganciclovir therapy. *American Journal of Hematology*, **51**, 104–111.

Marras, T.K., Chan, C.K., Lipton, J.H. *et al.* (2004) Long-term pulmonary function abnormalities and survival after allogeneic marrow transplantation. *Bone Marrow Transplantation*, **33**, 509–517.

Marras, T.K., Szalai, J.P., Chan, C.K. *et al.* (2002) Pulmonary function abnormalities after allogeneic marrow transplantation: a systematic review and assessment of an existing predictive instrument. *Bone Marrow Transplantation*, **30**, 599–607.

Mathew, P., Bozeman, P., Krance, R.A. *et al.* (1994) Bronchiolitis obliterans organizing pneumonia (BOOP) in children after allogeneic bone marrow transplantation. *Bone Marrow Transplantation*, **13**, 221–223.

Matulis, M. and High, K.P. (2002) Immune reconstitution after hematopoietic stem-cell transplantation and its influence on respiratory infections. *Seminars in Respiratory Infections*, **17**, 130–139.

McDonald, G.B., Sullivan, K.M. and Plumley, T.F. (1984) Radiographic features of esophageal involvement in chronic graft-vs.-host disease. *American Journal of Roentgenology*, **142**, 501–506.

McGaughey, D.S., Nikcevich, D.A., Long, G.D. *et al.* (2001) Inhaled steroids as prophylaxis for delayed pulmonary toxicity syndrome in breast cancer patients undergoing high-dose chemotherapy and autologous stem cell transplantation. *Biology of Blood and Marrow Transplantation*, **7**, 274–278.

Metcalf, J.P., Rennard, S.I., Reed, E.C. *et al.* (1994) Corticosteroids as adjunctive therapy for diffuse alveolar hemorrhage associated with bone marrow transplantation. University of Nebraska Medical Center Bone Marrow Transplant Group. *The American Journal of Medicine*, **96**, 327–334.

Monforte-Munoz, H., Kapoor, N. and Saavedra, J.A. (2003) Epstein-Barr virus-associated leiomyomatosis and posttransplant lymphoproliferative disorder in a child with severe combined immunodeficiency: case report and review of the literature. *Pediatric and Developmental Pathology*, **6**, 449–457.

Morales, I.J., Anderson, P.M., Tazelaar, H.D. and Wylam, M.E. (2003) Pulmonary cytolytic thrombi: unusual complication of hematopoietic stem cell transplantation. *Journal of Pediatric Hematology/Oncology*, **25**, 89–92.

Mossad, S., Kalaycio, M., Sobecks, R. *et al.* (2005) Steroids prevent engraftment syndrome after autologous hematopoietic stem cell transplantation without increasing the risk of infection. *Bone Marrow Transplantation*, **35**, 375–381.

Myers, J.L. and Colby, T.V. (1993) Pathologic manifestations of bronchiolitis, constrictive bronchiolitis, cryptogenic organizing pneumonia, and diffuse panbronchiolitis. *Clinics in Chest Medicine*, **14**, 611–622.

Noji, H., Shichishima, T., Ogawa, K. *et al.* (2004) Transfusion-related acute lung injury following allogeneic bone marrow transplantation in a patient with acute lymphoblastic leukemia. *Internal Medicine (Tokyo, Japan)*, **43**, 1068–1072.

Or, R., Gesundheit, B., Resnick, I. *et al.* (2007) Sparing effect by montelukast treatment for chronic graft versus host disease: a pilot study. *Transplantation*, **83**, 577–581.

Padilla, M.L., Schilero, G.J. and Teirstein, A.S. (2002) Donor-acquired sarcoidosis. *Sarcoidosis, Vasculitis, and Diffuse Lung Diseases*, **19**, 18–24.

Pastores, S.M., Papadopoulos, E., Voigt, L. and Halpern, N.A. (2003) Diffuse alveolar hemorrhage after allogeneic hematopoietic stem-cell transplantation: treatment with recombinant factor VIIa. *Chest*, **124**, 2400–2403.

Paz, H.L., Crilley, P., Patchefsky, A. *et al.* (1992) Bronchiolitis obliterans after autologous bone marrow transplantation. *Chest*, **101**, 775–778.

Pechet, T.V., de le, M.M., Mendeloff, E.N. *et al.* (2003) Lung transplantation in children following treatment for malignancy. *The Journal of Heart and Lung Transplantation*, **22**, 154–160.

Pedrazzoli, P., Ferrante, P., Kulekci, A. *et al.* (2003) Autologous hematopoietic stem cell transplantation for breast cancer in Europe: critical evaluation of data from the European Group for Blood and Marrow Transplantation (EBMT) Registry 1990–1999. *Bone Marrow Transplantation*, **32**, 489–494.

Peters, A., Manivel, J.C., Dolan, M. *et al.* (2005) Pulmonary cytolytic thrombi after allogeneic hematopoietic cell transplantation: a further histologic description. *Biology of Blood and Marrow Transplantation*, **11**, 484–485.

Peters, S.G. and Afessa, B. (2005) Acute lung injury after hematopoietic stem cell transplantation. *Clinics in Chest Medicine*, **26**, 561–569 vi.

Presneill, J.J., Nakata, K., Inoue, Y. and Seymour, J.F. (2004) Pulmonary alveolar proteinosis. *Clinics in Chest Medicine*, **25**, 593–613, viii.

Rabitsch, W., Deviatko, E., Keil, F. *et al.* (2001) Successful lung transplantation for bronchiolitis obliterans after allogeneic marrow transplantation. *Transplantation*, **71**, 1341–1343.

Redel-Montero, J., Santos-Luna, F., Lama-Martinez, R. *et al.* (2006) A lung transplant in a woman with bronchiolitis obliterans following an allogenic bone marrow transplant. *Archivos de Bronconeumologia*, **42**, 151–153.

Richard, C., Calavia, J., Loyola, I. *et al.* (1994) Chronic eosinophilic pneumonia in a patient treated with allogenic bone marrow transplantation. *Medicina Clinica (Barc)*, **102**, 462–464.

Robbins, R.A., Linder, J., Stahl, M.G. *et al.* (1989) Diffuse alveolar hemorrhage in autologous bone marrow transplant recipients [see comments]. *The American Journal of Medicine*, **87**, 511–518.

Roychowdhury, M., Pambuccian, S.E., Aslan, D.L. *et al.* (2005) Pulmonary complications after bone marrow transplantation: an autopsy study from a large transplantation center. *Archives of Pathology & Laboratory Medicine*, **129**, 366–371.

Sano, Y., Date, H., Nagahiro, I. *et al.* (2005) Living-donor lobar lung transplantation for bronchiolitis obliterans after bone marrow transplantation. *The Annals of Thoracic Surgery*, **79**, 1051–1052.

Schots, R., Kaufman, L., Van Riet, I. *et al.* (2003) Proinflammatory cytokines and their role in the development of major transplant-related complications in the early phase after allogeneic bone marrow transplantation. *Leukemia*, **17**, 1150–1156.

Shankar, S., Choi, J.K., Dermody, T.S. *et al.* (2004) Pulmonary hypertension complicating bone marrow transplantation for idiopathic myelofibrosis. *Journal of Pediatric Hematology/Oncology*, **26**, 393–397.

Sharma, S., Nadrous, H.F., Peters, S.G. *et al.* (2005) Pulmonary complications in adult blood and marrow transplant recipients: autopsy findings. *Chest*, **128**, 1385–1392.

Shoji, N., Ohyashiki, J.H., Suzuki, A. *et al.* (2003) Multiple pulmonary nodules caused by B-cell post-transplant lymphoproliferative disorder after bone marrow transplantation: monitoring Epstein-Barr virus viral load. *Japanese Journal of Clinical Oncology*, **33**, 408–412.

Sisson, J.H., Thompson, A.B., Anderson, J.R. *et al.* (1992) Airway inflammation predicts diffuse alveolar hemorrhage during bone marrow transplantation in patients with Hodgkin disease. *The American Review of Respiratory Disease*, **146**, 439–443.

Sloane, J.P., Depledge, M.H., Powles, R.L. *et al.* (1983) Histopathology of the lung after bone marrow transplantation. *Journal of Clinical Pathology*, **36**, 546–554.

St.John, R.C., Gadek, J.E., Tutschka, P.J. *et al.* (1990) Analysis of airflow obstruction by bronchoalveolar lavage following bone marrow transplantation. Implications for pathogenesis and treatment. *Chest*, **98**, 600–607.

Suratt, B.T., Lynch, D.A., Cool, C.D. *et al.* (2003) Interferon-gamma for delayed pulmonary toxicity syndrome resistant to steroids. *Bone Marrow Transplantation*, **31**, 939–941.

Thirman, M.J., Devine, S.M., O'Toole, K. *et al.* (1992) Bronchiolitis obliterans organizing pneumonia as a complication of allogeneic bone marrow transplantation [see comments]. *Bone Marrow Transplantation*, **10**, 307–311.

Thompson, A.M., Couch, M., Zahurak, M.L. *et al.* (2002) Risk factors for post-stem cell transplant sinusitis. *Bone Marrow Transplantation*, **29**, 257–261.

Todd, N.W., Peters, W.P., Ost, A.H. *et al.* (1993) Pulmonary drug toxicity in patients with primary breast cancer treated with high-dose combination chemotherapy and autologous bone marrow transplantation. *The American Review of Respiratory Disease*, **147**, 1264–1270.

Tolar, J., Coad, J.E., Ramsay, N.K. *et al.* (2001) Lymphoproliferative disorder presenting as pulmonary nodules after bone marrow transplantation. *Bone Marrow Transplantation*, **28**, 808–810.

Trisolini, R., Stanzani, M., Agli, L.L. *et al.* (2001) Delayed non-infectious lung disease in allogeneic bone marrow transplant recipients. *Sarcoidosis, Vasculitis, and Diffuse Lung Diseases*, **18**, 75–84.

Uberti, J.P., Ayash, L., Ratanatharathorn, V. *et al.* (2005) Pilot trial on the use of etanercept and methylprednisolone as primary treatment for acute graft-versus-host disease. *Biology of Blood and Marrow Transplantation*, **11**, 680–687.

Urahama, N., Tanosaki, R., Masahiro, K. *et al.* (2003) TRALI after the infusion of marrow cells in a patient with acute lymphoblastic leukemia. *Transfusion*, **43**, 1553–1557.

Vaksmann, G., Nelken, B., Deshildre, A. and Rey, C. (2002) Pulmonary arterial occlusive disease following chemotherapy and bone marrow transplantation for leukaemia. *European Journal of Pediatrics*, **161**, 247–249.

Wah, T.M., Moss, H.A., Robertson, R.J. and Barnard, D.L. (2003) Pulmonary complications following bone marrow transplantation. *British Journal of Radiology*, **76**, 373–379.

Wilczynski, S.W., Erasmus, J.J., Petros, W.P. *et al.* (1998) Delayed pulmonary toxicity syndrome following high-dose chemotherapy and bone marrow transplantation for breast cancer. *American Journal of Respiratory and Critical Care Medicine*, **157**, 565–573.

Wingard, J.R., Mellits, E.D., Jones, R.J. *et al.* (1989) Association of hepatic veno-occlusive disease with interstitial pneumonitis in bone marrow transplant recipients. *Bone Marrow Transplantation*, **4**, 685–689.

Wingard, J.R., Mellits, E.D., Sostrin, M.B. *et al.* (1988a) Interstitial pneumonitis after allogeneic bone marrow transplantation. Nine-year experience at a single institution. *Medicine (Baltimore)*, **67**, 175–186.

Wingard, J.R., Sostrin, M.B., Vriesendorp, H.M. *et al.* (1988b) Interstitial pneumonitis following autologous bone marrow transplantation. *Transplantation*, **46**, 61–65.

Witte, R.J., Gurney, J.W., Robbins, R.A. *et al.* (1991) Diffuse pulmonary alveolar hemorrhage after bone marrow transplantation: radiographic findings in 39 patients. *American Journal of Roentgenology*, **157**, 461–464.

Wojno, K.J., Vogelsang, G.B., Beschorner, W.E. and Santos, G.W. (1994) Pulmonary hemorrhage as a cause of death in allogeneic bone marrow recipients with severe acute graft-versus-host disease. *Transplantation*, **57**, 88–92.

Wong, R., Rondon, G., Saliba, R.M. *et al.* (2003) Idiopathic pneumonia syndrome after high-dose chemotherapy and autologous hematopoietic stem cell transplantation for high-risk breast cancer. *Bone Marrow Transplantation*, **31**, 1157–1163.

Woodard, J.P., Gulbahce, E., Shreve, M. *et al.* (2000) Pulmonary cytolytic thrombi: a newly recognized complication of stem cell transplantation. *Bone Marrow Transplantation*, **25**, 293–300.

Worthy, S.A., Flint, J.D. and Muller, N.L. (1997) Pulmonary complications after bone marrow transplantation: high-resolution CT and pathologic findings. *Radiographics*, **17**, 1359–1371.

Yanik, G., Hellerstedt, B., Custer, J. *et al.* (2002) Etanercept (Enbrel) administration for idiopathic pneumonia syndrome after allogeneic hematopoietic stem cell transplantation. *Biology of Blood and Marrow Transplantation*, **8**, 395–400.

Yotsumoto, S., Okada, F., Yotsumoto, S. *et al.* (2007) Bronchiolitis obliterans organizing pneumonia after bone marrow transplantation: association with human leukocyte antigens. *Journal of Computer Assisted Tomography*, **31**, 132–137.

Yousem, S.A. (1995) The histological spectrum of pulmonary graft-versus-host disease in bone marrow transplant recipients. *Human Pathology*, **26**, 668–675.

10

Pulmonary infections in patients on chronic glucocorticoid treatment

Ana Rañó and Carlos Agustí

Servei de Pneumologia Institut Clínic del Tòrax, Hospital Clínic, Barcelona, Spain

10.1   Introduction

In 1949 Hench *et al.* described the beneficial effect of treatment with cortisone in patients with rheumatoid arthritis. Since then, glucocorticoids (GC) have come to belong to the most widely and probably also most indiscriminately used drugs in the world.

The good results obtained with transplant techniques and the increase in the number of potential candidates requiring immunomodulative therapy to treat different chronic diseases may partially explain the extended use of these drugs over the last years. Glucocorticoids exert a decisive influence in the innate immune function of resident alveolar macrophages and granulocytes, the two major immunoregulatory cells in host defences against opportunistic and bacterial infections. The immunosuppressive effects of GC when used for long periods of time at relatively high doses may be devastating. Pneumonia in this scenario is a well known complication that must be dealt similarly to any other type of immunocompromised patient with pneumonia such as those recipients of solid organ transplantation or those receiving chemotherapy. The myriad of etiological factors and the potential complications and associated mortality of pneumonia in patients on chronic GC treatment support this assertion.

10.2   Associated inflammatory response in pneumonia

Under normal circumstances, microorganisms are prevented from reaching the alveoli by several anatomical defence mechanisms present in the upper airways. If these defence mechanisms are overwhelmed, the lung epithelial surface is still able to eliminate external agents through a complex mechanism aimed at ensuring a prompt protective response to microbiological invasion. The initiation, maintenance and resolution of this inflammatory response in the lungs will depend on the expression of a complex network of mediators.

Pulmonary Infection in the Immunocompromised Patient, Edited by Carlos Agustí and Antoni Torres
© 2009 John Wiley & Sons, Ltd.

In brief, activation of alveolar macrophages by bacterial products such as endotoxin from gram-negative bacilli and lipoteichoic acid and bacterial peptidoglycan from gram-positive bacteria (Jagger, Huo and Riches, 2002) will induce an inflammatory response characterized by the production of different cytokines. Cytokines are inter-cellular signalling polypeptides produced by activated cells. Cytokines generally have many different functions, depending on the target cells involved. Some cytokines are pro-inflammatory while others are anti-inflammatory, and it is believed that the balance between them determines the net effect of the inflammatory reaction in the lung (Antunes *et al.*, 2002). When this reaction is unbalanced, it may be deleterious for the host through a maladaptative or excessive release of endogenously generated inflam-matory compounds (Stevens, 1995).

Tumour necrosis factors-α (TNF-α) and interleukin-1β (IL-1β) are produced by activated alveolar macrophages and are considered the pro-inflammatory cytokines of the initial phase. These 'early response' cytokines trigger activation of other macro-phages and also mesenchymal cells, such as endothelial cells, epithelial cells and fibroblasts. The host response is further amplified by the expression of leukocyte chemoattractants (mainly IL-8), stimulators of the production of acute-phase proteins (mainly IL-6) (Gabay and Kushner, 1999), growth factors and adhesion molecules, resulting in an array of pro-inflammatory events.

10.3   Glucocorticoids: Mechanisms of action

Glucocorticoids inhibit the expression and action of many cytokines involved in the inflammatory response associated with pneumonia. Glucocorticoids are mainly trans-ported in the blood complexed to transcortin (corticosteroid-binding globulin) and albumin, although a small portion is in a free, metabolically activate state. The free GC molecules readily cross the plasma membrane into the cytoplasm. Once in the cytoplasm, GC bind to their specific receptor, the glucocorticoid receptor (GR). The GR exists as a heterocomplex located in the cytoplasm of nearly all human cells (Jantz and Sahn, 1999). The anti-inflammatory and immunosuppressive effects of GC are due to three molecular mechanisms. First, the ligand-activated GR binds as a homodimer to specific DNA sequences or so called GR responsive elements usually located in the promoter regions of target genes (De Bosscher, Vanden Berghe and Haegeman, 2003) to induce transcription, a phenomenon called transactivation. Second, an indirect negative regulation of gene expression (transrepression) is achieved by GR-protein interaction. The ligand activated receptor binds as a monomer to key pro-inflammatory transcription factors such as activator protein (AP)-1 and nuclear factor (NF)-κB. The resulting complex inhibits the initiation of transcription of relevant genes. This mechanism has been shown to be involved in the inhibition of different gene products that play a central role in inflamma-tion including IL-1, IL-2, IL-3, IL-6, IL-8, TNF-α, and GM-CSF. The third mechanism is GC signalling through membrane-associated receptors and second messengers (so-called non genomic pathways). The best-described non genomic mechanism involves the activation of endothelial nitric oxide synthetase (eNOS). Non-transcriptional activation of eNOS by GR represents a physiologically important signalling pathway by which GC exert their rapid, anti-inflammatory effects. Binding of GC to the GR stimulated phosphatidylinositol 3-kinase and protein kinase Akt, leading to eNOS activation and nitric oxide-dependent vasorelaxation (Hafezi-Moghadam *et al.*, 2002).

In summary, GC can reduce the expression and production of many cytokines by genomic mechanisms. But, GC can not select the specific type of cytokine, and leads to a global inhibition of pro-inflammatory cytokines of the 'initial phase' (IL-1β and TNF-α), the 'immunomodulatory' cytokines (IL-2, IL-3, IL-4, IL-6, IL-8, IL-12 and IFN-γ), and even the 'anti-inflammatory' mediators like IL-1ra and IL-10. Only some cytokines with 'reparatory' functions, such as TGF-β o PDGF, seem to be poorly affected by the effects of or even upregulated by the action of GCs.

The inflammatory actions of GC are not limited to interactions with cytokine expression and function. GCs also inhibit a variety of inflammatory mediators, such as phospolipase A2 and the subsequent arachidonic acid metabolites, or the gene transcription of the intercellular adhesion molecule-1 (ICAM-1) and E-selectin. In addition GC reduce gene expression of some inflammatory receptors such as taquicinin receptors (NK-1 and NK-2) or bradicinin receptors (B1 and B2) (Cosio, Torrego and Adcock, 2005).

Interestingly, the effects of GC over the inflammatory response in patients with pneumonia have been demonstrated in clinical studies. Agustí and collaborators (2003) evaluated the inflammatory response of patients with severe pneumonia having received GC treatment for long periods (more than 30 days). Results were compared to those from a group of patients with severe pneumonia without GC treatment and a third group of patients with pneumonia and GC treatment for a short period of time (9 ± 7 days, in most cases as a bronchodilator treatment). These authors observed that the local inflammatory response evaluated in bronchoalveolar lavage (BAL) measured by relevant cytokines such as IL-6 or TNF-alpha, was markedly diminished in patients having received GC for large periods of time compared to patients not having received such treatment. Furthermore, acute administration of GC had an intermediate effect on the suppression of the inflammatory response (Figure 10.1).

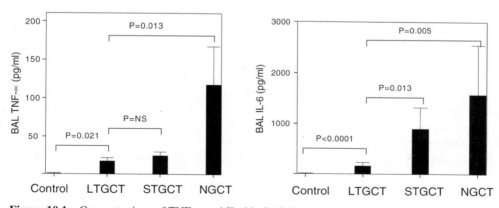

Figure 10.1 Concentrations of TNF-α and IL-6 in BAL from controls and patients receiving long term (LTGCT), short term (STGCT) or no (NGCT) GC treatment. Bars and error bars represent mean and standard error of the mean (SEM). Cytokines are expressed as pg/mL.

10.4   Glucocorticoid therapy in clinical practice

Glucocorticoids are one of the most widely used drugs in medicine with a broad myriad of indications. In this chapter, we will focus on two of the most common indications of GC in clinical practice. First, clinical conditions that cause severe immunosuppression such as transplant of solid organs or haematopoietic stem cells or oncologic patients treated with chemotherapy in whom GC are prescribed as adjuvant therapy. In this setting of profound immunosuppression, GC undoubtedly influences the incidence, severity and response to treatment of different pulmonary infections. The second scenario is the administration of GC (usually in small doses but for long periods of time), for the treatment of different chronic invalidating diseases, such as rheumatological or chronic pulmonary diseases (Chronic Obstructive Pulmonary Disease, COPD). In this setting and particularly in elderly patients with other co-morbid conditions such as diabetes mellitus, the administration of repetitive doses of GC can cause unexpected severe infections. High clinical suspicion and early diagnosis and treatment of the infection are mandatory in order to improve outcome.

Glucocorticoids in severe immunocompromised patients

Pulmonary infections represent the most common complication and one of the main causes of mortality in severe immunocompromised (IC) patients. Clinical management of these infections is complex since virtually any microorganism may be involved at any time in the evolution, mainly depending on the net state of immunosuppression. The most common groups of immunocompromised patients that a physician faces in clinical practice are: solid-organ transplant (SOT) and haematopoietic stem cell transplant (HSCT) recipients and cancer patients treated with intensive chemotherapy. Reasons for immunosupression in the IC patients are varied and differ depending on the group considered. Most probably, HSCT patients suffer the most severe immunousuppression. The conditioning regimen in these patients causes a complete destruction of haematopoietic cells including neutrophils, monocytes and macrophages. Also, damage of mucocutaneous barriers facilitates different infections. Allogeneic HSCT recipients may experience acute graft versus host disease (GVHD) that manifests as skin, gastrointestinal and liver injury. GVHD is associated with a delayed immunologic recovery and prolonged immundeficiency aggravated by the requirement of immuno-suppressive agents for its treatment. Additionally indwelling intravenous catheters are frequently placed and left *in situ* for weeks, acting as a portal of entry for opportunistic pathogens such as coagulase-negative *Staphylococci*, *Staphylococcus aureus*, *Candida* and *Enterococci*. In this clinical situation, the addition of GC may aggravate the net state of immunosuppression favouring the apparition of different pulmonary infections.

Bacterial Pneumonia

Bacterial infections and specifically, those caused by *S. Aureus* (mainly methicillin-resistant, MRSA) and multirresistant gram-negative bacilli (mainly *P. aeruginosa*,

Acinetobacter spp and *Stenotrophomonas maltophilia*) (BitMansour, Burns and Traver, 2002; Grasser *et al.*, 1993; Fujita *et al.*, 1996) are very common causes of pneumonia in severe IC patients. Many of these infections take place in the immediate post-transplant period when severe neutropenia occur. The use of GC in cases of chronic GVHD may facilitate the development of bacterial infections in later stages.

Fungal pneumonia

Allogeneic bone-marrow transplant recipients suffer profound immunosupression and these patients are particularly at risk for fungal infections (Marr *et al.*, 2002). Risk factors include host variables (age, underlying disease), transplant variables (stem cell source), cytomegalovirus disease, and late complications as acute and chronic graft-versus-host disease that requires GC treatment.

Pulmonary host defences against *A. fumigatus* are mediated by phagocytic cells of the innate immune system. Resident alveolar macrophages are thought to eliminate conidia by phagocytosis, whereas recruited polymorphonuclear neutrophils destroy hyphae by producing reactive oxygen species. If the immune defence system of the lung is weakened, then conidia germinate and produce hyphae that invade the surrounding lung tissues, leading to the development of invasive pulmonary aspergillosis (IPA). Invasive pulmonary aspergillosis is now the most common cause of infectious death in the late post-transplant period, accounting for 10% of these deaths in HSCT recipients. High cumulative doses of GC administered for prophylaxis or treatment of graft-versus-host-disease are associated with both risk of acquisition and poor outcome of invasive aspergillosis (Lionakis and Kontoyiannis, 2003). Besides the immune dysfunction that contributes to invasive aspergillosis, GC can induce alterations in the biology of *Aspergillus* species. Studies '*in vitro*' have shown increased growth of *A. fumigatus* and *A. flavus* on exposure to pharmacological doses of hydrocortisone (Ng, Robson and Denning, 1994). Furthermore, antifungals are known to be less effective in patients with neutropenia. Since neutrophils are defective in patients receiving GC, these drugs may hinder the efficacy of antifungals. In fact, neutropenia plus high cumulative GC administration is associated with worse invasive fungal infection diseases (Wiest *et al.*, 1989). Rapid GC tapering plus measures to abrogate neutropenia in patients with fungal infections should be attempted to improve therapeutic responses. In this sense, studies '*in vitro*' and in mice have demonstrated that interferon-γ and granulo-cyte-macrophage-colony stimulating factor (GM-CSF) prevented the suppression of PMN oxidative damage of *Aspergillus* hyphae in the presence of GC and the GC-induced suppression of cytokine production by alveolar macrophages after challenge with *A fumigatus* conidia (Roilides *et al.*, 1993; Brummer, Maqbool and Stevens, 2001; Brummer, Kamberri and Stevens, 2003).

Glucocorticoid therapy is also one of the most important factors favouring candida infections, including candidemia. In addition to their immunosuppressive effects, GC may also augment the virulence of both *Candida albicans* and nonalbicans *Candida* species (Lionakis and Kontoyiannis, 2003). For example, GC have been shown to enhance the adhesion of yeast cells to epithelia and constitutes one of the most common causes of blood stream infections in IC patients. Invasive fungal infections other than aspergillosis can be seen in immunocompromised patients taking glucocorticoids and include, zygomycosis, fusariosis, cryptococcosis and endemic micosis.

Viral pneumonia

Glucocorticoids not only favour the development of fungal infections, but also have a decisive influence on the apparition of other types of pulmonary infections in IC patients. Thus, and as already referred to in a previous chapter of this volume, the use of high dose GC is a well recognized risk factor for cytomegalovirus (CMV) pneumonia. CMV pneumonia represents one of the most common and lethal infections suffered by allogeneic bone marrow transplantation recipients and solid organ transplant patients, particularly those receiving heart/lung transplants. Recurrence of infectious virus from the latent viral genomes is the most common initiating event in the pathogenesis of CMV disease during states of immunodeficiency (Enright *et al.*, 1993). Negative CMV serology of the recipient, older age, total body irradiation, T cell-depleted marrow and high cumulative doses of GC administered for prophylaxis or treatment of GVHD are associated with risk of acquisition of CMV pneumonia.

Community respiratory viruses have also been recognized as a potential cause of pneumonia and death among haematopoietic stem cell transplantation recipients and patients with haematologic malignancies. The most frequently identified viruses are influenza, parainfluenza, respiratory syncitial virus, and adenovirus. Risk factors for developing pneumonia from these community respiratory viruses include: patients with leukemia, patients aged more than 65 years, and those with severe neutropenia or lymphopenia (Chemaly *et al.*, 2006). Nichols *et al.* (2004) demonstrated that among patients with influenza virus infection, pneumonia developed more commonly among those infected earlier after transplantation and those with concurrent lymphopenia. In addition, the duration of influenza virus shedding was longer in patients treated with GC doses of >1 mg/kg than among those treated with doses of more than 1 mg/kg (mean, 15 vs 9 days). These authors found that early antiviral therapy with neuraminidase inhibitors may prevent progression to pneumonia and decrease viral shedding.

Mycobacterium and nontuberculous mycobacterial infections

Although mycobacterium infections are relatively uncommon in transplant recipients in developed countries, the annualized rate of infection is 3–10 fold higher than that of the general population (Queipo *et al.*, 2003). A high level of suspicion is necessary to diagnose pulmonary tuberculosis in IC patients. The incidence of atypical mycobacterial infections, particularly *M. avium complex* and *M kansasii*, has dropped significantly among SOT recipients with the exception of lung transplant patients, and HSCT recipients. In a recent series by Weinstock *et al.* (2003), the reported infection rate of nontuberculous mycobacteria infections in allogenic HSCT was 5–20 fold higher than that of older series, probably in relation to immunosuppressive regimes (including corticosteroids). The authors suggested that nosocomial factors and improvement in detection techniques could partially explain this increase.

Pneumocystis jirovecii

Hughes *et al.* (1975), in their studies of *Pneumocystis jirovecii* pneumonia (PJP) in children with acute lymphoblastic leukemia, found an incidence ranging from 22 to 45%, depending on the chemotherapy used and the stage of leukemia. With the introduction of prophylaxis, the rate decreased to 0%. Without prophylaxis, rates approach 25% among patients with non-Hodgkin's lymphoma, severe combined immunodeficiency syndrome or rhabdomiosarcoma (Sepkowitz, Brown and Amstrong 1995). Generally, GC use is implicated when dosage is greater than 20 mg of prednisone equivalent for more than one month. Without prophylaxis, PJP develops in 5–15% of patients who undergo SOT or allogenic HSCT. Among heart-lung transplant, the rate is higher, approaching 25% in most series. Organ rejection and GC use may increase the risk.

Glucococorticoid therapy in mild immunosuppressive clinical settings

Classic immunosuppression as we know it is expanding to include apparently immuno-competent patients whose mild-moderate immune deficits are transiently worsened resulting in cumulative immunosuppression severe enough to cause life-threatening infections. Apparently immunocompetent hosts include patients with conditions such as cirrhosis, COPD, transfusion-associated haemosiderosis and diabetes mellitus. Certainly, recipients of long term GC doses represent one of the most representative groups of the so called 'apparently' immunocompetent host (Anaissie, 2008). The clinical use of GC with or without other immunosuppressive therapies has expanded over the last years in common diseases, such as COPD, asthma, idiopathic interstitial pneumonias, different chronic inflammatory diseases, systemic vasculitis, and different connective disorders. As a consequence, it might be expected that patients receiving long-term large doses of GC to have depressed resistance to a wide variety of infective agents. The association of long-term GC and cytotoxic treatments with fatal opportu-nistic infections (mainly *P. jirovecii* and *Candida sp*) (Hellmann, Petri and Whiting-O'Keefe, 1987; Sen *et al.*, 1991; Ognibene *et al.*, 1995) has been described in previous studies. Also, the use of GC therapy as the sole immunosuppressive drug has been recognized as an important factor for the incidence of multi-resistant bacterial and opportunistic pneumonia (Wiest *et al.*, 1989; Ullmer *et al.*, 2000; Meersseman *et al.*, 2004). Reports of serious pulmonary infections in patients with chronic lung diseases requiring permanent or repetitive doses of GC have been described. These include cases of invasive pulmonary aspergillosis, bacterial sepsis, herpes simplex, *P. jirovecii* or cytomegalovirus pneumonia (Conesa *et al.*, 1995; Palmer, Greenberg and Schiff, 1991; Wiest *et al.*, 1989). An anecdotic case of pulmonary infection by *S. stercoralis* is also described in a patient receiving chronic GC therapy (Namisato *et al.*, 2004). Table 10.1 shows the main etiological agents causing pulmonary infections in patients taking chronic GC treatment in the series by Agustí *et al.* (2003).

Table 10.1   Aetiology of pulmonary infiltrates and associated mortality.

	N. episodes	Mortality (%)
Bacterial		4/10 (40%)
Staphylococcus aureus oxacillin-sensitive	2	
Methicillin-resistant (MRSA)	3	
Enterococcus faecalis	1	
Gemella morbillorum	1	
Pseudomonas aeruginosa	1	
Legionella pneumophila	1	
Nocardia asteroids	1	
Fungal		6/9 (67%)
Aspergillus fumigatus	6	
Candida albicans	2	
Candida tropicalis	1	
Polymicrobial		2/3 (67%)
P. aeruginosa + A. fumigatus	1	
E. coli + A. niger + MRSA	1	
P. aeruginosa + Stenotrophomona m + A. fumigatus	1	
Viral		—
Varicella zoster virus	1	
Influenza A virus	1	
Other infections		2/4 (50%)
Pneumocystis jirovecci	2	
Mycobacterium tuberculosis	2	
Non-infectious		—
Chronic organizing pneumonia	1	—
Undetermined	4	—	1/4 (12%)

Bacterial pneumonia

Bacteria is one of the most frequent causes of pulmonary infections in patients with mild immunosuppressive conditions. The most common bacteria are gram-negative bacilli, particularly *P. aeruginosa*, *Acinetobacter spp*, multirresistant strains of *Stenotrophomona maltophilia*, *E. coli*, and *Klebsiella pneumoniae*.

In a series of 87 patients with systemic lupus erythematosus (Noël *et al.*, 2001), 40% of the patients had at least one infectious episode. Bacteria (mainly *Staphylococcus sp*), were responsible for 82% of the episodes, with 40% of them being infections of the lower respiratory tract. Five patients also developed tuberculous infection and nine viral infections (mainly varicella zoster virus). The only independent risk factor for infection and death in the multivariate analyses was treatment with intravenous GC and/or immunosuppressants.

Agustí *et al.* (2003), evaluated prospectively the etiology, clinical characteristics and prognostic factors for pulmonary complications in patients receiving long-term GC treatment. In this study the high prevalence of bacterial pneumonia was confirmed. The study included 33 patients (23 patients with different connective disorders and 10 with chronic pulmonary disorders) treated with prednisone at a dosage more than 30 mg/day for more than 30 days. Interestingly, bacterial infections were almost as prevalent as fungal infections, and particularly *S. aureus* constituted the most common bacteria isolated. This last finding is remarkable since, classically, GC treatment had not been considered as a risk factor for *Staphylococcus* pneumonia. In this study the associated mortality of pulmonary infections in patients taking chronic GC was high (45%), a percentage that is similar to what is observed in other immunosuppressive conditions. Based on this and on the high number of cases in which the empirical treatment did not cover the etiologic agent, antibiotics covering *Staphylococcus spp*, and gram-negative bacilli are recommended as first-line antibiotic treatment in patients taking high doses of GC for long periods of time.

Nocardia sp has also emerged as a potential opportunistic pathogen mainly in chronic respiratory patients. Different small series have described cases of pulmonary nocardiosis in COPD patients that received oral GC therapy for long periods of time. Mari *et al.* described 10 cases of pulmonary nocardiosis. Six out of 10 patients had COPD (Mari *et al.*, 2001). Mean time between onset of symptoms and diagnosis was five weeks and infections were restricted to the lung in 9/10 patients. Sputum culture was positive when performed (eight cases) and mortality was high (50%). Similarly, Menendez *et al.* (1997) evidenced that COPD and GC treatment were the main risk factors for acquiring this infection.

Fungal pneumonia

The number of cases of fungal pneumonia has increased as the use of GC expands in clinical practice (Ader *et al.*, 2005; Bulpa *et al.*, 2001; Rello *et al.*, 1998; Kontoyiannis and Bodey, 2002). In fact *Aspergillus spp* are one of the most frequent microorganisms causing pulmonary infiltrates in patients receiving long-term GC treatment in different clinical settings of apparent immunocompetent patients (Meersseman *et al.*, 2004). In our experience, *Aspergillus spp* and *Staphylococcus spp* were the most prevalent etiologic microorganisms accounting for more than 45% of the episodes of pulmonary infection (Agustí *et al.*, 2003). It is known that GC have profound effects on the distribution and function of neutrophils, monocytes and lymphocytes. Besides, GC can directly stimulate the growth of *Aspergillus fumigatus* 'in vitro' and decrease macrophages antifungal activity by inhibiting reactive oxidant intermediates (Philippe *et al.*, 2003).

Certainly, patients with chronic respiratory disorders, particularly COPD seem to be at special risk for *Aspergillus spp* infections. A series of factors may increase the susceptibility to suffer fungal infections in this group of patients other than the common requirement of long-term or repeated short-term GC treatment. Thus, the structural changes in lung architecture related to the pulmonary disease, the occurrence of frequent hospitalizations and antibiotic treatment, that leads to exposure to selected fungal pathogens or the common co-existence of comorbid conditions such as diabetes mellitus or malnutrition may also play an important role (Bulpa, Dive and Sibille, 2007). Assessing the incidence of IPA in this population is difficult due to the lack of a consistent case definition and the fact that colonization by *Aspergillus spp.* is often difficult to distinguish from IPA. In a review of 50 studies, COPD was the underlying condition in 36 out of 1941 (1,3%) patients with aspergillosis (Lin, Schranz and Teutsch,

2001). In one large study, 9% of 595 patients with IPA suffered from pulmonary disease, without distinguishing between respiratory disorders. A recent retrospective series (Agustí *et al.*, 2006) evaluating only patients on chronic GC treatment as a unique risk factor for pulmonary infections (excluding those patients also treated with another immunosuppressive drug), showed that eight out of the nine patients evaluated had chronic pulmonary disorders. The aetiology of the pulmonary infiltrates was a fungal pneumonia in eight patients and in one, it was multiresistant *Pseudomona aeruginosa* pneumonia. Glucocorticoids were given for the management of bronchial hyperresponsiveness, chronic asthma or diffuse interstitial involvement of the lung. Interestingly, IPA affected mainly patients with severe COPD, however cases of other chronic lung disorders such as chronic asthma, idiopathic pulmonary fibrosis or residual fibrotic post-TB lung lesions were also described. This finding suggests that is not the disease itself but rather the chronic alterations of the lung architecture that pose individuals at risk for fungal pneumonia if they require long term or repetitive doses of GC.

Establishing a diagnosis of IPA at an early stage of disease is necessary for successful treatment, but it is particularly challenging in mild immunosuppressive patients. Clinical findings of IPA in COPD patients on chronic GC treatment are non specific and a high degree of suspicion is required. The main clinical sign may be a non-specific antibiotic-resistant pneumonia associated with exacerbated dyspnoea (Bulpa, Dive and Sibille, 2007). Multiples episodes of breathlessness are characteristic of the infection and these exacerbations often occur after initial improvement of the respiratory symptoms. A significant bronchospastic component is documented in almost 80% of patients. Interestingly, only one third of the patients present with fever, probably due to the antipyretic effects of GC (Bulpa, Dive and Sibille, 2007). In non-neutropenic patients CT scan of the lungs shows low sensitivity for identification of specific signs of IPA. The halo sign is rarely seen or is a relatively late sign and its absence in this population has no negative predictive power (Gefter *et al.*, 1985).

Laboratory findings are non-specific. Definitive diagnosis of IPA requires demonstration of tissue invasion on biopsy specimen. However, several authors, in trying to achieve a provisional diagnosis, have required multiple cultures from respiratory specimens as an alternative. Interestingly, when the number of positive samples was examined in a hospital-based survey of aspergillosis, 61% of those with confirmed IPA had a single positive culture result and only 18% had three positive culture results (Perfect *et al.*, 2001). This suggests that requiring multiple positive results as a criterion for the diagnosis of IPA may underestimate the prevalence of this fungal infection (Denning, 2004). Although 10% of severe COPD patients may be colonized with *Aspergillus spp*, their presence in sputum or from samples obtained with bronchoscopy should not be trivialized, especially in cases of antibiotic-resistant pneumonia.

Galactomannan (GM) is a polysaccharide fungal cell wall component that is released during tissue invasion by *Aspergillus* hyphae and that can be detected in body fluids. Although the use of serum GM detection in HSCT recipients is very useful, its value in nonneutropenic patients is more controversial. The results obtained so far have been disappointing and suggest that serum GM is probably not a good marker for IPA in these patients. Thus, Meersseman *et al.* evaluated GM antigenaemia in critically ill COPD patients with suspected IPA. Among 25 patients tested, only 12 were positive (48%)

(Meersseman *et al.*, 2008). By contrast, these same authors, in a recent study evaluating a cohort of patients with ventilator-associated pneumonia caused by *Aspergillus* species in the intensive care unit setting, demonstrated that GM determination in bronchoalveolar lavage may be very useful with a diagnostic sensitivity of 88% and specificity of 87% compared with only 42% sensitivity for serum GM. In this study only 22% patients were neutropenic and 67% had underlying diseases other than haematologic cancer, including COPD.

Immediate initiation of antifungals should be considered when suspicion of IPA in COPD is strong since an early diagnosis and treatment is the only chance for cure. Small series and case reports demonstrate the extremely poor outcome of IPA in COPD patients with a mortality rate approaching 100% (Ader *et al.*, 2006). Different therapeutic approaches have been reported. Although Amphotericin B colloidal dispersion has been the most extensively antifungal treatment evaluated, the results of more recent studies suggest that voriconazole should be the first choice therapy (Bulpa, Dive and Sibille, 2007). As IPA mortality is so high, prevention of infection inside the hospital seems reasonable to eliminate obvious environmental sources of *Aspergillus spp.* In fact, some lethal cases of pulmonary aspergillosis in patients with COPD are described with nosocomial acquisition due to exposure to high concentrations or airbone *Aspergillus spp* related to air filter change. Such infection can be prevented by the establishment and application of guidelines for air filter replacement (Pittet *et al.*, 1996). Even hospital water is a frequently overlooked source of nosocomial aspergillosis (Anaissie and Costa, 2001).

COPD patients on chronic GC treatment may suffer invasion of the lung parenchyma causing fulminant, usually fatal IPA or may suffer a more indolent, cavitary, infectious process of the lung secondary to local invasion by *Aspergillus* species called chronic necrotizing or semi-invasive aspergillosis (Binder *et al.*, 1982). The clinical course is more indolent than IPA and definitive diagnosis requires demonstration of tissue invasion on biopsy specimen. Again, repetitive positive sputum or bronchial washings in patients with COPD or other underlying chronic lung diseases with a chronic indolent pneumonia may be sufficient to administer antifungal treatment. Interestingly, not only oral but also inhaled steroids might promote IPA in COPD patients. High doses of inhaled steroids have potential systemic effects causing some effects on immunity. Some reports of IPA in patients receiving high-potency inhaled GC (Leav, Fanburg and Hadley, 2000; Peter *et al.*, 2002) have been reported.

In summary, invasive pulmonary infections by *Aspergillus* should be considered in the differential diagnosis for a subset of severe COPD patients with long-term GC treatment. There should be a high level of suspicion for this fungal infection, given that definitive diagnosis is extremely difficult and the outcome is very poor and not improved by the maximal supportive care provided in the ICU (Kistemann *et al.*, 2002). Survival of patients with IPA depends largely on early diagnosis and the prompt institution of therapeutic measures.

Although the risk of GC therapy-associated infectious complications seems to be dose dependent, certainly, the minimum required GC exposure to be at risk for fungal pneumonia is difficult to quantify. This difficulty is further complicated by the frequent co-morbidities and additional risk factors for opportunistic infections that commonly affect these patients. Stuck *et al.*, by pooling data from 71 controlled clinical trials, evidenced that the rate of infections was not increased in patients given a daily dose lower than 10 mg/day or a cumulative dose of more than 700 mg of prednisone (Stuck, Minder and Frey, 1989). Moreover, treatment for less than five days or intermittent therapy appears to have less effect on immune function and predisposition of patients to infection than prolonged or continuous therapy. In a revision of autopsy-proven cases of opportunistic pneumonia in patients on chronic GC treatment, the overall mean prednisone equivalent dose at the time of admission was 34 ± 8 mg/d. In the hospital stay, the maximum daily dose of methylprednisolone varied from 60 mg/d to 1000 mg/d given for a mean of 26 days (Rodrigues et al., 1992). In particular, intravenous GC treatment in patients with COPD is associated with a rising incidence of invasive pulmonary aspergillosis (Crean et al., 1992; Jara-Palomares et al., 2007). Recently, Garnacho et al. (2005), in a multicentre prospective study including patients with an ICU stay longer than seven days, evidenced that both treatment with GC (OR 3.5) and COPD (OR 2.9) were significantly associated with Aspergillus spp isolation in respiratory secretions (Garnacho et al., 2005). Trof et al. (2007) consider as a risk factor for IPA in non-neutropenic patients, the combination of COPD with prolonged GC use or high-dose systemic GC longer than three weeks (for example, prednisone equivalent more than 20 mg/day).

Glucocorticoids have also been recognized as a risk factor for candidaemia and invasive candidiasis (Nucci and Colombo, 2002). The association of GC with candidaemia has been shown for *Candida albicans* and non-albicans Candida species. Invasive candidiasis has been demonstrated in patients with SLE. In this sense, Hellmann et al. (1987) demonstrated that invasive candidiasis is the most common deep-seated fungal infection in this group of patients.

Viral pneumonia

Pulmonary CMV infections have been rarely reported in immunocompetent patients (Eddleston et al., 1997; Kanno et al., 2001). Ikura et al. (2000) collected 34 cases identified in the literature and found no apparent risk factor. Another study evaluated seven histologically proven cases of CMV disease in patients with comorbid conditions (including GC treatment). Acute CMV infection may be more severe in some patients with lupus.

CMV pneumonitis, although rare, can affect patients with cancer. In a retrospective, autopsy-based study, 20 cases of CMV pneumonitis were identified among 9029 autopsies performed during 1964–1990. Cases were common among patients with multiple myeloma and brain tumour. All had received chemotherapy and 75% had received GC. Risk factors for CMV pneumonitis in cancer patients were use of GC, cyclophosphamide, methotrexate and fludarabine (Breathnach et al., 1999).

Pneumocystis jirovecii

Pneumocystis jirovecii pneumonia (PJP) is a recognized opportunistic pulmonary infection in GC-treated patients with rheumatologic diseases, especially SLE and

Wegener disease. Arend *et al.* (1995) retrospectively evaluated the underlying disorders and previous immunomodulatory treatments in patients with PJP. These authors observed that 22% of patients suffered from vasculitis or other immunologic disorders. Prednisone or other GC were employed in 92% out of the 78 patients evaluated. Quantification of previous GC treatment showed a large variability among patients, and the overall mortality rate for patients was 35%. A trend toward a higher mortality in patients with previous corticosteroid use was detected ($p = 0.6$).

Many cases with fatal progression are frequently associated with lymphopenia and low CD4 and CD8 cell counts. Since the time elapsed between the initiation of the immunosuppressive therapy and the identification of the infection is short in some patients and, due to the high associated mortality, some authors defend the need for a primary prophylaxis in patients with rheumatologic diseases treated with high dose GC therapy. Control of the CD4 and CD8 cell counts might help on this issue (Bachelez *et al.*, 1997).

Mycobacterium and nontuberculous mycobacterial infections

Patients treated with GC have an increased risk of developing tuberculosis. An interesting case-control study aimed to evaluate the association of GC and other risk factors with the development of tuberculosis, found that the adjusted odds ratio (OR) for current use of GC compared with no use was five. The adjusted ORs for using more than 15 mg or ≥15 mg daily dose of prednisone or its equivalent were 2.8 and 7.7, respectively. Obstructive pulmonary disorders also were important independent risk factors for tuberculosis in this series (Jick *et al.*, 2006). More recently, Mok *et al.* (2007) evaluated a long cohort of patients with systemic lupus erythematosus and mycobacterial infections. Interestingly, non-tuberculous mycobacterial infections were more likely to involve older patients with longer lupus disease duration, and who had a higher cumulative dose of prenisolone than mycobacterial infections.

Nagata *et al.* reported in a series of patients affected by lung cancer that the incidence of mycobacterial infection was significantly higher among those treated with antineoplastic therapy and GC than in those who received antineoplastic therapy alone. In this series, the administration of GC for relatively short periods (less than one month) could have led to a fatal mycobacterial infection with independence of the presence or absence of lymphocytopenia (Nagata *et al.*, 1993). Similarly, a post-mortem analysis evaluating the causes of death of almost 1000 consecutive patients treated for lung cancer with chemotherapy and GC during 14 years demonstrated an incidence of 5% of fatal infections. Fungal and bacterial infections were the most frequent aetiologies, closely followed by PJP and tuberculosis (Remiszewski *et al.*, 2001).

Slowly progressive pulmonary infection with *Mycobacterium avium complex* (MAC) has been described in middle-aged men with various comorbidities, particularly underlying lung disease, but GC use has been rarely associated with disseminated MAC infection (Prince *et al.*, 1989).

10.5   Diagnostic approach

The etiological diagnosis of pulmonary infiltrates in patients on long-term GC treatment is difficult. Clinical and radiological characteristics of pulmonary infections are often non specific and a high level of clinical suspicion is required for the diagnosis. Besides, the recognition of such infections may be delayed, since the anti-inflammatory properties of GC usually blunt the signs and symptoms of some opportunistic infections. Figure 10.2 represents a proposal for the management of pulmonary infiltrates in patients receiving long-term GC therapy.

Although sputum culture is considered a non-specific respiratory sample due to the potential of contamination by oral flora, it can be of help in guiding initial empirical treatment. Besides, the potential identification of microorganisms that occasionally infect patients on long-term GC treatment such as *aspergillus spp, nocardia spp*, or *mycobacteriae* might provide enough evidence to start specific treatment (Yu, Muder and Poorsattar, 1986). Based on that and on its availability, simplicity and cost-effectiveness, sputum culture is imperative as a first line diagnostic technique (Finch and Beaty, 1997). However, when the results of sputum culture are inconclusive and the initial response to empirical treatment is poor, fibreoptic bronchoscopy (FOB) should be promptly considered. Patients on long-term GC therapy may suffer opportunistic infections and there is risk for rapid dissemination of the disease with accompanying acute respiratory failure. The early use of FOB may add to the prompt identification of the specific etiologic agent, facilitating an etiology-guided treatment and avoiding unnecessary and potentially harmful additional treatment. FOB is a low-risk procedure that can be safely performed in most patients, including those with hypoxemia, with the application of supplemental oxygen or by means of a laryngeal mask in airways or during non-invasive ventilation. Different authors have shown evidence suggesting that the early use of FOB on immunocompromised patients may decrease mortality (Aisner, Scimpff and Wiernik, 1977). As previously shown in the chapter dealing with the diagnostic approach of immunocompromised patients, bronchoalveolar lavage (BAL) is a very reliable technique for detecting opportunistic infections, but also for bacteria, mycobacteria and other pathogens (Stover *et al.*, 1984; Jolis *et al.*, 1996; Sternberg, Baughman and Dohn, 1993). Bronchoalveolar lavage is particularly efficient in that it may still recover resistant pathogens after several days of empirical treatment allowing modifications of the primary regimen. Due to the potential benefits of BAL, this endoscopic technique should be used in patients on chronic GC treatment with pulmonary infiltrates that undergo FOB. The use of FOB in IC patients provides a specific diagnosis in 50–80% of the cases (Xaubet *et al.*, 1989; Hohenadel *et al.*, 2001). Particularly, the yield of BAL in a series of patients on chronic GC treatment was 56% (Agustí *et al.*, 2003). In this series, the protected specimen brush did not seem to add diagnostic information to BAL. By contrast, a simple, safe and cost-effective technique such as cuantitative cultures of tracheobronchial aspirates may constitute a good complement to BAL in the diagnosis of the etiology of pneumonia in different groups of immunocompromised patients including those on long-term GC treatment (Table 10.2).

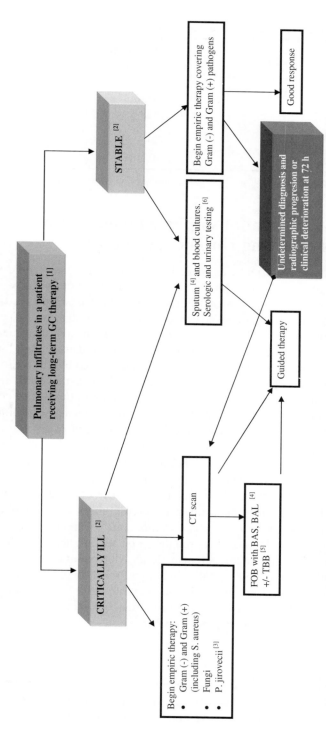

Figure 10.2 Proposed schema for diagnostic and treatment of patients receiving long-term GC therapy with suspected pneumonia. (1) Daily dose >10 mg or a cumulative dose >700 mg of prednisone. (2) Severity criteria based on modified ATS score by Ewig [presence of two or three minor criteria (systolic blood pressure <90 mmHg, multilobar involvement, PaO_2/FiO_2 <250] or one of two major criteria (requirement of mechanical ventilation, presence of septic shock)]. (3) If diffuse bilateral infiltrates. (4) Respiratory samples should qualitatively or quantitative cultured for bacterial pathogens, fungi and mycobacteria. (5) TBB in selected patients. (6) Serologic testing should include serum detection of *Aspergillus spp* galactomannan antigen and urinary antigen test for detection of *L. pneumophila* and *S. pneumoniae*. *Abbreviations:* AST: computed tomography; FOB: fibreoptic bronchoscopy; CT: computed tomography; BAS: bronchial aspirate; BAL: bronchoalveolar lavage; TBB: transbronchial biopsy.

Table 10.2 Diagnostic yield of the different procedures performed.

Procedures	Diagnostic yield n positive/total n (%)
Blood culture	3/31 (10%)
Sputum culture	10/19 (53%)
Bronchoscopy	14/22 (64%)
Bronchial aspirate	15/20 (75%)
Protected specimen brush	6/18 (33%)
Bronchoalveolar lavage	10/18 (56%)

Some microorganisms were simultaneously isolated with more than one procedure.

10.6 Empirical treatment of suspected pneumonia in patients receiving chronic GC therapy

The election of a particular empirical treatment in patients receiving chronic GC therapy should consider different factors. Among them, the specific underlying disease requiring steroid treatment, the dosage and total cumulative amount of GC received and the concomitant use of other immunosuppressive therapies (cytotoxic agents). Also, the assessment of the severity (presence of acute respiratory failure) can have an influence on the particular treatment a patient will receive. In general, patients receiving long-term GC treatment are prone to develop pulmonary infections caused by a diversity of microorganisms. Besides, the alarming increase in antimicrobial resistance as well as the prognostic implications of an inappropriate empirical treatment provides a compelling argument in favour of a combination therapy with broad spectrum antibiotics that include coverage for *Staphylococcus aureus* and that are adapted to local patterns of microbial resistance therapy (Ewig, Bauer and Torres, 2002). Lack of clinical stability and treatment failure should be assessed at 72 h. The absence of an early improvement with antibacterial treatment against *Staphylococcus aureus* and gram-negative bacilli (including *P. aeruginosa*) justify the early use of FOB and the consideration of an immediate use of an antifungal agent while waiting the microbiological results (Walsh *et al.*, 1991). Additional treatments for *P. jirovecci*, *M. tuberculosis*, and viruses should be considered, depending on the results of the bronchoscopic techniques. Similarly to what has been postulated in immunocompetent patients with pneumonia, the best approach for reducing infection related mortality in patients on chronic GC treatment should be the initial (and early) institution of a broad-spectrum antibiotic regime, the consideration of an early use of FOB and the institution of a de-escalating strategy when the results from microbiologic testing become available.

10.7 Prognosis

Mortality of pulmonary infections in patients receiving long-term GC therapy can be as high as 50% (Agustí *et al.*, 2003); a percentage that approaches that observed in patients with other types of immunosupressive conditions (Rano *et al.*, 2001). Thus, management of these patients should not differ considerably from that in other immunosuppressive settings. Different variables related to the severity of the pulmonary infection have prognostic significance. In particular, mechanical ventilation requirement is the strongest predictor of mortality confirming this variable as the most determinant in relation to mortality in different groups of immunocompromised patients (Rano et al., 2002). Other prognostic factors for mortality are ageing and variables related to the severity of the infection such as bilateral radiographic involvement or high severity index scores. Also, the inadequacy of the empirical antibiotic treatment is a very relevant prognostic variable since it is amenable to clinical intervention. This is of particular concern since it is demonstrated that in a high number of cases the empirical treatment does not cover the etiologic agent (Agustí et al., 2003). The implications of an excessive delay in establishing a specific diagnosis and the high diagnostic yield of BAS and BAL suggest that a bronchoscopy evaluation should be carried out early, once the pulmonary infiltrates have been identified.

10.8 Conclusions

Opportunistic pulmonary infections have emerged as an important cause of morbidity and mortality in patients receiving intensive chemotherapy, allogeneic HSCT, and solid organ transplantation. However, over the last years, reports have described a rising incidence of these infections in non-immunocompromised patients, even in the absence of an apparent predisposing immunodeficiency. The extensive use of GC to treat different chronic diseases seems to be the main risk factor. Moreover, there is mounting evidence that high doses and long durations of systemic GC therapy correlate with high risk and poor outcomes of some opportunistic infections (mainly due to *Aspergillus sp*). Several studies have shown that risk of opportunistic infection is lower when GC is administered on alternate days rather than a daily schedule.

The diagnosis of opportunistic lung infections is frequently delayed in patients taking GC, since an aggressive work-up for such infections is not always undertaken. An early detection of invasive fungal infection is mandatory due to the uniformly poor prognosis with late treatment. Based on this and on the high number of cases in which the empirical treatment did not cover the etiologic agent, antibiotics covering *Aspergillus*, *Staphylococcus spp* and gram-negative bacilli are recommended as first-line antibiotic treatment in patients taking high doses of GC for long periods of time. The prognostic implications of excessive delay in establishing a specific diagnosis and the high diagnostic yield of bronchoscopy favours the early employment of this technique once pulmonary infiltrates have been identified.

Once the pulmonary infection is detected, a rapid tapering of GC should be indicated in these patients. In transplant patients, the introduction of more selective immunosuppressive agents may help by decreasing the dose of GC needed to maintain graft function, producing fewer infectious complications. Restriction of GC administration to less than 21 days might reduce infection complications, since prolonged suppression of T-lymphocyte-mediated cellular immunity has been suggested to be essential for opportunistic infections.

Acknowledgement

Supported by Sociedad Española de Neumología y Cirugía Torácica (SEPAR), FIS 03/113 and CIBER 06/06/0028.

References

Agustí, C., Rañó, A., Aldabó, I. and Torres, A. (2006) Fungal pneumonia, chronic respiratory diseases and glucocorticoids. *Medical Mycology*, **44**, S207–S211.

Agustí, C., Rañó, A., Filella, X. *et al.* (2003) Pulmonary infiltrates in patients receiving long-term glucocorticoid treatment. Etiology, prognostic factors, and associated inflammatory response. *Chest*, **123**, 488–498.

Ader, F., Nseir, S., Le Berre, R. *et al.* (2005) Invasive pulmonary aspergillosis in chronic obstructive pulmonary disease: an emerging fungal pathogen. *Clinical Microbiology and Infection*, **11**, 427–429.

Ader, F., Nseir, S., Tillie-Leblond, I. and Guery, B. (2006) Acute invasive pulmonary aspergillosis in chronic lung diseases. A review. *Revue Des Maladies Respiratoires*, **23**, 6S11–6S16.

Aisner, J., Scimpff, S.C. and Wiernik, P.H. (1977) Treatment of invasive aspergillosis: relation to early diagnosis and treatment to response. *Annals of Internal Medicine*, **89**, 539–543.

Anaissie, E.J. (2008) A bad bug takes on a new role as a cause of ventilator-associated pneumonia. *American Journal of Respiratory and Critical Care Medicine*, **177**, 1–3.

Anaissie, E.J. and Costa, S.F. (2001) Nosocomial aspergillosis is waterbone. *Clinical Infectious Diseases*, **33**, 1546–1548.

Antunes, G., Evans, S.A., Lordan, J.L. and Frew, A.J. (2002) Systemic cytokine levels in community-acquired pneumonia and their association with disease severity. *The European Respiratory Journal*, **20**, 990–995.

Arend, S.M., Kroon, F.P. and van't Wout, J.W. (1995) Pneumocystis carinii pneumonia in patients without AIDS, 1980 through 1993. An analysis of 78 cases. *Archives of Internal Medicine*, **155**, 2436–2441.

Bachelez, H., Schremmer, B., Cadranel, J., *et al.* (1997) Fulminant Pneumocystis carinii pneumonia in 4 patients with dermatomyositis. *Archives of Internal Medicine*, **157**, 1501–1503.

Binder, R.E., Faling, L.J., Pugatch, R.D. *et al.* (1982) Chronic necrotizing pulmonary aspergillosis: a discrete clinical entity. *Medicine*, **61**, 109–124.

BitMansour, A., Burns, S.M. and Traver, D. (2002) Myeloid progenitors protect against invasive aspergillosis and *Pseudomonas aeruginosa* infection following hematopoietic stem cell transplantation. *Blood*, **100**, 4660–4667.

Breathnach, O., Donnellan, P., Collins, D. *et al.* (1999) Cytomegalovirus in a patient with breast cancer on chemotherapy. Case report and review of the literature. *Annals of Oncology*, **10**, 461–465.

Brummer, E., Kamberri, M. and Stevens, D.A. (2003) Regulation by granulocyte-macrophage colony-stimulating factor and/or steroids given in vivo of proinflammatory cytokine and chemokine production by bronchoalveolar macrophages in response to Aspergillus conidia. *The Journal of Infectious Diseases*, **187** (4), 705–709.

Brummer, E., Maqbool, A. and Stevens, D.A. (2001) Protection of bronchoalveolar macrophages by granucloyte-macrophage colony-stimulating factor (GM-CSF) against dexamethasone suppression of fungicidal activity for *Aspergillus fumigatus* conidia. *Medical Mycology*, **29**, 509–515.

Bulpa, P.A., Dive, A.M., Garrino, M.G. *et al.* (2001) Chronic obstructive pulmonary disease patients with invasive pulmonary aspergillosis: benefits of intensive care? *Intensive Care Medicine*, **27**, 59–67.

Bulpa, P., Dive, A. and Sibille, Y. (2007) Invasive pulmonary aspergillosis in patients with chronic obstructive pulmonary disease. *The European Respiratory Journal*, **30**, 782–800.

Chemaly, R.F., Ghosh, S. and Bodey, G.P., *et al.* (2006) Respiratory viral infections in adults with hematologic malignancies and human stem cell transplantation recipients: a retrospective study at a major cancer center. *Medicine*, **85**, 278–287.

Conesa, D., Rello, J., Valles, J. *et al.* (1995) Invasive aspergillosis: a life-threatening complication of short-term steroid treatment. *Annals of Pharmacotherapy*, **29**, 1235–1237.

Cosio, B.G., Torrego, A. and Adcock, I.M. (2005) Molecular mechanisms of glucocorticoids. *Archivos de Bronconeumologia*, **41**, 34–41.

Crean, J.M., Niederman, M.S., Fein, A.M. and Feinsilver, S.H. (1992) Rapidly progressive respiratory failure due to *aspergillus* pneumonia: a complication of short-term corticosteroid therapy. *Critical Care Medicine*, **20**, 148–150.

De Bosscher, K., Vanden Berghe, W. and Haegeman, G. (2003) The interplay between the glucocorticoid receptor and nuclear factor-kappa beta or activator protein-1: molecular mechanisms for gene repression. *Endocrine Reviews*, **24**, 488–522.

Denning, D.W. (2004) Aspergillosis in "nonimmunocompromised" critically ill patients. *American Journal of Respiratory and Critical Care Medicine*, **170**, 580–581.

Eddleston, M., Peacock, S., Juniper, M. and Warrell, D.A. (1997) Severe cytomegalovirus infection in immunocompetent patients. *Clinical Infectious Diseases*, **24**, 52–56.

Enright, H., Haake, R., Weisdorf, D. *et al.* (1993) Cytomegalovirus pneumonia after bone marrow transplantation. Risk factors and response to therapy. *Transplantation*, **55**, 1339–1346.

Ewig, S., Bauer, T.T. and Torres, A. (2002) The pulmonary physician in critical care: Nosocomial pneumonia. *Thorax*, **57**, 366–371.

Finch, D. and Beaty, C.D. (1997) The utility of a single sputum specimen in the diagnosis of tuberculosis. Comparison between HIV-infected and non-HIV-infected patients. *Chest*, **111**, 1174–1179.

Fujita, J., Yamadori, I., Xu, G. *et al.* (1996) Clinical features of *Stenotrophomonas maltophilia* pneumonia in immunocompromised patients. *Respiratory Medicine*, **90**, 35–38.

Gabay, C. and Kushner, I. (1999) Acute-phase proteins and other systemic responses to inflammation. *The New England Journal of Medicine*, **340**, 448–454.

Garnacho, J., Amaya, R., Ortiz, C. *et al.* (2005) Isolation of *Aspergillus spp* from the respiratory tract in critically ill patients: risk factors, clinical presentation and outcome. *Critical Care (London, England)*, **9**, 191–199.

Gefter, W.B., Albelda, S.M., Talbot, G.H. *et al.* (1985) Invasive pulmonary aspergillosis and acute leukemia: limitations in the diagnostic utility of the air crescent sing. *Radiology*, **157**, 605–610.

Grasser, Y., Klare, I., Halle, E. *et al.* (1993) Epidemiological study of an *Acinetobacter baumannii* outbreak by using polymerase chain reaction fingerprinting. *Journal of Clinical Microbiology*, **31**, 2417–2420.

Hafezi-Moghadam, A., Simoncini, T., Yang, Z. *et al.* (2002) Acute cardiovascular protective effect of corticosteroid are mediated by non-transcriptional activation of endothelial nitric oxide synthase. *Nature Medicine*, **8**, 473–479.

Hellmann, D.B., Petri, M. and Whiting-O'Keefe, Q. (1987) Fatal infections in systemic lupus erythematosis: the role of opportunistic organisms. *Medicine*, **66**, 341–348.

Hohenadel, I.A., Kiworr, M., Genitsariotis, R. *et al.* (2001) Role of bronchoalveolar lavage in immunocompromised patients with pneumonia treated with a broad spectrum antibiotic and antifungal regimen. *Thorax*, **56**, 115–120.

Hughes, W.T., Feldman, S., Aur, R.J. *et al.* (1975) Intensity of immunosuppressive therapy and the incidence of Pneumocystis carinii pneumonia. *Cancer*, **36**, 2004–2009.

Ikura, Y., Matsuo, T., Ogami, M. *et al.* (2000) Cytomegalovirus associated pancreatitis in a patient with systemic lupus erythematosus. *The Journal of Rheumatology*, **27**, 2715–2717.

Jagger, M.P., Huo, Z. and Riches, P.G. (2002) Inflammatory cytokine (interleukin-6 and tumor necrosis factor alpha) release in a human whole blood system in response to *Streptococcus pneumoniae* serotype 14 and its capsular polysaccharide. *Clinical and Experimental Immunology*, **130**, 467–474.

Jantz, M.A. and Sahn, S.A. (1999) Corticosteroids in acute respiratory failure. *American Journal of Respiratory and Critical Care Medicine*, **160**, 1079–1100.

Jara-Palomares, L., Mateos, I., Barrot, E. and Cisneros, J.M. (2007) *Aspergillus terreus* infection in COPD patients receiving corticoids. A report of three cases. *Enfermedades Infecciosas y Microbiología Clínica*, **25**, 415–420.

Jick, S.S., Lieberman, E.S., Rahman, M.U. and Choi, H. (2006) Glucocorticoid use, other associated factors, and the risk of tuberculosis. *Arthritis & Rheumatism*, **55**, 19–26.

Jolis, R., Castella, J., Puzo, C. *et al.* (1996) Diagnostic value of protected BAL in diagnosing pulmonary infections in immunocompromised patients. *Chest*, **109**, 601–607.

Kanno, M., Chandrasekar, P.H., Bentley, G. *et al.* (2001) Disseminated cytomegalovirus disease in hosts without acquired immunodeficiency syndrome and without an organ transplant. *Clinical Infectious Diseases*, **32**, 313–316.

Kistemann, T., Hunburg, H., Exner, M. *et al.* (2002) Role of increased environmental Aspergillus exposure for patients with chronic obstructive pulmonary disease (COPD) treated with corticosteroids in a intensive care unit. *International Journal of Hygiene and Environmental Health*, **204**, 347–351.

Kontoyiannis, D.P. and Bodey, G.P. (2002) Invasive aspergillosis in 2002: an update. *European Journal of Clinical Microbiology & Infectious Diseases*, **21**, 161–172.

Leav, B.A., Fanburg, B. and Hadley, S. (2000) Invasive pulmonary aspergillosis associated with high-dose inhaled fluticasone. *The New England Journal of Medicine*, **343**, 586.

Lin, S.J., Schranz, J. and Teutsch, S.M. (2001) Aspergillosis case-fatality rate: systematic review of the literature. *Clinical Infectious Diseases*, **32**, 358–366.

Lionakis, M.S. and Kontoyiannis, D.P. (2003) Glucocorticoids and invasive fungal infections. *Lancet*, **362**, 1828–1838.

Mari, B., Montón, C., Mariscal, D. *et al.* (2001) Pulmonary nocardiosis: clinical experience in ten cases. *Respiration; International Review of Thoracic Diseases*, **68**, 382–388.

Marr, K.A., Carter, R.A., Boeckh, M. *et al.* (2002) Invasive aspergillosis in allogenic stem cell transplant recipients: changes in epidemiology and risk factors. *Blood*, **100**, 4358–4366.

Meersseman, W., Lagrou, K., Maertens, J. *et al.* (2008) Galactomannan in bronchoalveolar lavage fluid: a tool for diagnosing aspergillosis in intensive care unit patients. *American Journal of Respiratory and Critical Care Medicine*, **177** (1), 27–34.

Meersseman, W., Vandecasteele, S.J., Wilmer, A. *et al.* (2004) Invasive aspergillosis in critically ill patients without malignancies. *American Journal of Respiratory and Critical Care Medicine*, **170**, 621–625.

Menendez, R., Cordero, P.J., Santos, M., Gobernado, M. and Marco, V. (1997) Pulmonary infection with Nocardia species, a report of 10 cases and review. *The European Respiratory Journal*, **10**, 1542–1546.

Mok, M.Y., Wong, S.S., Chan, T.M. *et al.* (2007) Non-tuberculous mycobaterial infection in patients with systemic lupus erythematosis. *Rheumatology*, **46**, 280–284.

Nagata, N., Nikaido, Y., Kido, M., Ishibashi, T. and Sueishi, K. (1993) Terminal pulmonary infections in patients with lung cancer. *Chest*, **103**, 1739–1742.

Namisato, S., Motomura, K., Haranaga, S. *et al.* (2004) Pulmonary strongyloidiasis in a patient receiving prednisolone therapy. *Internal Medicine*, **43**, 731–736.

Ng, T.T., Robson, G.D. and Denning, D.W. (1994) Hydrocortisone-enhanced growth of *Aspergillus spp*; implications for pathogenesis. *Microbiology (Reading, England)*, **140**, 2475–2479.

Nichols, W.G., Guthrie, K.A., Corey, L. and Boeckh, M. (2004) Influenza infections after hemato-poietic stem cell transplantation: risk factor, mortality, and effect of antiviral therapy. *Clinical Infectious Diseases*, **39**, 1300–1306.

Noël, V., Lortholary, O., Casassus, P. *et al.* (2001) Risk factor and pronostic influence of infection in a single cohort of 87 adults with systemic lupus erythematosis. *Annals of the Rheumatic Diseases*, **60**, 1141–1144.

Nucci, M. and Colombo, A.L. (2002) Risk factors for breakthrough candidemia. *European Journal of Clinical Microbiology & Infectious Diseases*, **21**, 209–211.

Ognibene, F.P., Shelhamer, J.H., Hoffman, G.S. *et al.* (1995) *Pneumocystis carinii* pneumonia: a major complication of immunosuppressive therapy in patients with Wegener's granulomatosis. *American Journal of Respiratory and Critical Care Medicine*, **151**, 795–799.

Palmer, L.B., Greenberg, H.E. and Schiff, M.J. (1991) Corticosteroid treatment as a risk factor for invasive aspergillosis in patients with lung disease. *Thorax*, **46**, 15–20.

Perfect, J.R., Cox, G.M., Lee, J.Y. *et al.*, Mycoses Study Group (2001) The impact of culture isolation of Aspergillus species: a hospital-based survey of Aspergillosis. *Clinical Infectious Diseases*, **33**, 1824–1833.

Peter, E., Bakri, F., Ball, D.M. *et al.* (2002) Invasive pulmonary filamentous fungal infection in a patient receiving inhaled corticosteroid therapy. *Clinical Infectious Diseases*, **35**, 54–56.

Philippe, B., Ibrahim-Granet, O., Prévost, M.C. *et al.* (2003) Killing of *Aspergillus fumigatus* by alveolar macrophages is mediated by reactive oxidant intermediates. *Infection and Immunity*, **71**, 3034–3042.

Pittet, D., Huguenin, T., Dharan, S. *et al.* (1996) Unusual cause of lethal pulmonary aspergillosis in patients with chronic obstructive pulmonary disease. *American Journal of Respiratory and Critical Care Medicine*, **154**, 541–544.

Prince, D.S., Peterson, D.D., Steiner, R.M. *et al.* (1989) Infection with mycobacterium avium complex in patients without predisposing conditions. *The New England Journal of Medicine*, **321**, 863–868.

Queipo, J.A., Broseta, E., Santos, M. *et al.* (2003) Mycobacterial infection in a series of 1261 renal transplant recipients. *Clinical Microbiology and Infection*, **9**, 518–525.

Rano, A., Agusti, C., Benito, N. *et al.* (2002) Prognostic factors of non-HIV immunocompromised patients with pulmonary infiltrates. *Chest*, **122**, 253–261.

Rano, A., Agusti, C., Jimenez, P. *et al.* (2001) Pulmonary infiltrates in non-HIV immunocompromised patients: a diagnostic approach using non-invasive and bronchoscopic procedures. *Thorax*, **56**, 379–387.

Rello, J., Esandi, M.E., Mariscal, D. *et al.* (1998) Invasive pulmonary aspergillosis in patients with chronic obstructive pulmonary disease: report of eight cases and review. *Clinical Infectious Diseases*, **26**, 1473.

Remiszewski, P., Slodkowska, J., Wiatr, E. *et al.* (2001) Fatal infection in patients treated for small lung cancer in the Institute of tuberculosis and Chest Diseases in the years 1980–1994. *Lung Cancer (Amsterdam, Netherlands)*, **31**, 101–110.

Rodrigues, J., Niederman, M., Fein, A. *et al.* (1992) Nonresolving pneumonia in steroid-treated patients with obstructive lung disease. *The American Journal of Medicine*, **93**, 29–34.

Roilides, E., Uhlig, K., Venzon, D. *et al.* (1993) Prevention of corticosteroid-induced suppression of human polymorphonuclear leukocyte-induced damage of *Aspergillus fumigatus* hypahe by granu-locyte-stimulating factor and gamma interferon. *Infection and Immunity*, **61**, 4870–4877.

Sen, R.P., Walsh, T.E., Fisher, W. and Brock, N. (1991) Pulmonary complications of combination therapy with cyclophosphamide and prednisone. *Chest*, **99**, 143–146.

Sepkowitz, K.A., Brown, A.E. and Amstrong, D. (1995) *Pneumocystis carinii* pneumonia without acquired immunodeficiency symdrome: more patients, same risk. *Archives of Internal Medicine*, **155**, 1125–1128.

Sternberg, R.I., Baughman, R.P. and Dohn, M.N. (1993) Utility of bronchoalveolar lavage in assessing pneumonia in immunosuppressed renal transplant recipients. *The American Journal of Medicine*, **95**, 358–364.

Stevens, D.L. (1995) Cytokines: an updated compendium. *Current Opinion in Infectious Diseases*, **8**, 175–180.

Stover, D.E., Zaman, M.B., Hajdu, S.I. *et al.* (1984) Bronchoalveolar lavage in diagnosis of diffuse pulmonary infiltrates in the immunocompromised host. *Annals of Internal Medicine*, **101**, 1–7.

Stuck, A.E., Minder, C.E. and Frey, F.J. (1989) Risk of infectious complications in patients taking glucocorticoids. *Reviews of Infectious Diseases*, **69**, 954–963.

Trof, R.J., Beishuizen, A., Debets-Ossenkopp, Y.J. *et al.* (2007) Management of invasive pulmonary aspergillosis in non-neutropenic critically ill patients. *Intensive Care Medicine*, **33**, 1694–1703.

Ullmer, E., Mayr, M., Bidet, I. *et al.* (2000) Granulomatous *Pneumocystis carinii* pneumonia in Wegener's granulomatosis. *The European Respiratory Journal*, **15**, 213–216.

Walsh, T., Lee, J., Lecciones, J. *et al.* (1991) Empiric therapy with amphotericin B in febrile granulocytopenic patients. *Reviews of Infectious Diseases*, **13**, 496–503.

Weinstock, D.M., Feinstein, M.B., Sepkowitz, K.A. *et al.* (2003) High rates of infection and colonization by nontuberculous mycobacteria after allogeneic hematopoietic stem cell transplantation. *Bone Marrow Transplant*, **31**, 1015–1021.

Wiest, P.M. Flanigan T., Salata, R.A. *et al.* (1989) Serious complications of corticosteroid therapy for COPD. *Chest*, **95**, 1180–1184.

Xaubet, A., Torres, A., Marco, F. *et al.* (1989) Pulmonary infiltrates in immunocompromised patients. Diagnostic value of telescoping plugged catheter and bronchoalveolar lavage. *Chest*, **95**, 130–135.

Yu, V.L., Muder, R.R. and Poorsattar, A. (1986) Significance of isolation of *aspergillus* from the respiratory tract in diagnosis of invasive pulmonary aspergillosis results from a three-year prospective study. *The American Journal of Medicine*, **81**, 249–254.

11

Intensive care management in the immunocompromised patient with pulmonary infiltrates

Gilles Hilbert, Didier Gruson and Frederic Vargas

Division of Medical Intensive Care, University Hospital, Bordeaux

In immunocompromised patients with acute respiratory failure (ARF), the recourse to mechanical ventilation remains associated with a raised mortality, even if the prognosis has improved during the last decade. Mechanical ventilation is an independent prognostic factor of mortality in immunocompromised patients; thus, to avoid intubation must remain a major objective in this pathology. After several studies showing the feasibility, two prospective randomized and controlled studies demonstrated that noninvasive ventilation (NIV) made it possible to improve the outcome in selected immunocompromised patients admitted to the intensive care unit. The method is mainly validated among patients of onco-haematology, and complementary studies would be useful among patients with other types of immunosuppression.

ARF in immunocompromised patients is a recognized indication of NIV, and according to recent international recommendations (of level I), NIV should be used whenever possible in this indication to reduce the risk of nosocomial pneumonia. Above all, NIV makes it possible to reduce the mortality of the patients of onco-haematology with ARF. The prognosis is still improved when a diagnosis of pneumonitis can be retained, and the bronchoscopy can be carried out directly under NIV among the more hypoxemic patients.

Undoubtedly, ARF in immunocompromised patients belongs to the indications of NIV which require experiment and a good control of the technique justifying, in this indication, to practice NIV in intensive care units.

11.1   Introduction

Pulmonary complications are an important cause of illness in immunocompromised patients and contribute substantially to the mortality associated with various types of

Pulmonary Infection in the Immunocompromised Patient, Edited by Carlos Agustí and Antoni Torres
© 2009 John Wiley & Sons, Ltd.

immunosuppression (Estopa *et al.*, 1984; Masur, Shelhamer and Parrillo, 1985). Pulmonary infiltrates commonly appear following chemotherapy, solid-organ transplant and haematopoietic stem-cell transplantation. With the increasing use of these treatment modalities and the growing potency of immunosuppressive regimens, physicians will more frequently be asked to evaluate and to care for these individuals. This, in particular, implies the physicians working in intensive care unit (ICU) when the respiratory failure occurs among these patients.

In ICU, strategies for management include both a specific approach, in terms of diagnosis tools and treatment regimens used, and a symptomatic approach, in terms essentially of treatment of acute respiratory failure (ARF). The diagnostic approach and the specific treatments of pulmonary infiltrates in the immunosuppressed patient are treated extensively elsewhere in the present book. Thus, we will discuss here the symptomatic approach of these patients with pulmonary infiltrates responsible for the ARF and requiring a management in ICU. Classically, these recipients frequently required intubation and mechanical ventilatory assistance. Too often, this intervention has been followed by further, ultimately fatal complications, including sepsis. Although invasive mechanical ventilation is highly effective and reliable in supporting alveolar ventilation, endotracheal intubation is associated with numerous risks of complications (Stauffer, 1994). Furthermore, in immunocompromised patients, mechanical ventilation is associated with a significant risk of death (Ewig *et al.*, 1998; Gruson *et al.*, 1999; Bach *et al.*, 2001; Kroschinsky *et al.*, 2002; Rano *et al.*, 2002). Thus, avoiding intubation should be an important objective in the management of hypoxemic acute ARF in immunosuppressed patients.

11.2   Invasive ventilation

Invasive ventilation concerns patients who are transferred to the ICU and who have been previously intubated and recipients who need a prompt intubation after admission and after a noninvasive ventilation (NIV) trial in other patients.

In immunocompromised patients, ARF has most often the features of acute lung injury (ALI) or acute respiratory distress syndrome (ARDS) mainly from pneumonia. Therefore, the ventilatory management of respiratory failure in these patients has to face one of the most severe lung diseases. Due to the lack of studies specifically dedicated to the treatment of ALI/ARDS in immunosuppressed patients, the general recommendations concern also this category of critically ill patients (Tobin, 2001; Anon, 2000). A recent study from the NIH demonstrated that the use of a low tidal volume (6 mL/kg of predicted body weight) reduces mortality compared to a traditional tidal volume (12 mL/kg of predicted body weight) (Anon, 2000). In this study, the positive end expiratory pressure (PEEP) level was individualized according to a predefined sequence correlated with the inspired fraction of oxygen. Briefly, several studies demonstrated that keeping the end-inspiratory plateau pressure below 30–35 cm H_2O and using low tidal volumes to avoid alveolar over distension are important goals of mechanical ventilation during ALI/ARDS; when low tidal volumes are used, the application of a high PEEP level keeping the end-inspiratory pressure below 30–35 cm H_2O, is needed to avoid lung derecruitment.

Although invasive mechanical ventilation is highly effective and reliable in supporting alveolar ventilation, endotracheal intubation is associated with numerous risks of complications. Complications of endotracheal intubation include upper-airway injuries, tracheal stenosis, tracheomalacia, sinusitis and ventilator-associated pneumonia (Stauffer, 1994). Furthermore, in immunocompromised patients, mechanical ventilation is associated with a significant risk of death (Ewig et al., 1998; Gruson et al., 1999; Bach et al., 2001; Kroschinsky et al., 2002; Rano et al., 2002; Soubani et al., 2004). Even if over the last years, overall survival rates of immunocompromised patients admitted to the ICU are improving, with, in part, the benefits of NIV in selected patients, leading the best experts to defend the concept to 'do everything that can be done', the negative impact of intubation and mechanical ventilation has been confirmed in several recent studies. In one particular study, in patients with haematological malignancy, the overall mortality in ICU was 44%, only 12% in patients without mechanical ventilation, but 74% among those under mechanical ventilation ($p < 0.001$); multivariate analysis revealed mechanical ventilation and SAPS II as independent prognostic factors of both ICU mortality and long-term survival (Kroschinsky et al., 2002). In their literature review, Soubani et al. evidenced clearly that the lower the percentage of patients receiving mechanical ventilation, the higher the survival rate (Soubani et al., 2004).

So, ARF was often seen by oncologists as the terminal stage of illness, this vision being based on these studies indicating a very low survival rate despite a heavy investment. On the other hand, a large proportion of these patients with ARF was refused by physicians of ICU, well aware that intubation with mechanical ventilation is a strong predictor of mortality in this population.

In the early 1990s, hospital survival for patients with human immunodeficiency virus (HIV)-related *Pneumocystis carinii* pneumonia and ARF, was very low, at around 20%. In a more recent study on 155 HIV patients intubated and mechanically ventilated for ARF, hospital mortality was 62% and still 80% in patients who received previously prophylaxis for *Pneumocystis carinii* (Randall Curtis et al., 2000).

Thus, avoiding intubation should remain a major objective in the management of hypoxemic ARF in immunocompromised patients.

11.3 Rationale for NIV

Above all, as detailed in the previous chapter, a major driving force behind the increasing use of NIV has been the desire to avoid the complications of invasive ventilation.

NIV uses a tight-fitting face mask as an alternative interface between the patient and the ventilator to avoid these complications. In contrast to invasive ventilation, NIV leaves the upper airway intact, preserves airway defence mechanisms, and allows patients to eat, drink, verbalize and expectorate secretions. The development of improved masks and ventilator technology made this mode of ventilation acceptable.

Several controlled studies have clearly demonstrated the benefits of NIV in acute exacerbations of chronic obstructive pulmonary disease (COPD) and, as stated in the conclusions
of the recent international consensus conference considering the role of NIV in ARF,
patients hospitalized for exacerbations of COPD with rapid clinical deterioration should be
considered for NIV to prevent further deterioration in gas exchange, respiratory workload,
and the need for endotracheal intubation (Anon, 2001). Starting from the good results
obtained in patients with acute exacerbations of COPD, NIV is now being used to support
those with hypoxemic ARF, certain of them with ALI or ARDS. Nevertheless, by contrast
with COPD patients with acute exacerbation who constitute a relatively homogeneous
group of patients, those with hypoxemic ARF constitute a much more heterogeneous group.
Overall, in patients with hypoxemic ARF, experience is less extensive than in COPD
patients. The consensus conference concluded that larger, controlled studies are required to
determine the potential benefit of adding NIV to standard medical treatment in the
avoidance of endotracheal intubation in hypoxemic ARF (Anon, 2001).

11.4   Mechanisms of improvement with NIV in immunocompromised patients with acute respiratory failure

In patients with hypoxemic ARF, intrapulmonary shunt and ventilation-perfusion
imbalances may cause life-threatening hypoxemia. Moreover, high work of breathing
from increased alveolar dead space and reduced respiratory system compliance may
cause ventilatory failure with hypercapnia and respiratory acidosis. When employed
during episodes of hypoxemic ARF, the goal of NIV is to ensure an adequate PaO_2 until
the underlying problem can be reversed.

Numerous case series and reports have shown that continuous positive airway pressure
(CPAP) (Greenbaum et al., 1976; Smith et al., 1980; Kesten and Rebuck, 1988; Gregg et al.,
1990; Brett and Sinclair, 1993; Hilbert et al., 2000; Covelli, Weled and Beekam, 1982) and
NIV (Confalonieri et al., 2002) improve oxygenation, reduce respiratory rate, and lessen
dyspnea in hypoxemic ARF. Kesten et al. applied 10 cm H_2O of nasal CPAP in nine subjects
with *Pneumocystis carinii* pneumonia and the acquired immunodeficiency syndrome
(AIDS), all of whom had presented with bilateral pulmonary infiltrates and hypoxemia
(Kesten and Rebuck, 1988). Twenty minutes of nasal CPAP without supplemental oxygen
increased mean PaO_2 from 56 to 68 mm Hg and decreased the calculated alveolar-arterial
oxygen gradient from 48 to 34 mm Hg. Confalonieri et al. have compared NIV vs. invasive
mechanical ventilation in AIDS patients with *Pneumocystis carinii* pneumonia (Confalonieri et al., 2002). Changes in arterial blood gas and respiratory rate were comparable in
the two groups of patients during the first 72 hours of the study.

Several prospective controlled studies, comparing CPAP or NIV with standard
medical treatment, have shown that use of these methods of ventilation in hypoxemic
ARF was associated with prompt improvement in pulmonary gas exchange as determined by arterial blood gases obtained within the first few hours (Antonelli et al., 1998;
Antonelli et al., 2000; Delclaux et al., 2000; Hilbert et al., 2001a). Antonelli et al.

conducted a prospective, randomized trial of NIV as compared with endotracheal intubation with conventional mechanical ventilation in 64 patients with hypoxemic ARF who required mechanical ventilation (Antonelli *et al.*, 1998). Seven (22%) of 32 patients randomized to NIV had ARDS of varied etiology. The patients in the two groups had a similar initial change in PaO_2/FiO_2: Within the first hour of ventilation, 20 patients (62%) in the NIV group and 15 (47%) in the conventional ventilation group had an improvement in PaO_2/FiO_2. Their PaO_2/FiO_2 ratios increased significantly from 116 ± 24 to 230 ± 76 mmHg with NIV and from 124 ± 25 to 211 ± 68 mmHg with conventional ventilation. In a study comparing NIV with standard treatment using supplemental oxygen administration in recipients of solid organ transplantation with hypoxemic ARF, 7 (22%) of 32 patients randomized to NIV had ARDS of varied etiology (Antonelli *et al.*, 2000). Within the first hour of treatment, 14 patients (70%) in the NIV group, and only 5 patients (25%) in the standard treatment group improved their ratio PaO_2/FiO_2. In another randomized controlled trial, the physiologic effects of CPAP vs. standard oxygen therapy were compared in 123 patients with hypoxemic ARF, and $PaO_2/FiO_2 \leq 300$ due to bilateral pulmonary oedema, 102 of them with ALI (Delclaux *et al.*, 2000). After one hour of treatment, median PaO_2/FiO_2 were greater with CPAP (203 vs. 151, $p = 0.02$). In a prospective, randomized trial of NIV, as compared with standard medical treatment with supplemental oxygen in immunosuppressed patients with hypoxemic ARF, initial improvement in PaO_2/FiO_2 was observed in 46% in the NIV group and in 15% in the standard group ($p = 0.02$) (Hilbert *et al.*, 2001a). Even if NIV was used intermittently, in a sequential mode, the protocol of NIV used in this study achieved significantly higher rates of improvement in gas exchange abnormalities, than in patients with standard treatment. Reducing the workload of breathing during noninvasive ventilation sessions may also allow respiratory muscles to be more efficient during non-assisted breaths.

NIV can improve the patho-physiology of hypoxemic respiratory failure. Mechanisms of improvement can include the beneficial effects of PEEP on distribution of extravascular lung water, on alveolar recruitment of under ventilated alveoli by increasing lung volume at end of expiration, and in early treatment of atelectasis. In addition, improvements in ventilation/perfusion ratios or even shunt undoubtedly occur in patients with ARDS, in whom the application of expiratory pressure should have an effect similar to that of PEEP in invasively ventilated patients. By lowering left ventricular transmural pressure, CPAP may reduce afterload and increase cardiac output, making it an attractive modality for therapy of acute pulmonary oedema. Even if CPAP alone is able to improve lung mechanics in patients with ARF and decrease work of breathing compared with unsupported ventilation (Katz and Marks, 1985), the addition of pressure-support (PS) has a positive effect in reducing work of breathing and maintaining a tidal volume compatible with adequate alveolar ventilation.

11.5 Clinical studies

The main studies on NIV in immunocompromised patients with hypoxemic ARF are reported in Table 11.1.

Table 11.1   Studies examining the efficacy of NIV in immunocompromised patients hypoxemic acute respiratory failure.

Refs	No. of patients	Particularities	Mask ventilatory mode	Intubation rate (%) NIV/Standard
Tognet *et al.*, 1994	18	Haematological + + Neutropenia	Nasal PS-PEEP	67
Conti *et al.*, 1998	16	Haematological Intubation criteria	Nasal PS-PEEP	31
Bedos *et al.*, 1999	66	*Pneumocystis carinii* pneumonia	Facial CPAP	32
Confalonieri *et al.*, 2002	24	*Pneumocystis carinii* pneumonia Case control study	Facial PS-PEEP	33
Azoulay *et al.*, 2001	48	Cancer (+ + Haematological)	PS-PEEP	56
Rocco *et al.*, 2004	38	Immunosuppressed patients Case control study	Helmet vs. Facial PS-PEEP	42
Hilbert *et al.*, 2000	64	Haematological Neutropenia	Facial CPAP	75
Antonelli *et al.*, 2000[a]	40	Solid organ transplantation $PaO_2/FiO_2 \leq 200$	Facial PS-PEEP	20/70
Hilbert *et al.*, 2001a[a]	52	Immunosuppressed patients $PaO_2/FiO_2 \leq 200$	Facial PS-PEEP	46/77

PS: Pressure Support; PEEP: positive end expiratory pressure; CPAP: continuous positive airway pressure; Standard: standard medical treatment related to the etiology of hypoxemic acute respiratory failure with O_2 supplementation.
[a]prospective, randomized, controlled studies.

Prospective nonrandomized studies

CPAP has been used successfully for years to correct severe hypoxemia in immuno-compromised patients with hypoxemic ARF (Kesten and Rebuck, 1988; Gregg *et al.*, 1990; Bedos *et al.*, 1999; Hilbert *et al.*, 2000). Gregg *et al.* studied the efficacy of CPAP in 10 AIDS patients with pneumonia and avoided intubation in seven of them (Gregg *et al.*, 1990). Bedos *et al.* reported data for 110 consecutive patients with ARF secondary to AIDS-related *Pneumocystis carinii* pneumonia and who were admitted to an ICU within 24 hrs after their hospital admission (Bedos *et al.*, 1999). CPAP was used initially in 66 (60%) patients and failed in 22 (32%) patients who received mechanical ventilation; 20 of these 22 patients died. These data suggest that CPAP with a face mask could be a safe and effective means of providing ventilatory support to patients with severe *Pneumocystis carinii* pneumonia and probably avoids intubation and its high mortality rate in a subgroup of less acutely ill patients. Among the 64 neutropenic patients with febrile acute hypoxemic normocapnic respiratory failure treated by CPAP in addition to standard therapy in the study by Hilbert *et al.*, CPAP was efficient in only 25% of cases (Hilbert *et al.*, 2000). The enrolled patients were critically ill, with a PaO_2/ FiO_2 ratio of 128 ± 32, and with a high SAPS II and more than two organ dysfunctions, explaining, in part, the poor results obtained. Nevertheless, all the responders and only four non responders survived their ICU stay. More recently, Confalonieri *et al.* have compared NIV vs. invasive mechanical ventilation in AIDS patients with *Pneumocystis carinii* pneumonia-related ARF needing mechanical ventilation (Confalonieri *et al.*, 2002). Twenty-four patients treated with NIV by a facial mask were matched with 24 patients treated with invasive ventilation by endotracheal intubation. Use of NIV avoided intubation in 67% of patients. Even if the existence of criteria of ARDS were not reported, all the patients were at a very advanced stage of ARF since they presented criteria of intubation. The NIV-treated group had a lower mortality in the ICU, the hospital and within two months of study entry. Differences in mortality between the two groups disappeared after six months. The findings of this study provide further support for applying NIV in AIDS patients with severe *Pneumocystis carinii* pneumonia-related ARF as a first-line therapeutic choice, but randomized controlled trials are required to confirm these results.

Tognet *et al.* have reported very early their experience of NIV in 18 hematological patients with ARF which occurred before, during or just after therapeutic aplasia (Tognet *et al.*, 1994). NIV, with a PS mode and preferably a nasal mask, was performed intermittently. Twelve patients were ultimately intubated and died. Seven needed intubation within three hours following admission (because of the inability of NIV to provide adequate ventilation in six patients). Six patients were not intubated and were discharged alive.

Conti *et al.* have evaluated treatment with NIV by nasal mask as an alternative to endotracheal intubation and conventional mechanical ventilation in 16 patients with haematological malignancies complicated by ARF and having intubation criteria (at inclusion, $PaO_2/FiO_2 = 87 \pm 22$) (Conti *et al.*, 1998). NIV was delivered via nasal mask by means of a BiPAP ventilator. Five patients died in the ICU following complications independent of the respiratory failure, while 11 were discharged from the ICU in stable condition after a mean stay of 4.3 ± 2.4 days and were discharged from the hospital. Thus, NIV proved to be feasible and appropriate for the treatment of respiratory failure in haematological patients who were at high risk of intubation-related complications.

Azoulay *et al.* found in a matched-pair analysis of cancer patients requiring MV support that the mortality among NIV patients was significantly lower than in conventionally ventilated patients (43.7% vs. 70.8%, $p = 0.008$) (Azoulay *et al.*, 2001).

More recently, a case-control study on a total of 34 patients was performed to evaluate the effectiveness of early administration of c-PAP through a helmet, in haematological malignancy patients with ARF (Principi *et al.*, 2004). Each patient was treated by c-PAP outside an ICU, righton the haematological ward. The authors described a success rate as high as possible in patients ventilated with the helmet, while eight NIV failures were registered in the group ventilated with a face mask because of an intolerance of this interface.

Prospective randomized controlled studies

Acute respiratory failure in patients undergoing solid organ transplantation

Organ transplantation has become a therapy for an increasing population of patients with end-stage organ failure. Although preventing rejection remains the principle focus in improving overall survival statistics, pulmonary complications following transplantation are responsible for most morbidity and contribute substantially to the mortality associated with various organ transplantation procedures.

Antonelli *et al.* studied solid organ transplant recipients with hypoxemic ARF and compared NIV delivered through a face mask with standard treatment using oxygen supplementation to avoid endotracheal intubation and decrease duration of ICU stay (Antonelli *et al.*, 2000). NIV resulted in lower intubation rates (20% vs. 70%, $p = 0.002$), fewer fatal complications (20% vs. 50%, $p = 0.05$), and reduced ICU stay and mortality (20% vs. 50%, $p = 0.05$). However, hospital mortality did not differ between NIV and standard therapy groups. In a subgroup analysis, patients with ARDS randomized to NIV had an intubation rate of 38% vs. 86% in the standard treatment group ($p = 0.08$).

Immunosuppressed patients with pulmonary infiltrates, fever and acute respiratory failure

Hilbert *et al.* hypothesized that the intermittent use of NIV at an early stage of hypoxemic ARF would reduce the need for endotracheal intubation and the incidence of complications. In a prospective, randomized, controlled study, we compared the efficacy of noninvasive ventilation delivered intermittently through a mask with that of standard medical treatment with supplemental oxygen and no ventilatory support in patients with immunosuppression from various causes in whom hypoxemic ARF had been precipitated by pulmonary infiltrates and fever (Hilbert *et al.*, 2001a).

The immunosuppression could have been caused by neutropenia after chemotherapy or bone marrow transplantation in patients with haematological cancers, drug-induced immunosuppression in organ-transplant recipients or as a result of corticosteroid or cytotoxic therapy for a nonmalignant disease, or AIDS.

The patients were selected and exclusion criteria were a requirement for emergent intubation for cardiopulmonary resuscitation, respiratory arrest, or a rapid deterioration in neurological status with a Glasgow Coma Scale ≤ 8; a haemodynamic instability or electrocardiogram instability; chronic obstructive pulmonary disease; a cardiac origin of the respiratory failure, which was established by physical signs, chest-X ray and echocardiogram; a partial pressure of arterial carbon dioxide ($PaCO_2$) more than 55 mm Hg, with acidosis (pH lesser than 7.35); failure of more than two new organs;

uncorrected bleeding diathesis; and tracheotomy, a facial deformity, or recent oral, oesophageal, or gastric surgery. Patients were randomly assigned to receive either standard treatment (26 patients) or standard treatment plus NIV through a face mask (26 patients). It is important to underline that randomization was made at an early stage of the respiratory failure, well before the patients were even headed for intubation.

NIV was delivered through a face mask, in a discontinuous mode, with a protocol close to that previously described in COPD patients; that is periods of NIV lasted at least 45 minutes and alternated every three hours with periods of spontaneous breathing (Hilbert *et al.*, 1997; Hilbert *et al.*, 1998). Between periods of ventilation, patients breathed oxygen spontaneously while SaO_2 was continuously monitored. NIV was automatically resumed when the arterial oxygen saturation was less than 85% or when dyspnea worsened, as evidenced by a respiratory rate of more than 30 breaths per minute.

During the first 24 hours, NIV was administered for a mean of 9 ± 3 hours. Subsequently, the mean duration of NIV was 7 ± 3 hours per day. The mean duration of NIV was 4 ± 2 days.

The rates of initial and sustained improvement in PaO_2/FiO_2 and other outcomes in both groups are reported in Table 11.2. In the NIV group, as compared with standard therapy, fewer patients required endotracheal intubation (12 vs. 20, $p = 0.03$) and there were fewer complications (13 vs. 21, $p = 0.02$). Overall, with NIV, there were improvements in mortality in the ICU (10 vs. 18, $p = 0.03$) and in total in-hospital mortality (13 vs. 21, $p = 0.02$).

Discussion

Neutropenia in patients with haematological malignancies was the most frequent type of immunosuppression in patients included in this last study (Hilbert *et al.*, 2001a). If NIV enabled us to avoid intubation in 'only' 47% of neutropenic patients, this rate was significantly higher than in the standard treatment group (7%, $p = 0.02$). Very high rates of mortality are recorded in patients with haematological malignancies admitted to an ICU, more particularly if they are neutropenic and if intubation and mechanical ventilation are necessary (Estopa *et al.*, 1984; Ewig *et al.*, 1998; Gruson *et al.*, 1999; Bach *et al.*, 2001; Rano *et al.*, 2002; Kroschinsky *et al.*, 2002; Soubani *et al.*, 2004; Rubenfeld and Crawford, 1996). The risk of complications of invasive mechanical ventilation is related to the duration of ventilatory support (Keenan, 1997). Recent prospective trials have shown the advantage of NIV in significantly reducing the incidence density of nosocomial pneumonia, by comparison with conventional intubation and positive pressure ventilation (Anon, 2005). It is important to note that ventilator-associated pneumonia was associated with in-ICU death in 100% of cases in both randomized controlled studies dealing with immunocompromised patients (Antonelli *et al.*, 2000; Hilbert *et al.*, 2001a).

In the study by Antonelli *et al.*, the eight ARDS patients randomized to NIV had an intubation rate of 37.5% and a mortality rate of 37% (Antonelli *et al.*, 2000). Few studies have reported on the application of NIV in ARDS. In another study by the same group,

Table 11.2   Outcome variables in the study by (Hilbert *et al.*, 2001a).

	Noninvasive ventilation group (*n* = 26)	Standard treatment group (*n* = 26)	*P* Value
Patients requiring intubation	12 (46%)	20 (77%)	0.03
Intubation by type of immunosuppression:			
Haematologic malignancy and neutropenia	8/15 (53%)	14/15 (93%)	0.02
Drug-induced immunodepression	3/9 (33%)	5/9 (56%)	0.32
Acquired Immuno deficiency Syndrome	1/2	1/2	
ICU^a deaths	10 (38%)	18 (69%)	0.03
ICU deaths per sub-population			
Haematologic malignancy and neutropenia	7/15 (47%)	13/15 (87%)	0.02
Drug-induced immunodepression	3/9 (33%)	4/9 (44%)	0.50
Acquired Immunodeficiency Syndrome	0/2	1/2	
Length of stay in ICU (in days)	7 ± 3	10 ± 4	0.06
Hospital deaths	13 (50%)	21 (81%)	0.02
Hospital deaths per sub-population			
Haematologic malignancy and neutropenia	8/15 (53%)	14/15 (93%)	0.02
Drug-induced immunodepression	4/9 (44%)	6/9 (67%)	0.32
Acquired Immunodeficiency Syndrome	1/2	1/2	

Values are presented as mean ± SD.
^{a}ICU: intensive care unit.

7 out of 32 patients randomized to NIV had ARDS. Four of the seven patients with ARDS avoided intubation and survived, while three patients required intubation and died. Only one trial enrolled exclusively patients with ALI/ARDS. Rocker *et al.*, in an uncontrolled study, reported the outcome of 12 episodes of ALI/ARDS in 10 patients treated with NIV (Rocker *et al.*, 1999). Overall success rate for NIV trials was 50%. In detail, avoidance of intubation was achieved on 6 out of 9 occasions (66%) when NIV was used as the initial mode of assisted ventilation; it failed after three episodes of planned (Masur, Shelhamer and Parrillo, 1985) or self (Estopa *et al.*, 1984) extubation. These encouraging results showed that NIV should be considered as a treatment option for patients in stable condition in the early phase of ALI/ARDS. The studies published to date should provide the rationale for prospective randomized studies.

Both trials showed that early application of NIV was well tolerated and helped avert the need for endotracheal intubation and improved the outcomes in selected immuno-compromised patients with hypoxemic ARF (Antonelli *et al.*, 2000; Hilbert *et al.*, 2001a). The authors used intermittent NIV, since the onset of management (Hilbert *et al.*, 2001a) or after the first 24 hours of treatment (Antonelli *et al.*, 2000), at a less advanced stage of hypoxemic ARF than in other studies that assessed the value of NIV in patients who met the criteria for intubation (Antonelli *et al.*, 1998; Conti *et al.*, 1998). On the basis of our previous experience, we use NIV in a sequential mode (Hilbert *et al.*, 2000; Hilbert *et al.*, 1997; Hilbert *et al.*, 1998). This mode is a discontinuous mode, with some specificity that is the predetermination of the duration of the ventilation sessions and of the time between the NIV sessions. One of the potential advantages of the sequential approach are a harmonious distribution of NIV sessions, a better acceptance and tolerance for the patients, and a better management by nursing staff. The protocol of sequential ventilation is appreciated by our staff and has contributed to the standardization of techniques of NIV in our ICU. It has not been necessary to modify the organization of our unit since the introduction of these new techniques.

Both randomized controlled studies dealing with immunocompromised patients have several limitations (Antonelli *et al.*, 2000; Hilbert *et al.*, 2001a). It is impossible to eliminate bias when a study cannot be blinded, and the studies included only selected patients with immunosuppression who were treated in a single ICU. Furthermore, all the patients in the study by Hilbert *et al.* were transferred to the ICU directly from medical wards. Some oncology units are set up as mini-ICUs and only patients whose condition is unstable are transferred to the typical ICU. Further studies are needed to refine the process of selecting patients for treatment with NIV.

NIV as a means of assisting ventilation during fibreoptic bronchoscopy

It is important to establish the specific causes of an immunocompromised patient's pulmonary disease so that specific therapy can be instituted. Furthermore, a positive diagnosis and a well adapted treatment could be the main determinants in the improved outcome of immunosuppressed patients managed with NIV (Hilbert *et al.*, 2001a). Consequently, fibreoptic bronchoscopy and bronchoalveolar lavage are major tools in diagnosing diffuse infiltrates that often occur in association with fever and new onset of respiratory symptoms in immunosuppressed patients (Hilbert *et al.*, 2001a; Stover *et al.*, 1984; Gruson *et al.*, 2000).

Nevertheless, although there is no absolute contraindication to this procedure, severe hypoxemia is an accepted contraindication to fibreoptic bronchoscopy in non intubated patients. The American Thoracic Society recommends avoiding bronchoalveolar lavage in patients who are breathing spontaneously with hypercapnia and/or hypoxemia that cannot be corrected to a PaO_2 of ≥ 75 mm Hg with supplemental oxygen.

In a study on eight immunosuppressed patients with suspected pneumonia and PaO_2/FiO_2 of ≤ 100, Antonelli *et al.* assessed the feasibility and safety of fibreoptic bronchoscopy with NIV (Antonelli *et al.*, 1996). They found that NIV during bronchoscopy was well-tolerated, significantly improved the PaO_2/FiO_2 ratio, and successfully avoided the need for endotracheal intubation. Another recent study, of 46 patients, suggests that the application of another non invasive interface that is the laryngeal mask airway, also appears to be a safe and effective alternative to intubation for accomplishing bronchoscopy with bronchoalveolar lavage in immunosuppressed patients with suspected pneumonia and severe hypoxemia ($PaO_2/FiO_2 \leq 125$) (Hilbert *et al.*, 2001b). In a recent prospective randomized trial on 26 patients, NIV was shown superior to conventional oxygen supplementation in preventing gas exchange deterioration, and with better haemodynamic tolerance, during fibreoptic bronchoscopy in patients with less severe forms of hypoxemia ($PaO_2/FiO_2 < 200$) (Antonelli *et al.*, 2002a). In this study, PS was 15 to 17 cm H_2O, PEEP was set at 5 cm H_2O and FiO_2 at 0.9; the session of NIV was started 10 minutes before the fibreoptic bronchoscopy and continued at least 30 minutes after the procedure. We currently have the same approach.

11.6   Equipment and techniques: particularities in immunocompromised patients

The time suitable to appreciate improvement or on the contrary NIV 'failure', may depend on many factors. The lack of ARF resolving at one to two hours makes it possible to individualize the patients for whom the efforts to try improving adaptation and outcome must be most important. Thus, consider if it could be possible to ameliorate several factors that can improve adaptation of the patient on NIV and the outcome of the technique. This reasoning is helpful within the first few hours of NIV when the patient needs to adapt, and also later when prolonged ventilation is required.

Many factors may be improved. Some of them are well known and similar to those we consider when PS with PEEP is used in intubated patients. Several others are more specific to NIV.

Interface

NIV can be administered to immunocompromised patients with different types of interface. The patient interface most commonly employed is a full-face or nasal mask secured firmly, but not tightly, with a head strap (Anon, 2001). The full-face mask delivers higher ventilation pressures with fewer leaks, requires less patient cooperation, and permits mouth breathing. However, it is less comfortable, increases the dead space, impedes communication, and limits oral intake. The nasal mask needs patent nasal passages and requires mouth closure to minimize air leaks. The leaks through the mouth decrease alveolar ventilation and may decrease the efficacy of NIV to reduce the work of breathing. Furthermore, high flows of gas passing through the nose in case of mouth leaks can markedly increase nasal resistance and thus further reduce the efficacy of nasal NIV (Richards et al., 1996).

Patients may develop complications related to the use of NIV such as skin necrosis, gastric distention, nosocomial pneumonia, or evidence of barotrauma (pneumothorax, pneumomediastinum, pneumoperitoneum, or pulmonary interstitial emphysema). Data from the literature, and observations from our practice, suggest a high incidence of facial-skin breakdown and/or intolerance of the interface in the subgroup of patients with hypoxemic ARF and hematological malignancies. The incidence of pressure necrosis of the skin over the nasal bridge reached 31% in an uncontrolled study (Conti et al., 1998). Three patients were excluded from the study by Hilbert et al. because they refused to keep the facial mask on during the first CPAP session (Hilbert et al., 2000). The reason was acute stress in one case and major painful mucositis in two cases. A bad tolerance of CPAP was reported in five other patients enrolled in this study and who were intubated. Mask intolerance because of pain, discomfort, or claustrophobia may require discontinuation of NIV and endotracheal intubation.

Various modifications are available to minimize this complication such as use of forehead spacers or the addition of a thin plastic flap that permits air sealing with less mask pressure on the nose. Straps that hold the mask in place are also important for patient comfort, and many types of strap assemblies are available. Most manufacturers provide straps that are designed for use with a particular mask. More points of attachment add to stability, and strap systems with Velcro fasteners are useful.

There is no evidence to support the use of particular patient interface devices in patients with hypoxemic ARF (Anon, 2001). Nevertheless, clinical experience suggests that full-face masks improve efficacy by reducing leaks and are more appropriate for use in the setting of severe hypoxemic ARF. As shown in Table 11.1, a facial mask was used preferentially in the studies examining the efficacy of NIV in immunocompromised patients with hypoxemic ARF.

The fact that most NIV failures are due to technical problems, justifies the recent studies which evaluated new interface devices. Attempting to improve tolerability of patients, Antonelli et al. adopted a transparent *helmet* made from latex-free polyvinyl chloride that allows patients to see, read and speak as an interface during NIV. They conducted a prospective trial, with a matched control group, in order to investigate the efficacy of NIV using the helmet to treat patients with hypoxemic ARF (Antonelli et al., 2002b). Six patients (18%) in the helmet group and nine patients (13%) in the facial mask group had ARDS. Eight patients (24%) in the helmet group and 21 patients (32%) in the facial mask group failed NIV and were intubated. No patients failed NIV because of intolerance of the technique in the helmet group in comparison with eight patients (38%) in the mask group ($p = 0.047$). Complications related to the technique (skin necrosis, gastric distension and eye irritation) were fewer in the helmet group compared with the standard mask group (no patients vs. 14 patients (21%), $p = 0.002$). The helmet allowed the continuous application of NIV for a longer period of time ($p = 0.05$). The authors concluded that NIV by helmet successfully treated hypoxemic ARF, with better tolerance and fewer complications than facial mask NIV. The helmet is very popular in Italy and excellent results have been reported with the administration of c-PAP through a helmet, in haematological malignancy patients with ARF (Principi et al., 2004). A better tolerance of the helmet, compared to a conventional interface, was also found in a case-control study (Rocco et al., 2004). However, this interface can be responsible for an increased work of breathing and dyspnea (Racca et al., 2005), a potential risk of CO_2 rebreathing, to be carefully weighed against the major benefits achieved respecting the integrity of the face. In practice, in many units, including ours, the helmet is used in the second or even third line, as an alternative to a face mask in case of intolerance causing skin lesions and promoting a risk of failure of the method.

Ventilatory modes

One of the main differences between management of COPD patients and of patients with hypoxemic ARF is the place of CPAP in the therapeutic armamentarium of physicians treating patients with hypoxemic ARF. Pressures commonly used to deliver CPAP to patients with hypoxemic ARF range from 5 to 15 cm H_2O. Such pressures can be applied using a wide variety of devices including CPAP valves connected to a compressed gas source, small portable units used for home therapy of obstructive sleep apnea, and ventilators designed for use in ICU. Depending on the critical care ventilator selected, CPAP may be administered using 'demand', 'flow-by', or 'continuous flow' techniques, with imposed work differing slightly between them. CPAP is widely used in the belief that it may reduce the need for intubation and mechanical ventilation in patients with acute hypoxemic respiratory insufficiency. Nevertheless, to our knowledge, although several studies have shown the ability of the method to improve hypoxemia, only one randomized study has demonstrated that the use of CPAP reduces the need for endotracheal intubation in patients with severe hypercapnic cardiogenic pulmonary oedema (Bersten et al., 1991). A recent study showed that, as compared with standard oxygen therapy, CPAP neither reduced the need for intubation nor improved outcomes in patients with hypoxemic ARF (Delclaux et al., 2000). On the contrary, positive results have been reported in randomized controlled studies where PS + PEEP were used (Antonelli et al., 2000; Hilbert et al., 2001a). During PS ventilation, the ventilator is triggered by the patient, delivers a set pressure for each breath and cycles to expiration either when it senses a fall in inspiratory flow rate below a threshold value, or at a preset time. Noninvasive PS ventilation offers the potential of excellent patient-ventilator synchrony, reduced diaphragmatic work, and improved patient comfort.

The choice of NIV with PS and PEEP, rather than CPAP, a technique previously systematically used in hypoxemic ARF in our ICU (Hilbert et al., 2000), has undoubtedly contributed to the good results recently reported in immunosuppressed patients

(Hilbert *et al.*, 2001a). In our practice, after the mask had been secured, the level of PS is progressively increased and adjusted for each patient to obtain an expired tidal volume of 7 to 10 ml per kilogram of body weight and a respiratory rate of fewer than 25 breaths per minute. PEEP is repeatedly increased by 2 cm H_2O, up to a level of 10 cm H_2O, until the FiO_2 requirement is 70% or less. The FiO_2 is adjusted to maintain SaO_2 above 90%. Ventilator settings are adjusted on the basis of continuous monitoring of SaO_2, clinical data, and measurements of arterial-blood gases. Studies comparing the impact on clinical outcome of CPAP and PS + PEEP, in patients with hypoxemic ARF, should be useful. For the moment, and looking forward to the results of further studies, PS ventilation + PEEP could be the ventilatory mode recommended for treatment with NIV of hypoxemic ARF.

Many factors must be considered when PS + PEEP are used. Some of them are well known (for instance: inspiratory trigger sensitivity, inspiratory flow) and close to those we consider when this ventilatory mode is used in intubated patients. Several others are more specific to NIV: for instance, the negative impact of leaks on workload of breathing with a risk of patient-ventilator asynchrony (Calderini *et al.*, 1999). Gas leaks around the mask or from the mouth limit the efficacy of the device, make monitoring of tidal volume difficult, may prevent adequate ventilatory assistance in patients who require high inspiratory airway pressures, and represent an important cause of failure. Leaks may also indicate low compliance or ventilation close to total lung capacity. Thus, a particular attention should be carried to the leaks during application of NIV in patients with hypoxic ARF. In a study on six patients with ALI due to AIDS-related opportunistic pneumonia, a time-cycled expiratory trigger provided a better patient-machine interaction than a flow-cycled expiratory trigger, in the presence of air leaks during NIV (Calderini *et al.*, 1999). Another possibility is to modify the threshold of flow cut-off.

We believe the first hours of delivering NIV, with careful attention to mask fit, patient comfort and patient-ventilator synchrony, represent a critical opportunity to improve outcome.

11.7   Predictive factors of NIV outcome

In the randomized study by Hilbert *et al.*, the effect on outcomes of the presence and the absence of a final diagnosis of the cause of pneumonitis with respiratory failure was studied (Hilbert *et al.*, 2001a). In the NIV group, the patients with a final diagnosis had significant lower rates for intubation ($p = 0.03$), death in the ICU ($p = 0.04$) or in the hospital ($p = 0.006$). So, a positive diagnosis and a well adapted treatment could be the main determinants in the improved outcome of immunosuppressed patients managed with NIV.

In a prospective study, variables predictive of NIV failure were investigated in 354 patients with hypoxemic ARF, 37 of them with immunosuppression (Antonelli *et al.*, 2001). Multivariate analysis identified age >40 years (OR 1.72, 95% CI 0.92–3.23), a higher SAPS II ≥ 35 (OR 1.81, 95% CI 1.07–3.06), the presence of ARDS or community-acquired pneumonia (OR 3.75, 95% CI 2.25–6.24), and a $PaO_2/FiO_2 \leq 146$

after 1 h of NIV (OR 2.51, 95% CI 1.45–4.35) as factors independently associated with failure of NIV.

Nevertheless, in practice, it can be difficult to predict an individual outcome and decide promptly to withdraw the noninvasive ventilatory support, keeping in mind the poor prognosis of intubation in numerous patients. On the other hand, it is crucial, in my opinion, to do all that can be made to try to optimize the technical aspects which are crucial for a successful application of NIV.

While learning techniques of NIV is described as simple in some studies, it is essential and especially must be continuous, allowing better indications of the technique, optimizing the technical aspects and monitoring, sole guarantors of the avoidance of a too delayed intubation when the method fails. Indeed, the use of NIV with a delay in reintubation can lead to excess mortality, and we should not delay the moment of reintubation if this last became necessary. Undoubtedly, ARF in immuno-compromised patients is one of the indications of NIV that require experience and a good control of the technique; in my opinion, this justifies, in this indication, the practice of NIV in ICU.

11.8 Conclusions

Starting from the good results obtained in patients with acute exacerbations of COPD, NIV is now being used to support those with hypoxemic ARF, certain of them with immunosuppression.

A reduction in the incidence of nosocomial infection is a consistent and important advantage of NIV compared with invasive ventilation and is probably one of the most important advantages of avoiding endotracheal intubation using NIV. ARF in immuno-compromised patients is a recognized indication of NIV, and according to recent international recommendations (of level I), NIV should be used whenever possible in this indication to reduce the risk of nosocomial pneumonia (Anon, 2005). Above all, NIV makes it possible to reduce the mortality of the patients of onco-haematology with ARF.

Given the risks of serious complications and death associated with intubation, the relative safety of appropriately applied NIV should change our approach to ventilation in immunocompromised patients with respiratory failure; patients in whom respiratory distress develops should be treated conventionally with oxygen and other indicated therapies and should be monitored closely; if moderate-to severe respiratory distress develops with tachypnea and hypoxemia, NIV should be initiated unless there are contraindications (Hill, 2001). The early involvement of intensivists in immuno-compromised patients' care, and the better definitions of patients who require ICU admission will probably play a major role in the future.

The experiences gradually acquired by the different units, the regular training of the personnel, further technological advances and future research, will position NIV more accurately in the therapeutic armamentarium of physicians dealing with immunocom-promised patients with ARF, and are likely to improve the conditions for performing NIV in the future.

References

Anon (2000) The ARDS Network. Ventilation with lower tidal volumes as compared with traditional tidal volumes for acute lung injury and the acute respiratory distress syndrome. *The New England Journal of Medicine*, **342**, 1301–1308.

Anon (2001) International consensus conferences in intensive care medicine: noninvasive positive pressure ventilation in acute respiratory failure. *American Journal of Respiratory and Critical Care Medicine*, **163**, 283–291.

Anon (2005) American Thoracic Society; Infectious Diseases Society of America. Guidelines for the management of adults with hospital-acquired, ventilator-associated, and healthcare-associated pneumonia. *American Journal of Respiratory and Critical Care Medicine*, **171**, 388–416.

Antonelli, M., Conti, G., Riccioni, L. *et al.* (1996) Noninvasive positive-pressure ventilation via face mask during bronchoscopy with BAL in high-risk hypoxemic patients. *Chest*, **110**, 724–728.

Antonelli, M., Conti, G., Rocco, M. *et al.* (1998) A comparison of noninvasive positive pressure ventilation and conventional mechanical ventilation in patients with acute respiratory failure. *The New England Journal of Medicine*, **339**, 429–435.

Antonelli, M., Conti, G., Bufi, M. *et al.* (2000) Noninvasive ventilation for treatment of acute respiratory failure in patients undergoing solid organ transplantation. A randomized trial. *The Journal of the American Medical Association*, **283**, 235–241.

Antonelli, M., Conti, G., Moro, M.L. *et al.* (2001) Predictors of failure of noninvasive positive pressure ventilation in patients with acute hypoxemic respiratory failure: a multi-center study. *Intensive Care Medicine*, **27**, 1718–1728.

Antonelli, M., Conti, G., Rocco, M. *et al.* (2002a) Noninvasive positive-pressure ventilation vs. conventional oxygen supplementation in hypoxemic patients undergoing diagnostic bronchoscopy. *Chest*, **121**, 1149–1154.

Antonelli, M., Conti, G., Pelosi, P. *et al.* (2002b) New treatment of acute hypoxemic respiratory failure: Noninvasive pressure support ventilation delivered by helmet – A pilot controlled trial. *Critical Care Medicine*, **30**, 602–608.

Azoulay, E., Alberti, C., Bornstain, C. *et al.* (2001) Improved survival in cancer patients requiring mechanical ventilatory support: impact of noninvasive mechanical ventilatory support. *Critical Care Medicine*, **29**, 519–525.

Bach, P.B., Schrag, D., Nierman, D.M. *et al.* (2001) Identification of poor prognostic features among patients requiring mechanical ventilation after hematopoietic stem cell transplantation. *Blood*, **98**, 3234–3240.

Bedos, J.P., Dumoulin, J.L., Gachot, B. *et al.* (1999) Pneumocystis carinii pneumonia requiring intensive care management: survival and prognostic study in 110 patients with human immuno‘-deficiency virus. *Critical Care Medicine*, **27**, 1109–1115.

Bersten, A.D., Holt, A.W., Vedig, A.E. *et al.* (1991) Treatment of severe cardiogenic pulmonary edema with continuous positive airway pressure delivered by face mask. *The New England Journal of Medicine*, **325**, 1825–1830.

Brett, A. and Sinclair, D.G. (1993) Use of continuous positive airway pressure in the management of community acquired pneumonia. *Thorax*, **48**, 1280–1281.

Calderini, E., Confalonieri, M., Puccio, P.G. *et al.* (1999) Patient-ventilator asynchrony during noninvasive ventilation: the role of expiratory trigger. *Intensive Care Medicine*, **25**, 662–667.

Confalonieri, M., Calderini, E., Terraciano, S. *et al.* (2002) Noninvasive ventilation for treating acute respiratory failure in AIDS patients with pneumocystis carinii pneumonia. *Intensive Care Medicine*, **28**, 1233–1238.

Conti, G., Marino, P., Cogliati, A. *et al.* (1998) Noninvasive ventilation for the treatment of acute respiratory failure in patients with hematologic malignancies: a pilot study. *Intensive Care Medicine*, **24**, 1283–1288.

Covelli, H.D., Weled, B.J. and Beekam, J.F. (1982) Efficacy of continuous positive airway pressure administered by face mask. *Chest*, **81**, 147–150.

Delclaux, C., L'Her, E., Alberti, C. *et al.* (2000) Treatment of acute hypoxemic nonhypercapnic respiratory insufficiency with continuous positive airway pressure delivered by a face mask: A randomized controlled trial. *The Journal of the American Medical Association*, **284**, 2352–2360.

Estopa, R., Torres-Marti, A., Kastanos, N. *et al.* (1984) Acute respiratory failure in severe hematologic disorders. *Critical Care Medicine*, **12**, 26–28.

Ewig, S., Torres, A., Riquelme, R. *et al.* (1998) Pulmonary complications in patients with haematological malignancies treated at a respiratory intensive care unit. *The European Respiratory Journal: Official Journal of the European, Society for Clinical Respiratory Physiology*, **12**, 116–122.

Greenbaum, D.M., Millen, J.E., Eross, B. *et al.* (1976) Continuous positive airway pressure without tracheal intubation in spontaneously breathing patients. *Chest*, **69**, 615–621.

Gregg, R.W., Friedman, B.C., Williams, J.F. *et al.* (1990) Continuous positive airway pressure by face mask in *Pneumocystis carinii* pneumonia. *Critical Care Medicine*, **18**, 21–24.

Gruson, D., Hilbert, G., Portel, L. *et al.* (1999) Severe respiratory failure requiring ICU admission in bone marrow transplant recipients. *The European Respiratory Journal: Official Journal of the European, Society for Clinical Respiratory Physiology*, **13**, 883–887.

Gruson, D., Hilbert, G., Valentino, R. *et al.* (2000) Utility of fiberoptic bronchoscopy in neutropenic patients admitted to intensive care unit with pulmonary infiltrates. *Critical Care Medicine*, **28**, 2224–2230.

Hilbert, G., Gruson, D., Gbikpi-Benissan, G. *et al.* (1997) Sequential use of noninvasive pressure support ventilation for acute exacerbations of COPD. *Intensive Care Medicine*, **23**, 955–961.

Hilbert, G., Gruson, D., Portel, L. *et al.* (1998) Non-invasive pressure support ventilation in COPD patients with postextubation hypercapnic respiratory insufficiency. *The European Respiratory Journal: Official Journal of the European, Society for Clinical Respiratory Physiology*, **11**, 1349–1353.

Hilbert, G., Gruson, D., Vargas, F. *et al.* (2000) Non-invasive continuous positive airway pressure in neutropenic patients with acute respiratory failure requiring intensive care unit admission. *Critical Care Medicine*, **28**, 3185–3190.

Hilbert, G., Gruson, D., Vargas, F. *et al.* (2001a) Noninvasive ventilation for treatment of acute respiratory failure in immunosuppressed patients with pulmonary infiltrates and fever, a randomized trial. *The New England Journal of Medicine*, **344**, 481–487.

Hilbert, G., Gruson, D., Vargas, F. *et al.* (2001b) Bronchoscopy with bronchoalveolar lavage via the laryngeal mask airway in high-risk hypoxemic immunosuppressed patients. *Critical Care Medicine*, **29**, 249–255.

Hill, N.S. (2001) Noninvasive ventilation for immunocompromised patients. *The New England Journal of Medicine*, **344**, 522–524.

Katz, J.A. and Marks, J.D. (1985) Inspiratory work with and without continuous positive airway pressure in patients with acute respiratory failure. *Anesthesiology*, **63**, 598–607.

Keenan, D.P. (1997) Effect of noninvasive positive pressure ventilation on mortality in patients admitted with acute respiratory failure: a meta-analysis. *Critical Care Medicine*, **25**, 1685–1692.

Kesten, S. and Rebuck, A.S. (1988) Nasal continuous positive airway pressure in *Pneumocystis carinii* pneumonia. *Lancet*, **ii**, 1414–1415.

Kroschinsky, F., Weise, M., Illmer, T. *et al.* (2002) Outcome and prognostic features of ICU treatment in patients with hematological malignancies. *Intensive Care Medicine*, **28**, 1294–1300.

Masur, H., Shelhamer, J. and Parrillo, J.E. (1985) The management of pulmonary infiltrates and fevers in immunocompromised patients. *The Journal of the American Medical Association*, **253**, 1769–1773.

Principi, T., Pantanetti, S., Catani, F. *et al.* (2004) Noninvasive continuous positive airway pressure delivered by helmet in hematological malignancy patients with hypoxemic acute respiratory failure. *Intensive Care Medicine*, **30**, 147–150.

Racca, F., Appendini, L., Gregoretti, C. *et al.* (2005) Effectiveness of mask and helmet interfaces to deliver noninvasive ventilation in a human model of resistive breathing. *Journal of Applied Physiology (Bethesda, Md.: 1985)*, **99**, 1262–1271.

Randall Curtis, J., Yarnold, P.R., Schwartz, D.N. *et al.* (2000) Improvements in outcomes of acute respiratory failure for patients with human immunodeficiency virus-related Pneumocystis carinii pneumonia. *American Journal of Respiratory and Critical Care Medicine*, **162**, 393–398.

Rano, A., Agusti, C., Benito, N. *et al.* (2002) Prognostic factors of non-HIV immunocompromised patients with pulmonary infiltrates. *Chest*, **122**, 253–261.

Richards, G.N., Cistulli, P.A., Ungar, R.G. *et al.* (1996) Mouth leak with nasal continuous positive airway pressure increases nasal airway resistance. *American Journal of Respiratory and Critical Care Medicine*, **154**, 182–186.

Rocco, M., Dell'Utri, D., Morelli, A. *et al.* (2004) Noninvasive ventilation by helmet or face mask in immunocompromised patients: a case-control study. *Chest*, **126**, 1508–1515.

Rocker, G.M., Mackenzie, M.G., Williams, B. *et al.* (1999) Noninvasive positive pressure ventilation: successful outcome in patients with acute lung injury/ARDS. *Chest*, **115**, 173–177.

Rubenfeld, G.D. and Crawford, S.W. (1996) Withdrawing life support from mechanically ventilated recipients of bone marrow transplants: a case for evidence based guidelines. *Annals of Internal Medicine*, **125**, 625–633.

Smith, R.A., Kirby, R.R., Gooding, J.M. *et al.* (1980) Continuous positive airway pressure (CPAP) by face mask. *Critical Care Medicine*, **8**, 483–485.

Soubani, A.O., Kseibi, E., Bander, J.J. *et al.* (2004) Outcome and prognostic factors of hematopoietic stem cell transplantation recipients admitted to a medical ICU. *Chest*, **126**, 1604–1611.

Stauffer, J.L. (1994) Complications of translaryngeal intubation, in *Principles and Practice of Mechanical Ventilation* (ed. M.J. Tobin), Marcel Dekker, Inc., New York, pp. 711–747.

Stover, D.E., Zaman, N.B., Hadjou, S.I. *et al.* (1984) Bronchoalveolar lavage in the diagnosis of diffuse pulmonary infiltrates in the immunosuppressed host. *Annals of Internal Medicine*, **101**, 1–7.

Tobin, M.J. (2001) Advances in mechanical ventilation. *The New England Journal of Medicine*, **344**, 1986–1996.

Tognet, E., Mercatello, A., Polo, P. *et al.* (1994) Treatment of acute respiratory failure with non-invasive intermittent positive pressure ventilation in haematological patients. *Clinical Intensive Care*, **5**, 282–288.

12

Current strategies and future directions in antibacterial treatment

Jan Jelrik Oosterheert and Andy I.M. Hoepelman

Department of Internal Medicine and Infectious Diseases, University Medical Center, Utrecht, The Netherlands

12.1   Introduction

Several conditions can lead to decreased defence mechanisms against bacterial infections, leading to an increased susceptibility for bacterial infections of the respiratory tract.

An important element in the care for patients with lower respiratory tract infections in these immunocompromised hosts is treatment with antimicrobial drugs. When initiating treatment for infectious diseases in general, an etiologic diagnosis is often not yet made. Therefore, initial treatment in respiratory infections is mostly empirical covering several suspected causative micro-organisms. Making a choice from available antibiotics should be based on consideration of several basic principles of antimicrobial treatment and the specifics defect in host defences. Since the first descriptions of correlations between an immunocompromised state and risk of infections, changes have occurred in initial antimicrobial strategy. Basic considerations of culture and molecular diagnostics based, targeted treatment regimens, were replaced by empirical antibacterial treatment strategies and antibacterial prophylaxis. In this chapter, we will discuss the possibilities for antibacterial treatment in pulmonary infections in the immunocompromised patient. First, we will describe basic considerations for antimicrobial treatment in general and options for antibacterial treatment. Subsequently, we discuss treatment strategies in immunocompromised patients and some specific patient groups.

12.2   Farmacokinetics and farmacodynamics

In general, the choice for an antimicrobial agent to treat pulmonary infection is based on the ability of the antimicrobial agent to reach adequate concentrations in lung tissue,

Pulmonary Infection in the Immunocompromised Patient, Edited by Carlos Agustí and Antoni Torres
© 2009 John Wiley & Sons, Ltd.

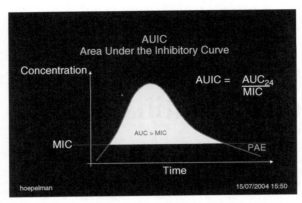

Figure 12.1 Pharmacokinetic and pharmacodynamic parameters that affect antibiotic therapy.

targeting the pathogens that have infected lung-tissue as well as the MIC of the infecting micro-organism. Important pharmacokinetic parameters are the drug's peak concentration, (Cmax), Area Under the Curve (AUC) or peak/MIC ratio and serum half-life. Important pharmacodynamic factors include the relationship between these pharmacokinetic parameters and the MIC of pathogens: the ratio of Cmax to MIC (Cmax: MIC), the ration of the drug's 24 hour AUC to MIC (AUC: MIC), the time the drug concentration exceeds the MIC (T > MIC). (Figure 12.1, Table 12.1) For β-lactams, which show time-dependent killing with minimal to no persistent effects, it has been shown that a time of free drug level above the MIC of more than 40% was required to achieve an 85–100% bacteriologic cure rate. The same holds true for macrolides, clindamydin and linezolid. Some other antimicrobial agents, such as aminoglycosides, are more effective when they have a high Cmax: MIC ratio. For aminoglycosides, Cmax: MIC ratio of more than 10, seems to result in the maximal potential for clinical response (Craig, 1998). Also for gram-negative pneumonia treated with aminoglycosides, it has been demonstrated that a Cmax/MIC ratio of 10 achieved within the first 48 h of aminoglycoside therapy is predictive of a favourable response (Kashuba *et al.*, 1999). Ketolides, azithromycin and fluoroquinolones display concentration-dependent bacterial killing, and tetracyclins and macrolides display time-dependent killing. In contrast to beta-lactam antibiotics they show no prolonged persistent effects (for example, post-antibiotic effect) that retard or prevent bacterial growth when free drug levels fall below the MIC. For azithromycin and the fluoroquinolones outcome is related to the AUC: MIC ratio (area under the inhibitory concentration (AUIC)). However, some investigators have claimed that Cmax/MIC is equally important (Craig, 1998). Maintenance of AUC:MIC greater than 100 optimizes the antibacterial killing of *S. pneumoniae* by fluoroquinolones (Nicolau, 2003). An AUC below this ratio only reduces cure rates, but may also select for resistance. Outcome for other agents, including the β-lactams, is best predicted by the T > MIC. A clear relationship between reduction in colony-forming units and T > MIC over 24 hours cefotaxime therapy was seen in pulmonary infections with *K. pneumoniae*. These pharmacodynamic and

Table 12.1 Pharmacokinetic and pharmacodynamc parameters correlating with antibacterial efficacy in animal infectio models.

Pharmacokinetic property	Cmax	Maximal serum concentration after single or multiple doses
	Tmax	Time after drug administration to reach Cmax
	AUC	Area under the concentration-time curve (relates to total drug exposure following a dose)
Pharmacodynamic property	Cmax/MIC, Peak/MIC (Aminoglycosides and fluoroquinolones)	Ratio of the maximum serum concentration to the MIC (predicts activity of concentration dependent bactericidal antibiotics)
	AUC/MIC (AUIC) (Aminoglycosides, fluoroquinolones, azithromcin, tetracycline, vancomycin)	Ratio of the area under the concentraion-time curve to the MIC (also predicts activity of concentration dependent bactericidal antibiotics)
	$T > MIC$, t_{eff} (Penicillins, cephalosporins, carbapenems, aztreonam, macrolides, clindamycin)	Time above the MIC; the duration of time during a dosing interval that serum concentration remains above the MIC (predicts activity of time-dependent bactericidal antibiotics)

pharmacokinetic features are important to determine whether concentration or time of exposure are clinically preferable (Nicolau, 2003). In addition to the prediction of efficacy, the Cmax/MIC ratio has been used *in vitro* and *in vivo* to predict the development of resistance (Blaser *et al.*, 1987). Especially for fluoroquinolones, it has been shown that for efficacy an $AUC > 125$ is needed and for prevention of resistance development an AUC of >100 is needed (Craig, 2001) (Table 12.2)

Bacterial growth may be inhibited following exposure to antibiotics even after the drug concentration has fallen far below the MIC. This is referred to as post-antibiotic effect (PAE) and can be demonstrated *in vitro* by observing bacterial growth kinetic after a drug is removed. Post-antibiotic effects vary with different drugs and micro-organisms, ranging from prolonged post-antibiotic effects for gram-negative bacilli after exposure to antibacterials inhibiting protein synthesis or nucleid acid synthesis, (e.g. aminoglycosides, fluoroquinolones, tetracyclins, macrolides, chlampheciol and rifampin) to short PAEs or no PAEs for gram-negative bacilli after exposure to β-lactam antibiotics. It has been reported that PAEs in animal models may be longer than those measured *in vivo* (Gudmundsson *et al.*, 1993).

Table 12.2   Frequently used antibiotics for respiratory infections and their activities against common respiratory pathogens.

Agent	Active against respiratory micro-organism	Remarks
Penicillins Benzylpenicillins	Small spectrum of activity: gram-positive and some gram-negative bacteria: S. aureus (MSSA), streptococci, B. antracis, *H. influenzae*. No activity against penicillinase producing micro-organisms, Chlamydia, mycobacteria, Mycoplasma. Resistance is common for S. aureus and B. anthracis.	Cheap Resistance is common in some areas
Amoxicillin	Aminopenicillin. Broad spectrum of activity against gram-positive and gram-negative bacteria. No activity against penicillinase producing staphylococci, some proteus strains, pseudomonas, klebsiella and enterobacter.	
Amoxicillin + clavulanic acid	Clavulanic acid enhances the spectrum of activity of amoxicillin to penicillinase producing staphylococci, klebsiella, P. mirabilis, *H. influenzae* Chromosomal β-lactamases as in enterobacteriacea and *P. aeruginosa* are insensitive to clavulanic acid.	
Flucloxacilline	Small spectrum of activity against gram-positive micro-organisms, mainly penicillinase producing strains.	
Piperacillin	Broad spectrum of activity against gram-positive and gram-negative micro-organisms. Pseudomonas and Proteus are also sensitive.	
Carbapenems	Broad spectrum of activity against gram-positive and gram-negative micro-organisms, including enterobacteriaceae and pseudomonas. Mycoplasma, chlamydia are not sensitive. Carbapenems are insensitive to most β-lactamases	

Table 12.2   (*Continued*)

Agent	Active against respiratory micro-organism	Remarks
Cephalosporins		
Second generation (e.g. cefuroxime)	S. pneumoniae, S. aureus Hae mophilus (para)influenzae, Moraxella catarrhalis. Insensitive are Pseudomonas, Proteus vulgaris, Enterobacter Legionella, Listeria monocytogenes, meticillin resistant, Staphylococcus aureus- and epidermidis epidermidis Cefuroxim is insensitive to β-lactamases and staphylococcal pennicellinase.	
Third generation (e.g. ceftriaxone)	Spectrum of activity includes gram-positive, *S. pneumoniae* and S. aureus; gram-negative and anaerobic bacteria. Insensitive are methicillin resistant staphy lococci, mycoplamsa, mycobacterium spp. Ceftriaxone is resistant to most β-lactamases.	
Macrolides		
Erythromycin	Streptococci and staphylococci (including penicillinase producing strains) are sensitive as re Mycoplasma pneumoniae, Legionella pneumophila, Chlamydia and Haemophilus influenzae.	Gastro-intestinal side effects
Clarithromycin	Gram-positive micro-organisms as streptococci and staphylococci are sensitive and gram-negative micro-organisms as *H. influenzae*, *M. catharralis*, and *L. pneumophila*. Chlamydia and Mycoplasma are also sensitive.	
Azithromycin	Gram-positive micro-organisms as streptococci and staphylococci are sensitive and gram-negative micro-organisms as *H. influenzae*, *M. catharralis*, and *L. pneumophila*. Chlamydia and Mycoplasma are also sensitive as are M. avium complex. Pseudomonas is not sensitive.	Once daily dosing, high tissue concentrations
Quinolones		Resistance develops easily in all quinolones

(*continued*)

Table 12.2   (*Continued*)

Agent	Active against respiratory micro-organism	Remarks
Ciprofloxacin	Broad spectrum of activity including gram-negative (Pseudomonas aeruginosa) and gram-positive aerobic micro-organisms. Streptococci and Mycoplasma are moderately sensitive. Entero-bacteriaceae, other gram-negatives, limited against gram-positive bacteria.	
Levofloxacin	Broad spectrum of activity against most relevant gram-positive and gram-negative (Pseudomonas aeruginosa) bacteria. Also active against atypical micro-organisms as Chlamydia and Mycoplasma. MRSA is not sensitive	
Moxifloxacin	Spectrum of activity includes gram-positive, gram-negative and atypical micro-organisms. Extending activity, including against anaerobes. and atypical micro-organisms. Somewhat less active against Staphylococcus aureus(MIC90 of 0.12 µg/mL; Burkholderia cepacia, Pseudomonas aeruginosa, *Pseudomonas fluorescens* and Stenotrophomonas maltophilia.)	
Aminoglycosides	Gram-negatives: some proteus species, pseudomonas, klebsiella, *E. coli*. Gram-positives: some staphylococci (S. aureus, including penicillin and methicillin resistant strains)	Small therapeutic window
Tetracyclins (doxycyclin)	Broad spectrum of activity including gram-positive, gram-negative microorganisms and Rickessiae, Mycoplasma	Not to be used inpregnancy and childhood
Clindamycin	Activity against most aerobic gram-positive cocci, as *S. pneumoniae* and other streptococci. Mycoplasma is also sensitive.	
Vancomycin	Sensitive are a lot of gram-positive micro-organisms including staphylococci and streptococci being resistant against other antibiotics. No activity against gram-negative micro-organisms, vancomycin resistant enterococci and vancomycin resistant MRSA and mycobacteria.	

Table 12.2 (*Continued*)

Agent	Active against respiratory micro-organism	Remarks
Trimethoprim/ sulfamethoxazole	Most gram-positive and gram-negatives are sensitive. No activity against Pseudomonas aeruginsa, myocplasma, M. tuberculosis.	
Linezolid	Gram-positives including VRE, MRSA	
Daptomycin	S. aureus (including MRSA), Group A, B, C, G streptococci, Amoxicillin resistant enterococci, vancomycin resistant enterococci	
Ketolides	Streptococcus pneumoniae, Hae mophilus influenzae, Moraxella catarrhalis, Chlamydophila pneumoniae, or Mycoplasma pneumoniae	Telithromycin can induce severe hepatic dysfunction and is contra-indicated for use in patients with myastenia gravis.

When two antibiotics are given together, they may interact additively (when the activity of the drugs in combination is equal to the sum (or a partial sum) of their independent activities), synergistically, (when the combined effect is greater than the sum of their independent activities) antagonistically, (if the activity of the combination is less than the sum of their independent effects) or there may be no interaction. *In vitro* time-kill curves comparing the rate of bactericidal activity of each antibiotic alone with that of the combination are used to asses these interactions. In addition to synergism, combinations of antibiotics can be used for prevention of the emergence of resistant pathogens (for example, in the treatment of pulmonary tuberculosis), increased spectrum of activity, for example, treatment of polymicrobial infections (for example, the treatment of a combined 'typical' and 'atypical' infection in community-acquired pneumonia) and to diminish toxicity. (If lower dosages can be used when combinations are given.) Possible disadvantages of the use of combinations of antibiotics are interactions, antagonism and increased side-effects.

12.3 Antibacterial treatment options

Beta-lactams are frequently used in respiratory tract infections. All antibiotics in this class contain a cyclic amide called a β-lactam. Main classes are the penicillins containing a five-membred ring, the carbapenems with a five membred ring with a double bond, the cephalosporins containing a six membred unsaturated ring with a sulfur atom and the monobactams with cyclic amides in a four membred ring. The common feature of the penicillins is the possession of a thiazolidine, a β-lactam ring. Penicillins inhibit a transpeptidation reaction in the bacterial cell-wall synthesis, through binding to penicillin binding penicillins. (PBPs). The spectrum of the penicillins varies from narrow-spectrum agents with activity largely limited to gram-positive cocci (for example penicillin G) to broad-spectrum agents with activity against many gram-negative bacilli (for example, piperacillin). For penicillins, absorption after oral administration is variable, especially in older patients. After absorption, penicillins are distributed in the extracellular fluid, excretion is largely via the kidney. Side-effects are uncommon and mostly mild, however allergic reactions can occur. The therapeutic window of penicillins is large, dose alterations in renal insufficiency are mostly not necessary. Penetration in lung tissue is good, which is an important feature for the treatment of respiratory infections. Discussion exists whether pneumonia caused by resistant *S. pneumoniae* strains has implications for clinical outcome. A prospective study in 884 patients showed no differences in clinical outcome for patients with infections with penicillin susceptible and penicillin resistant strains (Appelbaum, 2002; Yu *et al.*, 2003). Pharmacodynamic studies have shown that a time above the MIC of about 40% of the dosing interval is predictive of bacteriological efficacy for beta-lactams (Craig, 1998).

Of the penicillins, parenteral penicillin G, or oral amoxicillin are the drugs of choice for treating infections with *S. pneumoniae*, with penicillin MICs < 1.0 μg/mL (Heffelfinger *et al.*, 2000). Ampicillin, cefotaxime and ceftriaxone can be used for infections with *S. pneumoniae* strains resistant to penicillin (MIC, <2 μg/mL) (Bartlett *et al.*, 2000). Penicillins combined with β-lactamase inhibitors (for example, amoxicillin-clavulanate) are active against β-lactamase-producing organisms, such as *H. influenzae*, beta-lactamase producing anaerobes, and *M. catarrhalis*, but these combinations offer no advantage over penicillin G against *S. pneumoniae*. Penicillins are inactive against *M. pneumoniae* and *C. pneumoniae*, and ineffective in the treatment of *Legionella* (Bartlett *et al.*, 2000).

When penicillins were first available, all *S. aureus* strains were susceptible to penicillins. Now, 90–95% of *S. aureus* strains are penicillin resistant by producing beta-lactamases. Therefore, in the treatment of *S. aureus* infections, beta-lactamase resistant penicillins such as flucloxacillin are an option. However, resistance has also emerged against these antibiotics. *S. aureus* strains that are resistant to methicillin should be considered to be resistant to all other beta-lactam antibiotics, including the cephalosporins and carbapenems, even if *in vitro* testing suggests otherwise. These methicillin resistant *S. areus* strains can be treated with glycopeptide antibiotics such as vancomycin, daptomycin or linezolid and perhaps the newer cephalosporins (Falagas, Siempos and Vardakas, 2008; Lentino, Narita and Yu, 2008).

The general feature of cephalosporins is the possession of a β-lactam ring fused to a six membered dihydrothizine ring, to form the cephem nucleus of cephalosporins. Modifications of side chains have resulted in different generations of cephalosporins. The mode of action is comparable to the penicillins, cephalosporins are bactericide antibiotics through inhibition of the cell wall synthesis, the target being penicillin binding sites. Toxicity is mostly mild, there is cross-reactivity to penicillins for allergic reactions.

Three factors are important in the development of resistance to cephalosporins. Alterations in the target site (PBP), production of β-lactamases and prevention of the antibiotic to reach the target site. Often combinations occur. Cephalosporins are excreted via the kidney, which mandates caution in use in the presence of renal failure. Ceftriaxone has a half-life of about eight hours and therefore generally a once daily dosing regimen is sufficient, resulting in a cheap and effective treatment of serious bacterial infections as compared to cefuroxime in combination with gentamicin (Hoepelman, Rozenberg-Arska and Verhoef, 1988).

Important for the treatment of pulmonary infections: the penetration in lung tissue is excellent. First generation cephalosporins are active against most gram-positive microorganisms, but are relatively sensitive to β-lactamases. Second generation cephalosporins cefuroxim are more stable to β-lactamase and are active against gram-negative bacteria. Third generation cephalosporins such as ceftriaxone are less active against staphylococci, but are generally stable to β-lactamase and are active against gram-negative bacteria, some others (for example, Ceftazidime) are also active against *P. Aeruginosa*. Newer generation cephalosporins such as cefipime exhibit broad spectrum activity against both gram-positive and gram-negative bacteria, and is recommended in guidelines for the treatment of febrile neutropenia. The probability of reaching a time above the MIC of at least 70% in extended spectrum beta-lactamase infections, is highest for cefipime. However, its use has been associated with an increase in mortality (Yahav *et al.*, 2007; Ramphal and Ambrose, 2006). The carbapenems meropenem, ertapenem and imipenem exhibit the same mode of action as the other penicillins and can be used against a broad spectrum of aerobic and anaerobic gram-positive and gram-negative organisms and are frequently used in patients with febrile neutropenia: most strains of *S. pneumoniae*, *P. aeruginosa*, and virtually all strains of *H. influenzae*, *M. catarrhalis*, anaerobes and methicillin-susceptible *S. aureus* are susceptible. Activity against penicillin-resistant *S. pneumoniae* is generally adequate. Long-term treatment with these agents can lead to secondary fungal infections.

Of the monobactams, Aztreonam is a monocyclic b-lactam antibiotic and therefore classified as a monobactum. It has no activity against gram-positive or anaerobic bacteria because it does not bind to PBPs in these species. It does bind to PBP3 in Enterobacteriaceae, Pseudomonades and other gram-negative aerobic organisms. Resistance mechanisms include failure to penetrate the outer membrane, destruction by b-lactamases or a failure to bind to PBPs. Aztreonam is not absorbed from the gastrointestinal tract, and should be administered intramuscularly or intravenously. Therapeutic are reached in sputum, bronchial secretions, and pericardial, pleural, peritoneal, fluids. Serum concentrations of aztreonam are higher and the serum half-life is prolonged in patients with renal impairment. No major adverse reactions to aztreonam have been reported. Because of its lack of cross-reactivity with other b-lactam antibiotics, aztreonam can be used safely in patients with serious allergy to penicillins or cephalosporins. Because aztreonam has a spectrum of activity limited to aerobic gram-negative bacteria, the drug should not be used alone for empiric therapy in seriously ill patients. Aztreonam has been used safely and effectively in conjunction with clindamycin, erythromycin, metronidazole, penicillins and vancomycin.

The chemical basis of the macrolides is a macrocyclic lactone ring. Azithromycin is a member of the azalides, a subgroup of the macrolides. Macrolides reversibly bind to the 50 S ribosomal subunit, resulting in blockage of transpeptidation and translocation reactions in chain elongation thereby inhibiting bacterial cell-wall synthesis. Absorption after oral administration varies between patients. Macrolides also exhibit anti-inflammatory reactions (Wales and Woodhead, 1999). Whether these anti-inflammatory reactions are of importance in pulmonary infections is not known. To protect macrolides from gastric acid breakdown after oral administration, several coatings have been developed. Clarithromycin and azithromycin have long half-lives and all macrolides penetrate well in all tissues. Erythromycin is poorly tolerated because of gastrointestinal side effects and phlebitis. Newer macrolides such as azithromycin and clarithromycin are better tolerated but also more expensive. Drug interactions can occur through interacting with the cytochrome p450 in the liver. There are two mechanisms of macrolide resistance by *S. pneumoniae*. First, the M phenotype, because of an efflux mechanism, is associated with MICs of 2–8 µg/mL and, in theory, may be overcome by high doses; this mechanism is prevalent in the United States. Second, the ERM phenotype, due to ribosomal alterations, is associated with MICs > 64 µg/mL; this mechanism predominates in Europe. Erythromycin, Clarithromycin and Azithromycin all appear to be effective for treating pulmonary infections caused by *M. pneumoniae*, *C. pneumoniae*, and *Legionella*. For macrolides bacteriological efficacy correlates with T > MIC. Higher survival rates are seen in animal models if T > MIC is 40–50% of the dosage interval. Human studies in otitis media and sinusitis support these findings (Andes, 2001).

In the past few years, quinolones have become a popular class of antimicrobials to treat various diseases, with the ability to treat serious infections orally as well as parenterally. The first antibiotic representing this class of antimicrobials, nalixidinic acid, had only activity against gram-negative micro-organisms and had no activity against *Pseudomonas spp*, gram-positive infections or anaerobic microorganisms. Modification of the structure led to the synthesis of norfloxacin, which exhibited activity against *Pseudomonas spp*, but adequate serum levels were hardly reached and could predominantly only be used in urinary tract infections. Further modifications led to the development of ciprofloxacin which mend a revolution in the treatment of a number of infectious diseases. This agent combines a broad spectrum of activity for example against *P. aeruginosa*, *Staphylococcus aureus* and *Legionella Pneumophila*, a better pharmacokinetic profile, adequate serum and tissue concentrations, even after oral administration and low toxicity levels. Unfortunately for the treatment of lower respiratory tract infections, the activity against *S. pneumonia* is limited. Even further modifications have led to the development of the newer fluoroquinolones as levofloxacin and moxifloxacin. These agents are characterized by an increased activity against gram-positive micro-organisms, however at the expense of activity against *P. aeruginosa*. Quinolones show bactericidal activity through inhibition of bacterial topoisomerase enzymes (DNA gyrase and topoisomerase IV) thereby influencing DNA-synthesis. Examples of currently available agents in this class for pulmonary infections are ciprofloxacin, ofloxacin, levofloxacin and moxifloxacin. These drugs show a wide range of activity, being active *in vitro* against most clinically significant aerobic gram-positive cocci, gram-negative bacilli, *H. influenzae*, *M. catarrhalis*, *Legionella*, *M. pneumoniae*, and *C. pneumoniae*. One study showed clinical outcomes with levofloxacin were significantly better than with a cephalosporin regimen for empirical treatment of CAP (File *et al.*, 1997). A matter of concern is the rapid development of resistance to fluoroquinolones, which can develop even during treatment (Davidson *et al.*, 2002; Low and Ambrose, 2004). Resistance develops by mutations in bacterial DNA resulting in the target enzymes being more difficult to inhibit by fluoroquinolones or by alterations in the bacterial cell membrane or active efflux of the drug resulting in low intrabacterial concentrations. Antimicrobial activity is dependent of the AUC: MIC ratio. A ratio of more than 25 is indicative of clinical success for gram-positive infections (Florea *et al.*, 2004). Oral absorption for the newer quinolones is generally excellent, and high concentrations in lung tissues are reached. Moxifloxacin is less prone for the development of resistance, probably because two mutations instead of one are needed for resistance development. Ciprofloxacin-induced mutations in the topoisomerase IV gene hardly increase Moxifloxacin MICs. Not until there also is a mutation in the gyrA gene, MIC increases up to 2 mg/l suggesting a complex target interaction of Moxifloxacin (Pestova *et al.*, 2000). Furthermore, the molecule is large and can therefore probably be less easily be effluxed from the bacterium. This means an extra barrier against resistance development. In addition, resistance development of *S. pneumoniae* for Moxifloxacin depends on two mutations.

The aminoglycosides (gentamicin, tobramycin) are bactericidal antibiotics and influence bacterial mRNA. They have a concentration-dependent bactericidal effect and can generally be dosed once daily. These agents are active *in vitro* against aerobic and facultative gram-negative bacilli, including *P. aeruginosa*. The risk for ototoxicity and nefrotoxicity mandate careful dosing. The most frequently used tetracyclin in clinical practice is doxycyclin. Tetracyclins inhibit bacterial protein synthesis and are bacteriostatic. Doxycyclin is well tolerated, can be dosed twice daily, has good bioavailability and a low price. The tetracyclines are active against the 'atypical' organisms, (*M. pneumoniae*, *C. pneumoniae*, and *Legionella*). About 15% of pneumococci are resistant to doxycyclin. As mentioned previously, tetracyclins should not be used in pregnancy or in young children because of their adverse effects on osteogenesis and dentition.

Vancomycin and teicoplanin show universal activity against *S. pneumoniae*. It is also active against other gram-positive organisms, including methicillin-resistant *S. aureus*. Excessive use of vancomycin promotes the development of vancomycin resistant enterococci and of *S. aureus* strains that are only intermediately susceptible and should therefore not be used as a first-line agent in respiratory infections.

Clindamycin has good activity against gram-positive cocci, including efflux pump mediated macrolide resistant pneumococci and most methicillin-susceptible *S. aureus*. Clindamycin is the preferred drug for anaerobic pulmonary infections, such as aspiration pneumonia and lung abscess. It is, however, inactive against *H. influenzae* and the atypical pathogens.

Trimethoprim-Sulfamethoxazole (TMP-SMZ) inhibits the bacterial synthesis of dihydrofolic acid and is active against a broad spectrum of gram-positive and gram-negative organisms. However, about 20–25% of *S. pneumoniae* strains are resistant, and more than 70% of penicillin-resistant *S. pneumoniae* isolates are not susceptible to TMP-SMZ. TMP-SMZ is active against *P. carinii* an infection which can occur in HIV infected patients with CD4 < 200 µl.

Antiviral agents that can be used for treatment or preventions of influenza infections are amantadine and rimantadine (inhibitors of hemagglutinin) and Relenza (aero-solized) and oseltamivir (neuraminidase inhibitors). To be effective in treatment, these agents should be administered within 48 hours after onset of symptoms. Doing so, a reduction in the duration of symptoms of about one day can be established and viral shedding diminishes. The use of these agents is advised for treating influenza by IDSA (Bartlett *et al.*, 2000).

Chloramphenicol is no longer the drug of choice for any specific infection. The availability of other agents has dramatically reduced the need for this antibiotic. However, because it is effective, readily available and inexpensive, it is still used as first-line therapy in many parts of the world. Chloramphenicol inhibits protein synthesis by binding to the larger 50 and 70 s ribosome of the bacterium and is bactericidal against *H. influenzae*, S pneumoniae and has activity against chlamydiae and mycoplasms. Chloramphenicol is metabolized by the liver and the physician should be on alert for toxicity from other agents that are metabolized by the liver when administering chloramphenicol. Because of the narrow therapeutic/toxic ratio, it is important to monitor serum levels of this antibiotic. The most important toxic effects include reversible bone marrow depression and aplastic anemia.

12.4   Resistance

Macrolide resistance is either due to modification of the target site, encoded by the erm B gene, or an active efflux pump that removes macrolides from the cell, encoded by the mef gene. In *S. pneumoniae*, the erm gene is associated with high levels of resistance to all macrolides. Over 50% of macrolide resistance in Europe is caused by mutations in the erm B gene (Johnston *et al.*, 1998), whereas presence of an efflux pump is the predominant resistance mechanism of *S. pneumoniae* to macrolides in the USA (Garau, 2002). Erythromycin resistance based upon efflux mechanisms can be overcome by the use of newer macrolides, such as azithromycin (Garau, 2002).

The newer fluoroquinolones, such as levofloxacin and moxifloxacin, are active, *in vitro*, against most relevant significant aerobic gram-positive cocci, the enterobac-teriaceae, *H. influenzae, M. catarrhalis, Legionella species, M. pneumoniae* and *C. pneumoniae*, which make them attractive compounds for treatment of CAP. Development of resistance to fluoroquinolones, which can occur even during treatment, however, is a matter of serious concern (Davidson *et al.*, 2002; Low and Ambrose, 2004). Resistance to fluoroquinolones results from mutations in the target enzymes (DNA gyrase and topoisomerase IV), thereby reducing the inhibitory effects of fluoroquinolones on bacterial DNA-synthesis. Strains usually become fully resistant when both target genes are mutated. Other resistance mechanisms include alterations in the bacterial cell membrane and active efflux of the drug (Davidson *et al.*, 2002; Low and Ambrose, 2004).

Importantly, prevalence of antibiotic resistance varies geographically. For instance, prevalence of reduced susceptibility to penicillin among *S. pneumoniae* is around 40% in Spain and less than 1% in the Netherlands (http://www.earss.rivm.nl), and is probably related to the usage of these agents. Therefore, decisions on empirical antimicrobial treatment should be based on local antibiotic resistance rates.

Recently, an emergence of infections, mostly skin infection but sporadically severe CAP, caused by so-called Community-Associated methicillin-resistant S. aureus (CA-MRSA) have been reported from the US and Europe (Miller *et al.*, 2005; Bradley, 2005) CA-MRSA are resistant to all β-lactam antibiotics, but are frequently still susceptible to clindamycin, co-trimoxazole and fluoroquinolones.

Recommended initial antibacterial treatment in pulmonary infections

In the initial treatment of suggested pulmonary infection in immunocompromised patients, initial therapy is predominantly based on the clinical presentation rather than the presumed causative pathogen. (Table 12.3) For pulmonary infections in immuno-compromised hosts, basic considerations for empirical treatment are no different from other infections: possible causative micro-organisms, epidemiological features, host-factors, resistance patterns of micro-organisms and farmacokinetic and farmaco-dynamic features of antibiotics should all be taken into consideration. Combinations of β-lactam antibiotics are frequently used. Synergystic effects of this combination for the treatment for *S. pneumoniae* infections have been described (Darras-Joly *et al.*, 1996). However, a meta-analysis of 64 sepsis trials, showed that the addition of an aminoglycoside to β-lactam treatment did not change fatality, but increased the risk for adverse events (Paul *et al.*, 2004).

In a model study, it was shown that combination therapy may be required to prevent the emergence of resistant *P. aeruginosa* in neutropenic patients (Dudley *et al.*, 1987).

The most commonly used two-drug therapy in neutropenic patients with cancer, excluding regimens with vancomycin, includes an aminoglycoside (gentamicin, tobramycin, or amikacin) with an antipseudomonal carboxypenicillin or ureidope-nicillin (ticarcillin-clavulanic acid or piperacillin-tazobactam); an aminoglycoside with an antipseudomonal cephalosporin, such as cefepime or ceftazidime; and an aminoglycoside plus a carbapenem (imipenem-cilastatin or meropenem). Generally, the different two-drug combinations yield similar results when variations in experi-mental design, definitions, end points and underlying primary diseases are taken into consideration.

Advantages of combination therapy are potential synergistic effects against gram-negative bacilli and minimal emergence of drug-resistant strains during treatment (Sepkowitz, Brown and Armstrong, 1994). The major disadvantages are the lack of activity of these combinations against some gram-positive bacteria, and nephrotoxicity, ototoxicity and hypokalemia associated with aminoglycosides and carboxypenicillins.

Table 12.3   Most likely pathogens and preferred empirical therapy in lower respiratory tract infections.

Respiratory infection	Most likely pathogens	Preferred empirical therapy
CAP, outpatients	S. pneumoniae, M. pneumoniae, C. pneumoniae	Amoxicillin, Macrolide, fluoroquinolone
CAP, inpatients	S, pneumoniae, H. influenzae, M. pneumoniae, C. pneumoniae, L. pneumophila	Extended spectrum cephalosporin plus a macrolide, β-lactam/β-lactamase inhibitor plus a macrolide, or a fluoroquinolone alone if not severe and admitted for other reasons: amoxicillin
CAP, ICU	S. pneumoniae, Legionella spp, H. influenzae, enteric gram-negative bacilli, S. aureus, aspiration	Extended spectrum cephalosporin plus macrolide, β-lactam/β-lactamase inhibitor plus either fluoroquinolone or macrolide. In structural lung disease: antipseudomonal agents. Aspiration: fluoroquinolone with or without clindamycin, metronidazole or a β-lactam/β-lactamase inhibitor.
HAP including ventilator associated pneumonia	Severity	Second generation cephalosporin or nonpseudomonal third generation/beta-lactam beta-lactamase inhibitor combination
	Mild-to-moderate/no unusual risk factors and onset any time/severe early onset: Enteric gram-negative bacilli, enterobacter species, e coli, klebsiella, proteus, serratioa, H. influenzae, methicillin sensitive s. aureus	
	Risk factors or mild-to-moderate:	Clindamycin ± vancomycin, (if possible MRSA)
	Anaerobes, S. aureus, Legionella,	Erytyromycin
	P. aeruginosa	Treat as severe HAP
	Severe	
	P. aeruginosa Acinetobacter MRSA	Aminoglycosice or ciprofloxacin plus antipseudomonal penicillin/augmentin/imipenem/aztreonam/ceftazidime/cefoperazone ± vancomycin

Based on the recommendations of ATS, BTS and IDSA guidelines for community-acquired pneumonia (Bartlett *et al.*, 2000; American Thoracic Society, 2001; Anon, 2001) and the ATS guidelines for hospital acquired pneumonia (Anon, 1996).

Limited studies show that a single daily dose of an aminoglycoside with ceftriaxone is as effective as multiple daily doses of these drugs and as effective as monotherapy with ceftazidime (Rubinstein, Lode and Grassi, 1995). Another disadvantage is the need for monitoring serum levels of aminoglycosides in patients with impaired renal function with adjusting the dosage until optimal therapeutic concentrations are achieved. Combinations of quinolones with beta-lactams or glycopeptides are an option for initial therapy for patients not receiving quinolone prophylaxis. Newer fluoroquinolones such as moxifloxacin, or levofloxacin have been used selectively to treat patients who have cancer. One study showed that ciprofloxacin plus piperacillin-tazobactam is as effective as tobramycin and piperacillin-tazobactam (Peacock *et al.*, 2002). Any initial antibiotic regimen should include drugs with antipseudomonal activity (Chatzinikolaou *et al.*, 2000).

Combinations including vacomycin should be used with care, because of the emergence of vancomycin-resistant organisms. Several studies have evaluated vancomycin drug combinations for the treatment of neutropenic patients with fever. However, guidelines recommend the inclusion of vancomycin in initial empirical therapy only for selected patients with clinically suspected serious catheter-related infections, known colonization with penicillin- and cephalosporin-resistant pneumococci or methicillin-resistant *S. aureus*, positive results of blood culture for gram-positive bacteria before final identification and susceptibility testing, or hypotension or other evidence of cardiovascular impairment (Hughes *et al.*, 2002).

Linezolid, an oxazolidinone, offers promise for treatment of drug-susceptible and -resistant gram-positive bacterial infections, including those due to vancomycin-resistant enterococci, but myelosuppression associated with its use is less attractive in the treatment of immunocompromised patients (Rubinstein *et al.*, 2001).

12.5 HIV related bacterial pulmonary infections

Although bacterial pneumonias can occur throughout the course of HIV infection, they tend to develop more frequently in individuals with advanced immunosuppression (Hirschtick *et al.*, 1995; Farizo *et al.*, 1992). A direct relation between the CD4 count and the incidence of bacterial pneumonia was noted in a 1995 report: 2.3, 6.8 and 10.8 episodes per 100 patient years with respective CD4 counts of more than 500, 200 to 500, and less than 200 cells/microL(Hirschtick *et al.*, 1995). HIV infection is also a risk factor for recurrent pneumococcal pneumonia and bacteremia (Turett, Blum and Telzak, 2001). Bacterial pneumonia is a common cause of HIV related morbidity. Infection with *S. pneumoniae* is 150–300 times more common among patients with HIV infection than in age-matched HIV-uninfected populations (Caiaffa, Graham and Vlahov, 1993; Wallace *et al.*, 1997). Despite relatively normal CD4$^+$ T lymphocyte counts, patients can develop serious pneumococcal infections. This may be due to qualitative B-cell defects that impair the ability to produce pathogen-specific antibody, hypergammaglobulinemia leading to opsonization defects, or impaired neutrophil function or numbers or both. However, the most consistent predictor of infections is the absolute CD4$^+$ T lymphocyte count (Redd *et al.*, 1990; Gilks, 1993; Boschini *et al.*, 1996).

Bacterial causes of pulmonary infections include *Streptococcus pneumoniae*, *Haemophilus influenzae*, *Pseudomonas aeruginosa*, and *Staphylococcus aureus*. *Legionella pneumophila*, *Mycoplasma pneumoniae*, *Chlamydia pneumoniae* and *M. tuberculosis* are less frequently isolated (Benson *et al.*, 2004).

Because pneumocystis carinii pneumonia is also common in HIV positive patients and can co-exist with bacterial pneumonia, an induced sputum examination or bronchoalveolar lavage for *P. jiroveci* staining in patients with CD4$^+$ T lymphocyte count <200 cells μL, other signs of advanced immunodeficiency, a previous history of PCP or other AIDS-related condition, or diffuse infiltrates on chest radiograph is recommended. Usually, these patients have elevated LDH levels and are hypoxic. For patients with CD4 counts below 200 and not receiving PCP profylaxis, initial therapy should also cover PCP with high dose co-trimoxazol, which is also effective against most other pathogens. In severe PCP infection, (pa02 < 70 mm Hg) concomitant use of corticosteroids has been showing to improve outcomes (Benson *et al.*, 2004). Obviously, initial therapy for HIV-related bacterial pneumonia should at least target the most commonly identified pathogens, particularly *S. pneumoniae* and *H. influenzae*. Therefore, treatment guidelines appropriate for HIV-uninfected patients are applicable to those with HIV infection (Bartlett *et al.*, 2000; Mandell *et al.*, 2007; Heffelfinger *et al.*, 2000). (Table 12.4, Table 12.5) In line with this, combination therapy with a

Table 12.4 Preferred antimicrobial therapy when causative micro-organisms are known.

Micro-organism	Preferred targeted therapy, duration
S. pneumoniae	
Penicillin susceptible	Penicillin G, Amoxicillin
Penicillin resistant (MIC < 2 μg/mL)	Agents based on *in vitro* susceptibility tests, including cefotaxime and ceftriaxone, fluoroquinolone, vancomycin
H. Influenzae	Cephalosporin (second or third generation) doxycyclin, β-lactam + β-lactamase inhibitor, azithromycin, TMP-SMX
M. pneumoniae	Doxycyclin, macrolide
C. pneumoniae	Doxycyclin, macrolide
L. pneumophila	Macrolide ± rifampin; fluoroquinolone
S. aureus	Nafcillin/oxacillin ± rifampin or gentamicin; (BTS)
Methicillin susceptible	Flucloxacillin ± rifampicin
Methicillin resistant	Vancomycin ± rifampin or gentamicin
M. catharralis	Cephalosprin (2/3) TMP/SMZ, macrolide
Anaerobes	β-lactam + β-lactamase inhibitor, clindamycin
P. aeruginosa	Aminoglycoside + for example Piperacillin or carbapenem
C. psittacci	Doxycyclin
Coxiella burnetii	Tetracyclin
Influenzavirus	oseltamivir or zanamavir

Based on the recommendations of ATS, BTS and IDSA guidelines for community-acquired pneumonia (Bartlett *et al.*, 2000; American Thoracic Society, 2001; Anon, 2001) and the ATS guidelines for hospital acquired pneumonia (Anon, 1996).

Table 12.5 Epidemiologic conditions or host factors related to specific pathogens in patients with community-acquired pneumonia.

Feature	Possible pathogens
Alcoholism	*S. pneumoniae*, anaerobes, gram-negative bacilli, *Mycobacterium Tuberculosis*
COPD/smoker	*S. pneumoniae*, *H. influenzae*, *M. catharralis*, *L. pneumophila*
Nursing home residency	*S. pneumoniae*, gram-negative bacilli, *H. influenzae, s. aureus*, anaerobes, *c. pneumoniae, Mycobacterium Tuberculosis*
Poor dental hygiene	Anaerobes
Exposure to birds	*C. psittaci, C. neoformans, H. capsulatum*
Exposure to rabbits	Francisella tularensis
Exposure to farm animals or parturient cats	Coxiella burnetii
Influenza activity in community	*Influenza, S. pneumoniae, S. aureus, H. influenzae*
Aspiration	Anaerobes
Structural disease of the lung	*P. aeruginosa, S. aureus*
Injection drug use	*S. aureus*, anaerobes, *M. tuberculosis, pneumocystis carinii*
Recent antibiotic therapy	Drug resistant pneumococci, *P. aeruginosa*
Cooling towers, air conditioning and so on	*Legionella pneumophila*
Shelter for homeless/jail	*S. pneumoniae, M. tuberculosis*
Diabetic ketoacidosis	*S. pneumoniae, S. aureus*
Solid organ transplantation	*S. pneumoniae, H. influenzae, Legionella spp, P. carinii, strongyloides stercoralis*
Sickle cell	*S. pneumoniae*
HIV cd4 < 200/µL	*P. carinii, S. pneumoniae, H. influenzae, C. neoformans, M. tuberculosis, rhodococcus equi*
Granulocytopenia	Aerobic gram-negative rod-like bacteria such as *E. coli* or *K. pneumoniae, Aspergillus spp.*

Based on the recommendations of the ATS and the CTS for the management of community-acquired pneumonia (American Thoracic Society, 2001; Mandell *et al.*, 2000).

macrolide or quinolone plus a cephalosporin should be considered for those with severe illness. For high-level penicillin-resistant isolates (MIC > 4.0 mg/mL), therapy should be guided by susceptibility results. Among patients with severe immunodeficiency (CD4$^+$ T lymphocyte counts <50/ml), a known history of previous *Pseudomonas* infection, bronchiectasis, or relative or absolute neutropenia, broadening empiric coverage to include *P. aeruginosa* and other gram-negative bacilli should be considered, which may include treatment with ceftazidime, cefepime, piperacillin-tazobactam, a carbapenem, or high dose ciprofloxacin or levofloxacin. The strategy most effective in preventing bacterial pneumonia in HIV-infected patients is to optimize anti-retroviral therapy (Benson *et al.*, 2004). No well-documented benefit has been determined for secondary prophylaxis after successful completion of antibiotic treatment for bacterial respiratory tract infections, but adults with CD4$^+$ counts of >200 cells/µL could be administered a single dose of 23-valent polysaccharide pneumococcal vaccine. Annual administration of influenza vaccine might be useful in preventing pneumococcal superinfection of influenza respiratory tract infections (Benson *et al.*, 2004; Mandell *et al.*, 2007; Heffelfinger *et al.*, 2000). However, administration of antibiotic profylaxis should be considered in patients who have frequent recurrences of serious bacterial respiratory infections. TMP-SMX, administered for PCP prophylaxis and clarithromycin or azithromycin, administered for mycobacterium avium complex prophylaxis, are appropriate for drug-sensitive organisms.

12.6 Length of treatment

Controlled trials that specifically have addressed the question how long pulmonary infections should be treated are lacking. This decision is usually based on the pathogen, response to treatment, comorbid illness and complications. In neutropenic patients, the most important determinant of successful discontinuation of antibiotics is the neutrophil count. Several approaches, based on common sense, are often used. For example, if no infection is identified after three days of treatment, if the neutrophil count is >500 cells/mm^3 for two consecutive days, and if the patient is afebrile for >48 hours, antibiotic therapy may be stopped at that time. If the patient becomes afebrile but remains neutropenic, the proper antibiotic course is less well defined. Some specialists recommend continuation of antibiotics, given intravenously or orally, until neutropenia is resolved (Freifeld and Pizzo, 1997; Hughes and Patterson, 1984). It is reasonable for neutropenic patients who appear healthy clinically, who were in a low risk category at onset of treatment, who have no discernible infectious lesions, and who have no radiographic or laboratory evidence of infection, to have their use of systemic antibiotics stopped after five to seven days without fever, or sooner, if haematologic recovery occurs (Hughes *et al.*, 2002). If use of antibiotics is stopped while the patient still is neutropenic, close monitoring and immediate restart of intravenous antibiotics when fever comes back is recommended (Joshi *et al.*, 1984). Continuous administration of antibiotics throughout the neutropenic episode for patients with profound neutropenia (<100 cells/mm^3), mucous membrane lesions, unstable vital signs, or other identified risk factors is recommended (Joshi *et al.*, 1984; Hughes *et al.*, 2002). In patients with prolonged neutropenia in whom haematologic recovery cannot be anticipated, one can consider stopping antibiotic therapy after two weeks, if no site of infection has been identified and the patient can be observed carefully.

For patients who remain febrile after recovery of the neutrophil count to >500 cells/mm^3 and despite receipt of broad-spectrum antibacterial therapy, reassessment for undiagnosed infection directed at fungal (especially chronic systemic candidiasis, aspergillosis, histoplasmosis and trichosporonosis), mycobacterial, or viral infections is advised (Talbot, Provencher and Cassileth, 1988). Antibiotic therapy can generally be stopped despite persistent fever four to five days after the neutrophil count reaches more than 500 cells/mm^3 if no infectious lesions are identified.

If a causative microbe is identified, the antibiotic regimen may be changed, if necessary, to provide optimal treatment with minimal adverse effects and lowest cost, but broad-spectrum coverage should be maintained to prevent breakthrough bacteremia (Hughes *et al.*, 2002). In the absence of evident infectious disease and positive culture results, treatment for compliant adults may be changed after two days of intravenous therapy to an oral antibiotic combination of ciprofloxacin and amoxicillin-clavulanic acid (Freifeld *et al.*, 1999; Kern *et al.*, 1999). If patients are without fever, the advice is to modify antibiotic therapy for specific organisms, if identified, and to continue the use of broad-spectrum antibiotics for seven days or longer, until cultures have become sterile and the patient has clinically recovered. If the causative organism is not found and the patient is receiving drugs intravenously and was at low risk at the onset of treatment, treatment may be changed to oral ciprofloxacin plus amoxicillin-clavulanate. If evidence of progressive disease becomes apparent during the initial antibiotic course, consideration should be given to either the addition of appropriate antibiotics or a change to different antibiotics. Whether a change is indicated will also depend on the initial antibiotic regimen (Hughes *et al.*, 2002).

12.7 Conclusions

Initial treatment for suggested pulmonary infections in the immunocompromised host is mostly empiric and broad spectrum. The initial treatment regimens are dependent of host factors, possible causative micro-organisms and their resistance spectrum and the pharmacodynamic and pharmacokinetic profiles of available drugs. How long patients should be treated is a difficult question, but the recommended length of treatment is dependent of the isolated micro-organism and recovery of the immunocompromised state. Future directions are aimed at vaccination strategies and the development of new antimicrobials drugs, aimed at resistant pathogens such as MRSA or VRE.

References

American Thoracic Society (2001) Guidelines for the management of adults with community acquired pneumonia. *American Journal of Respiratory and Critical Care Medicine*, **163**, 1730–1754.

Andes, D. (2001) Pharmacokinetic and pharmacodynamic properties of antimicrobials in the therapy of respiratory tract infections. *Current Opinion in Infectious Diseases*, **14** (2), 165–172.

American Thoracic Society (2005) 'Guidelines for the Management of Adults with Hospital-acquired, Ventilator-associated, and Healthcare-associated Pneumonia'. *American Journal of Respiratory and Critical Care Medicine*, **171**, 388–416.

Appelbaum, P.C. (2002) Resistance among Streptococcus pneumoniae: Implications for drug selection. *Clinical Infectious Diseases: An Official Publication of the Infectious Diseases Society of America*, **34** (12), 1613–1620.

Bartlett, J.G., Dowell, S.F., Mandell, L.A., File, TM., Jr, Musher, D.M. and Fine, M.J. (2000) Practice guidelines for the management of community-acquired pneumonia in adults. Infectious Diseases Society of America. *Clinical Infectious Diseases: An Official Publication of the Infectious Diseases Society of America*, **31** (2), 347–382.

Benson, C.A., Kaplan, J.E., Masur, H., Pau, A. and Holmes, K.K. (2004) Treating opportunistic infections among HIV-infected adults and adolescents: recommendations from CDC, the National Institutes of Health, and the HIV Medicine Association/Infectious Diseases Society of America. *MMWR Recommendations Reports*, **53** (RR-15), 1–112.

Blaser, J., Stone, B.B., Groner, M.C. and Zinner, S.H. (1987) Comparative study with enoxacin and netilmicin in a pharmacodynamic model to determine importance of ratio of antibiotic peak concentration to MIC for bactericidal activity and emergence of resistance. *Antimicrobial Agents and Chemotherapy*, **31** (7), 1054–1060.

Boschini, A., Smacchia, C., Di, F.M, Schiesari, A., Ballarini, P., Arlotti, M. *et al.* (1996) Community-acquired pneumonia in a cohort of former injection drug users with and without human immunodeficiency virus infection: incidence, etiologies, and clinical aspects. *Clinical Infectious Diseases: An Official Publication of the Infectious Diseases Society of America*, **23** (1), 107–113.

Bradley, S.F. (2005) Staphylococcus aureus pneumonia: Emergence of MRSA in the community. *Seminars in Respiratory and Critical Care Medicine*, **26** (6), 643–649.

Caiaffa, W.T., Graham, N.M. and Vlahov, D. (1993) Bacterial pneumonia in adult populations with human immunodeficiency virus (HIV) infection. *American Journal of Epidemiology*, **138** (11), 909–922.

Chatzinikolaou, I., Abi-Said, D., Bodey, G.P., Rolston, K.V., Tarrand, J.J. and Samonis, G. (2000) Recent experience with Pseudomonas aeruginosa bacteremia in patients with cancer: Retrospective analysis of 245 episodes. *Archives of Internal Medicine*, **160** (4), 501–509.

Craig, W.A. (1998) Pharmacokinetic/pharmacodynamic parameters: rationale for antibacterial dosing of mice and men. *Clinical Infectious Diseases: An Official Publication of the Infectious Diseases Society of America*, **26** (1), 1–10.

Craig, W.A. (2001) Does the dose matter? Clinical infectious diseases: An official publication of the Infectious Diseases Society of America, **33** (Suppl 3), S233–S237.

Darras-Joly, C., Bedos, J.P., Sauve, C., Moine, P., Vallee, E., Carbon, C. *et al.* (1996) Synergy between amoxicillin and gentamicin in combination against a highly penicillin-resistant and -tolerant strain of Streptococcus pneumoniae in a mouse pneumonia model. *Antimicrobial Agents and Chemotherapy*, **40** (9), 2147–2151.

Davidson, R., Cavalcanti, R., Brunton, J., Bast, D.J., de Azavedo, J.C.S., Kibsey, P. *et al.* (2002) Resistance to levofloxacin and failure of treatment of pneumococcal pneumonia. *The New England Journal of Medicine*, **346**, 747–749.

Dudley, M.N., Mandler, H.D., Gilbert, D., Ericson, J., Mayer, K.H. and Zinner, S.H. (1987) Pharmacokinetics and pharmacodynamics of intravenous ciprofloxacin. Studies *in vivo* and in an *in vitro* dynamic model. *The American Journal of Medicine*, **82** (4A), 363–368.

Falagas, M.E., Siempos, I.I. and Vardakas, K.Z. (2008) Linezolid versus glycopeptide or beta-lactam for treatment of Gram-positive bacterial infections: meta-analysis of randomised controlled trials. *Lancet Infectious Diseases*, **8** (1), 53–66.

Farizo, K.M., Buehler, J.W., Chamberland, M.E., Whyte, B.M., Froelicher, E.S., Hopkins, S.G.M. *et al.* (1992) Spectrum of disease in persons with human immunodeficiency virus infection in the United States. *The Journal of the American Medical Association*, **267** (13), 1798–1805.

File, TM. Jr, Segreti, J., Dunbar, L., Player, R., Kohler, R., Williams, R.R. *et al.* (1997) A multicenter, randomized study comparing the efficacy and safety of intravenous and/or oral levofloxacin versus ceftriaxone and/or cefuroxime axetil in treatment of adults with community-acquired pneumonia. *Antimicrobial Agents and Chemotherapy*, **41** (9), 1965–1972.

Florea, N.R., Tessier, P.R., Zhang, C., Nightingale, C.H. and Nicolau, D.P. (2004) Pharmacodynamics of moxifloxacin and levofloxacin at simulated epithelial lining fluid drug concentrations against Streptococcus pneumoniae. *Antimicrobial Agents and Chemotherapy*, **48** (4), 1215–1221.

Freifeld, A. and Pizzo, P. (1997) Use of fluoroquinolones for empirical management of febrile neutropenia in pediatric cancer patients. *The Pediatric Infectious Disease Journal*, **16** (1), 140–145.

Freifeld, A., Marchigiani, D., Walsh, T., Chanock, S., Lewis, L., Hiemenz, J. *et al.* (1999) A double-blind comparison of empirical oral and intravenous antibiotic therapy for low-risk febrile patients with neutropenia during cancer chemotherapy. *The New England Journal of Medicine*, **341** (5), 305–311.

Garau, J. (2002) Treatment of drug-resistant pneumococcal pneumonia. *Lancet Infectious Diseases*, **2** (7), 404–415.

Gilks, C.F. (1993) Pneumococcal disease and HIV infection. *Annals of Internal Medicine*, **118** (5), 393.

Gudmundsson, S., Einarsson, S., Erlendsdottir, H., Moffat, J., Bayer, W. and Craig, W.A. (1993) The post-antibiotic effect of antimicrobial combinations in a neutropenic murine thigh infection model. *The Journal of Antimicrobial Chemotherapy*, **31** (Suppl D), 177–191.

Heffelfinger, J.D., Dowell, S.F., Jorgensen, J.H., Klugman, K.P., Mabry, L.R., Musher, D.M. *et al.* (2000) Management of community-acquired pneumonia in the era of pneumococcal resistance: a report from the Drug-Resistant Streptococcus pneumoniae Therapeutic Working Group. *Archives of Internal Medicine*, **160** (10), 1399–1408.

Heffelfinger, J.D., Dowell, S.F., Jorgensen, J.H., Klugman, K.P., Mabry, L.R., Musher, D.M. *et al.* (2000) Management of community-acquired pneumonia in the era of pneumococcal resistance: a report from the Drug-Resistant Streptococcus pneumoniae Therapeutic Working Group. *Archives of Internal Medicine*, **160** (10), 1399–1408.

Hirschtick, R.E., Glassroth, J., Jordan, M.C., Wilcosky, T.C., Wallace, J.M., Kvale, P.A. *et al.* (1995) Bacterial pneumonia in persons infected with the human immunodeficiency virus. Pulmonary Complications of HIV Infection Study Group. *The New England Journal of Medicine*, **333** (13), 845–851.

Hoepelman, I.M., Rozenberg-Arska, M. and Verhoef, J. (1988) Comparison of once daily ceftriaxone with gentamicin plus cefuroxime for treatment of serious bacterial infections. *Lancet*, **1** (8598), 1305–1309.

Hughes, W.T. and Patterson, G. (1984) Post-sepsis prophylaxis in cancer patients. *Cancer*, **53** (1), 137–141.

Hughes, W.T., Armstrong, D., Bodey, G.P., Bow, E.J., Brown, A.E., Calandra, T. *et al.* (2002) 2002 guidelines for the use of antimicrobial agents in neutropenic patients with cancer. *Clinical Infectious Diseases: An Official Publication of the Infectious Diseases Society of America*, **34** (6), 730–751.

Hughes, W.T., Armstrong, D., Bodey, G.P., Bow, E.J., Brown, A.E., Calandra, T. *et al.* (2002) 2002 guidelines for the use of antimicrobial agents in neutropenic patients with cancer. *Clinical Infectious Diseases: An Official Publication of the Infectious Diseases Society of America*, **34** (6), 730–751.

Johnston, N.J., De Azavedo, J.C., Kellner, J.D. and Low, D.E. (1998) Prevalence and characterization of the mechanisms of macrolide, lincosamide, and streptogramin resistance in isolates of Strepto-coccus pneumoniae. *Antimicrobial Agents and Chemotherapy*, **42** (9), 2425–2426.

Joshi, J.H., Schimpff, S.C., Tenney, J.H., Newman, K.A. and De Jongh, C.A. (1984) Can antibacterial therapy be discontinued in persistently febrile granulocytopenic cancer patients? *The American Journal of Medicine*, **76** (3), 450–457.

Kashuba, A.D., Nafziger, A.N., Drusano, G.L. and Bertino, J.S., Jr (1999) Optimizing aminoglycoside therapy for nosocomial pneumonia caused by gram-negative bacteria. *Antimicrobial Agents and Chemotherapy*, **43** (3), 623–629.

Kern, W.V., Cometta, A., De Bock, R., Langenaeken, J., Paesmans, M. and Gaya, H. (1999) Oral versus intravenous empirical antimicrobial therapy for fever in patients with granulocytopenia who are receiving cancer chemotherapy. International Antimicrobial Therapy Cooperative Group of the European Organization for Research and Treatment of Cancer. *The New England Journal of Medicine*, **341** (5), 312–318.

Lentino, J.R., Narita, M. and Yu, V.L. (2008) New antimicrobial agents as therapy for resistant gram-positive cocci. European Journal of Clinical Microbiology & Infectious Diseases: Official Publication of the European Society of Clinical Microbiology, **27** (1), 3–15.

Low, D.E. (2004) Quinolone resistance among pneumococci: therapeutic and diagnostic implications. *Clinical Infectious Diseases: An Official Publication of the Infectious Diseases Society of America*, **38** (Suppl 4), S357–S362.

Mandell, L.A., Marrie, T.J., Grossman, R.F., Chow, A.W. and Hyland, R.H. (2000) and the Canadian community-acquired pneumonia working group. Canadian guidelines for the initial management of community-acquired pneumonia: an evidence-based update by the Canadian Infectious Diseases Society and the Canadian Thoracic Society. *Clinical Infectious Diseases: An Official Publication of the Infectious Diseases Society of America*, **31**, 383–421.

Mandell, L.A., Wunderink, R.G., Anzueto, A., Bartlett, J.G., Campbell, G.D., Dean, N.C. *et al.* (2007) Infectious Diseases Society of America/American Thoracic Society consensus guidelines on the management of community-acquired pneumonia in adults. *Clinical Infectious Diseases: An Official Publication of the Infectious Diseases Society of America*, **44** (Suppl 2), S27–S72.

Miller, L.G., Perdreau-Remington, F., Rieg, G., Mehdi, S., Perlroth, J., Bayer, A.S. *et al.* (2005) Necrotizing fasciitis caused by community-associated methicillin-resistant Staphylococcus aureus in Los Angeles. *The New England Journal of Medicine*, **352** (14), 1445–1453.

Nicolau, D.P. (2003) Optimizing outcomes with antimicrobial therapy through pharmacodynamic profiling. *Journal of Infection and Chemotherapy: Official Journal of the Japan Society of Chemotherapy*, **9** (4), 292–296.

Paul, M., Benuri-Silbiger, I., Soares-Weiser, K. and Leibovici, L. (2004) Beta lactam monotherapy versus beta lactam-aminoglycoside combination therapy for sepsis in immunocompetent patients: systematic review and meta-analysis of randomised trials. *British Medical Journal (Clinical Research ed.)*, **328** (7441), 668.

Peacock, J.E., Herrington, D.A., Wade, J.C., Lazarus, H.M., Reed, M.D., Sinclair, J.W. *et al.* (2002) Ciprofloxacin plus piperacillin compared with tobramycin plus piperacillin as empirical therapy in febrile neutropenic patients. A randomized, double-blind trial. *Annals of Internal Medicine*, **137** (2), 77–87.

Pestova, E., Millichap, J.J., Noskin, G.A. and Peterson, L.R. (2000) Intracellular targets of moxifloxacin: a comparison with other fluoroquinolones. *The Journal of Antimicrobial Chemotherapy*, **45** (5), 583–590.

Ramphal, R. and Ambrose, P.G. (2006) Extended-spectrum beta-lactamases and clinical outcomes: current data. *Clinical Infectious Diseases: An Official Publication of the Infectious Diseases Society of America*, **42** (Suppl. 4), S164–S172.

Redd, S.C., Rutherford, G.W., III, Sande, M.A., Lifson, A.R., Hadley, W.K, Facklam, R.R. *et al.* (1990) The role of human immunodeficiency virus infection in pneumococcal bacteremia in San Francisco residents. *The Journal of Infectious Diseases*, **162** (5), 1012–1017.

Rubinstein, E., Lode, H. and Grassi, C. (1995) Ceftazidime monotherapy vs. ceftriaxone/tobramycin for serious hospital-acquired gram-negative infections. Antibiotic Study Group. *Clinical Infectious Diseases: An Official Publication of the Infectious Diseases Society of America*, **20** (5), 1217–1228.

Rubinstein, E., Cammarata, S., Oliphant, T. and Wunderink, R. (2001) Linezolid (PNU-100766) versus vancomycin in the treatment of hospitalized patients with nosocomial pneumonia: a randomized, double-blind, multicenter study. *Clinical Infectious Diseases: An Official Publication of the Infectious Diseases Society of America*, **32** (3), 402–412.

Sepkowitz, K.A., Brown, A.E. and Armstrong, D. (1994) Empirical therapy for febrile, neutropenic patients: persistence of susceptibility of gram-negative bacilli to aminoglycoside antibiotics. *Clinical Infectious Diseases: An Official Publication of the Infectious Diseases Society of America*, **19** (4), 810–811.

Talbot, G.H., Provencher, M. and Cassileth, P.A. (1988) Persistent fever after recovery from granulocytopenia in acute leukemia. *Archives of Internal Medicine*, **148** (1), 129–135.

Turett, G.S., Blum, S. and Telzak, E.E. (2001) Recurrent pneumococcal bacteremia: risk factors and outcomes. *Archives of Internal Medicine*, **161** (17), 2141–2144.

Wales, D. and Woodhead, M. (1999) The anti-inflammatory effects of macrolides. *Thorax*, **54** (Suppl 2), S58–S62.

Wallace, J.M., Hansen, N.I., Lavange, L., Glassroth, J., Browdy, B.L., Rosen, M.J. *et al.* (1997) Respiratory disease trends in the Pulmonary Complications of HIV Infection Study cohort. Pulmonary Complications of HIV Infection Study Group. *American Journal of Respiratory and Critical Care Medicine*, **155**, 72–80.

Yahav, D., Paul, M., Fraser, A., Sarid, N. and Leibovici, L. (2007) Efficacy and safety of cefepime: a systematic review and meta-analysis. *Lancet Infectious Diseases*, **7** (5), 338–348.

Yu, V.L., Chiou, C.C., Feldman, C., Ortqvist, A., Rello, J., Morris, A.J. *et al.* (2003) An international prospective study of pneumococcal bacteremia: correlation with *in vitro* resistance, antibiotics administered, and clinical outcome. *Clinical Infectious Diseases: An Official Publication of the Infectious Diseases Society of America*, **37** (2), 230–237.

13

Current strategies in the treatment of fungal infections in the intensive care unit setting

Mitchell Goldman[1] and George A. Sarosi[2]

[1]Indiana University School of Medicine, Department of Medicine, Division of Infectious Diseases, Indianapolis, Indiana, USA [2]Indiana University School of Medicine, Department of Medicine, Indianapolis, Indiana, USA

13.1   Introduction

Fungal infections in the intensive care unit (ICU) should not be viewed as a single set of diseases differing only in the causative organism. Broadly speaking there are two groups of patients with fungal infections who need care in an ICU setting – patients infected with agents of the endemic mycoses and patients with severe underlying and immuno-compromising diseases infected with opportunistic fungi. Patients infected with endemic fungi are usually otherwise healthy, while patients who develop opportunistic fungal infections are sick with their underlying illness and have received interventions and treatments that predispose them to these infections. It should be noted that these two groups may not always be entirely separate, as the endemic fungi may complicate the course of immunosuppressed patients, especially those with advanced human immunodeficiency virus infection or the acquired immune deficiency syndrome (HIV/AIDS) (Sarosi, 2006).

During the last decade, increasing use of haematopoetic stem cell transplantation (HSCT), solid organ transplantation and immunosuppressant therapies for rheumato-logic as well as a number of other inflammatory conditions has led to an increase in the number of those at risk for opportunistic fungal infections. The manifestations of fungal infections in immunocompromised patients are often more severe than those seen in persons with intact immune systems.

Fortunately, over the last 15 years we have witnessed the development of new anti-fungal medications with differential activity against a wide variety of fungal pathogens and improved safety profiles. We have also seen the development of non-invasive tests

Pulmonary Infection in the Immunocompromised Patient, Edited by Carlos Agustí and Antoni Torres
© 2009 John Wiley & Sons, Ltd.

for various fungal pathogens. This chapter will provide an update of the current strategies in the treatment of serious fungal infections encountered in the critical care setting.

13.2   Antifungal therapies

A patient's underlying health has a major impact on the potential treatment options. The distinction between the two groups was not important when the only available antifungal agent was the polyene agent, amphotericin B deoxycholate (AMB-d). Even though this drug was toxic, one had to use it since there were really no other choices. This situation has improved markedly with the arrival of the lipid preparations of amphotericin B (AMB-L) and parenterally available azoles, fluconazole first, than itraconazole. During the past five years our therapeutic choices expanded to include new, advanced azoles and an entirely new class of antifungal agents, the echinocandins. At present there are only three echinocandins approved for use against fungal infections. In general we view these drugs as having equivalent efficacy (Dismukes, 2006).

A few words need to be said about the expected toxicities of the various antifungal agents. AMB is nephrotoxic, which severely limits its use. The nephrotoxicity of AMB is dose dependent and is influenced by the renal function at the inception of therapy. The kidney damage attributed to AMB occurs through the development of renal tubular acidosis, which in turns leads to massive loss of potassium and magnesium, which may be exacerbated by intravascular volume contraction. With careful management of the volume status and ion loss, the nephrotoxicity of AMB-d can be ameliorated and the drug can usually be administered in adequate amounts long enough to achieve a cure (Mayer et al., 2002). Nevertheless, the drug is difficult to use and it is toxic, and recently AMB-L has largely replaced the parent compound. AMB-d is still a highly effective drug and can be used with care. The current practice of starting directly with AMB-L is understandable even though the few studies that looked at the head-to-head comparisons of the two agents have not found large differences between AMB-d and AMB-L (Leenders et al., 1997; Sharkey et al., 1996; Johnson et al., 2002).

The toxicity of the azoles is milder. Fluconazole is well tolerated, even in very high doses. The most feared toxicity is the rare occurrence of drug-induced hepatitis. One advantage of fluconazole is the ability to use oral fluconazole following improvement on the intravenous formulation. Itraconazole was also available in both intravenous and oral formulations, though the intravenous formulation will no longer be manufactured. The oral itraconazole capsule formulation has major absorption problems while an itraconazole solution formulation that does not require an acidic environment for absorption achieves more reliable drug levels. Voriconazole is also well tolerated, but it may cause visual disturbances, which resolve after the drug is stopped. It is also available in both intravenous and oral formulations. Posaconazole, a new and powerful agent, is available only in oral form and it requires a high fat intake to aid absorption (Pappas et al., 2004). The echinocandins have very few serious side effects. This class was developed entirely in the laboratory and its therapeutic target, β–D-glucan, does not exist in mammalian cells (Kurtz and Rex, 2001).

13.3 The endemic fungi in the critical care unit

The endemic fungi are of interest predominantly in North America, the Caribbean basin and certain areas of South America. However, with a highly mobile population, with increasing leisure time, and with rapid transportations across distances these patients may turn up at unexpected locations far removed from their endemic areas (Gutierrez *et al.*, 2005; Antinori *et al.*, 2006).

Histoplasmosis

Epidemiology, microbiology and pathogenesis

Histoplasmosis is the most frequently encountered illness among the endemic mycoses and is the best understood among them. *Histoplasma capsulatum var. capsulatum* is the agent in the New World, while *H. capsulatum var. dubosii* is seen in West Africa and will not be dealt with in this chapter. The fungus is a soil-dwelling, temperature-dependent, dimorphic organism. The endemic area in North America extends from the eastern edge of North Dakota down to West Texas and all points east of this line, except Florida and New England. In Canada, the endemic area involves the Saint Lawrence Valley. The entire Caribbean basin is endemic and so are the areas of South America abutting on the Caribbean (Goodwin, Loyd and DePrez, 1981; Wheat, 2006). Indigenous infections have been seen in other areas of the world but their apparent frequency is minimal.

The organism lives in soil enriched by organic nitrogen, usually under large bird roosts or in bat-caves. When the soil is disturbed, the spores become airborne and are inhaled. The portal of entry for all the endemic fungi is the lung. Following inhalation, the infecting spores reach the alveoli where they immediately convert from the saprophytic phase to the tissue invasive form, which for both histoplasmosis and blastomycosis is a single budding yeast. This rapid conversion allows the infecting particles to elude phagocytosis and multiply. The yeasts are eventually ingested by macrophages and within these macrophages, the fungus disseminates throughout the body prior to the establishment of T cell-dependent immunity. All organs may be involved in the process of dissemination, but organs of the reticuloendothelial (RE) system are most likely to be involved. With the advent of T cell-mediated immunity the macrophages are able to contain the infection by the formation of granulomas. Analogous to tuberculosis some organisms remain alive in these granulomas and may reactivate with the waning of cell-mediated immunity, usually secondary to development of an illness such as HIV/AIDS with degradation of T-cell-mediated immune function or as the result of the administration of cytotoxic agents used in cancer chemotherapy or in transplantation as well as those treated with tumour necrosis factor alpha (TNF-α) blocking agents often for rheumatologic or other autoimmune disorders (Lee *et al.*, 2002; Wood *et al.*, 2003; Rychly and DiPiro, 2005).

Clinical manifestations

The vast majority of infected, immunologically intact individuals will have no clinically detectable illness and the only residual may be the development of a positive skin test to histoplasmin. When illness does develop, it tends to be a mild, influenza-like illness with cough and frequent myalgias. Rarely, especially after inhaling a large infecting dose in a closed space such as a storm-cellar, a rapidly progressive and potentially lethal disease develops. These patients develop rapidly progressive air-space disease and will often require mechanical ventilation (Figure 13.1).

Rapid diagnosis is critical since the tempo of the disease may be overwhelming. In the right environment of the endemic area, a compatible clinical illness with an abnormal chest radiograph is highly suggestive but not diagnostic of histoplasmosis. The radiologic picture is that of a rapidly moving micronodular infiltrate involving all areas of the lung. This clinical picture usually develops within 10–14 days after exposure. Extensive pulmonary disease may also develop in HIV/AIDS patients when the previously dormant infection is reactivated under the pressure of decreased T cell function (Wheat *et al.*, 1990; Johnson, Hamill and Sarosi, 1989). The radiographic picture in these cases often appears indistinguishable from primary infection.

Diagnosis

The most important part of rapid diagnosis is a high index of suspicion. A careful history including travel and exposure to potential sources of aerosol in areas known to be

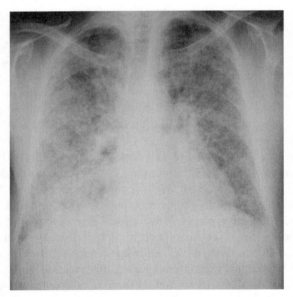

Figure 13.1   Admission radiograph of an archeologist just before intubation. Note the diffuse and multiple small lesions characteristic of acute overwhelming histoplasmosis.

endemic is critical. While blood cultures may be positive, especially in patients with HIV/AIDS (Wheat *et al.*, 1990), growth may take three–five days.

When histoplasmosis is considered, fungal blood cultures should be obtained. The best rapid diagnostic test is the determination of the histoplasma polysaccharide antigen (HAg) in both blood and urine (Wheat, 2003). While this test is readily available in North America, it is usually sent to far-away consulting laboratories with considerable delay in diagnosis. The test reflects the number of organisms present in infected individuals and is usually negative in the mild illnesses seen in most infected subjects. Multiple other serologic tests exist for the diagnosis of histoplasmosis. All of these tests measure either IGM or IGG antibodies. Interpretation is difficult and a single titre is seldom diagnostic, only suggestive. Perhaps the only time an antibody-based test is diagnostic is if one can show a fourfold increase or decrease in the titre. Since two tests four to six weeks apart are needed the antibody based tests are seldom useful during an acute illness (Wheat *et al.*, 1992).

When the HAg is not readily available, bronchoscopy with bronchoalveolar lavage (BAL) should be done. The small yeasts of *H. capsulatum* can often be recognized within phagocytes, but because of their small size they may be confused with the yeasts of *Candida spp.* BAL fluid may also be used for measurement of HAg. When disseminated disease is suspected, a bone marrow biopsy can often yield the diagnosis within minutes (Davies, Mckenna and Sarosi, 1979). Similarly, examination of the peripheral blood smear may rarely allow rapid identification of the fungus as it circulates in phagocytes.

Treatment

Treatment of severe histoplasmosis begins with a polyene – either AMB-L or AMB-d. In a small randomized trial AMB-L was slightly more effective. The dose needs to be escalated rapidly and maintained at 5 mg/kg of AMB-L or 0.7 mg/kg AMB-d until clinical stability after which the patient should receive 200 mg itraconazole twice daily for at least 6–12 months. We recommend continuing polyene treatment as long as air-exchange problems remain and the patient is still ventilated (Wheat *et al.*, 2007).

Repeated measurements of the HAg are recommended when treating an immuno-suppressed patient with disseminated histoplasmosis. Decreases in the Hag titre are seen with effective therapy and relapses of infection are associated with subsequent increases in the Hag titre.

Blastomycosis

Epidemiology, microbiology and pathogenesis

Traditionally blastomycosis is mentioned in the same breath as histoplasmosis, but the two diseases are very different clinically and epidemiologically. While histoplasmosis is a disease of the RE system, and always leads to a granulomatous histopathologic picture, blastomycosis begins as a pyogenic infection and only later will granulomas appear. Moreover, the pyogenic picture never completely disappears and blastomycosis should be thought of as a pyogranulomatous process (Sarosi and Davies, 1979).

The endemic area of blastomycosis is less well defined than the endemic area for histoplasmosis, since reliable skin tests for *Blastomyces dermatitidis* were never deployed. *The suggested endemic area* is an area derived by listing the patient's residence, without clear proof that the infection occurred in that location. Using this method, the proposed endemic area of blastomycosis overlaps most of the endemic area of histoplasmosis and extends farther north and west into the prairie provinces of Canada. The endemic areas with the highest rates of infection include the states of Arkansas and Mississippi in the Southern United States, and the northern states of the Great Lakes, including Wisconsin, Michigan and Minnesota (Davies and Sarosi, 1997).

Blastomyces dermatitidis is a soil-dwelling, temperature dependent, dimorphic fungus. Unlike epidemics of histoplasmosis, which often involved entire communities, blastomycosis outbreaks are smaller and involve only a handful of individuals. Men are more frequently involved among sporadically occurring cases, but in epidemics there is no sex or age preference. Most patients had extensive involvement with outdoor pursuits, such as hunting, fishing or construction.

Clinical manifestations

The acute infection often begins as an influenza-like syndrome with fever, cough and myalgias. The nonproductive cough will become productive of purulent sputum and early on the chest radiograph resembles community acquired pneumonia though infiltrates will progress rapidly if diagnosis and treatment are delayed (Davies and Sarosi, 1997) (Figure 13.2).

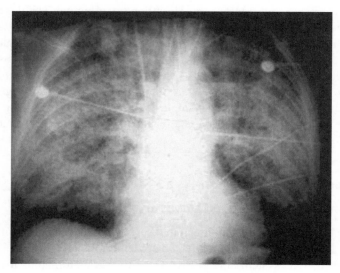

Figure 13.2   Rapidly fatal blastomycosis.

Often patients are seen after two or more courses of broad-spectrum oral antibiotics have failed.

Diagnosis

A travel and exposure history will often point toward blastomycosis, but the mainstay of diagnosis remains a high index of suspicion. The most rapid diagnosis is examination of freshly expectorated sputum (or other biologic specimen, such as pus from a skin lesion) after digestion with 10% potassium hydroxide (KOH) (Sarosi and Davies, 1979; Lemos, Guo and Baliga, 2000; Martynowicz and Prakash, 2002). In expert hands this method is highly accurate. While sputum culture is very helpful, it is time consuming and may take as long as 30 days. When the tempo of the disease is rapid, BAL will often show the fungus (Figure 13.3).

Since *B. dermatitidis* is not found in RE tissues, bone marrow examination is not helpful. Up to 20–25% of patients will have dissemination, mostly to the skin, bones, brain or prostate, often providing easy access to diagnostic material. In spite of the frequency of extra-pulmonary spread, blood cultures are seldom positive. A recently developed blood and urine test, measuring antigen shows promise (Durkin *et al.*, 2004; Mongkolrattanothai *et al.*, 2006). Measurement of antibody by various methods is less well developed than in histoplasmosis; it may have some utility in diagnosis when the tempo of the infection is slow enough to allow collection of acute and convalescent specimens.

Treatment

Treatment follows a similar path to histoplasmosis – when the disease is extensive and either requires mechanical ventilation or threatens to – treatment must begin with a polyene identical to our recommendation for histoplasmosis. If the meninges, brain or

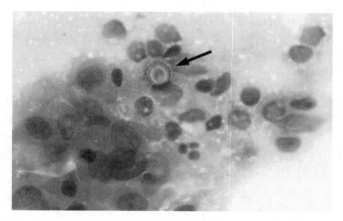

Figure 13.3 After intubation for respiratory failure, BAL shows the *Blastomyces dermatitidis* fungus (Giemsa X 400).

spinal cord are involved, even when there is no gas-exchange problem, polyenes are recommended as therapy. Following stabilization of the infiltrate and with improvement of gas-exchange oral itraconazole should be used for 6–12 months (Chapman *et al.*, 2000). Following the response to treatment, repeated measurement of the antigen may be useful, but this method has not been well studied (Mongkolrattanothai *et al.*, 2006).

Coccidioidomycosis

Epidemiology, microbiology and pathogenesis

Although the fungus *Coccidioides immitis* was originally described in Argentina, the vast majority of infections occur in the southwestern states of the US and adjacent areas of Mexico. In the US, the endemic area involves the Central Valley of California, the low desert area of Arizona and parts of New Mexico, and the desert area of Utah, all below 3500 feet elevation. This area is the Lower Sonoran Life Zone with hot weather and very low rainfall.

Coccidioides immitis is also a soil-dwelling dimorphic fungus, but the tissue-invasive form is the giant spherule, rather than a yeast form. Similar to histoplasmosis and blastomycosis, the portal of entry is the lung. After inhalation of the infecting arthrospore, the organism converts into the tissue invasive form, leading to the formation of a giant spherule containing many spherules. With maturation, the giant spherule ruptures, releasing the multitude of spherules, propagating the infection. Not all infected individuals develop a clinical illness following exposure, but up to 40–50% will have some symptoms (Galgiani, 1993; Stevens, 1995).

Clinical manifestations

The extent of the disease is probably related to the infecting dose. Similar to blastomycosis but not to histoplasmosis, coccidioidomycosis will often present as community acquired pneumonia (CAP) and in a recent small study almost a third of the patients with CAP in the Tucson, Arizona area had acute coccidioidomycosis (Valdivia *et al.*, 2006). The chest radiograph may show a lobar infiltrate or a diffuse nodular infiltrate (Figure 13.4).

The tempo of the disease is highly variable but it tends to move very fast in AIDS patients.

In addition to the severe pulmonary disease ICU physicians need to be aware of the tropism of *C. immitis* to the meninges. Meningeal involvement may occur without evidence of the disease at any other site or it may occur with pulmonary involvement. The meningitis usually has no acute meningeal signs and the most frequent presentation is headache and confusion (Johnson and Einstein, 2006).

Diagnosis

Diagnosis is difficult but the correct tests need to be employed. The 'gold standard' remains the recovery in culture of the infecting fungus. The process is slow, may take

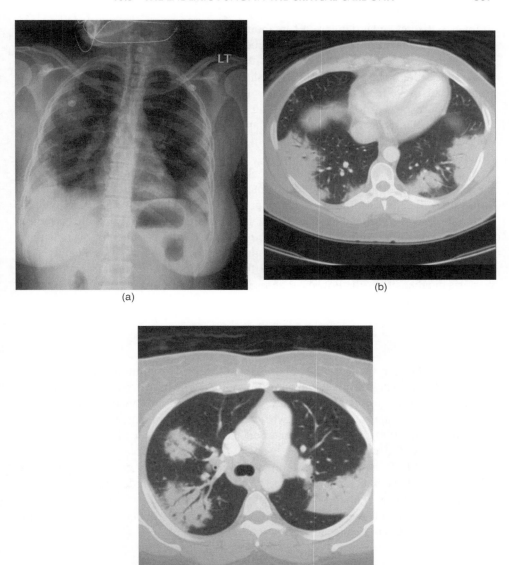

Figure 13.4 (a) Admission radiograph of a graduate student with 'community acquired pneumonia' after a five-day course of azythromycin and 10-day course of levofloxacin (turned out to be coccidioidomycosis). (b) Chest CT showing multiple lesions of dense consolidation. (c) Chest CT two days later showing progression of disease.

as long as 30 days and is dangerous for laboratory personnel due to the very high risk of infection when handling cultures. When coccidioidomycosis is suspected, laboratory personnel must be notified in order for them to take additional precautions. The material should not be plated on a Petri dish and should only be placed into slants. The minimal air-movement that accompanies the opening of a Petri dish is enough to create an aerosol. Serologic tests have long been the mainstay of diagnosis and in this disease these tests are well developed and validated. The height of the titre as measured in some laboratories may be roughly indicative of the extent of the disease (Pappagianis, 2001).

In a recent publication, investigators applied the HAg to patients with coccidioidomycosis with some success, suggesting potential applicability (Kuberski *et al.*, 2007). In critically ill patients with gas-exchange problems BAL may be useful. Staining of the material should be with the Papanicolau stain. When meningitis is suspected a lumbar puncture will show evidence for chronic meningitis with a mononuclear cell pleocytosis, elevated protein and decreased glucose. The culture is often negative and antibody tests need be done. Frequently the presence of documented coccidioidomycosis in other sites will allow the diagnosis of coccidioidomycotic meningitis purely on the base of the pleocytosis.

Treatment

For acutely ill patients with severe pulmonary involvement, we initiate treatment with a polyene. Unfortunately, even polyenes are not reliably effective in coccidioidomycosis. In the more chronic forms of the disease both fluconazole and itraconazole have been used. Itraconazole appears to be somewhat better in bone involvement than fluconazole (Galgiani *et al.*, 2000). The recently licensed azole, posaconazole also appears to have excellent activity against the fungus (Stevens *et al.*, 2007; Catanzaro *et al.*, 2007; Nagappan and Deresinski, 2007). Meningitis in patients without coma may be treated with fluconazole (Johnson and Einstein, 2006); in patients with decreased sensorium, polyenes may be used both intravenously as well as intrathecally (Stevens and Shatsky, 2001). After apparent recovery, fluconazole should be continued for the life of the patient to prevent late recurrences (Dewsnup *et al.*, 1996).

13.4   Other yeast infections in the critical care unit

Cryptococcosis

Epidemiology, microbiology and pathogenesis

Cryptococcal disease is caused by infection with *Cryptococcus neoformans* a fungus with a worldwide distribution. Like other fungi discussed in this chapter, the route of infection for this disease is inhalational. The most frequent form of cryptococcal disease seen in ICUs is cryptococcal meningitis, although cryptococcal pulmonary disease may become fulminant, especially in those with HIV/AIDS. Cryptococcal meningitis was a well described, but rare infection prior to the widespread use of solid organ transplantation and vigorous use of cytoreductive chemotherapy. With the onset of the HIV pandemic, cryptococcal meningitis emerged as the most common fungal agent causing opportunistic infections in this group of patients. An estimated 5% of patients in the US developed cryptococcal meningitis prior to the availability of HAART; while in sub-Saharan Africa this figure reached 30%.

Clinical manifestations

Clinical manifestations are non-specific and patients may show either subtle or at times no clinical evidence of meningismus. Patients with cryptococcal meningitis not infrequently present with fever and confusion without focal neurological findings. Cryptococcal pulmonary disease is less well studied than the meningeal infection. The majority of patients with pulmonary cryptococcal infection present with a subacute to chronic course and are seldom seen in the ICU. The presentation of cryptococcal pneumonia is often dependent upon the degree of immunosuppression in a given host. Those with no recognizable immune suppression often present with a solitary infiltrate or nodule whereas those with severe immunosuppression present diffuse infiltrates and hypoxemia.

Diagnosis

For cryptococcal meningitis, lumbar puncture will establish the diagnosis, especially since the availability of the test kit for measurement of the cryptococcal antigen (CrAg) in either cerebrospinal fluid (CSF) or in blood. The CSF formula will usually show elevated WBCs with mononuclear cell preponderance, elevated protein and reduced glucose. Nevertheless, measurement of CrAg is important, since the CSF cell counts may be completely normal in HIV/AIDS and the diagnosis is most frequently established with a positive CrAg titre. In patients with HIV/AIDS and cryptococcal meningitis, the serum CrAg is frequently positive and may provide a diagnosis awaiting the performance of a lumbar puncture. That said, the availability of serum CrAg testing should not delay a lumbar puncture if the index of suspicion is high for cryptococcal disease. Pulmonary infections are best diagnosed by examination and culture of bronchoalveolar lavage or biopsy specimens.

Given the improved sensitivity of routine blood cultures for the detection of C. neoformans, a diagnosis of cryptococcal infection can at times be made from a positive routine blood culture. This is particularly true for those with profound cellular immune defects as seen in HIV/AIDS or transplantation. It is important to recognize the possibility of cryptococcal infection in this setting, as care providers may incorrectly assume that all positive cultures demonstrating yeast in a blood culture are Candida spp. and choose an echinocandin drug which has no significant activity against C. neoformans, as empiric therapy.

Treatment

Treatment guidelines for cryptococcal meningitis are well established and are based on well-designed, high quality randomized trials (van der Horst *et al.*, 1997). All the trials were performed on HIV infected patients prior to the availability of highly active antiretroviral therapy (HAART). Although the trials did not include pulmonary disease most experts agree that the application of data from meningeal studies is appropriate (Saag *et al.*, 2000). It is clear that the mainstay of therapy is still an AMB containing product administered until clinical stability occurs, followed by fluconazole therapy. Fluconazole therapy alone is not as efficacious for severe cryptococcal meningitis. The echinocandins have no role in the treatment of cryptococcosis.

Since the availability of HAART, the prevalence of cryptococcal meningitis has declined though this infection is still seen in minimally immunocompromised patients, where the prognosis is unfortunately poorer than in the much younger population with HIV/AIDS (Ecevit *et al.*, 2006).

Invasive candidiasis

Epidemiology, microbiology and pathogenesis

Candidemia represents a major problem in hospitals, especially in the ICU setting (Fridkin, 2005; Trick *et al.*, 2002; Garbino *et al.*, 2002). *Candida spp* blood stream invasion is now the fourth most common cause of all nosocomial blood stream infections in the United States, with similar high rates in other countries (Marchetti *et al.*, 2004). As healthcare technologies advance, more critically ill patients are surviving for longer periods of time and are exposed to an increasing number of invasive procedures. This process has led to a very large number of highly susceptible critically ill patients in ICU care (Ostrosky-Zeichner and Pappas, 2006).

Candida spp. are normal inhabitants of the mouth and gastrointestinal tract and C. albicans is the most common colonizing *Candida* spp. As such, the most common *Candida* spp recovered from bloodstream infections is *C. albicans*. Risk factors for candidemia include the presence of a central venous catheter, length of hospitalization, prior bacteremia, receipt of antibacterials, receipt of parenteral nutrition, chronic renal failure or dialysis use and neutropenia (Wenzel, 1995; Bassetti *et al.*, 2007). It is difficult to imagine today that a positive blood culture for *Candida albicans* was frequently disregarded in the 1950s and was referred to as 'self limited'. For many years the issue of 'contamination' versus 'infection' was unresolved and the isolation of *Candida spp* was often regarded as 'normal flora'. Finally, a consensus conference by experienced clinical investigators laid the controversies surrounding positive *Candida spp* blood cultures to rest – all positive blood cultures were meaningful and all should be treated (Edwards *et al.*, 1997).

During the last 15 years, the incidence of *C. albicans* has been declining and there has been an increase in non-albicans *Candida spp* in bloodstream infections in most but not all institutions (Ostrosky-Zeichner and Pappas, 2006; Garbino *et al.*, 2002). Some of the increase in non-albicans *Candida* spp and fall in *C. albicans* can be attributed to fluconazole exposure which can favour the overgrowth of certain non-albicans species, particularly *C. glabrata* (Marr, 2004; Diekema *et al.*, 2002; Abi-Said *et al.*, 1997). In one study, colonization with *C. glabrata* and susceptibility to fluconazole were monitored serially in patients receiving fluconazole (Bennett, Izumikawa and Marr, 2004). In those with repeated *C. glabrata* colonization while receiving fluconazole, the recovered *C. glabrata* isolates showed reduced susceptibility to fluconazole that worsened over time. The mechanism of this resistance was an increase in efflux of the drug from these organisms (Bennett, Izumikawa and Marr, 2004).

Of importance to care in the ICU is the understanding of the breakthrough pathogens, pathogens unlikely to respond to specific antifungal therapies as well as the potential for cross-resistance to other antifungals. For patients exposed to fluconazole, *C. glabrata* and *C. krusei* are well described non-albicans *Candida* spp causing clinical infection (Marr, 2004). Fluconazole may be ineffective against many *C. glabrata* isolates and is clearly ineffective for *C. krusei*, a less commonly recovered organism. Of additional importance is the observation that voriconazole may be less active against *C. glabrata* isolates demonstrating fluconazole resistance (Pfaller *et al.*, 2003). Regarding the echinocandins, *C. parapsilosis* (Cheung *et al.*, 2006; Barchiesi *et al.*, 2006) is generally less susceptible to this drug class. Infection with *C. parapsilosis* has been reported to develop in patients while receiving an echinocandin (Cheung *et al.*, 2006) and an increased incidence of *C. parapsilosis* infections has been reported in association with increased echinocandin use in a tertiary care unit setting (Forrest, Weekes and Johnson, 2008). Finally, *C. lusitaniae*, a rarely isolated yeast, is often unresponsive to AMB (Pappagianis *et al.*, 1979; Guinet *et al.*, 1983).

Clinical manifestations

The clinical manifestations of invasive candidiasis or *Candida* spp bloodstream infections are generally non-specific and cannot be differentiated from bacterial infections based on clinical findings. The organism readily produces a biofilm that adheres to vascular and other catheter related materials resulting in bloodstream catheter associated infections as well as peritoneal dialysis catheter associated infections. *Candida* spp bloodstream infections may present as isolated fungemia or disseminated infection. Dissemination to almost any site can occur including the brain, joints, vertebral discs, pericardium and pleural space. Infection of the eye or endophthalmitis may also occur (Brooks, 1989). Cutaneous rashes may occur and may be most often seen in neutropenic patients. A shock-like picture may be present in those with candidemia, though this appears to be relatively rare (Hadley *et al.*, 2002a). In patients with candidemia presenting in shock, the mortality rate is nearly 60% (Hadley *et al.*, 2002a).

Another important point to understand, in the care of critically ill patients, is the relative rarity of *Candida* spp as a cause of primary pneumonia. Pulmonary involvement if present is most commonly a result of disseminated infection from a fungemia. Practically speaking, it is important to realize that *Candida* spp colonization of ICU patients receiving antibacterial agents is extremely common and unlikely to represent primary *Candida* spp pneumonia.

Diagnosis

While the majority of invasive *Candida* spp infections are detected via positive blood cultures, reliance on blood culture isolation as the only criterion for treatment initiation may be insufficient (Berenguer *et al.*, 1993). At the same time, interpreting the potential importance of *Candida* spp isolation from non-sterile sites in individual patients has been difficult. The widespread acceptance of new culture methodologies using special media that allow for faster identification of species of *Candida* spp has helped (Horvath *et al.*, 2003), but the intrinsic problem of separating significant from insignificant isolates from non-sterile sites remains. Generations of experts have tried to create a reproducible and reliable serologic test for the diagnosis of *Candida spp* infections. The recent emergence of the serologic test for β-D-glucan for the first time allows some hope for the development of sensitive and specific serodiagnostic test – that may aid in the early diagnosis of invasive candidiasis in susceptible patients (Odabasi *et al.*, 2004).

Fungal susceptibility testing has lagged behind bacterial susceptibility tests until recently and such testing is now readily available (Rex and Pfaller, 2002). Studies of real-time fungal susceptibility results and the effect of such testing on patient care are generally lacking (Magiorakos and Hadley, 2004) though such testing may be valuable in the care of immunosuppressed populations (Hadley *et al.*, 2002b; Magiorakos and Hadley, 2004). More importantly, newer techniques have allowed more rapid speciation of yeasts recovered in cultures, which is perhaps even more useful than the determination of the minimum inhibitory concentration of an antifungal agent to the isolate. In fact, once speciation is available, one can make a highly accurate prediction of susceptibility to the given drug (Pappas *et al.*, 2004).

For patients with documented *Candida* spp bloodstream infection, clinicians should maintain a high index of suspicion for the development of disseminated sites of infection. Even subtle back pain should prompt evaluation for vertebral osteomyelitis (Miller and Mejicano, 2001) and any decrease in vision should prompt an evaluation for endophthalmitis, a complication that may require intraocular antifungal therapy and at times surgical intervention (Brooks, 1989). Concern for the development of endophthalmitis, which may not be associated with symptoms in ICU patients who are intubated and sedated, has led to the recommendation that at least one careful dilated funduscopic examination be performed on all patients with candidemia (Pappas *et al.*, 2004; Brooks, 1989).

Treatment

In addition to offering specific antifungal therapy, there are certain general principles that should be followed when one encounters a patient with an invasive *Candida* spp infection. Most authorities agree that *whenever possible*, all foreign objects should be removed. These include all lines of vascular access as well as other implants or foreign materials that may be implicated or in contact with the infection. Clearly, this is not always feasible and as tunnelled catheters are at a lower risk of becoming contaminated, these may be left *in situ* for a trial of therapy in patients who are clinically stable and without obvious distant foci of infection.

Drug therapy recommendations have been made by the Infectious Disease Society of America (IDSA) in 2004 and this set of recommendations will be replaced soon to accommodate the new agents that have been approved since its original publication (Pappas *et al.*, 2004). According to these guidelines (Pappas *et al.*, 2004), initial therapy may use AMB-d, fluconazole (Rex *et al.*, 1994), or and caspufungin (Mora-Duarte *et al.*, 2002). The recently approved echinocandins, anidulofungin and micafungin should be viewed as being biologically equivalent to caspofungin, while voriconazole has a more broad-spectrum activity against *Candida* spp than fluconazole. All of these agents have been found to be effective in the treatment of candidemia (Reboli *et al.*, 2007; Pappas *et al.*, 2007). Similarly, most investigators view AMB-d and AMB-L as equipotent in the doses recommended. Since AMB-L is far less nephrotoxic than AMB-d the patients renal function should dictate the choice.

Local circumstances play an essential role in choosing the drug before sensitivities become available. In a patient who is receiving fluconazole prophylaxis, when yeast consistent with *Candida* spp is isolated from blood, a non-azole drug should be picked. Although voriconazole is effective in the treatment of *Candida* spp blood stream infections we do not recommend it in those previously exposed to prior fluconazole because of the potential for cross-resistance.

Preemptive antifungal therapy is antifungal therapy provided to a patient at risk for invasive candidiasis in the absence of evidence of *Candida* spp infection. For ICU patients with risk factors who remain febrile despite antibacterial agents preemptive therapy has been given serious consideration given the reduced sensitivity of culture techniques in improved tolerability of newer antifungal agents. While a number of studies evaluating such an approach have been underpowered, a recent cost-effectiveness analysis supports the use of preemptive fluconazole if the likelihood of invasive candidiasis is greater than 2.5% or fluconazole resistance less than 24.0%. In the setting of greater resistance levels to fluconazole, empirical echinocandin therapy may be preferred (Golan *et al.*, 2005). We believe that such an approach is reasonable.

13.5 Invasive mould infections in the critical care unit

Aspergillosis

Epidemiology, microbiology and pathogenesis

Invasive aspergillosis is a serious and potentially life-threatening fungal infection most often caused by the filamentous organism *Aspergillus fumigatus*. Invasive pulmonary aspergillosis usually affects individuals with haematologic malignancies with prolonged deficits of neutrophil number or function, those with graft-versus-host disease following haematopoetic stem-cell transplantation (HSCT) and following prolonged corticosteroid use or recipients of solid organ transplantation (Singh and

Paterson, 2005). In recent years there have been increasing reports of invasive aspergillosis in critical care unit settings, not only in patients with haematologic malignancies or organ transplantation, but also in patients receiving steroids for chronic obstructive pulmonary disease, asthma, rheumatoid arthritis or vasculitides and in patients with cirrhosis (Meersseman *et al.*, 2004; Cornillet *et al.*, 2006; Meersseman *et al.*, 2008). Infection has also been associated with the receipt of tumour necrosis factor-alpha (TNF-α) blocking therapies (De Rosa *et al.*, 2003; Warris, Bjorneklett and Gaustad, 2001).

Aspergillus species are classified as moulds and are found with a worldwide distribution. These organisms are ubiquitous, are usually found in soil and decaying matter and produce conidia (spores) between 2 and 5 μ in diameter that easily becomes airborne (Kwon-Chung and Bennett, 1992a). *Aspergillus* species can be easily isolated from air from the outside environment as well as from hospital air (Kwon-Chung and Bennett, 1992a). While most infections have been attributed to inhalation of conidia travelling through air, exposure to and inhalation of contaminated water may also be a source of this infection in nosocomial settings (Warris *et al.*, 2003; Anaissie and Costa, 2001). *Aspergillus fumigatus* is the most common species implicated in human disease while infections due to *A. flavus*, *A. terreus*, *A. nidulans* and *A. niger* are less common. As responses to the presently available antifungal agents may differ by *Aspergillus* spp, it is important if at all possible to identify these organisms to the species level following recovery in culture (Lass-Flörl *et al.*, 2005).

Clinical manifestations

The most frequent clinical manifestation of aspergillosis in immunosuppressed patients is invasive pulmonary aspergillosis, seen in about 80–90% of those infected. The paranasal sinuses may also represent an initial site of infection in immunosuppressed hosts. Aspergillosis is an angioinvasive infection and disseminated disease involving other tissues distant to the lung occurs in about approximately 5–25% of cases (Singh and Paterson, 2005; Denning, 1998). Sites of dissemination can include almost any tissues with the most feared being central nervous system (CNS) infection as it is associated with a worse prognosis, particularly in the setting of multi-focal CNS disease (Figure 13.5).

While pulmonary infection may initially be asymptomatic, common symptoms include a dry cough, dull or pleuritic chest pain, and at times haemoptysis. Haemoptysis while not present in the majority of cases ranges from mild to quite severe. Dyspnea may be seen as well in association with pleuritic pain or in the presence of more diffuse pulmonary infiltrates. The course of disease is frequently very rapid once recognized, particularly in the setting of persistent severe neutropenia.

There are a number of characteristic radiographic findings associated with pulmonary aspergillosis, best identified through the use of computed tomography (CT) scanning. In a recent evaluation of a multicentre study of aspergillosis over 90% of patients with acute invasive pulmonary aspergillosis were reported to have had at least one macronodular lesion with approximately 60% also demonstrating a halo sign (Greene *et al.*, 2007). Other radiographic findings, included consolidations (30%),

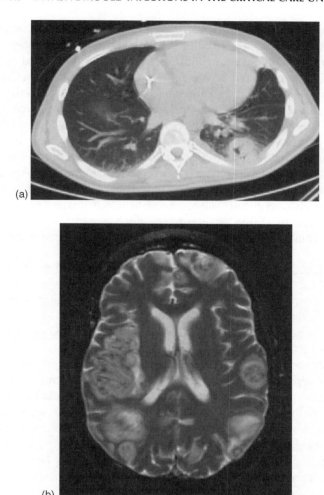

Figure 13.5   (a) Chest CT in a patient with graft versus host disease presenting with chest pain and aphasia following haematopoetic stem cell transplant. Biopsy revealed aspergillosis. (b) Brain MRI T2 weighted image with multiple lesions indicative of CNS aspergillosis in the same patient.

infarct-shaped nodules (27%), cavitary lesions (20%) and air-crescent signs (10%) (Greene *et al.*, 2007). Patients presenting with a halo sign may have significantly better responses to treatment and greater survival than patients with other radiographic findings (Greene *et al.*, 2007).

Diagnosis

Historically, the diagnosis of aspergillosis has required an appropriate patient at risk, a compatible syndrome and a tissue specimen demonstrating the organism recovered from a normally sterile site or evidence of invasion of tissues accompanied by the identification of *Aspergillus* spp in culture. Several criteria for the diagnosis of proven, probable and possible invasive fungal infections have been proposed by the European Organization for Research and Treatment of Cancer/Mycosis Study Group (EORTC/MSG) (Ascioglu *et al.*, 2002; de Pauw and Patterson, 2005) The criteria for proven disease have included (1) host factors (including neutropenia, prolonged use of steroids within the last 60 days, fever and graft-versus-host disease); (2) microbiologic (positive culture, direct microscopic evaluations for mould); and (3) major clinical/radiologic criteria (CT imaging halo sign, air-crescent sign, or cavity within area of consolidation and (4) minor clinical criteria that include symptoms (cough, chest pain, haemoptysis). While it is always desirable to have the highest level of information in order to have a diagnosis of proven aspergillosis and to be able to clearly distinguish colonization with *Aspergillus* spp from true infection, in patients with haematologic malignancies and low platelet counts it may be difficult to obtain appropriate tissue specimens in a timely manner.

Regarding clinical decision making, a recent study assessing the applicability of the 2002 EORTC/MSG definitions (Ascioglu *et al.*, 2002) for proven aspergillosis, found that in autopsy proven cases of invasive pulmonary aspergillosis in patients with haematologic malignancies, that only about 10% of such cases were classified as having proven aspergillosis while alive (Subira *et al.*, 2003). Radiographic features and clinical factors including underling leukemia, profound neutropenia, pleuritic chest pain, and cavitary or nodular lesions detected on CT scan have all been associated with aspergillosis as opposed to other infectious etiologies for pneumonia in patients with cancer (Hachem *et al.*, 2006). Such predictive factors can be used to aid decisions on early prophylactic and therapeutic antifungal medications while diagnostic evaluations are ongoing. It is important to recognize that the decision to initiate antifungal therapy for invasive aspergillosis should not depend upon meeting the criteria for proven aspergillosis, but rather should be done with an understanding of the patient risk and clinical presentation and supported by diagnostic testing. It is also important to recognize that other fungi such as *Fusarium* species, *Pseudoallescheria boydii* and the Zygomcytes (agents of zygomycosis) may have a similar histological appearance in stained tissue specimens and these organisms should be distinguished from *Aspergillus* spp if at all possible in order to best direct antifungal therapies.

Given the difficulties in obtaining adequate diagnostic samples through the use of invasive tests, there has long been an interest in non-invasive tests for the diagnosis of invasive aspergillosis. A double-sandwich ELISA test for detection of the fungal cell wall constituent, galactomannan, has been approved in a number of countries as a diagnostic aid for aspergillosis. The *Aspergillus* galactomannan test can be performed using serum or other body fluids in order to support the diagnosis of invasive aspergillosis. This test has demonstrated the greatest utility when used to serially monitor serum of patients at high risk, such as those undergoing chemotherapy for haematologic malignancies or those undergoing HSCT (Maertens *et al.*, 2001). The test has been evaluated in a number of clinical settings and an understanding of reasons for false-positive tests results, as well as the test sensitivity and specificity are crucial in order to best utilize this test. In a recent meta-analysis, the overall galactomannan assay test performance had a sensitivity of 71% and specificity of 89% for proven cases of invasive aspergillosis (Pfeiffer, Fine and Safdar, 2006). In our experience, the serum galactomannan test has been valuable, particularly in patients with low platelets or other contraindications to biopsy presenting with a syndrome compatible with invasive aspergillosis. In instances when the galactomannan *Aspergillus* antigen is strongly positive, we have been able to avoid tissue biopsies while maintaining enough confidence in our diagnosis to optimize our treatment targeting aspergillosis (Figure 13.6).

Recent case definition proposals for invasive aspergillosis have allowed *Aspergillus* antigen testing in BAL fluid, CSF and or serum to support the diagnosis of probable or possible invasive aspergillosis (Ascioglu *et al.*, 2002; de Pauw and Patterson, 2005). A recently published prospective study assessed the utility of galactomannan testing of BAL fluid in a critical care unit setting in 110 patients with recognized risk factors for aspergillosis as well as those with cirrhosis or HIV who had two of the three features including: new pulmonary infiltrates, signs or symptoms suggestive of invasive mycoses or fever recurrent or refractory to treatment with antibacterial agents. Post mortem examinations were performed on 69 of 73 (95%) persons who died in this

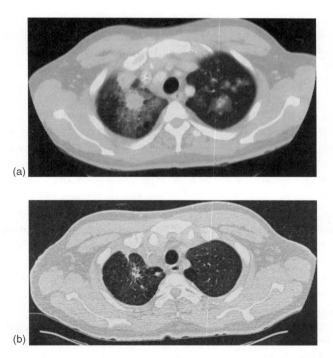

(a)

(b)

Figure 13.6   (a) Chest CT in a patient with leukemia, neutropenia and fever despite antibacterials. Thrombocytopenia precluded biopsy. Serum *Aspergillus* gallactomannan antigen was strongly positive. (b) Improvement documented following eight weeks of voriconazole and neutrophil recovery.

study. Using a cutoff index of 0.5, the sensitivity and specificity of galactomannan detection *in BAL fluid* was 88 and 87% respectively, whereas the sensitivity of *serum* galactomannan testing was only 42%. In 11 of 26 cases of proven aspergillosis, BAL cultures and serum galactomannan studies remained negative while the BAL galactomannan was positive.

Treatment

Single agent therapy

Despite advances in diagnostic modalities, and improved therapeutic options, invasive aspergillosis continues to be a life-threatening infection, with the highest rate of mortality observed in patients with recipients of allogeneic HSCT. In allogeneic HSCT recipients with invasive aspergillosis, the attributable mortality ranges from 22% (Upton *et al.*, 2007) to as high as 77% (Pagano *et al.*, 2007). All cause mortality has been reported to be as high as 70–87% in these patients (Upton *et al.*, 2007; Lin, Schranz and Teutsch, 2001). Mortality rates in patients undergoing less intensive regimens are lower.

Following the completion of a large, multi-centre randomized, trial comparing initial therapy voriconazole to standard AMB-d for proven and probable invasive aspergillosis, voriconazole has become the standard of care for this disease (Herbrecht *et al.*, 2002). Voriconazole was associated with higher response rates, improved survival and better tolerability (Herbrecht *et al.*, 2002). The use of voriconazole for invasive aspergillosis has been independently associated with a reduced risk of death from aspergillosis compared to those receiving other antifungal therapies outside of the clinical trial setting (Upton *et al.*, 2007). In addition to demonstrating efficacy in invasive pulmonary infections, voriconazole has been effective in CNS infections (Schwartz *et al.*, 2005). In a limited number of patients infected with *Aspergillus terreus*, an emerging pathogen resistant to AMB, voriconazole appeared to be effective (Steinbach *et al.*, 2004). Given the large-scale comparative trial results and performance of voriconazole in a vast number of clinical settings, in our opinion, voriconazole is the treatment of choice for invasive aspergillosis. This viewpoint is consistent with the recently published IDSA treatment guidelines for aspergillosis (Walsh *et al.*, 2008).

The echinocandin antifungal agents, caspofungin, micafungin and anidulofungin all have *in vitro* activity against *Aspergillus* spp and echinocandins are effective in animal models of aspergillosis (Petraitiene *et al.*, 2002; Petraitis *et al.*, 2003). In *Aspergillus* spp *in vitro* culture systems, echinocandins demonstrate only fungistatic activity. In a neutropenic rabbit model, caspofungin was associated with comparable survival to AMB, though animals treated with caspofungin had lesser reductions in both fungal burden and serum galactomannan when compared to AMB (Petraitiene *et al.*, 2002). The most significant support for the use of echinocandins for treatment of aspergillosis is the results of a trial evaluating the use of caspofungin in 83 patients failing or intolerant to other antifungal agents (Maertens *et al.*, 2004). Favourable responses were seen in 45% of patients, including 50% with pulmonary infection and

23% with disseminated infection. This study was completed before the widespread availability of voriconazole limiting the ability to generalize these results in patients who may have failed voriconazole primary therapy. Responses to micafungin, when used alone or in combination with other antifungal agents, have also been reported when used as primary or salvage treatment for invasive aspergillosis (Denning *et al.*, 2006).

Due to the lack of fungicidal activity against *Aspergillus* spp as well as the lack of large-scale clinical trials supporting the use of these agents for aspergillosis, we do not recommend echinocandins as single agents for initial therapy for invasive aspergillosis. These agents may have a role in salvage therapy particularly in combination with other antifungal agents as well as a role in primary therapy for aspergillosis when combined with other agents (see discussion of combination therapy).

Posaconazole, a broad-spectrum azole antifungal agent, presently only available in an oral formulation, is the most recently approved antifungal azole. Posaconazole has activity against *Aspergillus* spp as well as significant activity against a number of fungal pathogens responsible for clinical zygomycosis. In animal models, posaconazole has demonstrated activity in pulmonary and CNS aspergillosis (Imai *et al.*, 2004). Posaconazole has also been evaluated as salvage therapy in aspergillosis and when compared to historical controls, the overall success rate for posaconazole was 42% and compared to 26% for those treated with other salvage antifungals (prior to availability of voriconazole or echinocandins) (Walsh *et al.*, 2007). Posaconazole like voriconazole and itraconazole has *in vitro* activity against *A. terreus*. Posaconazole is active in animal models of invasive aspergillosis due *A. terreus* and as described for voriconazole a limited number of patients with *A. terreus* infections have been successfully treated with posaconazole (Hachem *et al.*, 2004). For posaconazole, given the limited number of patients with invasive aspergillosis treated to date, lack of comparative trial data and availability only as an oral suspension, this agent should not be considered as first line therapy for invasive aspergillosis. Posaconazole may be considered as part of a salvage regimen for aspergillosis pending additional trial data.

Treatment

Combined antifungal therapies

While the availability of voriconazole has been associated with improved outcomes for invasive aspergillosis, mortality for this disease remains high, particularly in patients who have undergone HSCTs. Various experimental models have demonstrated enhanced efficacy of dual therapies when compared to single agent therapies. Following the development of the newer triazoles and echinocandins, well-tolerated agents with significant activity against *Aspergillus* spp, there has been renewed interest in using combination antifungal therapies to treat aspergillosis. In animal models of aspergillosis, combinations of echinocandins with newer triazoles agent have demonstrated superior activity when compared to either agent alone (Petraitis *et al.*, 2003; Maccallum, Whyte and Odds, 2005). Models utilizing combinations of AMB with echinocandins have also shown greater efficacy for the combination than that for either agent alone (Dennis *et al.*, 2006). The results of combining a triazole with AMB however have been mixed (Meletiadis *et al.*, 2006).

To date, there have been no adequately powered controlled randomized clinical trials using combination antifungal therapies for aspergillosis in humans. Over the last six years there have been a number of centres reporting their experience with combinations of antifungal agents (Marr *et al.*, 2004; Maertens *et al.*, 2006), one small randomized controlled pilot study (Caillot *et al.*, 2006) and one prospective multi-centre observational study (Singh *et al.*, 2006). In a series of 48 patients with haematological malignancies treated with caspofungin plus AMB-L for possible or documented invasive aspergillosis, the combination was associated with a response rate of 42% overall with only a 18% response rate in those with documented infections who received the combination antifungals after failing single AMB-L. A 30-patient pilot study in patients with haematological malignancies evaluating the combination of low-dose (3 mg/kg/d) AMB-L plus standard dose caspofungin versus high dose AMB-L (10 mg/kg/d) as initial treatment for invasive aspergillosis showed a trend towards improved survival in the combination group (Caillot *et al.*, 2006). As salvage therapy following failure of AMB-d, in 16 patients with haematologic malignancies, the combination of voriconazole with caspofungin was associated with reduced mortality, when compared to 31 historical controls treated in a previous study with single-agent voriconazole (Marr *et al.*, 2004). Finally, a prospective multi-centre observational study of primary treatment of invasive aspergillosis in 40 solid organ transplant recipients, compared the combination of voriconazole plus caspofungin to 47 historical controls who had received single agent AMB-L (Singh *et al.*, 2006). In this study the 90-day survival with combination therapy was 67.5% compared to a 51% survival in the historical single agent control group. While these survival differences did not achieve statistical significance, in those patients with renal failure and in those with *A. fumigatus* infection, combination therapy was independently associated with improved survival.

As has been stated in previous reviews of combination antifungal therapy (Chamilos and Kontoyiannis, 2006; Johnson and Perfect, 2007), we need large randomized clinical trials in order to determine that combination antifungal therapy is superior to single agent therapy for these life-threatening infections. While it is clear that such studies would be extremely expensive and difficult to complete, such studies in our opinion are justified. While the data from these small series of patients receiving combinations of antifungal agents may be encouraging, such studies do not provide a sufficient basis to accept combination antifungal therapies as a standard of care for primary or for that matter salvage treatment of invasive aspergillosis.

Zygomycosis

Epidemiology, microbiology and pathogenesis

The Zygomycete fungi are moulds that are the etiologic agents of zygomycosis. The Zygomcyete class includes organisms in the order Mucorales, responsible for the clinical infections often referred to as mucormycosis attributed to infection secondary to *Mucor* species. The Zygomycyte class also includes non-*Mucor* species in the order Mucorales that cause similar infections, referred to as zygomcyosis. The Zygomycete class also includes the order Entomophthorales, and the *Conidiobolus* and *Basidiobolus* species, most commonly found in Africa and South-East Asia. These organisms cause infections characteristically different from infections attributed to Mucorales and will not be discussed in this section as they are not encountered with any significant frequency in the ICU setting.

Of importance are a number or organisms in the Zygomycete class included in the genera, *Absidia, Apophysomyces, Cokeromyces, Cunninghamella, Mucor, Rhizomucor, Rhizopus, Saksenaea, Syncephalastrum*, all known causes of human disease (Kwon-Chung and Bennett, 1992b). The most common pathogens causing zygomycosis are *Rhizopus* spp, followed by *Mucor* spp. Together, these two species are responsible for approximately 70% of cases (Roden *et al.*, 2005). These organisms are commonly recovered throughout the environment and may be especially concentrated in and sporulate after growth in decaying vegetables, seeds and fruits, old bread, compost material, soil and animal excreta (Kwon-Chung and Bennett, 1992b).

Most clinical disease is attributed to the inhalational route with deposition of airborne conidia in the upper or lower airways resulting in invasion of the nasal or paranasal sinus structures or invasion of the lung as a primary site of infection. Gastrointestinal disease has been described and likely is the result of the invasion of the gastrointestinal tract after ingestion of food contaminated by spores. Primary cutaneous disease has been described following exposure to contaminated bandages and in the absence of such an exposure in patients with extensive burns. Finally, infection has been associated with injectable drug use presumably through injection of contaminated materials directly into the bloodstream.

Clinically, zygomycosis or mucormycosis (terms often used interchangeably) are infections characterized by invasion of tissues and blood vessels including the nasal and sinus cavities, lung, brain and skin (Roden *et al.*, 2005). Dissemination disease is seen in about 25% of cases (Roden *et al.*, 2005). Infections caused by the Zygomycetes are serious infections associated with considerable morbidity and mortality (Roden *et al.*, 2005). These infections are mainly found in those with diabetic ketoacidosis, prolonged neutropenia complicating haematologic malignancies or those immunosuppressed as a result of anti-rejection therapies following solid organ or haematopoetic stem cell transplantation (Roden *et al.*, 2005). Those receiving deferoximine therapy are also at risk for these infections (Roden *et al.*, 2005). In some cases no known immunologic deficits are noted (Roden *et al.*, 2005).

Clinical manifestations

The most common clinical presentation of zygomycosis is invasive sinus disease, which may be complicated by extension into local tissues such as the orbits, brain (referred to as rhinocerebral zygomycosis), oral cavity or other facial structures (Figure 13.7).

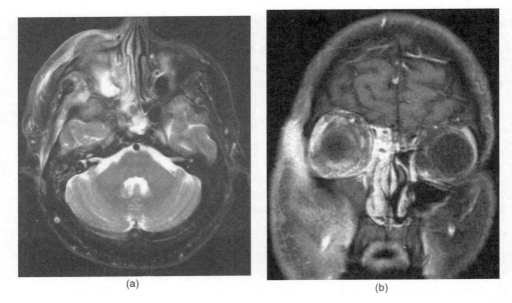

(a)   (b)

Figure 13.7   (a and b) Zygomycosis presenting as facial swelling and proptosis. T2 weighted MRI images showing disease invading right sinuses, right orbit and soft tissues of the head and neck. Tissue debridement and high-dose lipid amphotericin resulted in a cure.

This infection is angioinvasive and associated with tissue necrosis and thrombosis of vascular structures. Direct invasion of the brain can occur and is seen most commonly as a direct extension from sphenoid sinus infection. Neurologic complications may also occur following haematogenous dissemination or following cavernous sinus thrombosis, as the cavernous sinus vascular receives venous drainage from the nose, paranasal sinuses, upper lip, orbits and pharynx. Invasive sinus disease is the form of zygomycosis seen most commonly in diabetics where as pulmonary disease is the most common form of the infection in those with haematologic malignancies (Roden *et al.*, 2005). These infections often take quite an aggressive course and are associated with significant morbidity and mortality. Mortality for sinus infections ranges from 16% for sinus infection alone to approximately 60% when presenting as rhinocerebral disease (Roden *et al.*, 2005). Cerebral infections are associated with mortality rates of 80% or greater (Roden *et al.*, 2005).

Pulmonary disease most often presents in a manner similar to that of invasive aspergillosis and is characterized by consolidation, cavitary lesions and at times air crescent signs (Figure 13.8).

Extension of infection from the lung to other structures in the mediastinum may occur. Mortality for pulmonary zygomycosis is about 75%, demonstrating the seriousness of these infections and severely compromised hosts. Cutaneous infections may occur following inoculation at intravenous or other access sites, zygomycosis involving extensive wounds as is seen in burn patients may be quite severe.

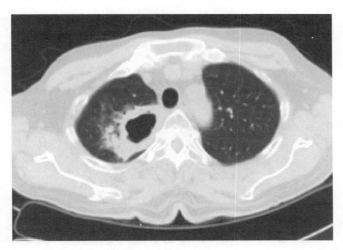

Figure 13.8 Cavitary lesion on chest CT in a patient one year after liver transplant. Fine needle aspirate histology demonstrated mould with aseptate hyphae consistent with zygomycosis. *Mucor* species grew in culture.

Diagnosis

In tissue, the Zygomycetes produce hyphae, that appear very broad (7–15 um) and typically lack regular septations (Kwon-Chung and Bennett, 1992b). Invasion of blood vessels and tissue necrosis are often seen in infected tissues. Branching of the hyphal elements occur at irregular angles with irregular spacing. The hyphal walls may be quite thin and irregular, which, not uncommonly, results in an appearance in tissue characterized twisting, collapse or folding of the hyphae along the long axis (Kwon-Chung and Bennett, 1992b). These histopathologic features are characteristic enough in the majority of cases to differentiate infection with the zygomycetes from *Aspergillus* spp or *Fusarium* spp in a good tissue specimen (Figure 13.9).

Treatment

Recognition of the clinical syndromes associated with zygomycosis, a prompt diagnosis and a combined approach of medical and surgical therapies are often required to provide a patient with the highest probability of response to therapy (Roden *et al.*, 2005). In our experience delays in diagnosis attributed to a less aggressive approach to obtaining appropriate tissue biopsy specimens can result in delays in definitive treatment leading to poor outcomes. It is our belief that early surgical intervention is of prime importance in the management of this disease.

Given the increasing number of antifungal therapies available it is important to understand the antimicrobial susceptibility patterns of the most common fungi responsible for zygomycosis. AMB is active against most of the agents of zygomycosis and the newer triazole posaconazole has significant activity against many of the Zygomycetes

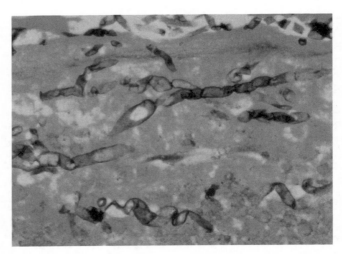

Figure 13.9   Gomori methanamine silver (GMS) stain of sinus tissue demonstrating irregular folded hyphae indicative of zygomycosis.

(Sun *et al.*, 2002a). While itraconazole has demonstrated some *in vitro* activity against these organisms, itraconazole is less active than posaconazole or AMB and not widely accepted as a therapeutic option (Sun *et al.*, 2002b). Voriconazole and fluconazole have no activity against the Zygomycetes (Sun *et al.*, 2002a). It is important to recognize that infections attributed to the Zygomycetes have been identified as an important cause of 'breakthrough' infections in those exposed to voriconazole (Kontoyiannis *et al.*, 2005; Chamilos *et al.*, 2005). In recent years, the incidence of zygomycosis has increased mainly due to the increasing use of haematopoetic stem cell transplants (Roden *et al.*, 2005).

Standard AMB-d has significant activity against the Zygomycete fungi and this agent was previously considered to be the agent of choice in the treatment of zygomycosis. Debridement of infected and devitalized tissues along with high doses AMB-d (1 mg/kg daily) have been effective in controlling invasive rhinocerebral disease in patients with underlying diabetes as well as those with other immunologic defects. Following the development of the less nephrotoxic lipid formulations of amphotericin, it has been accepted that high-dose AMB-L formulations using either liposomal amphotericin B or amphotericin B lipid complex (5 mg/kg daily) along with surgical debridement are now considered to be the agents of choice for initial treatment of these infections.

Pulmonary infections have similarly been treated with high doses of AMB containing preparations. Surgical resection of involved lung tissue has not generally been pursued as an initial adjunct to medical therapy, however, surgical resection of involved pulmonary tissues is often considered after an initial response to medical therapy for those who will require additional chemotherapy. As discussed previously, the newer azole antifungal posaconazole has significant activity against many of the agents of zygomycosis. Posaconazole orally at a dose of 800 mg daily has demonstrated promising results in patients with proven or probable zygomycosis who were refractory to or intolerant of AMB containing therapies. The response rate with posaconazole (including complete or partial response rates) was 60% in a report of salvage therapy. Adjunctive surgical therapies were commonly used in this patient population. Of note was that responses were seen in 72% of patients with cerebral involvement. In our opinion posaconazole is a promising agent for treatment of zygomycosis and should be considered in patients who are refractory to or intolerant of high dose AMB-L preparations. Posaconazole may also be considered as step down therapy after a response to AMB containing therapy though the use of posaconazole in this setting has not been adequately studied.

13.6 Summary

Advances in medicine as a whole and increasing use of immunosuppressive treatments have led to increased numbers of patients at risk for serious and invasive fungal infections. During the last decade we have witnessed many advances in antifungal treatment with the development of whole new classes of agents active against a wide variety of pathogens that effect critically ill patients. Optimal care of this patient group requires a high index of suspicion for fungal infections and knowledge of the ever-expanding therapeutic options. We look forward to the development of cost-effective diagnostic tests as well as the development of additional antifungal therapies available for use in the critical care setting.

References

Abi-Said, D., Anaissie, E., Uzun, O. *et al.* (1997) The epidemiology of hematogenous candidiasis caused by different Candida species. *Clinical Infectious Diseases*, **24**, 1122–1128.

Anaissie, E.J. and Costa, S.F. (2001) Nosocomial aspergillosis is waterborne. [see comment]. *Clinical Infectious Diseases*, **33**, 1546–1548.

Antinori, S., Magni, C., Nebuloni, M. *et al.* (2006) Histoplasmosis among human immunodeficiency virus-infected people in Europe: report of 4 cases and review of the literature. *Medicine (Baltimore)*, **85**, 22–36.

Ascioglu, S., Rex, J.H., De Pauw, B. *et al.* (2002) Defining opportunistic invasive fungal infections in immunocompromised patients with cancer and hematopoietic stem cell transplants: an international consensus. *Clinical Infectious Diseases*, **34**, 7–14.

Barchiesi, F., Spreghini, E., Tomassetti, S. *et al.* (2006) Effects of caspofungin against Candida guilliermondii and Candida parapsilosis. *Antimicrobial Agents & Chemotherapy*, **50**, 2719–2727.

Bassetti, M., Trecarichi, E.M., Righi, E. *et al.* (2007) Incidence, risk factors, and predictors of outcome of candidemia. Survey in 2 Italian university hospitals. *Diagnostic Microbiology & Infectious Disease*, **58**, 325–331.

Bennett, J.E., Izumikawa, K. and Marr, K.A. (2004) Mechanism of increased fluconazole resistance in Candida glabrata during prophylaxis. *Antimicrobial Agents & Chemotherapy*, **48**, 1773–1777.

Berenguer, J., Buck, M., Witebsky, F. *et al.* (1993) Lysis-centrifugation blood cultures in the detection of tissue-proven invasive candidiasis. Disseminated versus single-organ infection. *Diagnostic Microbiology and Infectious Disease*, **17**, 103–109.

Brooks, R.G. (1989) Prospective study of Candida endophthalmitis in hospitalized patients with candidemia. *Archives of Internal Medicine*, **149**, 2226–2228.

Caillot, D., Thiebaut, A., Herbrecht, R. *et al.* (2006) Liposomal Amphotericin B in combination with caspofungin versus liposomal Amphotericin B high dose regimen for the treatment of invasive aspergillosis in immunocompromised patients: Randomized pilot study (Combistrat trial). 16th Congress of the International Society for Human and Animal Mycology (Focus on Fungal Infections 16); 8–10 March, 2006, Las Vegas, Nevada, USA.

Catanzaro, A., Cloud, G.A., Stevens, D.A. *et al.* (2007) Safety, tolerance, and efficacy of posaconazole therapy in patients with nonmeningeal disseminated or chronic pulmonary coccidioidomycosis. *Clinical Infectious Diseases*, **45**, 562–568.

Chamilos, G. and Kontoyiannis, D.P. (2006) The rationale of combination antifungal therapy in severely immunocompromised patients: empiricism versus evidence-based medicine. *Current Opinion in Infectious Diseases*, **19**, 380–385.

Chamilos, G., Marom, E.M., Lewis, R.E. *et al.* (2005) Predictors of pulmonary zygomycosis versus invasive pulmonary aspergillosis in patients with cancer. *Clinical Infectious Diseases*, **41**, 60–66.

Chapman, S.W., Bradsher, R.W., Jr, Campbell, G.D., Jr *et al.* (2000) Practice guidelines for the management of patients with blastomycosis. Infectious Diseases Society of America. *Clinical Infectious Diseases*, **30**, 679–683.

Cheung, C., Guo, Y., Gialanella, P. and Feldmesser, M. (2006) Development of candidemia on caspofungin therapy: a case report. *Infection*, **34**, 345–348.

Cornillet, A., Camus, C., Nimubona, S. *et al.* (2006) Comparison of epidemiological, clinical, and biological features of invasive aspergillosis in neutropenic and nonneutropenic patients: a 6-year survey. *Clinical Infectious Diseases*, **43**, 577–584.

Davies, S.F., Mckenna, R.W. and Sarosi, G.A. (1979) Trephine biopsy of the bone marrow in disseminated histoplasmosis. *The American Journal of Medicine*, **67**, 617–622.

Davies, S.F. and Sarosi, G.A. (1997) Epidemiological and clinical features of pulmonary blastomycosis. *Seminars in Respiratory Infections*, **12**, 206–218.

De Pauw, B.E. and Patterson, T.F. (2005) Should the consensus guidelines' specific criteria for the diagnosis of invasive fungal infection be changed? *Clinical Infectious Diseases*, **41** (Suppl 6), S377–S380.

De Rosa, F.G., Shaz, D., Campagna, A.C. *et al.* (2003) Invasive pulmonary aspergillosis soon after therapy with infliximab, a tumor necrosis factor-alpha-neutralizing antibody: a possible healthcare-associated case? [see comment]. *Infection Control & Hospital Epidemiology*, **24**, 477–482.

Denning, D.W. (1998) Invasive aspergillosis. *Clinical Infectious Diseases*, **26**, 781–803.

Denning, D.W., Marr, K.A., Lau, W.M. *et al.* (2006) Micafungin (FK463), alone or in combination with other systemic antifungal agents, for the treatment of acute invasive aspergillosis. *Journal of Infection*, **53**, 337–349.

Dennis, C.G., Greco, W.R., Brun, Y. *et al.* (2006) Effect of amphotericin B and micafungin combination on survival, histopathology, and fungal burden in experimental aspergillosis in the p47phox−/− mouse model of chronic granulomatous disease. *Antimicrobial Agents & Chemotherapy*, **50**, 422–427.

Dewsnup, D.H., Galgiani, J.N., Graybill, J.R. *et al.* (1996) Is it ever safe to stop azole therapy for Coccidioides immitis meningitis? *Annals of Internal Medicine*, **124**, 305–310.

Diekema, D.J., Messer, S.A., Brueggemann, A.B. *et al.* (2002) Epidemiology of candidemia: 3-year results from the emerging infections and the epidemiology of Iowa organisms study. *Journal of Clinical Microbiology*, **40**, 1298–1302.

Dismukes, W.E. (2006) Antifungal therapy: lessons learned over the past 27 years. *Clinical Infectious Diseases*, **42**, 1289–1296.

Durkin, M., Witt, J., Lemonte, A. *et al.* (2004) Antigen assay with the potential to aid in diagnosis of blastomycosis. *Journal of Clinical Microbiology*, **42**, 4873–4875.

Ecevit, I.Z., Clancy, C.J., Schmalfuss, I.M. and Nguyen, M.H. (2006) The poor prognosis of central nervous system cryptococcosis among nonimmunosuppressed patients: a call for better disease recognition and evaluation of adjuncts to antifungal therapy. *Clinical Infectious Diseases*, **42**, 1443–1447.

Edwards, J.E., Jr, Bodey, G.P., Bowden, R.A. *et al.* (1997) International conference for the development of a consensus on the management and prevention of severe candidal infections. *Clinical Infectious Diseases*, **25**, 43–59.

Forrest, G.N., Weekes, E. and Johnson, J.K. (2008) Increasing incidence of Candida parapsilosis candidemia with caspofungin usage. *Journal of Infection*, **56**, 126–129.

Fridkin, S.K. (2005) The changing face of fungal infections in health care settings. *Clinical Infectious Diseases*, **41**, 1455–1460.

Galgiani, J.N. (1993) Coccidioidomycosis. *The Western Journal of Medicine*, **159**, 153–171.

Galgiani, J.N., Catanzaro, A., Cloud, G.A. *et al.* (2000) Comparison of oral fluconazole and itraconazole for progressive, nonmeningeal coccidioidomycosis. A randomized, double-blind trial. Mycoses Study Group. *Annals of Internal Medicine*, **133**, 676–686.

Garbino, J., Kolarova, L., Rohner, P. *et al.* (2002) Secular trends of candidemia over 12 years in adult patients at a tertiary care hospital. *Medicine (Baltimore)*, **81**, 425–433.

Golan, Y., Wolf, M.P., Pauker, S.G. *et al.* (2005) Empirical anti-Candida therapy among selected patients in the intensive care unit: a cost-effectiveness analysis. *Annals of Internal Medicine*, **143**, 857–869.

Goodwin, R.A., Loyd, J.E. and Des Prez, R.M. (1981) Histoplasmosis in normal hosts. *Medicine (Baltimore)*, **60**, 231–266.

Greene, R.E., Schlamm, H.T., Oestmann, J.W. *et al.* (2007) Imaging findings in acute invasive pulmonary aspergillosis: clinical significance of the halo sign. [see comment]. *Clinical Infectious Diseases*, **44**, 373–379.

Guinet, R., Chanas, J., Goullier, A. *et al.* (1983) Fatal septicemia due to amphotericin B-resistant Candida lusitaniae. *Journal of Clinical Microbiology*, **18**, 443–444.

Gutierrez, M.E., Canton, A., Sosa, N. *et al.* (2005) Disseminated histoplasmosis in patients with AIDS in Panama: a review of 104 cases. *Clinical Infectious Diseases*, **40**, 1199–1202.

Hachem, R., Sumoza, D., Hanna, H. *et al.* (2006) Clinical and radiologic predictors of invasive pulmonary aspergillosis in cancer patients: should the European Organization for Research and Treatment of Cancer/Mycosis Study Group (EORTC/MSG) criteria be revised? *Cancer*, **106**, 1581–1586.

Hachem, R.Y., Kontoyiannis, D.P., Boktour, M.R. *et al.* (2004) Aspergillus terreus: an emerging amphotericin B-resistant opportunistic mold in patients with hematologic malignancies. *Cancer*, **101**, 1594–1600.

Hadley, S., Lee, W.W., Ruthazer, R. and Nasraway, S.A. Jr (2002a) Candidemia as a cause of septic shock and multiple organ failure in nonimmunocompromised patients. *Critical Care Medicine*, **30**, 1808–1814.

Hadley, S., Martinez, J.A., Mcdermott, L. *et al.* (2002b) Real-time antifungal susceptibility screening aids management of invasive yeast infections in immunocompromised patients. *Journal of Antimicrobial Chemotherapy*, **49**, 415–419.

Herbrecht, R., Denning, D.W., Patterson, T.F. *et al.* (2002) Voriconazole versus amphotericin B for primary therapy of invasive aspergillosis. *New England Journal of Medicine*, **347**, 408–415.

Horvath, L.L., Hospenthal, D.R., Murray, C.K. and Dooley, D.P. (2003) Direct isolation of Candida spp. from blood cultures on the chromogenic medium CHROMagar Candida. *Journal of Clinical Microbiology*, **41**, 2629–2632.

Imai, J.K., Singh, G., Clemons, K.V. and Stevens, D.A. (2004) Efficacy of posaconazole in a murine model of central nervous system aspergillosis. [erratum appears in Antimicrob Agents Chemother. 2004 Dec; 48(12):4931]. *Antimicrobial Agents & Chemotherapy*, **48**, 4063–4066.

Johnson, M.D. and Perfect, J.R. (2007) Combination antifungal therapy: what can and should we expect? *Bone Marrow Transplantation*, **40**, 297–306.

Johnson, P.C., Hamill, R.J. and Sarosi, G.A. (1989) Clinical review: progressive disseminated histoplasmosis in the AIDS patient. *Seminars in Respiratory Infections*, **4**, 139–146.

Johnson, P.C., Wheat, L.J., Cloud, G.A. *et al.* (2002) Safety and efficacy of liposomal amphotericin B compared with conventional amphotericin B for induction therapy of histoplasmosis in patients with AIDS. *Annals of Internal Medicine*, **137**, 105–109.

Johnson, R.H. and Einstein, H.E. (2006) Coccidioidal meningitis. *Clinical Infectious Diseases*, **42**, 103–107.

Kwon-Chung, K.J. and Bennett, J.E. (1992a) Medical Mycology (eds K.J. Kwon-Chung and J.E. Bennett), Lea & Febiger, Philadelphia.

Kwon-Chung, K.J. and Bennett, J.E. (1992b) Medical Mycology (eds K.J. Kwon-Chung and J.E. Bennett), Lea & Febiger, Philadelphia.

Kontoyiannis, D.P., Lionakis, M.S., Lewis, R.E. *et al.* (2005) Zygomycosis in a tertiary-care cancer centre in the era of Aspergillus-active antifungal therapy: a case-control observational study of 27 recent cases. [see comment]. *Journal of Infectious Diseases*, **191**, 1350–1360.

Kuberski, T., Myers, R., Wheat, L.J. *et al.* (2007) Diagnosis of coccidioidomycosis by antigen detection using cross-reaction with a Histoplasma antigen. *Clinical Infectious Diseases*, **44**, e50–e54.

Kurtz, M.B. and Rex, J.H. (2001) Glucan synthase inhibitors as antifungal agents. *Advances in Protein Chemistry*, **56**, 423–475.

Lass-Flörl, C., Griff, K., Mayr, A. *et al.* (2005) Epidemiology and outcome of infections due to Aspergillus terreus: 10-year single centre experience. *British Journal of Haematology*, **131**, 201–207.

Lee, J.H., Slifman, N.R., Gershon, S.K. *et al.* (2002) Life-threatening histoplasmosis complicating immunotherapy with tumor necrosis factor alpha antagonists infliximab and etanercept. *Arthritis & Rheumatism*, **46**, 2565–2570.

Leenders, A.C., Reiss, P., Portegies, P. *et al.* (1997) Liposomal amphotericin B (AmBisome) compared with amphotericin B both followed by oral fluconazole in the treatment of AIDS-associated cryptococcal meningitis. *AIDS*, **11**, 1463–1471.

Lemos, L.B., Guo, M. and Baliga, M. (2000) Blastomycosis: organ involvement and etiologic diagnosis. A review of 123 patients from Mississippi. *Annals of Diagnostic Pathology*, **4**, 391–406.

Lin, S.J., Schranz, J. and Teutsch, S.M. (2001) Aspergillosis case-fatality rate: systematic review of the literature. *Clinical Infectious Diseases*, **32**, 358–366.

Maccallum, D.M., Whyte, J.A. and Odds, F.C. (2005) Efficacy of caspofungin and voriconazole combinations in experimental aspergillosis. *Antimicrobial Agents & Chemotherapy*, **49**, 3697–3701.

Maertens, J., Glasmacher, A., Herbrecht, R. *et al.* (2006) Multicenter, noncomparative study of caspofungin in combination with other antifungals as salvage therapy in adults with invasive aspergillosis. *Cancer*, **107**, 2888–2897.

Maertens, J., Raad, I., Petrikkos, G. *et al.* (2004) Efficacy and safety of caspofungin for treatment of invasive aspergillosis in patients refractory to or intolerant of conventional antifungal therapy. *Clinical Infectious Diseases*, **39**, 1563–1571.

Maertens, J., Verhaegen, J., Lagrou, K. *et al.* (2001) Screening for circulating galactomannan as a noninvasive diagnostic tool for invasive aspergillosis in prolonged neutropenic patients and stem cell transplantation recipients: a prospective validation. *Blood*, **97**, 1604–1610.

Magiorakos, A.P. and Hadley, S. (2004) Impact of real-time fungal susceptibility on clinical practices. *Current Opinion in Infectious Diseases*, **17**, 511–515.

Marchetti, O., Bille, J., Fluckiger, U. *et al.* (2004) Epidemiology of candidemia in Swiss tertiary care hospitals: secular trends, 1991–2000. *Clinical Infectious Diseases*, **38**, 311–320.

Marr, K.A. (2004) Invasive Candida infections: the changing epidemiology. *Oncology (Williston Park)*, **18**, 9–14.

Marr, K.A., Boeckh, M., Carter, R.A. *et al.* (2004) Combination antifungal therapy for invasive aspergillosis. [see comment]. *Clinical Infectious Diseases*, **39**, 797–802.

Martynowicz, M.A. and Prakash, U.B. (2002) Pulmonary blastomycosis: an appraisal of diagnostic techniques. *Chest*, **121**, 768–773.

Mayer, J., Doubek, M., Doubek, J. *et al.* (2002) Reduced nephrotoxicity of conventional amphotericin B therapy after minimal nephroprotective measures: animal experiments and clinical study. *The Journal of Infectious Diseases*, **186**, 379–388.

Meersseman, W., Lagrou, K., Maertens, J. *et al.* (2008) Galactomannan in bronchoalveolar lavage fluid: a tool for diagnosing aspergillosis in intensive care unit patients. *American Journal of Respiratory & Critical Care Medicine*, **177**, 27–34.

Meersseman, W., Vandecasteele, S.J., Wilmer, A. *et al.* (2004) Invasive aspergillosis in critically ill patients without malignancy. *American Journal of Respiratory & Critical Care Medicine*, **170**, 621–625.

Meletiadis, J., Petraitis, V., Petraitiene, R. *et al.* (2006) Triazole-polyene antagonism in experimental invasive pulmonary aspergillosis: in vitro and in vivo correlation. *Journal of Infectious Diseases*, **194**, 1008–1018.

Miller, D. and Mejicano, G. (2001) Vertebral osteomyelitis due to Candida species: case report and literature review. *Clinical Infectious Diseases*, **33**, 523–530.

Mongkolrattanothai, K., Peev, M., Wheat, L.J. and Marcinak, J. (2006) Urine antigen detection of blastomycosis in pediatric patients. *Pediatric Infectious Disease Journal*, **25**, 1076–1078.

Mora-Duarte, J., Betts, R., Rotstein, C. *et al.* (2002) Comparison of caspofungin and amphotericin B for invasive candidiasis. *New England Journal of Medicine*, **347**, 2020–2029.

Nagappan, V. and Deresinski, S. (2007) Reviews of anti-infective agents: posaconazole: a broad-spectrum triazole antifungal agent. *Clinical Infectious Diseases*, **45**, 1610–1617.

Odabasi, Z., Mattiuzzi, G., Estey, E. *et al.* (2004) Beta-D-glucan as a diagnostic adjunct for invasive fungal Infections: validation, cutoff development, and performance in patients with acute myelogenousleukemia and myelodysplastic syndrome. *Clinical Infectious Diseases*, **39**, 199–205.

Ostrosky-Zeichner, L. and Pappas, P.G. (2006) Invasive candidiasis in the intensive care unit. *Critical Care Medicine*, **34**, 857–863.

Pagano, L., Caira, M., Nosari, A. *et al.* (2007) Fungal infections in recipients of hematopoietic stem cell transplants: results of the SEIFEM B-2004 study – Sorveglianza Epidemiologica Infezioni Fungine Nelle Emopatie Maligne. *Clinical Infectious Diseases*, **45**, 1161–1170.

Pappagianis, D. (2001) Serologic studies in coccidioidomycosis. *Seminars in Respiratory Infections*, **16**, 242–250.

Pappagianis, D., Collins, M.S., Hector, R. and Remington, J. (1979) Development of resistance to amphotericin B in Candida lusitaniae infecting a human. *Antimicrobial Agents & Chemotherapy*, **16**, 123–126.

Pappas, P.G., Rex, J.H., Sobel, J.D. *et al.* (2004) Guidelines for treatment of candidiasis. *Clinical Infectious Diseases*, **38**, 161–189.

Pappas, P.G., Rotstein, C.M., Betts, R.F. *et al.* (2007) Micafungin versus caspofungin for treatment of candidemia and other forms of invasive candidiasis. *Clinical Infectious Diseases*, **45**, 883–893.

Petraitiene, R., Petraitis, V., Groll, A.H. *et al.* (2002) Antifungal efficacy of caspofungin (MK-0991) in experimental pulmonary aspergillosis in persistently neutropenic rabbits: pharmacokinetics, drug disposition, and relationship to galactomannan antigenemia. *Antimicrobial Agents & Chemotherapy*, **46**, 12–23.

Petraitis, V., Petraitiene, R., Sarafandi, A.A. *et al.* (2003) Combination therapy in treatment of experimental pulmonary aspergillosis: synergistic interaction between an antifungal triazole and an echinocandin. *Journal of Infectious Diseases*, **187**, 1834–1843.

Pfaller, M.A., Diekema, D.J., Messer, S.A. *et al.* (2003) Activities of fluconazole and voriconazole against 1,586 recent clinical isolates of Candida species determined by Broth microdilution, disk diffusion, and Etest methods: report from the ARTEMIS Global Antifungal Susceptibility Program, 2001. *Journal of Clinical Microbiology*, **41**, 1440–1446.

Pfeiffer, C.D., Fine, J.P. and Safdar, N. (2006) Diagnosis of invasive aspergillosis using a galacto-mannan assay: a meta-analysis. *Clinical Infectious Diseases*, **42**, 1417–1727.

Reboli, A.C., Rotstein, C., Pappas, P.G. *et al.* (2007) Anidulafungin versus fluconazole for invasive candidiasis. *New England Journal of Medicine*, **356**, 2472–2482.

Rex, J.H., Bennett, J.E., Sugar, A.M. *et al.* (1994) A randomized trial comparing fluconazole with amphotericin B for the treatment of candidemia in patients without neutropenia. Candidemia Study Group and the National Institute. *New England Journal of Medicine*, **331**, 1325–1330.

Rex, J.H. and Pfaller, M.A. (2002) Has antifungal susceptibility testing come of age? *Clinical Infectious Diseases*, **35**, 982–989.

Roden, M.M., Zaoutis, T.E., Buchanan, W.L. *et al.* (2005) Epidemiology and outcome of zygomy-cosis: a review of 929 reported cases. *Clinical Infectious Diseases*, **41**, 634–653.

Rychly, D.J. and DiPiro, J.T. (2005) Infections associated with tumor necrosis factor-alpha antago-nists. *Pharmacotherapy*, **25**, 1181–1192.

Saag, M.S., Graybill, R.J., Larsen, R.A. *et al.* (2000) Practice guidelines for the management of cryptococcal disease. Infectious Diseases Society of America. *Clinical Infectious Diseases*, **30**, 710–718.

Sarosi, G.A. (2006) Fungal infections and their treatment in the intensive care unit. *Current Opinion in Critical Care*, **12**, 464–469.

Sarosi, G.A. and Davies, S.F. (1979) Blastomycosis. *American Review of Respiratory Diseases*, **120**, 911–938.

Schwartz, S., Ruhnke, M., Ribaud, P. *et al.* (2005) Improved outcome in central nervous system aspergillosis, using voriconazole treatment. *Blood*, **106**, 2641–2645.

Sharkey, P.K., Graybill, J.R., Johnson, E.S. *et al.* (1996) Amphotericin B lipid complex compared with amphotericin B in the treatment of cryptococcal meningitis in patients with AIDS. *Clinical Infectious Diseases*, **22**, 315–321.

Singh, N., Limaye, A.P., Forrest, G. *et al.* (2006) Combination of voriconazole and caspofungin as primary therapy for invasive aspergillosis in solid organ transplant recipients: a prospective, multicenter, observational study. *Transplantation*, **81**, 320–326.

Singh, N. and Paterson, D.L. (2005) Aspergillus infections in transplant recipients. *Clinical Micro-biology Reviews*, **18**, 44–69.

Steinbach, W.J., Perfect, J.R., Schell, W.A. *et al.* (2004) In vitro analyses, animal models, and 60 clinical cases of invasive Aspergillus terreus infection. *Antimicrobial Agents & Chemotherapy*, **48**, 3217–3225.

Stevens, D.A. (1995) Coccidioidomycosis. *New England Journal of Medicine*, **332**, 1077–1082.

Stevens, D.A., Rendon, A., Gaona-Flores, V. *et al.* (2007) Posaconazole therapy for chronic refractory coccidioidomycosis. *Chest*, **132**, 952–958.

Stevens, D.A. and Shatsky, S.A. (2001) Intrathecal amphotericin in the management of coccidioidal meningitis. *Seminars in Respiratory Infections*, **16**, 263–269.

Subira, M., Martino, R., Rovira, M. *et al.* (2003) Clinical applicability of the new EORTC/MSG classification for invasive pulmonary aspergillosis in patients with hematological malignancies and autopsy-confirmed invasive aspergillosis. *Annals of Hematology*, **82**, 80–82.

Sun, Q.N., Fothergill, A.W., Mccarthy, D.I. *et al.* (2002a) In vitro activities of posaconazole, itraconazole, voriconazole, amphotericin B, and fluconazole against 37 clinical isolates of zygomycetes. *Antimicrobial Agents & Chemotherapy*, **46**, 1581–1582.

Sun, Q.N., Najvar, L.K., Bocanegra, R. *et al.* (2002b) In vivo activity of posaconazole against Mucor spp. in an immunosuppressed-mouse model. *Antimicrobial Agents & Chemotherapy*, **46**, 2310–2312.

Trick, W.E., Fridkin, S.K., Edwards, J.R. *et al.* (2002) Secular trend of hospital-acquired candidemia among intensive care unit patients in the United States during 1989–1999. *Clinical Infectious Diseases*, **35**, 627–630.

Upton, A., Kirby, K.A., Carpenter, P. *et al.* (2007) Invasive aspergillosis following hematopoietic cell transplantation: outcomes and prognostic factors associated with mortality. *Clinical Infectious Diseases*, **44**, 531–540.

Valdivia, L., Nix, D., Wright, M. *et al.* (2006) Coccidioidomycosis as a common cause of community-acquired pneumonia. *Emerging Infectious Diseases*, **12**, 958–962.

van Der Horst, C.M., Saag, M.S., Cloud, G.A. *et al.* (1997) Treatment of cryptococcal meningitis associated with the acquired immunodeficiency syndrome. National Institute of Allergy and Infectious Diseases Mycoses Study Group and AIDS Clinical Trials Group. *New England Journal of Medicine*, **337**, 15–21.

Walsh, T., Anaissie, E., Denning, D. *et al.* (2008) Treatment of Aspergillosis: Clinical Practice Guidelines of the Infectious Diseases Society of America. *Clinical Infectious Diseases*, **46**, 327–360.

Walsh, T.J., Raad, I., Patterson, T.F. *et al.* (2007) Treatment of invasive aspergillosis with posaconazole in patients who are refractory to or intolerant of conventional therapy: an externally controlled trial. *Clinical Infectious Diseases*, **44**, 2–12.

Warris, A., Bjorneklett, A. and Gaustad, P. (2001) Invasive pulmonary aspergillosis associated with infliximab therapy. *New England Journal of Medicine*, **344**, 1099–1100.

Warris, A., Klaassen, C.H., Meis, J.F. *et al.* (2003) Molecular epidemiology of Aspergillus fumigatus isolates recovered from water, air, and patients shows two clusters of genetically distinct strains. *Journal of Clinical Microbiology*, **41**, 4101–4106.

Wenzel, R.P. (1995) Nosocomial candidemia: risk factors and attributable mortality. *Clinical Infectious Diseases*, **20**, 1531–1534.

Wheat, L.J. (2003) Current diagnosis of histoplasmosis. *Trends in Microbiology*, **11**, 488–494.

Wheat, L.J. (2006) Histoplasmosis: a review for clinicians from non-endemic areas. *Mycoses*, **49**, 274–282.

Wheat, L.J., Connolly-Stringfield, P., Williams, B. *et al.* (1992) Diagnosis of histoplasmosis in patients with the acquired immunodeficiency syndrome by detection of Histoplasma capsulatum polysaccharide antigen in bronchoalveolar lavage fluid. *American Review of Respiratory Diseases*, **145**, 1421–1424.

Wheat, L.J., Connolly-Stringfield, P.A., Baker, R.L. *et al.* (1990) Disseminated histoplasmosis in the acquired immune deficiency syndrome: clinical findings, diagnosis and treatment, and review of the literature. *Medicine (Baltimore)*, **69**, 361–374.

Wheat, L.J., Freifeld, A.G., Kleiman, M.B. *et al.* (2007) Clinical practice guidelines for the management of patients with histoplasmosis: 2007 update by the Infectious Diseases Society of America. *Clinical Infectious Diseases*, **45**, 807–825.

Wood, K.L., Hage, C.A., Knox, K.S. *et al.* (2003) Histoplasmosis after treatment with anti-tumor necrosis factor-alpha therapy. *American Journal of Respiratory & Critical Care Medicine*, **167**, 1279–1282.

14

Current strategies and future directions in cytomegalovirus (CMV) pneumonitis

Julio C. Medina Presentado[1] and José M. Aguado[2]

[1]Cátedra de Enfermedades Infecciosas, Universidad de la República, Uruguay
[2]Unit of Infectious Diseases, University Hospital 12 de Octubre, Madrid, Spain

14.1 Effects of CMV infection in immunocompromised patients

Cytomegalovirus (CMV) is a β herpes virus with a double stranded DNA genome of 240 kbp. It is a ubiquitous virus that causes an infection that persists for life. The majority of these infections are subclinical in healthy subjects, nevertheless CMV infections is an important cause of morbidity and mortality in immunocompromised patients (Sia and Patel, 2000; Wingard, 1999).

The CMV genome is composed of lineal, double stranded DNA, surrounded by a protein lining, called matrix, that contains phosphoproteins (pp65, pp150 etc.) highly immunogenic that are capable of deregulating the cellular cycle of the host cell. This lining is surrounded by glycoproteins (gB, gN, gO, gH, gM, gL), necessary for the virus infectivity: entrance to the host cell, cell to cell dissemination and maturing. The main reservoir of CMV contains the fibroblasts, myeloid cells and endothelial cells (Rowshani *et al.*, 2005).

As with other herpes virus, the CMV invades the host cell, inhibits protein synthesis and liberates viral DNA to the nuclei where the replication starts immediately. A strategy that shares with other herpes virus, is the ability of stopping the immune response of the host by inhibiting the RNA formation, blocking the presentation of antigenic peptides of the cell surface and blocking the apoptosis. These mechanisms prompt to a latent infection that may be reactivated in immunosuppressed subjects.

The potential of CMV infection and disease is also influenced by the interaction with other viruses. The current evidence suggests that there is a temporal relation between the

Pulmonary Infection in the Immunocompromised Patient, Edited by Carlos Agustí and Antoni Torres
© 2009 John Wiley & Sons, Ltd.

detection of HHV-6 and HHV-7 and the appearance of CMV infection and also with CMV disease (Medina, Pérez-Sartori and Aguado, 2007).

The effects of CMV on the immunocompromised patient can be divided into two categories: direct effects (causing viral syndrome or organ compromise) and indirect effects of the virus due to mediators produced by the host in response to the viral invasion (Rubin, 2007) (Medina *et al.*, 2008). There are three types of indirect effects: (a) *immunomodulation*: CMV contributes to immunosuppression and in this way favours the development of diseases caused by other pathogens; (b) *allograft injury*: CMV seems to promote classical rejection in transplant recipients, as well as a vasculopathy of the allograft, and (c) *oncogenesis*: CMV promotes Epstein-Barr virus related B cell lymphoproliferative disease.

14.2   Pathophysiology of CMV pneumonitis

Pneumonitis is one of the most important diseases related to CMV, specially in solid organ transplant (SOT) recipients (Rubin, 1990). To understand the pathogenic role of CMV on the lung it is important to analyze which are the effects of CMV on endothelial cells, alveolar epithelial cells, antigen presenting dendritic cells and monocyte/macrophages (Langhoff and Siegel, 2006). The endothelial infection has a complex and not completely clear role in the pathophysiology of pneumonitis. The infection of the endothelial cells has been demonstrated and is probably responsible for passing the virus to transmigrating monocytes and macrophages. Furthermore cytomegalic endothelial cells may detach and circulate by the blood infecting the lung tissue.

The alveolar epithelium is a target of the inflammatory response and could play a role by its capacity of modulating the initiation and resolution of the inflammatory processes in the alveolar space. Seventy-five per cent of the alveolar cells infected by CMV in pneumonitis are epithelial cells, and the infection is associated with the absence of expression of the major histocompatibility complex (MHC) class II in the alveolar epithelium. Because of this, the infected alveolar cells without the MHC class II have a very limited capacity of processing and presenting alveolar antigens. This may contribute to the immunosuppression associated with CMV and with the virus persistence.

The dendritic cells in the airway form an extended network throughout the pulmonary epithelium, lung parenchyma and alveolar spaces. CMV may be transmitted to dendritic cells by infected monocytes/macrophages or by contact with the endothelial cells. It is possible that activated macrophages are the primary cell source of viral production which subsequently infects resident lung dendritic cells (Langhoff and Siegel, 2006).

When tumour necrosis factor (TNF) binds to the CMV receptors of latently infected cells, the virus is reactivated and clinical disease occurs as direct infection causing pneumonia, and indirect infection in which cytokines are released by the host, and produce the same effect as the rejection in lung transplant recipients. The presence of multiple gB genotypes, rather than the presence of a single gB genotype, could be a critical factor associated with severe clinical manifestations of pneumonitis in immunocompromised patients (Coaquette *et al.*, 2004).

Table 14.1 Risk factors for CMV in solid organ transplant recipients.

Primary infection (donor positive/recipient negative)
Allograft rejection
Anti-CD3 monoclonal antibody (OKT3)
Antihuman lymphocyte globulin (ALG), Antihuman thymocyte globulin (ATG)
Daclizumab
High-dose steroids
mycophenolate mofetil
Inadequate cytotoxic response
Type of organ transplant (lung, heart-lung > heart $\geq$ liver > kidney)
High viral load
Allogenic stimulation
Viral co-infections (HHV-6 and HHV-7)
Other immunosuppressive drugs, intraoperative hypotermia
Adaptive immune defects (T cells)

14.3   Risk factors for CMV pneumonitis

Solid organ transplant recipients

Many factors could increase the incidence of CMV pneumonia in SOT recipients (Table 14.1). The patients at greatest risk for CMV pneumonia are those donor positive/ recipient negative who have a reactivation of a latent infection due to increased immunosuppression (rejection and use of boluses of steroids or anti-CD3 monoclonal antibodies) (Langhoff and Siegel, 2006).

Patients receiving heart/lung or lung transplants are at high risk for CMV infections. The higher frequency of CMV pneumonitis in lung transplant may be due to the fact that the lung harbours latent CMV and therefore great amounts of CMV can be transmitted in the allograft. Others risk factors identified include the use of potent immunosuppressive agents such as antilymphocyte antibodies and daclizumab. The use of antilymphocyte antibody therapy for immunosuppression increases both the risk for infection and the severity of the disease.

Haematological stem cell transplant (HSCT) recipients

HSCT recipients are at high risk for developing CMV pneumonia. Risk factors for CMV disease in HSCT are resumed in Table 14.2. The risk for CMV pneumonia without

Table 14.2 Risk factors for CMV in haematopoietic stem cell transplantation.

Positive CMV serology
Antithymocyte globulin
Cyclosporine A
FK506
Older age
Graft-vs-host disease (GVHD)
Allogenic graft

prophylaxis is greater in allogenic (20–35%) compared to autologous transplantation (1–6%). The majority of cases are due to reactivation of latent CMV in seropositive recipients. Seronegative recipients who receive stem cells from a seropositive donor have less risk of developing CMV disease post transplant than seropositive recipients; this contrasts with SOT recipients. The patients who develop graft-versus-host disease are particularly predisposed to develop CMV pneumonia. Cyclosporine A and tacrolimus scarcely have a role in viral reactivation, but could perpetuate the replication after reactivation. Both antithymocyte globulin and OKT3 antibodies induce viral reactivation due to the sharp decrease in the cellular immunity caused by the elimination of circulating T lymphocytes (Rovira and Ruiz-Camps, 2007).

Other immunosuppressed patients

The incidence of CMV pneumonia in patients with cancer or AIDS is much lower than in the transplantation setting (Sepkowitz, 2002). Introduction of highly active antiretroviral therapy (HAART) has resulted in a decrease in the number of cases in patients with AIDS.

CMV disease is rare in patients with cancer. In a retrospective, autopsy-based study only 20 cases of CMV pneumonia were identified among 9029 autopsies performed during 1964–1990 in adults without transplanted organs or HIV-AIDS (Mera *et al.*, 1996). Cases were more common among patients with multiple myeloma and brain tumour. All had received chemotherapy and 75% had received corticosteroids. The risk factors for CMV pneumonitis in cancer patients are use of steroids, cyclophosphamide, methotrexate and fludarabine (Breathnach *et al.*, 1999; Shimada *et al.*, 2004; Manna *et al.*, 2003).

14.4   Pulmonary manifestations of CMV infection

CMV pneumonitis contributes directly and indirectly to both morbidity and mortality, particularly in transplant recipients. CMV not only causes overt pulmonary manifestations as pneumonitis; careful studies have also documented subtle abnormalities in pulmonary function in the majority of the patients with CMV infection. So, almost all kidney transplant patients with CMV infection have subclinical involvement when measuring carbon monoxide diffusion capacity. Subclinical pneumonitis could also render the lungs more susceptible to opportunistic infections (de Maar *et al.*, 2003).

Among SOT recipients, lung transplant recipients have the highest incidence of CMV pneumonitis (Langhoff and Siegel, 2006). HSCT recipients are also at particular risk for developing severe CMV pneumonitis. Approximately one half of marrow graft recipients develop interstitial pneumonia, usually after successful engraftment; nearly one half of these cases are associated with CMV infection. The attack rate is higher for those with underlying malignancy than for those with aplastic anemia, and the mortality rate approaches 90% (Jeffery *et al.*, 1974).

Clinical manifestations of pneumonitis are primarily seen one to four months posttransplant. Symptoms usually begin insidiously with anorexia, malaise and fever, often accompanied by myalgias and arthralgias. Afterwards a cough appears. Initially, dyspnea and tachypnea are not noted, but over several days progressive respiratory distress can appear, although most patients with CMV pneumonia have little respiratory distress at rest. Auscultation of the lungs is usually unrevealing, and the best correlate on physical examination with the degree of respiratory embarrassment, hypoxemia and extension of pneumonia on chest radiography, is the respiratory rate (Aguado, 2004). Although CMV pneumonia progresses rapidly to respiratory failure in some kidney, heart or liver transplant recipients, in most individuals the lung involvement is relatively minor at onset. The severe form of pneumonia is far more common in lung and heart-lung transplant patients (Patel and Paya, 1997). In lung transplantation CMV pneumonitis could be confused with acute rejection. Both may present with low-grade fever, shortness of breath, nonproductive cough, and changes in measured pulmonary function.

The chest radiograph may demonstrate perihilar infiltrates, interstitial oedema, focal consolidation affecting the lower lobes, pleural effusions, lung nodules or a combination of these patterns (Lee et al., 2004).

It is important to take into account the possibility of coinfection of CMV with other microorganisms. Approximately 10–20% of patients with CMV pneumonitis have dual or sequential infection. CMV has been described in association with miliary tuberculosis (Cheng et al., 2007), Aspergillus (Kuboshima et al., 2007), Pneumocystis jiroveci pneumonia (Scemama et al., 2007), Candida sp. (Forslöw et al., 2006), Pseudomonas aeruginosa (Catalla and Leaf, 2000), and Cryptococcus or Nocardia (Rubin, 2007).

14.5   Indirect respiratory effects of CMV infection

CMV has been implicated in causing increased immunosuppression and secondary opportunistic lung infections in SOT recipients (Rubin, 1986) (Rubin, 1989). CMV induces alveolar macrophage dysfunction that favours the development of superinfection with these organisms. It also facilitates the colonization of the upper respiratory tract with gram-negative bacilli, and this could be the reservoir for latter pulmonary infection. Another risk factor for pulmonary superinfection appears to be CMV-induced leukopenia. As with other clinical manifestations of CMV, pulmonary superinfection appears to be more common in patients with primary as opposed to reactivation disease (Ho, 1991).

Some of the most compelling evidence linking CMV infection with allograft injury comes from lung and heart-lung transplantation (Scott et al., 1991). Some authors clearly linked bronchiolitis obliterans (BOS) in the allograft to both symptomatic and asymptomatic infection with the virus. On the other hand, other authors demonstrated that histopathologically confirmed CMV pneumonia treated with ganciclovir is not a risk factor for BOS or patient survival (Tamm et al., 2004).

14.6   Diagnosis of CMV pneumonitis

The diagnosis of CMV pneumonia requires the identification of the virus from the lower respiratory tract by bronchoalveolar lavage (BAL), transbronchial or surgical lung biopsy. BAL has shown itself to be useful in different groups of immunosuppressed patients: patients with cancer or HIV infection, SOT and HSCT recipients, and others (Joos *et al.*, 2007).

The diagnosis of CMV pneumonitis is based on the presence of viral intranuclear inclusions characteristic of CMV lung infection on cytopathologic study, associated with the demonstration of the presence of CMV antigen by monoclonal antibody staining or CMV DNA by PCR, or in the isolation of the organism from lung tissue. The utility of CMV PCR on BAL fluid has been recently studied in immunosuppressed patients with haematological malignancy and pneumonia. In these patients the qualitative PCR for CMV in BAL was not clinically useful. Among 18 of 134 patients (13.4%) with PCR positive for CMV in BAL, only 4 of them had a definite or probable diagnosis of CMV pneumonia, but the other 14 had other alternative diagnosis (Hohenthal *et al.*, 2005). Some authors suggest that PCR is too sensitive for the diagnosis of CMV and should not be used on BAL samples (Langhoff and Siegel, 2006). Quantitative PCR of BAL, especially when epithelial lining fluid is analyzed, may offer advantages over qualitative assays, but the data are scanty and need further confirmation (Drew, 2007).

An early intervention with an aggressive diagnostic approach such as surgical lung biopsy by minithoracotomy could be beneficial for patients who require mechanical ventilation (Suh *et al.*, 2006). Lung biopsy may show alveolar thickening, acute alveolar oedema, haemorrhage and inflammatory cell infiltration with positive immuno-histochemical stains for CMV. High-resolution CT aids in planning for lung biopsy. Findings in CMV pneumonitis include areas of dense consolidation, reticulation, nodules and bronchiectasis (Catalla and Leaf, 2000). CT is also useful to predict the patient's outcome. The prognosis is poor in those forms of disease beginning bilaterally as diffuse or patchy ground-glass opacity followed by progressive air-space consolidation. A change in the CT pulmonary lesions toward diffuse ground-glass opacity seems to correlate with an unfavourable course (Horger *et al.*, 2006).

The diagnosis of CMV pneumonitis could be considered probable or definite (Preiksaitis *et al.*, 2005) (Ljungman *et al.*, 2002). *Probable pneumonia*: signs and/or symptoms of pulmonary disease in the absence of other documented causes, plus evidence of CMV in blood and/or bronchoalveolar lavage fluid by viral culture, antigenemia or a DNA/RNA-based assay. *Definite pneumonia*: signs and/or symptoms of pulmonary disease, plus detection of CMV in lung tissue by immunohistochemical analysis or *in situ* hybridization (the presence of typical CMV inclusions could be considered definitive disease).

Isolation of the CMV or antigen in BAL is evidence of viral shedding, but it does not confirm that clinical and radiologic findings are due to CMV pneumonitis, for the definitive diagnosis of CMV pneumonia it is necessary to find CMV in a lung biopsy.

14.7   Antiviral agents against CMV

Ganciclovir and Valganciclovir

Ganciclovir (GCV) was the first antiviral agent approved for treatment of CMV disease and has become the gold standard for management. It is an acyclic nucleoside analogue of 2'-deoxyguanosine (Merigan *et al.*, 1992; Goodrich *et al.*, 1993). Oral GCV has a low bioavailability (approximately 5%) and it is considered insufficient for induction therapy. So the development of new drugs with better bioavailability was necessary. Valganciclovir (VGCV) is the l-valyl ester of ganciclovir and is rapidly metabolized to the active form, ganciclovir. It has a bioavailability of approximately 60%. Once-daily administration of VGCV 900 mg produces systemic exposure to GCV that is equivalent to that produced with once-daily administration of IV GCV 5 mg/kg (Biron, 2006; Wiltshire *et al.*, 2005; Pescovitz *et al.*, 2000).

Paya *et al.* compared VGCV to oral ganciclovir in a randomized, double-blind, double-dummy study of 364 D + /R−SOT recipients. Patients were randomized to receive VGCV 900 mg once-daily or oral GCV 1000 mg t.i.d. for 100 days posttransplant. The incidence of CMV disease at 12 months was comparable in the two treatment groups, and the safety profiles were similar (Paya *et al.*, 2004).

Foscarnet

Foscarnet (FOS) is the trisodium salt of phosphormophonic acid, a pyrophosphonate analogue. FOS is considered a second-line therapy, but it is the preferred drug for patients who are failing GCV therapy due to viral resistance, or those who cannot be treated with GCV due to neutropenia or leucopenia (Razonable and Emery, 2004). The major dose-limiting toxicity of FOS is renal impairment. Adequate hydration and frequent monitoring of serum creatinine levels in patients receiving FOS is necessary.

Cidofovir

It is an acyclic nucleoside phosphonate. Cidofovir (CDV) is available only as an IV formulation; its oral bioavailability is less than 5%. It is not a recommended drug for treating CMV pneumonitis and it has the disadvantage of renal toxicity.

Valacyclovir

This is the l-valyl ester of acyclovir. It is useful for prophylaxis in SOT recipients and it has been shown to reduce the risk of CMV disease even in seronegative receptors (Hodson *et al.*, 2005).

New Anti-CMV Drugs

The development of new drugs is necessary to achieve a better cure rate of CMV pneumonitis and to fight against resistance to GCV because FOS, the alternative to GCV, has several toxic effects. New drugs could also be useful to improve prophylaxis.

Many molecules are being tried. Maribavir (1-(β-L-ribofuranosyl)-2-isopropylamino-5,6-dichlorobenzimidazole) also known as GW1263W94, is one of the most promising anti-CMV drugs in clinical development. It is a potent and selective, orally bioavailable, drug with a novel mechanism of action against CMV. A phase 3 study is taking place to compare the efficacy, safety and tolerability of maribavir versus oral ganciclovir in the prophylaxis of CMV in liver transplant recipients with high risk to develop CMV disease (ViroPharma Inc., 2007). Other molecules in pre-clinical stages of development are: Benzimidazol, Adefovir, Lobucavir, CMV423, GW275175X, Alkoxyalkyl-cidofovir esters o BAY 38-4766. Table 3 shows the dosage of anti-cytomegalovirus antiviral agents in therapy and prevention.

14.8   Treatment of CMV pneumonia

In SOT recipients

A typical course of treatment is three to four weeks of acute therapy followed by two to four months of buffer therapy. However, duration of treatment should be guided by molecular methods. Standard treatment consists of a course of intravenous GCV 5 mg/kg twice daily, adjusted for renal insufficiency. Some authors add CMV hyperimmune globulin when treating severe disease, but there is scarce evidence for this. The benefit of the therapy with GCV depends on the severity of the CMV pneumonia. GCV diminishes the mortality from 90 to 60% in patients with severe respiratory insufficiency that need mechanical ventilation; in less severe pneumonias it reduces mortality from 50 to 20%.

The classic treatment for pneumonitis is IV GCV, but it has the inconvenience of long-term IV catheter access and it is expensive. On the other hand, VGCV results in a simpler alternative. Recently Äsberg A and the VICTOR Study Group (Äsberg *et al.*, 2007) published the results of a randomized, open-label, parallel-group, active drug-controlled, multicentre noninferiority trial in adult SOT recipients with CMV disease. A total of 321 patients received at least one dose of assigned medication; the 164 patients randomized to treatment with 900 mg twice daily VGCV and 157 patients to 5 mg/kg twice daily IV GCV were the intention-to-treat population. The success rate of viremia eradication at day 21 was 45.1% for VGCV and 48.4% for GCV (95% CI -14.0 to $+8.0\%$), and at day 49; 67.1 and 70.1%, respectively ($p=$ NS). Treatment success, as assessed by investigators, was 77.4% versus 80.3% at day 21 and 85.4% versus 84.1% at day 49 ($p=$ NS). There were not differences between the two groups with respect to adverse effects: total patients with adverse event; 70.1% vs. 63.7% respectively ($p=0.221$). The authors concluded that oral VGCV shows comparable safety and is not inferior to IV GCV for treatment of CMV disease in organ transplant recipients and provides a simpler treatment strategy. One of the limitations of this study was that the treatment allocation was not blinded. Nevertheless, this excellent study gives the best evidence so far to support the VGCV use in SOT recipients with CMV disease. Unfortunately, CMV pneumonia constituted only the 6,7% ($n=11$) in the VGCV group and the 10,2% ($n=16$) in the GCV IV group, and lung and heart transplants represented only approximately 10% in both groups; it is well known that in these transplant recipients CMV pneumonia is more severe. The small number of CMV pneumonias evaluated prompt us to be cautious when indicating VGCV in this entity and in this group of patients. It is probable that many patients get benefit from VGCV, but others, with the most severe pneumonias could require IV GCV. There is a need for prospective,

Table 14.3 Dosage of anti-cytomegalovirus antiviral agents in therapy and prevention.

Drug	Bioavailability	Excretion	Creatinine clearance	Dose/route	Frequency in therapy or preemptive therapy	Frequency in prophylaxis
Ganciclovir	Poor	Renal	>70	5 mg /kg/IV	q12h	q24h
			50–69	2,5 mg/kg/IV	q12h	q24h
			25–49	1,25 mg/kg/IV	q12h	q24h
			10–24	0625 mg/kg/IV	q12h	q24h
			<10	0625 mg/kg/IV	After hemodialysis	After hemodialysis
Valganciclovir	Good	Renal	>60	900 mg/po	q12h	q24h
			40–59	450 mg/po	q12h	q24h
			25–39	450 mg/po	q24h	q48h
			10–24	450 mg/po	q48h	q72h

randomized studies, with a bigger number of patients with CMV pneumonia to clarify this point.

Although primary drug resistance in the absence of previous drug exposure is very unusual (Rubin, 2007), appearance of GCV resistance is an emergent problem and it has been described in 2.2–15.2% of SOT recipients, depending on the type of transplant (Lurain *et al.*, 2002; Bhorade *et al.*, 2002). Resistance to GCV could be due to the mutation of the gene UL97, UL54 or both. The mutation of UL54 could also determine resistance to other drugs like CDV or FOS. GCV-resistant CMV disease has been significantly associated with D + /R− serostatus (Li *et al.*, 2007; Limaye *et al.*, 2000). Other risk factors for GCV-resistant CMV disease are: high viral replication, multiple episodes of CMV disease, suboptimal tissue-plasma drug concentrations, lung and kidney-pancreas transplant recipients, prolonged antiviral drug administration and use of potent immunosuppression (Razonable and Paya, 2003).

FOS is the agent of choice for treatment of GCV-resistant disease. Unfortunately, nephrotoxicity is common when FOS is given in combination with cyclosporine or tacrolimus. The major toxicity of this agent is renal failure and reduced levels of magnesium, calcium and phosphate. FOS is recommended for patients who persist to how symptoms under GCV treatment or when symptoms appear in patients receiving long-term prophylaxis with GCV or VGCV; also in patients with severe leukopenia that precludes the use of GCV. Several studies show that the association of GCV plus FOS is synergic *in vitro* against CMV (Manischewitz *et al.*, 1990) and also has the best clinical response in case of GCV resistance (Mylonakis, Kallas and Fishman, 2002; Langhoff and Siegel, 2006). The combination of GCV plus FOS or leflunomide may be useful in the setting of GCV-resistant CMV disease (Montoya, 2007). In the case of GCV and FOS resistance CDV is recommended. Nevertheless, the appearance of a high grade of resistance to GCV is associated with cross resistance to CDV. In the case of resistance to the three drugs, combination strategies should be considered (Torre-Cisneros *et al.*, 2005). Finally, immunosuppression management is an important aspect of CMV strategies. Exogenous immunosuppression should be significantly reduced in the face of severe CMV pneumonitis (Rubin, 2007).

In HSCT recipients

In this group of patients the treatment of CMV pneumonitis with IV GCV did not achieve a reduction in the mortality rate. When immunoglobulin is added to this treatment the survival rate improves (50–70% compared to 0–15% of the historic controls). Nevertheless, there are no randomized studies that support this association. Improvement in the mortality rate could be due to an earlier diagnosis of CMV pneumonitis and an earlier treatment. Forslöw *et al.* analyzed retrospectively 997 HSCT recipients to evaluate the change over time in the incidence, etiology and risk factors for death related to pneumonia within three months after HSCT. Death related to pneumonia occurred in 56 (5.6%) patients. Cytomegalovirus (37%) was the main pathogen involved, especially during the first two decades studied. In patients receiving bone marrow transplantation during the last decade, the incidence of death related to pneumonia was 2.8% compared to 8.9% during the first decade. The authors concluded that the rate of mortality related to pneumonia (including CMV pneumonia) had decreased over time, possibly as a result of improved diagnostic, prophylactic and therapeutic methods and treatment (Forslöw *et al.*, 2006).

The introduction of prophylaxis against CMV in HSCT recipients led to a decline in the incidence of CMV disease within the first 100 days since transplantation, nevertheless prophylaxis predispose to a later onset of CMV pneumonia after 100 days post transplant, after finishing prophylaxis (Kotloff, Ahya and Crawford, 2004).

Although there are no controlled studies about CMV pneumonitis treatment, therapeutic guidelines propose a combination of 5 mg/kg bid of IV GCV plus high dose of unspecific IV gammaglobulin (500 mg/kg every other day, total 7–10 doses) (Forman and Zaia, 1994). There is no evidence that support a superiority of hiperimmune CMV gammaglobulin over the unspecific one, and the former is more expensive.

The recommended duration of treatment is 21–28 days for the induction therapy, followed by maintenance therapy (GCV 5 mg/kg once a day + gammaglobulin 500 mg/kg per week) for four weeks. Monitoring the response to the treatment is recommended, at least weekly. The decrease of the antigenemia and DNAemia is not immediate after beginning treatment; an increase is also possible within the first week of treatment. This increase of the values does not mean treatment failure. The objective is to obtain negative antigenemia or DNAemia after two or three weeks.

14.9   Prevention of CMV pneumonia

Prophylaxis versus preemptive therapy

Many efforts have been directed to prevention of CMV pneumonitis, but it is not clear which is the best strategy. Prophylaxis consists of giving an antiviral to prevent the development of CMV infection or disease in a patient without clinical or viral markers of active infection. Preemptive therapy consists of giving antiviral treatment when viral markers turn positive, which indicates active infection in patients still asymptomatic. Whether prophylactic therapy or preemptive therapy should be used in a different setting is under discussion (Puius and Snydman, 2007).

Preemptive therapy is initiated by virologic markers. It minimizes the drug exposure because it is not initiated immediately after transplant and the number of patients who are treated is smaller. But it may not eliminate the indirect effects of CMV and some episodes may escape detection. On the other hand, prophylaxis is universal, eliminates direct and indirect effects of CMV. The problems with this strategy are toxicity, overtreatment, delayed immune reconstitution, and risk of late onset CMV disease after prophylaxis.

An excellent metanalysis recently published, clearly documents the benefit of prophylaxis. Hodson E.M. *et al.* evaluated the benefits and risks of antiviral drugs to prevent CMV disease in the SOT recipients. They evaluated 32 trials (3737 participants). Prophylaxis with ACV, GCV or VGCV, compared with placebo or no treatment, reduced significantly the risk of CMV disease, infection and mortality mainly due to the decrease in related CMV mortality. In the direct comparative trials, GCV was more effective than ACV in preventing CMV disease. VGCV and IV GCV were as effective as oral GCV. The authors concluded that prophylaxis with antivirals reduces CMV disease and the related mortality in SOT.

With respect to the duration of prophylaxis there is a consensus of a duration of 90–100 days post transplant; nevertheless Doyle *et al.* recently documented that a course of six months could be more beneficial than the classic three months (Doyle *et al.*, 2006). In one study, late-onset CMV disease was more prevalent in D+/R− liver transplant recipients who had received prophylaxis versus preemptive therapy, suggesting that perhaps prophylactic treatment with a potent antiviral agent interfered with development of cell-mediated immune response (Singh, 2006). Late-onset CMV pneumonitis constitutes a problem not elucidated (Meylan and Manuel, 2007). Extending the duration of prophylaxis beyond 100 days has been proposed as a strategy to avoid late-onset CMV disease, however, this increases the costs substantially.

Two meta-analysis (Strippoli *et al.*, 2006; Small, Lau and Snydman, 2006) and two prospective trials (Khoury *et al.*, 2006; Diaz-Pedroche *et al.*, 2006) recently compared prophylactic versus preemptive therapy with dissimilar results. Both meta-analysis concluded that universal prophylaxis and preemptive therapy are equally effective in reducing the incidence of CMV disease. Khoury J. A. *et al.* concluded that prophylaxis was more effective in reducing the occurrence of CMV infection, but possibly less effective in preventing symptomatic disease in high risk D+/R− patients.

Our group (Diaz-Pedroche *et al.*, 2006) prospectively followed 301 seropositive SOT recipients to assess the efficacy and safety of VGCV in the prevention of CMV disease in high-risk patients. Asymptomatic patients with an antigenemia test ≥ 25 positive cells/ 2×10^5 polymorphonuclear cells received VGCV 900 mg twice a day as preemptive therapy until resolution of antigenemia (minimum 14 days). Additionally, patients treated with antilymphocytic drugs for more than six days received prophylaxis with VGCV 900 mg once a day during 90 days. No patient developed CMV disease during the follow-up. Viral load (antigenemia) decreased a mean of 78% from baseline after seven days of VGCV therapy ($p = 0.024$) and 98% at day 14 ($p = 0.029$). The authors concluded that VGCV is safe and highly efficacious in the prevention of CMV disease in high-risk seropositive organ transplant recipients.

Use of vaccines

The development of a vaccine to prevent CMV disease is still a challenge. Over the past 30 years many attempts have been made to design a vaccine able to prevent symptomatic congenital disease and disease in immunocompromised individuals, particularly transplant patients. However, few vaccines progressed to clinical studies and no one has been licensed yet. The candidate CMV vaccines are discussed below.

Whole virus live attenuated vaccines (Towne strain vaccine and recombinant Towne and Toledo strain vaccine) The Towne vaccine was the first vaccine developed. This is a live attenuated form of the CMV Towne strain, and has been extensively evaluated since 1975. It induces humoural and cellular immunity to the virus in healthy immunocompetent subjects but only gives modest protection against CMV diseases and it is not able to prevent the infection (Zhong and Khanna, 2007; Gandhi and Khana, 2004). Another live attenuated vaccine is a chimerical one based on Towne strain and Toledo strain. An ongoing trial with this vaccine on CMV-seropositive adults showed strong T-cell immunity, but preexisting immunity made it difficult to analyze the results. Phase I trials showed that both Towne and Town/Toledo vaccines are safe, but extensive long-term clinical trials are necessary to rule out risks regarding the use of live replicating-competent vaccines: prenatal damage, and the problem of latency and reactivation in immunocompromised patients.

Subunit vaccines. Made of the most relevant antigens, either combined with adjuvant or vectored vaccines, they could overcome the possible problems of long-term safety. They are based on the assumption that immunity directed toward a limited number of antigens is sufficient to induce protective immunity. Purified glycoprotein B plus different adjuvants are being evaluated in animal models and in humans (adults, toddlers, postpartum women and soon with transplant patients). Another form of subunit vaccine is the vectored one: the gene for the CMV antigen is expressed in a non replicating vector. The vectors used for these vaccines are canarypox, adenovirus and vaccine virus Ankara. Canarypox-gB induces both T-cell responses and neutralizing antibodies in animals but it does not induce sufficient neutralizing antibodies in humans. Recent trials are studying a prime boosting approach combined with other vaccines: two doses of canarypox-gB followed by a dose of Towne vaccine. This trial showed a strong anti-CMV neutralizing antibodies response and significant and long lasting CD4 and CD8 responses.

Other vaccines made with other vectors

(a) *DNA vaccines* A bivalent DNA vaccine (pp65 and gB) induces gB-specific neutralizing antibodies and virus specific cytotoxic T lymphocyte responses in a murine model. It also induces antibody and T-cell immunity in CMV seronegative humans. A trivalent DNA vaccine based on pp65, gB and, that is, -1 in combination with Towne vaccine is recently being tested.

(b) *Other vaccines* (Dense bodies based vaccines and peptide based vaccines). Dense bodies are enveloped, replication defective subviral particles formed during replication in cell culture. They contain the dominant CMV antigens. Dense bodies are a novel promising approach. Animal studies showed that immunization with DBs could induce humoural and cellular responses. Another approach is a peptide-based vaccine with synthetic inmunodominant CTL epitopes and/or   T-helper epitopes. This vaccine is safe in animal testing and can induce CD8 and CTL response. Finally, a polyepitope technology is being investigated (multiple epitopes from eight different CMV antigens) (Zhong and Khanna, 2007; Gandhi and Khana, 2004).

Immune based treatment

The recovery of CMV specific T cell immunity decreases the risk of developing disease. Many attempts have been made to passively restore CMV cellular immunity by infusion of either virus specific CD8 or a combination of CD4 and CD8. Adoptive immunotherapy is still confined to research centres. Immunomodulatory therapy of CMV pneumonia after liver transplantation has been assayed with good results (Wang *et al.*, 2006).

In a recent review Hodson *et al.* assessed the benefits and harms of immunoglobulins (IgG), vaccines or interferon for preventing symptomatic CMV disease in SOT recipients. They conclude that currently there are no indications for IgG or interferon in the prophylaxis of CMV disease in recipients of SOT. Although IgG reduced the risk of death from CMV disease in six trials, there was no difference in the risk of CMV disease, infection or all-cause mortality when comparing antiviral medication combined with IgG and antiviral medication alone. There was no significant difference in the risk of CMV disease with anti CMV vaccine or interferon compared with placebo or no treatment (Hodson *et al.*, 2007).

Acknowledgements

To Graciela Pérez-Sartori MD, for the revision of the English version of the manuscript.

References

Aguado, J.M. (2004) Cytomegalovirus Infection in Transplant Patients. PCCU-Lesson 14, Volume 15. Sistema de educación continua del American College of Chest Physicians.

Äsberg, A., Humar, A., Rollag, H., Jardine, A.G., Mouas, H., Pescovitz, M.D. *et al.*, on behalf of the VICTOR Study Group (2007) Oral valganciclovir is noninferior to intravenous ganciclovir for the treatment of cytomegalovirus disease in solid organ transplant recipients. *American Journal of Transplantation*, **7**, 2106–2113.

Bhorade, S.M., Lurain, N.S., Jordan, A., Leischner, J., Villanueva, J., Durazo, R. *et al.* (2002) Emergence of ganciclovir-resistant cytomegalovirus in lung transplant recipients. *The Journal of Heart and Lung Transplantation*, **21**, 1274–1282.

Biron, K.K. (2006) Antiviral drugs for cytomegalovirus diseases-Mini-review. *Antiviral Research*, **71**, 154–163.

Breathnach, O., Donnellan, P., Collins, D. *et al.* (1999) Cytomegalovirus pneumonia in a patient with breast cancer on chemotherapy: Case report and review of the literature. *Annals of Oncology*, **10**, 461–465.

Catalla, R. and Leaf, H.L. (2000) Aspects of pulmonary infections after solid organ transplantation. *Current Infectious Disease Reports*, **2**, 201–206.

Cheng, J.W., Chen, Y.C., Tian, Y.C., Fang, J.T. and Yang, C.W. (2007) Coinfection of cytomegalovirus and miliary tuberculosis in a post-renal transplant recipient. *Journal of Nephrology*, **20** (1), 114–118.

Coaquette, A., Bourgeois, A., Dirand, C., Varin, A., Chen, W. and Herbein, G. (2004) Mixed cytomegalovirus glycoprotein B genotypes in immunocompromised patients. *Clinical Infectious Disease*, **39**, 155–161.

de Maar, E.F., Verschuuren, E.A.M., Harmsen, M.C., The, T.H. and van Son, W.J. (2003) Pulmonary involvement during cytomegalovirus infection in immunosuppressed patients. *Transplant Infectious Disease*, **5**, 112–120.

Diaz-Pedroche, C., Lumbreras, C., San Juan, R. *et al.* (2006) Valganciclovir preemptive therapy for the prevention of cytomegalovirus disease in high-risk seropositive solid-organ transplant recipients. *Transplantation*, **82**, 30–35.

Doyle, A.M., Warburton, K.M., Goral, S. *et al.* (2006) 24-week oral ganciclovir prophylaxis in kidney recipients is associated with reduced symptomatic cytomegalovirus disease compared to a 12-week course. *Transplantation*, **81**, 1106–1111.

Drew, W.L. (2007) Laboratory diagnosis of cytomegalovirus infection and disease in immuno-compromised patients. *Current Opinion in Infectious Diseases*, **20**, 408–411.

Forman, S.J. and Zaia, J.A. (1994) Treatment and prevention of cytomegalovirus pneumonia after bone marrow transplantation: where do we stand? *Blood*, **83**, 2392–2398.

Forslöw, U., Mattsson, J., Ringden, O., Klominek, J. and Remberger, M. (2006) Decreasing mortality rate in early pneumonia follow hematopoietic stem cell transplantation. *Scandinavian Journal of Infectious Diseases*, **38**, 970–976.

Gandhi, M.K. and Khana, R. (2004) Human citomegalovirus: clinical aspects, immune regulation and emerging treatments. *Lancet Infectious Diseases*, **4**, 725–738.

Goodrich, J.M., Bowden, R.A., Fisher, L., Keller, C., Schoch, G. and Meyers, J.D. (1993) Ganciclovir prophylaxis to prevent cytomegalovirus disease after allogeneic marrow transplant. *Annals of Internal Medicine*, **118**, 173–178.

Ho, M.(ed.) (1991) *Cytomegalovirus: Biology and Infection*, Plenum, New York, NY.

Hodson, E.M., Jones, C.A., Webster, A.C., Strippoli, G.F.M., Barclay, B.G., Kable, K. *et al.* (2005) Antiviral medications to prevent cytomegalovirus disease and early death in solid-organ transplant recipients: a systematic review of randomised controlled trials. *Lancet*, **365** (9477), 2105–2115.

Hodson, E.M., Jones, C.A., Strippoli, G.F.M., Webster, A.C. and Craig, J.C. (2007). Immunoglobulins, vaccines or interferon for preventing citomegalovirus disease in solid organ transplant recipients [Reviews]. *The Cochrane Database of Systematic Reviews*. Date of mot recent update: 20 Feb (3) (2007).

Hohenthal, U., Itala, M., Salonen, J. *et al.* (2005) Bronchoalveolar lavage in immunocompromised patients with haematological malignancy: value of new microbiological methods. *European Journal of Haematology*, **74**, 203–211.

Horger, M.S., Pfannenberg, C., Einsele, H., Beck, R., Hebart, H., Lengerke, C. *et al.* (2006) Cytomegalovirus pneumonia after stem cell transplantation: correlation of CT findings with clinical outcome in 30 patients. *American Journal of Roentgenology*, **187**, W636–W643.

Jeffery, J.R., Guttmann, R.D., Becklade, M.R. *et al.* (1974) Recovery from severe cytomegalovirus pneumonia in a renal transplant patient. *The American Review of Respiratory Disease*, **109**, 129–133.

Joos, L., Chhajed, P.N., Wallner, J., Battegay, M., Steiger, J. and Gratwohl, A. (2007) Pulmonary infections diagnosed by BAL: a 12-year experience in 1066 immunocompromised patients. *Respiratory Medicine*, **101**, 93–97.

Khoury, J.A., Storch, G.A., Bohl, D.L. *et al.* (2006) Prophylactic versus preemptive oral valganciclovir for the management of cytomegalovirus infection in adult renal transplant recipients. *American Journal of Transplantation*, **6**, 2134–2143.

Kotloff, R.M., Ahya, V.N. and Crawford, S.W. (2004) Pulmonary complications of solid organ and hematopoietic stem cell transplantation. *American Journal of Respiratory and Critical Care Medicine*, **170**, 22–48.

Kuboshima, S., Tsuruoka, K., Shirai, S., Sasaki, H., Sakurada, T., Miura, H. *et al.* (2007) An autopsy case of microscopic polyangiitis complicated with pulmonary aspergilloma and cytomegalovirus pneumonia. *Nippon Jinzo Gakkai Shi*, **49** (2), 125–129.

Langhoff, E. and Siegel, R.E. (2006) Pneumonitis in human cytomegalovirus infection. *Current Infectious Disease Reports*, **8**, 222–230.

Lee, P., Minai, O.A., Mehta, A.C., DeCamp, M.M. and Murthy, S. (2004) Pulmonary nodules in lung transplant recipients: etiology and outcome. *Chest*, **125**, 165–172.

Li, F., Kenyon, K.W., Kirby, K.A., Fishbein, D.P., Boeckh, M. and Limaye, A.P. (2007) Incidence and clinical features of ganciclovir-resistant cytomegalovirus disease in heart transplant recipients. *Clinical Infectious Diseases*, **45**, 439–447.

Limaye, A.P., Corey, L., Koelle, D.M., Davis, C.L. and Boeckh, M. (2000) Emergence of ganciclovir-resistant cytomegalovirus disease among recipients of solid organ-transplants. *The Lancet*, **356**, 645–649.

Ljungman, P., Griffiths, P. and Paya, C. (2002) Definitions of cytomegalovirus infection and disease in transplant recipients. *Clinical Infectious Diseases*, **34**, 1094–1097.

Lurain, N.S., Bhorade, S.M., Pursell, K.J., Avery, R.K., Yeldandi, V.V., Isada, C.M. *et al.* (2002) Analysis and characterization of antiviral drug-resistant Cytomegalovirus isolates from solid organ transplant recipients. *The Journal of Infectious Diseases*, **186**, 760–768.

Manischewitz, J.F., Quinnan, G.V., Lane, H.C. and Wittek, A.E. (1990) Synergistic effect of ganciclovir and foscarnet on cytomegalovirus replication in vitro. *Antimicrobial Agents and Chemotherapy*, **34**, 373–375.

Manna, A., Cordani, S., Canessa, P. and Pronzato, P. (2003) CMV infection and pneumonia in hematological malignancies. *Journal of Infection and Chemotherapy*, **9**, 265–267.

Medina, J., Pérez-Sartori, G. and Aguado, J.M. (2007) Interactions between Cytomegalovirus and other viruses (HHV6, HHV7, HCV and EBV) in transplantation [Review]. *Trends in Transplantation*, **1**(3), 129–136.

Medina, J., Pérez-Sartori, G., Raúl Caltenco-Serrano and Aguado, J.M. (2008) Response and Pathogenic Mechanisms of Cytomegalovirus Infection in Transplant Recipients [Review]. *Trends in Transplantation*, **2**(3) (In Press).

Mera, J.R., Whimbey, E., Elting, L. *et al.* (1996) Cytomegalovirus pneumonia in adult nontransplantation patients with cancer: review of 20 cases occurring from 1964 through 1990. *Clinical Infectious Diseases*, **22**, 1046–1050.

Merigan, T.C., Renlund, D.G., Keay, S., Bristow, M.R., Starnes, V., O'Connell, J.B. *et al.* (1992) A controlled trial of ganciclovir to prevent cytomegalovirus disease after heart transplantation. *The New England Journal of Medicine*, **326**, 1182–1186.

Meylan, P.R. and Manuel, O. (2007) Late-onset cytomegalovirus disease in patients with solid organ transplant. *Current Opinion in Infectious Diseases*, **20**, 412–418.

Montoya, J.G. (2007) Improving the tools in the fight against cytomegalovirus or strengthening David to defeat goliath. *Current Opinion in Infectious Diseases*, **20**, 397–398.

Mylonakis, E., Kallas, W.M. and Fishman, J.A. (2002) Combination antiviral therapy for ganciclovir-resistant cytomegalovirus infection in solid-organ transplant recipients. *Clinical Infectious Diseases*, **34**, 1337–1341.

Patel, R. and Paya, C.V. (1997) Infections in solid-organ transplant recipients. *Clinical Microbiology Reviews*, **10**, 86–124.

Paya, C., Humar, A., Dominguez, E., Washburn, K., Blumberg, E., Alexander, B. *et al.*, Valganciclovir Solid Organ Transplant Study Group (2004) Efficacy and safety of valganciclovir vs. oral ganciclovir for prevention of cytomegalovirus disease in solid organ transplant recipients. *American Journal of Transplantation*, **4**, 611–620.

Pescovitz, M.D., Rabkin, J., Merion, R.M. *et al.* (2000) Valganciclovir results in improved oral absorption of ganciclovir in liver transplant recipients. *Antimicrobial Agents and Chemotherapy*, **44**, 2811–2815.

Preiksaitis, J.K., Brennan, D.C., Fishman, J. and Allen, U. (2005) Canadian society of transplantation consensus workshop on cytomegalovirus management in solid organ transplantation final report. *American Journal of Transplantation*, **5**, 218–227.

Puius, Y.A. and Snydman, D.R. (2007) Prophylaxis and treatment of cytomegalovirus disease in recipients of solid organ transplants: current approach and future challenges. *Current Opinion in Infectious Diseases*, **20**, 419–424.

Razonable, R.R. and Emery, V.C. (2004) Management of CMV infection and disease in transplant patients [consensus article—IHMF® management recommendations]. *Herpes*, **11**, 77–86.

Razonable, R.R. and Paya, C.V. (2003) Herpesvirus infections in transplant recipients: current challenges in the clinical management of cytomegalovirus and Epstein-Barr virus infections. *Herpes*, **10** (3), 60–65.

Rovira, M. and Ruiz-Camps, I. (2007) Infecciones en el transplante de progenitors hematopoyéticos. *Enfermedades Infecciosas y Microbiología Clínica*, **25** (7), 477–486.

Rowshani, A.T., Bemelman, F.J., van Leeuwen, E.M., van Lier, R.A. and ten Berge, I.J. (2005) Clinical and immunologic aspects of cytomegalovirus infection in solid organ transplant recipients. *Transplantation*, **79**, 381–386.

Rubin, R.H. (1989) The indirect effects of cytomegalovirus infection on the outcome of organ transplantation. *The Journal of the American Medical Association*, **261**, 3607–3609.

Rubin, R.H. (1990) Impact of cytomegalovirus infection on organ transplant recipients. *Reviews of Infectious Diseases*, **12** (Suppl 7), S754–S766.

Rubin, R.H. (2007) The pathogenesis and clinical management of cytomegalovirus infection in the organ transplant recipient: the end of the 'silo hypothesis'. *Current Opinion in Infectious Diseases*, **20**, 399–407.

Scemama, J., Amathieu, R., Tual, L., Fessenmeyer, C., Stirnemann, J. and Dhonneur, G. (2007) Cotrimoxazole Pneumocystis jiroveci pneumonia treatment failure: co-infection cytomegalovirus role? *Annales Françaises D'Anesthèsie et de Rèanimation*, **26** (6), 604–607.

Scott, J.P., Higenbottam, T.W., Sharples, L. *et al.* (1991) Risk factors for obliterative bronchiolitis in heart-lung transplant recipients. *Transplantation*, **51**, 813–817.

Sepkowitz, K.A. (2002) Opportunistic infections in patients with and patients without acquired immunodeficiency syndrome. *Clinical Infectious Diseases*, **34**, 1098–1107.

Sharma, S., Nadrous, H.F., Peters, S.G., Tefferi, A., Litzow, M.R., Aubry, M.-C. *et al.* (2005) Pulmonary complications in adult blood and marrow transplant recipients: autopsy findings. *Chest*, **128**, 1385–1392.

Shimada, A., Koga, T., Shimada, M. *et al.* (2004) Cytomegalovirus pneumonitis presenting small nodular opacities. *Internal Medicine*, **43**, 1198–1200.

Shorr, F.A., Susla, G.M. and O'Grady, N.P. (2004) Pulmonary infiltrates in the non-HIV-infected immunocompromised patient: etiologies, diagnostic strategies, and outcomes. *Chest*, **125**, 260–271.

Sia, I.G. and Patel, R. (2000) New strategies for prevention and therapy of cytomegalovirus infection and disease in solid-organ transplant recipients. *Clinical Microbiology Reviews*, **13**, 83–121.

Singh, N. (2005) Late-onset cytomegalovirus disease as a significant complication in solid organ transplant recipients receiving antiviral prophylaxis: a call to heed the mounting evidence. *Clinical Infectious Diseases*, **40**, 704–708.

Singh, N. (2006) Cytomegalovirus infection in solid organ transplant recipients: new challenges and their implications for preventive strategies. *Journal of Clinical Virology*, **35**, 474–477.

Small, L.N., Lau, J. and Snydman, D.R. (2006) Preventing postorgan transplantation cytomegalovirus disease with ganciclovir: a meta-analysis comparing prophylactic and preemptive therapies. *Clinical Infectious Diseases*, **43**, 869–880.

Stratta, R.J., Shaeffer, M.S., Markin, R.S. *et al.* (1992) Cytomegalovirus infection and disease after liver transplantation: an overview. *Digestive Diseases and Sciences*, **37**, 673–688.

Strippoli, G.F., Hodson, E.M., Jones, C. and Craig, J.C. (2006) Preemptive treatment for cytomegalovirus viremia to prevent cytomegalovirus disease in solid organ transplant recipients. *Transplantation*, **81**, 139–145.

Suh, G.Y., Kang, E.H., Chung, M.P., Lee, K.S., Han, J., Kataichi, M. *et al.* (2006) Early intervention can improve clinical outcome of acute interstitial pneumonia. *Chest*, **129**, 753–761.

Tamm, M., Aboyoun, C.L., Chhajed, P.N., Rainer, S., Malouf, M.A. and Glanville, A.R. (2004) Treated cytomegalovirus pneumonia is not associated with bronchiolitis obliterans syndrome. *American Journal of Respiratory and Critical Care Medicine*, **170**, 1120–1123.

Torre-Cisneros, J., Fortún, J., Aguado, J.M. *et al.* (2005) Recomendaciones GESITRA-SEIMC y RESITRA sobre prevención y tratamiento de la infección por citomegalovirus en pacientes trasplantados. *Enfermedades Infecciosas y Microbiología Clínica*, **23** (7), 424–437.

ViroPharma Inc. (2007) ViroPharma announces presentation of Phase 3 clinical data for maribavir. Available: http://www.viropharma.com/ (accessed September 7).

Wang, G.-S., Chen, G.-H., Lu, M.-Q., Yang, Y., Cai, C.-J., Yi, H.-M. *et al.* (2006) Immunomodulatory therapy of cytomegalovirus pneumonia after liver transplantation. *Chinese Medical Journal*, **119** (17), 1430–1434.

Wiltshire, H., Hirankarn, S., Farrell, C. *et al.* (2005) Pharmacokinetic profile of ganciclovir after its oral administration and from its prodrug, valganciclovir, in solid organ transplant recipients. *Clinical Pharmacokinetics*, **44**, 495–507.

Wingard, J.R. (1999) Opportunistic infections after blood and marrow transplantation. *Transplant Infectious Disease*, **1**, 3–20.

Zhong, J. and Khanna, R. (2007) Vaccine strategies against human citomegalovirus infection. *Expert Review of Anti-Infective Therapy*, **5** (3), 449–459.

15

Antiviral agents against respiratory viruses

Michael G. Ison

Transplant & Immunocompromised Host Infectious Diseases Service, Northwestern University Feinberg School of Medicine, Chicago, Illinois, USA

There are a wide range of viruses that affect the respiratory tree in immunocompromised individuals. Typically these represent viruses that are primarily involving the respiratory tract (the community respiratory viruses, including influenza, respiratory syncycial virus (RSV), parainfluenza virus (PIV), human metapneumovirus (hMPV), rhinovirus, coronavirus and adenovirus) and those who's respiratory involvement is typically a sequellae of systemic infection (such as the herpes viruses (herpes simplex virus (HSV), cytomegalovirus (CMV), and varicella-zoster virus (VSV)) and measles). The community respiratory viruses (CRVs) are the most common viral infections of the lung among transplant recipients and are thus the focus of this chapter; data on management of herpes virus pulmonary infections is discussed elsewhere.

The incidence of these community respiratory viruses is just now being understood thanks to prospective studies using contemporary molecular techniques (Ison, 2005). The community respiratory viruses appear to occur with the same seasonal variation in immunocompromised and immunocompetent patients, but immunocompromised patients may have atypical clinical presentations, prolonged viral shedding, and increased morbidity (acute and chronic rejection, persistent airflow obstruction, in addition to bacterial, fungal and viral infections) and mortality (Ison, 2005). Prevention is the cornerstone to management of CRVs in immunosuppressed patients. There are numerous reports of large outbreaks of CRVs in transplant populations (Abdallah *et al.*, 2003; Chui *et al.*, 2004; Garcia *et al.*, 1997; Jones *et al.*, 2000; Malavaud *et al.*, 2001; Nichols *et al.*, 2004a; Taylor, Vipond and Caul, 2001; Weinstock *et al.*, 2000). As such, a low threshold should be held for considering CRVs in the differential diagnosis when patients present with respiratory symptoms. When a CRV is being considered, the patient should be placed in appropriate isolation until an alternative cause is identified or replication has been reported to have ceased (Anon, 2000, Dykewicz, 2001).

Pulmonary Infection in the Immunocompromised Patient, Edited by Carlos Agustí and Antoni Torres
© 2009 John Wiley & Sons, Ltd.

Table 15.1   Agents used to prevent and treat community respiratory viruses.

Virus	Vaccine	Antivirals

Influenza	Injectable	M2 inhibitors
		    Amantadine
		    Rimantadine

	Live, Attenuated[a]
	    Intranasal
		Neuraminidase Inhibitors
		    Oseltamivir
		    Zanamivir

RSV	NA	Ribavirin ± IgIV, RSV Ig[b], Palivizumab
PIV	NA	No antiviral with proven efficacy
hMPV	NA	Ribavirin ± IgIV[c]
Rhinovirus	NA	Pleconaril[d]
Coronavirus	NA	
Adenovirus	NA	Cidofovir Ganciclovir, ddC[b], Vidarabine[b]

NA = Not Available. Vaccines for RSV, PIV, hMPV and adenovirus in development;
many are live, attenuated vaccines and therefore of limited applicability to this population.
[a]Contraindicated in highly immunosuppresed individuals.
[b]Limited availability.
[c]Based on *in vitro* data only.
[d]Available as investigational agent only. Studied in immunocompetent patients but not
FDA approved for this indication.

There is a vaccine to prevent influenza but none of the other CRVs (see Table 15.1) (Ison, 2005; Smith *et al.*, 2006). Although the injectable influenza vaccine has been documented to be safe among immune suppressed individuals and does not appear to predispose transplant recipients to rejection, its efficacy is nearly universally less than when applied to healthy immune competent patients (Avetisyan *et al.*, 2005; Blumberg *et al.*, 1996; Cavdar *et al.*, 2003; Dengler *et al.*, 1998; Duchini *et al.*, 2001; Engelhard *et al.*, 1993; Hayney *et al.*, 2004; Kumar, Ventura and Vanderwerf, 1978; Lawal *et al.*, 2004; Machado *et al.*, 2005; Mack *et al.*, 1996; Magnani *et al.*, 2005; Mazzone *et al.*, 2004; Sanchez-Fructuoso *et al.*, 2000; Smith *et al.*, 2006; Soesman *et al.*, 2000; White-Williams *et al.*, 2006). It should be noted that the live attenuated intra-nasal formulation is contraindicated in immunocompromised individuals (Smith *et al.*, 2006).

15.1   M2 inhibitors

Overview

Amantadine (Symmetrel) and rimantadine (Flumadine) are M2 inhibitors which pose antiviral activity against influenza A viruses alone. Unfortunately, resistance to M2 inhibitors has recently developed and spread globally (Bright *et al.*, 2005). As a result, this class of antiviral currently has limited activity.

Mode of action

Amantadine (Symmetrel) and rimantadine (Flumadine) inhibit the replication of influenza A viruses at low concentrations (<1.0 µg/mL) by blocking the action of the M2 protein (Hayden and Aoki, 1999). M2, an acid-activated ion channel found only in influenza A viruses, is a membrane protein required for efficient nucleocapsid release after viral fusion with the endosomal membrane (Bui, Whittaker and Helenius, 1996). Low concentrations of the drugs inhibit the ion channel function of the M2 protein, which inhibits viral uncoating or disassembly of the virion during endocytosis and, in H7-subtypes, alters HA maturation during viral assembly (Dolin et al., 1982; Hayden and Aoki, 1999). Amantadine and rimantadine also increase the lysosomal pH, which in turn may inhibit virus-induced membrane fusion events for several enveloped viruses (Hayden and Aoki, 1999).

Pharmacokinetics

Amantadine is rapidly absorbed, with a 53–100% bioavailability, and reaches peak plasma levels within 4.5 hours (Aoki and Sitar, 1988). The drug is predominately excreted unchanged in the urine by glomerular filtration and tubular secretion and has a plasma elimination half-life is about 11–15 hours (Aoki and Sitar, 1988). Elimination is markedly prolonged in patients with renal impairment and decreases about twofold in the elderly (Aoki and Sitar, 1988). Amantadine is widely distributed with salivary levels equivalent to those of blood and nasal mucus comparable to plasma at eight hours after dosing (Aoki and Sitar, 1988; Hayden et al., 1985). Amantadine crosses the placenta and blood-brain barrier with CSF levels equal to 56–96% of serum levels and distributes in breast milk (Hayden and Aoki, 1999; Aoki and Sitar, 1988).

Rimantadine has nearly complete oral bioavailability and achieves maximal plasma concentration three to five hours after ingestion (Hayden and Aoki, 1999; Jefferson et al., 2006; Wills et al., 1987b). The plasma half-life ranges from 24 to 36 hours. Rimantadine levels in nasal secretions average 1.5 times those of plasma levels (Hayden and Aoki, 1999; Jefferson et al., 2006; Wills et al., 1987b). Rimantadine undergoes extensive metabolism, including hydroxylation, conjugation and glucuronidation in the liver before being excreted in the urine. Only 25% of the parent drug is excreted unchanged in the urine (Hayden and Aoki, 1999; Jefferson et al., 2006; Wills et al., 1987b).

Indications

Amantadine and rimantadine are indicated for the prevention and treatment of influenza A virus illness (Dolin et al., 1982). Most placebo-controlled studies of these drugs in the management of influenza have been conducted in previously healthy persons (Jefferson et al., 2006). Amantadine and rimantadine come as 100 mg tablets and a syrup formulation (50 mg/5 mL) (Jefferson et al., 2006).

Prophylaxis

Prophylaxis with amantadine or rimantadine is approximately 70–90% effective in preventing symptomatic influenza A infections (Hayden and Aoki, 1999; Jefferson *et al.*, 2006). The standard dose is 100 mg twice daily for the prevention of influenza; this is continued while the patient is presumed to be at risk (Hayden and Aoki, 1999; Jefferson *et al.*, 2006).

Treatment

Amantadine or rimantadine therapy reduces duration of fever and symptoms in patients with documented influenza A by about one day compared to placebo if the medication is initiated within 48 hours of symptom onset in otherwise healthy patients (Dolin *et al.*, 1982; Hayden and Aoki, 1999; Jefferson *et al.*, 2006). Treatment is also associated with more rapid functional recovery (Hayden and Aoki, 1999; Jefferson *et al.*, 2006) and resolution of small airways functional abnormalities. Studies comparing the therapeutic activity of amantadine and rimantadine are few but generally show comparability (Hayden and Aoki, 1999; Jefferson *et al.*, 2006). Amantadine appears safe and efficacious in reducing length of fever and illness in children older than two. (Hayden and Aoki, 1999; Jefferson *et al.*, 2006; Thompson *et al.*, 1987; Nahata and Brady, 1986; Committee on Infectious, 2007). Paediatric studies have found variable clinical benefits relative to acetaminophen controls and document the frequent emergence of drug-resistant variants (Jefferson *et al.*, 2006; Thompson *et al.*, 1987; Nahata and Brady, 1986). Controlled data to support the use of M2 inhibitors in treating severe influenza or in preventing complications is lacking; one retrospective study found no important differences in duration of illness or hospitalization between the amantadine-treated and untreated patients hospitalized with influenza (Kaiser and Hayden, 1999). One retrospective study of nursing home residents suggested that early treatment might reduce lower respiratory complications (Bowles *et al.*, 2002).

In haematopoietic stem cell transplant and acute leukemia patients who received therapy with one of the M2 inhibitors, a reduced risk of progression to pneumonia (35% vs. 76%) was found compared to no treatment (La Rosa *et al.*, 2001b). However, resistance emergence is common in such patients (Englund *et al.*, 1998).

Dosage in special situations

In adults, the usual dose for treatment or prevention of influenza A infection is 100 mg q12hr for both drugs (see Table 15.2) (Hayden and Aoki, 1999; Jefferson *et al.*, 2006; Smith *et al.*, 2006). Dosing of amantadine and rimantadine should be adjusted in the setting of renal failure (Table 15.2) (Capparelli *et al.*, 1988). Neither M2 inhibitor is cleared by haemodialysis (Hayden and Aoki, 1999; Jefferson *et al.*, 2006). Patients who are over 65 years of age should have the dose of both medications reduced to 100 mg once daily to avoid side effects (Hayden and Aoki, 1999; Jefferson *et al.*, 2006). Rimantadine needs dose adjustment to 100 mg QD for serious hepatic insufficiency

Table 15.2 Dosage of anti-influenza agents.

Compound	Population	Prophylaxis	Treatment
M2 Inhibitors			
Amantadine	Paediatric	1–9 yo	2–4 mg/lb/day (not to exceed 150 mg/d)
		≥9 yo	
	Adult	100 mg BID	100 mg BID
	Elderly (≥65 yo)	100 mg QD	100 mg QD
	Renal dysfunction	Cr Cl <15 mL/min	200 mg ×1 then 100 mg QD
		Cr Cl 15–29 mL/min	200 mg ×1 then 100 mg QOD
		Cr Cl 30–50 mL/min	200 mg Q 7 d
Rimantadine	Paediatric	>10 yo	5 mg/kg QD (not to exceed 150 mg/d)
		≥10 yo	100 mg BID
	Adult	100 mg BID	100 mg BID
	Elderly	100 mg QD	100 mg QD
	Renal dysfunction	Cr Cl ≤10 mL/min	100 mg QD
Neuraminidase inhibitors			
Oseltamivir	Paediatric[a]	≤15 kg	30 mg QD	≤15 kg	30 mg BID
		15–23 kg	45 mg QD	15–23 kg	45 mg BID
		23–40 kg	60 mg QD	23–40 kg	60 mg BID
		≥40 kg	75 mg QD	≥40 kg	75 mg BID
	Adult	75 mg QD	75 mg BID
	Renal dysfunction Cr Cl: 10–30 mL/min	75 mg QOD or 30 mg QD	75 mg QD
Zanamivir	Paediatric[b]	10 mg (2 inhalations) QD	10 mg (2 inhalations) BID
	Adult	10 mg (2 inhalations) QD	10 mg (2 inhalations) BID

Approved for the prevention and treatment of influenza in children ≥1 years old.
Approved for the prevention of influenza in children ≥5 years old and for the treatment of influenza in children ≥7 years old.

(Wills *et al.*, 1987a). The recommended paediatric dosage of both amantadine and rimantadine is 5 mg/kg/day to a maximum of 150 mg/day divide BID in children younger than 10 (Hayden and Aoki, 1999; Jefferson *et al.*, 2006; Smith *et al.*, 2006; Committee on Infectious, 2007). Amantadine and rimantadine are embryotoxic and teratogenic in preclinical tests and amantadine may be associated with birth defects (Hayden and Aoki, 1999; Jefferson *et al.*, 2006).

Adverse effects

The most common side effects of the M2 inhibitors are minor CNS complaints (anxiety, difficulty concentrating, insomnia, dizziness, headache and jitteriness) and gastrointestinal upset (Hayden and Aoki, 1999; Jefferson *et al.*, 2006). Patients who receive amantadine may develop antimuscarinic effects, orthostatic hypotension and congestive heart failure at low frequencies (Hayden and Aoki, 1999; Jefferson *et al.*, 2006). Particularly in the elderly or those with renal failure, serious central nervous system (CNS) side-effects due to amantadine and less often rimantadine, include confusion, disorientation, mood alterations, memory disturbances, delusions, nightmares, ataxia, tremors, seizures, coma, acute psychosis, slurred speech, visual disturbances, delirium, occulogyric episodes and hallucinations (Hayden and Aoki, 1999; Jefferson *et al.*, 2006). Amantadine causes CNS side effects in about 15 to 30% of persons, as well as dose-related abnormalities in psychomotor testing (Hayden and Aoki, 1999; Jefferson *et al.*, 2006). The incidence and severity of CNS adverse effects are less common with rimantadine (Keyser *et al.*, 2000).

Concomitant ingestion of antihistamines or anticholinergic drugs increases the CNS effects of amantadine (Hayden and Aoki, 1999; Jefferson *et al.*, 2006). Trimethoprim-sulfamethoxazole and triamterene-hydrochlorothiazide decrease the renal clearance of amantadine, which enhances the risk of CNS toxicity (Hayden and Aoki, 1999; Jefferson *et al.*, 2006). Quinine and quinidine likewise reduce the clearance of amantadine. Coadministration with monoamine oxidase inhibitors may precipitate life threatening hypertension. The drug does not appear to interact with the cytochrome P450 system (Hayden and Aoki, 1999; Jefferson *et al.*, 2006). Cimetidine is associated with 15 to 20% increases and aspirin or acetaminophen with 10% decreases in plasma rimantadine concentrations, but such changes are unlikely to be of clinical significance (Hayden and Aoki, 1999; Jefferson *et al.*, 2006). Patients receiving either amantadine or rimantadine along with drugs affecting CNS function, such as antihistamines, antidepressants, minor tranquillizers, should be monitored closely.

Resistance

M2 inhibitor resistance occurs from changes in the amino acids that constitute the protein and results in cross-resistance among all M2 inhibitors (Hayden, 2006). M2 inhibitor resistance appears to be stable and persistent (Bright *et al.*, 2006; Englund *et al.*, 1998). These features have contributed to the rapid and widespread emergence of M2 inhibitors that currently limits the effectiveness of this class of drugs (Bright *et al.*, 2006; Hayden,

2006; Smith *et al.*, 2006). M2 inhibitor resistance among A/H3N2 viruses in the Asia, Europe and the United States is very high (Bright *et al.*, 2005); regions, such as Australia and New Zealand, which have lower rates are noting increased prevalence of resistant virus over time (Barr, 2007). Even among A/H1N1 viruses, there is increasing prevalence of resistance to M2 inhibitors, globally (Barr, 2007; Hayden, 2006; Smith *et al.*, 2006). In patients with susceptible wild type virus initially, up to a third will shed resistant variants within two to four days after the start of therapy (Hayden and Aoki, 1999; Jefferson *et al.*, 2006). Emergence of resistant virus does not appear to cause a rebound in illness in immunocompetent adults but may be associated with protracted illness and shedding in immunocompromised hosts (Englund *et al.*, 1998; Ison *et al.*, 2006). Importantly, resistant virus can be spread to others and has caused failures of antiviral prophylaxis under close contact conditions, as in nursing homes and households (Hayden, 1996a). The resistant virus appears to retain wild-type pathogenicity and causes an influenza illness indistinguishable from susceptible strains (Ison *et al.*, 2006). Use of combinations of antivirals may result in a lower risk of resistant virus emergence; the impact of tested antiviral combinations has not been studied in the current era of M2 inhibitor resistance (Bright *et al.*, 2006; Ison *et al.*, 2003).

15.2 Neuraminidase inhibitors

Overview

Oseltamivir (Tamiflu, a prodrug of the active carboxylate) and zanamivir (Relenza) are sialic acid analogues that potently and specifically inhibit influenza A and B neuraminidases by competitively and reversibly interacting with the active enzyme site (Moscona, 2005). These drugs are active against all nine neuraminidase subtypes in nature including most of the avian strains of influenza A H5N1 and H9N2 that infected humans (Hayden, 2006).

Mode of action

Influenza A and B viruses possess a surface glycoprotein with neuraminidase activity whereas influenza C viruses do not. This enzyme cleaves terminal sialic acid residues and destroys the receptors recognized by viral haemagglutinin. This activity is essential for release of virus from infected cells, for prevention of viral aggregates, and for viral spread within the respiratory tract (Colman, 1994).

Available compounds

Oseltamivir

Pharmacokinetics

Oral oseltamivir ethyl ester is well absorbed and rapidly cleaved by esterases in the gastrointestinal tract, liver, or blood. The bioavailability of the active metabolite, oseltamivir carboxylate, is estimated to be approximately 80% in previously healthy persons (He, Massarella and Ward, 1999; Oo *et al.*, 2001). Peak oseltamivir carboxylate concentrations are reached at five hours after oral administration and the plasma elimination half-life is 6–10 hours (He, Massarella and Ward, 1999; Oo *et al.*, 2001). Both the prodrug and parent are eliminated primarily unchanged through the kidney by glomerular filtration and anionic tubular secretion (He, Massarella and Ward, 1999). Distribution is not well characterized in humans, but peak bronchoalveolar lavage levels are similar to plasma levels in animals (McClellan and Perry, 2001). Drug levels in middle ear fluid and sinus aspirates are similar to those in the blood (McClellan and Perry, 2001).

Indications

Oseltamivir is indicated for the prevention and treatment of uncomplicated acute illness due to influenza infection in patients one year and older. Oseltamivir comes as 30, 45 and 75 mg tablets and as a white tutti-frutti–flavoured suspension.

Prophylaxis

Once daily oseltamivir (see Table 15.2) is 80–92% effective in reducing the incidence of influenza in treated individuals (Hayden *et al.*, 1999; Hayden *et al.*, 2004; Peters *et al.*, 2001; Welliver *et al.*, 2001; Moscona, 2005). Oseltamivir prophylaxis provided additional benefit in addition to influenza vaccination among frail elderly patients (0.5% vs. 5.0%; 91% protective efficacy) (Peters *et al.*, 2001). Oseltamivir prophylaxis appeared to be safe and well tolerated in preventing influenza among HSCT recipients (Vu *et al.*, 2007; Chik *et al.*, 2004). In a case-control study, an influenza outbreak was controlled by the use of oseltamivir in an outpatient residential facility for patients undergoing HSCT. Patients received oseltamivir for a median of 17 days (10–81); none of the 45 patients who took oseltamivir developed influenza (Vu *et al.*, 2007). There was no significant difference in adverse effects between patient cases and controls (Vu *et al.*, 2007). Among 32 paediatric HSCT recipients, oseltamivir 75 mg daily was 100% effective in preventing laboratory-confirmed influenza and use was associated with a low rate of side effects (16%, mostly gastrointestinal upset) (Chik *et al.*, 2004). To expand on these findings, a prospective, randomized, placebo-controlled study of oseltamivir for seasonal prophylaxis is currently being conducted among HSC, kidney and liver transplant recipients.

Treatment

Oseltamivir 75 mg twice daily (Table 15.2) for five days when started within the first two days of symptoms, was associated with a shorter time to alleviation of illness (29–35 hours shorter) and with reductions in severity of illness (0.5–4.1 days shorter) (Moscona, 2005), duration of fever, time to return to normal activity, quantity of viral shedding, duration of impaired activity and complications leading to antibiotic use, particularly bronchitis, compared to placebo in previously healthy adults (Moscona,

2005; Cooper *et al.*, 2003; Aoki *et al.*, 2003; Kaiser *et al.*, 2003; Nicholson *et al.*, 2000; Treanor *et al.*, 2000). The earlier the medication is started, the greater the clinical response (Aoki *et al.*, 2003). In a paediatric study enrolling children between the ages of 1 and 12 years, oseltamivir 2 mg/kg BID for five days significantly reduced illness duration and severity, time to resumption of full activities, and the occurrence of complications leading to antibiotic use, particularly acute otitis media (Whitley *et al.*, 2001).

There is limited data on the safety, efficacy and optimal dosing of oseltamivir among patients hospitalized for influenza and in patients with altered immune systems (Ison, 2005; Ison and Hayden, 2002; Kaiser and Hayden, 1999). These patients typically have muted symptoms and prolonged shedding of virus; likewise, they may be at increased risk for infectious and non-infectious complications of influenza (Ison, 2005; Ison and Hayden, 2002; Kaiser and Hayden, 1999). As a result, some have advocating starting therapy beyond 48 hours after symptom onset and using oseltamivir at higher doses (150 mg vs. 75 mg BID) and for a longer duration (Ison, 2005; Ison *et al.*, 2006). Many of the registration studies of oseltamivir compared 75 mg BID with 150 mg BID; in general, there was a trend to more rapid virologic clearance without an increased incidence or severity of adverse effects (Aoki *et al.*, 2003; Moscona, 2005; Nicholson *et al.*, 2000; Treanor *et al.*, 2000). Likewise, there is limited data to suggest that later onset of antiviral medication among hospitalized adults may have clinical benefit (Ison *et al.*, 2003).

Among immunocompromised patients, there is emerging data, from predominantly retrospective studies, suggesting that oseltamivir is both safe and effective in these populations. Oseltamivir for the treatment of influenza in HSCT recipients is associated with reduced morbidity, a reduced risk of progression to lower track disease and reduced mortality (Ison *et al.*, 2006; La Rosa *et al.*, 2001b; Nichols *et al.*, 2004b; Machado *et al.*, 2004). Since shedding is prolonged, some recommend that oseltamivir should be continued until viral shedding has ceased (Ison, 2005; Ison and Hayden, 2002; Nichols *et al.*, 2004b). A prospective, dose-ranging study of oseltamivir for the treatment of influenza among HSC, kidney and liver transplant recipients is currently under way.

Dosage in special situations

Oseltamivir dose should be reduced by 50%–75 mg once a day for treatment and 75 mg every other day or 30 mg of suspension daily for prophylaxis when a patient has a creatinine clearance of less than 30 mg/dL (Table 15.2) (Moscona, 2005). Doses of oseltamivir should be given after haemodialysis. The safety and pharmacokinetics in patients with hepatic impairment have not been evaluated (Moscona, 2005). Oseltamivir should not be used in pregnant women unless the benefits of therapy clearly outweigh the potential risks (pregnancy category C) (Moscona, 2005). Although drug concentrations over time are 25–35% higher in the elderly at steady state, no dose adjustment is deemed necessary (He, Massarella and Ward, 1999).

Adverse effects

Oral oseltamivir is generally well tolerated (Moscona, 2005). Oseltamivir is associated with nausea, discomfort and, less often, emesis in a minority of treated patients

(Moscona, 2005). Nausea and vomiting occurs at approximately 10–15% excess in oseltamivir recipients (Moscona, 2005). Gastrointestinal complaints are usually mild-to-moderate in intensity, usually resolve despite continued dosing, and ameliorated by administration with food (Moscona, 2005). Postmarketing reports suggest that oseltamivir may be associated rarely with skin rash, hepatic dysfunction, and neuropsychiatric events. The post-marketing reports of self-injury and delirium, mostly among Japanese paediatric patients, has not been studied prospectively, but close monitoring of these individuals is recommended (Roche, 2007).

No clinically significant drug interactions have been recognized. However, probenecid blocks tubular secretion and doubles the half-life of the oseltamivir (He, Massarella and Ward, 1999). No interactions with the cytochrome P450 enzymes occur *in vitro*. Protein binding is below 10% (He, Massarella and Ward, 1999).

Zanamivir

Pharmacokinetics

The oral bioavailability of zanamivir is low (<5%), and most clinical trials have used intranasal or dry powder inhalation delivery. The current dry powder formulation is mixed with lactose (5 mg zanamivir per 20 mg lactose) (Moscona, 2005). Following inhalation of the dry powder, approximately 7–21% is deposited in the lower respiratory tract and the remainder in the oropharynx (Cass *et al.*, 1999a; Cass, Efthymiopoulos and Bye, 1999b). Median zanamivir concentrations are above 1000 ng/mL in induced sputum six hours after inhalation and remain detectable up to 24 hours (Cass, Efthymiopoulos and Bye, 1999b). The peak plasma concentration averages 46 µg/L after a single 16 mg inhalation of zanamivir, suggesting minimal systemic exposure to the drug (Cass, Efthymiopoulos and Bye, 1999b).

Indications

Zanamivir is indicated for the treatment (seven years and older) and prophylaxis (five years and older) of influenza in adults and children. Zanamivir is delivered by inhalation with a proprietary breath-activated device (DISKHALER).

Prophylaxis

Once daily inhaled zanamivir for four weeks was 69–81% efficacious in preventing laboratory-confirmed influenza illness (Cooper *et al.*, 2003; Monto *et al.*, 1999). In nursing homes experiencing influenza outbreaks, inhaled zanamivir was more effective for prevention of influenza A illness than oral rimantadine, in part because of frequent resistance emergence to the M2 inhibitor (Dunn and Goa, 1999). There is no data about the use of zanamivir for prophylaxis in immunosuppressed patients. Zanamivir is not recommended for patients with underlying airways disease due to risk of serious bronchospams (Moscona, 2005).

Treatment

Inhaled zanamivir in adults has consistently shown at least one less day of disabling influenza symptoms, and most studies have found a reduction in the number of nights of disturbed sleep, in length of time to resumption of normal activities, and in the use of symptom relief medications when therapy is started within 48 hours of symptom onset (Moscona, 2005). Similar therapeutic benefits have also been shown in children ages 5 to 12 years old (Hedrick *et al.*, 2000). Greatest benefit was noted in patients who were febrile at the time of enrolment, those started on therapy within 30 hours after the onset of symptoms, and in adults aged 50 years and older (Dunn and Goa, 1999; Moscona, 2005). Zanamivir has also been associated with a 40% reduction in lower respiratory tract complications of influenza leading to antibiotics, particularly bronchitis and pneumonia (Lalezari *et al.*, 2001).

Zanamivir appears generally well tolerated and effective in treating influenza in patients with mild to moderate asthma or chronic obstructive pulmonary disease (Lalezari *et al.*, 2001; Murphy *et al.*, 2000). An uncontrolled study found zanamivir to be safe and possibly effective in allogeneic stem cell transplant recipients, although viral shedding persisted an average of two weeks into therapy (Johny *et al.*, 2002). The combination of a non-FDA approved formulation of zanamivir plus rimantadine found that there was a trend to more rapid cessation of cough in dual therapy patients and M2 resistant virus was only noted in patients who received rimantadine monotherapy; none was noted in the combined therapy arm (Ison *et al.*, 2003). Although this data suggests that dual therapy may be associated with a lower risk of resistance and possibly enhanced efficacy, the current high rate of M2 inhibitor resistance makes this combination unappealing (Bright *et al.*, 2006; Ison *et al.*, 2003; Smith *et al.*, 2006).

Dosage in special situations

Although the plasma elimination half-life increases with creatinine clearance ≤ 70 mL/min, drug accumulation is negligible after inhalation and dose adjustment is not necessary for renal or hepatic dysfunction. Certain populations, particularly very young, frail, or cognitively impaired patients, may have difficulty using the drug delivery system (Diggory *et al.*, 2001). Zanamavir is classified as a category C drug in pregnancy but it has poor bioavailability and lack of documented teratogenic effects in preclinical studies.

Adverse effects

Topically applied zanamivir is generally well tolerated in controlled studies, including those involving patients with asthma and COPD (Murphy *et al.*, 2000). Post-marketing reports indicate that bronchospasm been may be an uncommon but potentially severe problem, particularly in patients with acute influenza and underlying reactive airways disease (Kent, 2000). Anecdotal reports of hospitalization and fatality indicate that inhaled zanamivir should be used cautiously in such patients. Current guidelines advise against the use of zanamivir in patients with underlying airway disease, unless the patient is closely monitored and has a fast-acting inhaled bronchodilator available when inhaling zanamivir (Smith *et al.*, 2006). No difference in adverse events between zanamivir and placebo (lactose) recipients have been found (Murphy *et al.*, 2000). Less than 5% zanamivir recipients have reported diarrhorea, nausea, sinusitis, nasal signs and symptoms, bronchitis, cough, headache, dizziness and ear, nose and throat infections. Low bioavailability is associated with low exposure to circulating zanamivir, and no clinically significant drug interactions have been recognized. *In vitro* studies suggest that zanamivir does not inhibit or induce cytochrome p450 enzymes.

Resistance

Zanamivir and oseltamivir carboxylate resistance results from mutations in the viral haemagglutinin and/or neuraminidase (Gubareva, 2004; McKimm-Breschkin, 2000; Zambon *et al.*, 2001). In the hemagglutinin variants, mutations in or near the receptor binding site make the virus less dependent on neuraminidase action, whereas neuraminidase mutations directly affect interaction with the inhibitors (Gubareva, 2004; McKimm-Breschkin, 2000; Zambon *et al.*, 2001). The particular neuraminidase mutation determines the degree of resistance and cross-resistance (that is, R229K causes high level resistance in oseltamivir but not zanamivir) (Gubareva, 2004; Ison *et al.*, 2006; McKimm-Breschkin, 2000). Oseltamivir resistant variants have been recovered from less than 1% of treated adults and about 4–18% of treated children (Aoki, Boivin and Roberts, 2007). The possible clinical and epidemiologic significance of such variants requires study and a global Neuraminidase Inhibitor Susceptibility Network has been established to address these concerns (Zambon *et al.*, 2001). Use of combinations of antivirals may result in a lower risk of resistant virus emergence; the impact of tested antiviral combinations has not been studied in the current era of M2 inhibitor resistance (Bright *et al.*, 2006; Ison *et al.*, 2003).

15.3   Cidofovir

Overview

Cidofovir is a cytosine analogue that has activity against most herpes viruses as well as adenovirus.

Mode of action

Cidofovir is a cytosine analogue that competitively inhibits dCTP and slows chain elongation via inhibition of viral DNA polymerase (Ison, 2006).

Pharmacokinetics

Cidofovir has low bioavailability (less than 5%) and is therefore only available as an intravenous solution. The compound is widely distributed and cleared renally via filtration and active secretion. As a result, propenicid reduces clearance and increases blood levels (Hayden, 2000).

Indications

Cidofovir is indicated for the treatment of CMV retinitis in patients with AIDS, but is often used off label for the treatment of adenovirus infections. Cidofovir is active against all serotypes of adenovirus *in vitro* (de Oliveira *et al.*, 1996; Morfin *et al.*, 2005). Animal models of ocular infection have clearly demonstrated virologic and clinical efficacy (Ison, 2006). In humans, however, data are still mostly retrospective in nature but suggest that cidofovir use is associated with significantly lower mortality compared to historical controls or other antivirals (Baldwin *et al.*, 2000; Bordigoni *et al.*, 2001; Carter *et al.*, 2002; Fanourgiakis *et al.*, 2005; Hatakeyama *et al.*, 2003; Hoffman *et al.*, 2001; Howard *et al.*, 1999; Lankester *et al.*, 2004; Legrand *et al.*, 2001; Leruez-Ville *et al.*, 2004; Ljungman *et al.*, 2003; Muller *et al.*, 2005; Nagafuji *et al.*, 2004). Typically, one of two regimens is used for the management of adenoviral disease: 5 mg/kg Q1–2 weeks or 1 mg/kg TIW (Hoffman *et al.*, 2001; Legrand *et al.*, 2001). Although the 1 mg/kg TIW is associated with less nephrotoxicity (Hoffman *et al.*, 2001), the efficacy of the two regimens have not been directly compared. Additionally, the 1 mg/lg TIW regimen is associated with breakthrough CMV and HSV infections (Guzman-Cottrill *et al.*, 2005; Nagafuji *et al.*, 2004). Two recent studies of immunosuppressed patients with adenoviremia and invasive adenovirus disease were monitored by quantitative PCR to determine their response to cidofovir (5 mg/kg Q week for two weeks then every other week) (Leruez-Ville *et al.*, 2004; Neofytos *et al.*, 2007). Most clearly responded virologically and clinically to cidofovir; the remaining 4/14 patients had persistent viral replication and eventually died. Of note, there was a significant delay between onset of symptoms and institution of therapy in these fatal cases (median 18 days). A decline in viral load of 1 log or greater in the 7–10 days after the first dose was predictive of a successful outcome (Leruez-Ville *et al.*, 2004).

Dosage in special situations

There is limited data on how to dose cidofovir with advanced renal insufficiency. Use is contraindicated with serum creatinine >1.5 mg/dL, creatinine clearance <55 mL/min, or greater than 2 + protein (Hayden, 2000).

Adverse effect

The most frequent severe adverse reactions associated with cidofovir include nephrotoxicity, cytopenias and ocular toxicity. Because of the risk of ocular hypotony, it is recommended that intraocular pressures be closely monitored in patients being treated with cidofovir. Nephrotoxicity should be screened for in all patients before infusions by checking serum creatinine and urine for protein. Likewise, nephrotoxicity can be minimized by giving 2 gm of probenecid and a litre of normal saline three hours before the cidofovir infusion and giving additional saline and 1 gm of probenecid at two and eight hours post-infusion (Hayden, 2000; Ison, 2006).

15.4   Ribavirin

Overview

Ribavirin (Virazole, Rebetol) is a guanosine analogue with a wide range of antiviral activity including influenza viruses, respiratory syncytial virus, parainfluenza viruses, and adenovirus.

Mode of action

Ribavirin is rapidly phosphorylated by intracellular enzymes and the triphosphate inhibits influenza virus RNA polymerase activity and competitively inhibits the guanosine triphosphate–dependent 5′-capping of influenza viral messenger RNA. In addition, ribavirin depletes cellular guanine pools (Wray, Gilbert and Knight, 1985a; Wray et al., 1985b). Ribavirin also shows anti-proliferative and immunomodulatory effects.

Pharmacokinetics

Oral ribavirin has a bioavailability of 33–45% in adults and children and achieves peak plasma concentration of 0.6 µg/mL one to two hours after ingestion of a 400 mg dose in adults. Ribavirin has a short initial (0.3–0.7 hours) and long terminal-phase half-life (18–36 hours) and is eliminated by hepatic metabolism and renal clearance (Connor et al., 1993; Connor, Hintz and Vandyke, 1984; Laskin et al., 1987; Paroni et al., 1989). After aerosol administration, plasma levels increase with exposure and range from 0.2–1 µg/ml. Respiratory secretions have levels of up to 1000 µg/mL, which declines with a half-life of 1.4–2.5 hours (Paroni et al., 1989).

Indictations

Ribavirin is only indicated for the treatment of respiratory syncytial virus (RSV) and hepatitic C infection. Ribavirin has also been used off-label for the management of parainfluenza (PIV) and adenovirus infections; the efficacy of this compound for these infections has not been documented, as discussed below. Ribavirin is available in 200 mg capsules, oral solution (40 mg/mL) and 6 gm powder for inhalational solution; intravenous formulations must be formulated by individual pharmacies using good manufacturing practices (Ventre and Randolph, 2007). The inhalational solution must be delivered by a proprietary nebulizer (Viratek small particle aerosol generator (SPAG-2)) (Ventre and Randolph, 2007).

Anti-influenza treatment

There is extensive in vitro data suggesting that ribavirin alone or in combination with other anti-influenza agents is active against most human strains of influenza. High oral doses (8.4 gm over two days) provided moderate symptom relief in acute influenza (Stein *et al.*, 1987). There is limited additional data in clinical practice (Hayden, 1996b).

Anti-RSV treatment

Trials of aerosolized ribavirin for the treatment of severe respiratory syncytial virus in infants have shown no consistent effect on duration of hospitalization time or mortality (Ventre and Randolph, 2007). Likewise, long term follow-up of ribavirin recipients has likewise found no consistent benefits on pulmonary function (Ventre and Randolph, 2007). Current guidelines recommend that decisions regarding the use of ribavirin administration should be made on the basis of particular clinical circumstances and clinician experience (Pediatrics, 2006). Administration of a more concentrated aerosol solution (60 mg/mL) over two hours three times daily appears well tolerated and easier to administer (Englund *et al.*, 1994).

Ribavirin has also been studied for the treatment of RSV infections in immuno-compromised patients. One prospective study in HSCT recipients with upper respiratory RSV infection who received preemptive aerosolized ribavirin found acceptable tolerance and a trend to reduction of viral load (Boeckh *et al.*, 2007). Retrospective reports suggest that aerosolized ribavirin is superior to IV ribavirin in stem cell transplant recipients (Ison, 2005; Ison and Hayden, 2002). Survival is improved when treatment is started before respiratory failure or when infection was limited to the upper respiratory tract (Ison, 2005; Ison and Hayden, 2002). Intravenous ribavirin has been shown to be effective for the management of RSV in lung transplant recipients (Glanville *et al.*, 2005). The use of oral ribavirin has been studied in patients with RSV and appears to have some degree of efficacy (Chakrabarti *et al.*, 2001), and some centres use oral ribavirin plus immunoglobulin preparations for the treatment of RSV. Further studies of oral ribavirin are needed. Addition of intravenous antibodies appears to have the greatest benefit in reducing mortality (Ison, 2005; Ison and Hayden, 2002). Although the retrospective data suggests that palivizumab is the preparation associated with the lowest mortality when combined with aerosolized ribavirin (Boeckh *et al.*, 2001), RSV Ig or IgIV plus aerosolized ribavirin have improved mortality relative to aerosolized ribavirin alone (Cortez *et al.*, 2002; De Vincenzo *et al.*, 1996; Ghosh *et al.*, 2000; Ghosh *et al.*, 2001; Glanville *et al.*, 2005). There is insufficient data to determine which antibody preparation is superior. From the available data, use of aerosolized ribavirin plus an antibody preparation should be considered the preferred regimen for managing serious RSV infections in immunocompromised patients (Ison, 2005; Ison and Hayden, 2002).

Anti-PIV treatment

Although aerosolized and intravenous ribavirin and IgIV have been tried, neither has been shown to reduce viral titers or mortality in HSCT recipients (Nichols *et al.*, 2004a; Nichols, Gooley and Boeckh, 2001). Among lung transplant recipients, response to oral, aerosolized and intravenous ribavirin is more promising (McCurdy, Milstone and Dummer, 2003; Wendt, Fox and Hertz, 1995).

Anti-adenovirus treatment

Ribavirin only has *in vitro* activity against subgroup C viruses for which there is a wide variation in the $IC_{50}s$ (Morfin *et al.*, 2005; Naesens *et al.*, 2005; Potter *et al.*, 1976), and few studies have shown a mortality benefit with the use of this agent (61–77% mortality) (Abe *et al.*, 2003; Baldwin *et al.*, 2000; Bertrand *et al.*, 2000; Bordigoni *et al.*, 2001; Buchdahl, Taylor and Warner, 1985; Cassano, 1991; Chakrabarti *et al.*, 1999; Emovon *et al.*, 2003; Gavin and Katz, 2002; Hromas *et al.*, 1994; Jurado Chacon *et al.*, 1998; Jurado *et al.*, 1995; Kapelushnik *et al.*, 1995; La Rosa *et al.*, 2001a; Lankester *et al.*, 2004; Liles *et al.*, 1993; Mann *et al.*, 1998; McCarthy *et al.*, 1995; Miyamura *et al.*, 2000; Murphy *et al.*, 1993; Sabroe *et al.*, 1995; Schleuning *et al.*, 2004; Shetty *et al.*, 2000; Whimbey, Englund and Couch, 1997). In one recent study, despite receiving ribavirin, all four immunocompromised children with disseminated adenoviral disease (three with subgroup C viruses (1, 2 and 5)) died and only one had a slight reduction in the level of viral DNA measured by quantitative PCR (Lankester *et al.*, 2004). Overall, there is not convincing evidence that ribavirin significantly reduces viral load and its use is not associated with a meaningful reduction in mortality (Ison, 2006).

Dosage in special situations

Systemic ribavirin is contraindicated in patients with creatinine clearance of less than 50 mg/min and the dose should be reduced by one-third for patients under the age of 10 years. Dose adjustment is needed if there is a substantial decline in hematocrit and the drug should be discontinued if the haematocrit drops below 8.5 gm/dL. Ribavirin is contraindicated in pregnant women and in male partners of women who are pregnant because of teratogenicity of the drug. Pregnancy should be avoided during therapy and six months after completion of therapy in both female patients and in female partners of male patients taking ribavirin (Pregnancy category X).

Adverse effects

Systemic ribavirin can cause a dose-related extravascular haemolytic anemia and at higher doses, suppression of bone marrow release of erythroid elements. Severe anemia may require dose adjustment or cessation or use of erythropoitin. Aerosolized ribavirin can cause bronchospasm, mild conjunctival irritation, rash, psychologic distress if administered in an oxygen tent, and rarely, acute water intoxication. Bolus intravenous administration may cause rigours. Antagonism of both drugs may occur when ribavirin is combined with zidovudine.

Resistance

Resistance for the respiratory viruses has not been described.

15.5 Investigational agents

Anti-influenza agents

With the threat of pandemic influenza growing, there has been significant research into new anti-influenza agents. Many of the agents are neuraminidase inhibitors that have either enhanced activity against resistant viruses, intravenous formulations, or prolonged half-lives (Ong and Hayden, 2007). DAS181 (NexBio, San Diego, California) is a topically applied conjugated sialidase that is entering testing in humans (Ong and Hayden, 2007; Malakhov *et al.*, 2006). Several topical haemaglutinin inhibitors, including cyanovirin-N are being investigated as are several oral and topical polymerase inhibitors, including T-705 (Toyama Chemical Company, Toyama, Japan) (Ong and Hayden, 2007; Sidwell *et al.*, 2007).

Anti-adenovirus agents

A lipid-ester analog of cidofovir, CMX0001 (Chimerix, Durham, North Carolina) is currently undergoing phase I testing. It appears to be orally bioavailable with reduced nephrotoxicity compared to cidofovir. *In vitro*, the lipid ester derivatives of cidofovir are 5- to 2500-fold more potent against adenovirus than the parent compound (Hartline *et al.*, 2005; Ison, 2006).

Anti-RSV agents

One of the most advanced anti-RSV agents is RSV604 (Arrow Therapeutics Ltd, London, UK), a novel oral benzodiazepine analogue that targets the nucleocapsid protein (Chapman *et al.*, 2007). In a small randomized, double-blind, placebo-controlled phase II study in adult stem cell transplant recipients with proven RSV infection, RSV604 was found to be well tolerated but had widely variable absorption. Antiviral efficacy correlated with peak drug exposure. A reformulated version of the drug is undergoing further testing (Marty *et al.*, 2007). Additionally, there is a new anti-RSV monoclonal antibiody (mortavizumab, MedImmune, Gaithersburg, Maryland) that appears to have a longer half-life and stronger binding affinity to RSV than palivizumab (Young, 2007).

Anti-parainfluenza agents

Two new haemagglutinin-neuraminidase inhibitors, BCX2798 and BCX2855 (Bio-Cryst, Birmingham, Alabama) show significant anti-PIV activity *in vitro* and *in vivo*, but have not been tested in humans to date (Alymova *et al.*, 2004).

Anti-rhinovirus agents

Pleconaril (Schering-Plough, Kenilworth, New Jersey) was studied extensively in healthy adults with rhinoviral colds, was well tolerated, and led to faster resolution of symptoms, to more rapid improvement in symptom scores, and to clearance of virus from nasal mucous (Hayden *et al.*, 2003). Pleconaril was not approved by the FDA and is therefore not commercially available. Because of its induction of the CyP-450 enzymes (Hayden *et al.*, 2003), interaction with common immunosuppressants should be expected. The compound has been reformulated into an intranasal formulation which is currently undergoing study; it is unclear what role this formulation would play in a patient with severe disease or if it can safely be nebulized to deliver the drug to the lower respiratory tract. Several other novel antivirals, including 3C proteases, are either too early in development to determine their safety and efficacy or are not being actively developed (Patick, 2006). In immunocompetent patients, serum neutralizing antibodies correlate with protection and topical interferon may have efficacy in preventing and in moderating viral shedding and symptoms (Anzueto and Niederman, 2003); their role in transplant recipients has not been studied. Systemic interferon may predispose solid organ transplant rejection and should be used with extreme care.

References

Abdallah, A., Rowland, K.E., Schepetiuk, S.K., To, L.B. and Bardy, P. (2003) An outbreak of respiratory syncytial virus infection in a bone marrow transplant unit: effect on engraftment and outcome of pneumonia without specific antiviral treatment. *Bone Marrow Transplantation*, **32**, 195–203.

Abe, S., Miyamura, K., Oba, T., Terakura, S., Kasai, M., Kitaori, K., Sasaki, T. and Kodera, Y. (2003) Oral ribavirin for severe adenovirus infection after allogeneic marrow transplantation. *Bone Marrow Transplantation*, **32**, 1107–1108.

Alymova, I.V., Taylor, G., Takimoto, T., Lin, T..-H., Chand, P., Babu, Y.S., Li, C., Xiong, X. and Portner, A. (2004) Efficacy of novel hemagglutinin-neuraminidase inhibitors BCX 2798 and BCX 2855 against human parainfluenza viruses in vitro and in vivo. *Antimicrobial Agents and Chemotherapy*, **48**, 1495–1502.

Anon (2000) Guidelines for preventing opportunistic infections among hematopoietic stem cell transplant recipients. *Morbidity and Mortality Weekly Report*, **49**, 1–128.

Anzueto, A. and Niederman, M.S. (2003) Diagnosis and Treatment of Rhinovirus Respiratory Infections. *Chest*, **123**, 1664–1672.

Aoki, F.Y., Boivin, G. and Roberts, N. (2007) Influenza virus susceptibility and resistance to oseltamivir. *Antiviral Therapy*, **12**, 603–616.

Aoki, F.Y., Macleod, M.D., Paggiaro, P., Carewicz, O., El Sawy, A., Wat, C., Griffiths, M., Waalberg, E. and Ward, P. (2003) Early administration of oral oseltamivir increases the benefits of influenza treatment. *The Journal of Antimicrobial Chemotherapy*, **51**, 123–129.

Aoki, F.Y. and Sitar, D.S. (1988) Clinical pharmacokinetics of amantadine hydrochloride. *Clinical Pharmacokinetics*, **14**, 35–51.

Avetisyan, G., Ragnavolgyi, E., Toth, G.T., Hassan, M. and Ljungman, P. (2005) Cell-mediated immune responses to influenza vaccination in healthy volunteers and allogeneic stem cell transplant recipients. *Bone Marrow Transplantation*, **36**, 411–415.

Baldwin, A., Kingman, H., Darville, M., Foot, A.B., Grier, D., Cornish, J.M., Goulden, N., Oakhill, A., Pamphilon, D.H., Steward, C.G. and Marks, D.I. (2000) Outcome and clinical course of 100 patients with adenovirus infection following bone marrow transplantation. *Bone Marrow Transplantation*, **26**, 1333–1338.

Barr, I. (2007) The Emergence of Adamantane Resistance in Influenza A (H1) Viruses in Australia and Regionally in 2006. IX International Symposium on Respiratory Virus Infections, Hong Kong.

Bertrand, P., Faro, A., Cantwell, P. and Tzakis, A. (2000) Intravenous ribavirin and hyperammonemia in an immunocompromised patient infected with adenovirus. *Pharmacotherapy*, **20**, 1216–1220.

Blumberg, E.A., Albano, C., Pruett, T., Isaacs, R., Fitzpatrick, J., Bergin, J., Crump, C. and Hayden, F. G. (1996) The immunogenicity of influenza virus vaccine in solid organ transplant recipients. *Clinical Infectious Diseases*, **22**, 295–302.

Boeckh, M., Berrey, M.M., Bowden, R.A., Crawford, S.W., Balsley, J. and Corey, L. (2001) Phase 1 evaluation of the respiratory syncytial virus-specific monoclonal antibody palivizumab in recipients of hematopoietic stem cell transplants. *Journal of Infectious Diseases*, **184**, 350–354.

Boeckh, M., Englund, J., Li, Y., Miller, C., Cross, A., Fernandez, H., Kuypers, J., Kim, H., Gnann, J. and Whitley, R.J., NIAID Collaborative Antiviral Study Group (2007) Randomized controlled multicenter trial of aerosolized ribavirin for respiratory syncytial virus upper respiratory tract infections in hematopoietic cell transplant recipients. *Clinical Infectious Diseases*, **44**, 245–249.

Bordigoni, P., Carret, A.S., Venard, V., Witz, F. and Le Faou, A. (2001) Treatment of adenovirus infections in patients undergoing allogeneic hematopoietic stem cell transplantation. *Clinical Infectious Diseases*, **32**, 1290–1297.

Bowles, S.K., Lee, W., Simor, A.E., Vearncombe, M., Loeb, M., Tamblyn, S., Fearon, M., Li, Y. and Mcgeer, A. Oseltamivir Compassionate Use Program, G. (2002) Use of oseltamivir during influenza outbreaks in Ontario nursing homes, 1999–2000. *Journal of the American Geriatrics Society*, **50**, 608–616.

Bright, R.A., Medina, M.J., Xu, X., Perez-Oronoz, G., Wallis, T.R., Davis, X.M., Povinelli, L., Cox, N. J. and Klimov, A.I. (2005) Incidence of adamantane resistance among influenza A (H3N2) viruses isolated worldwide from 1994 to 2005: a cause for concern. *Lancet*, **366**, 1175–1181.

Bright, R.A., Shay, D.K., Shu, B., Cox, N.J. and Klimov, A.I. (2006) Adamantane resistance among influenza A viruses isolated early during the 2005–2006 influenza season in the United States. *The Journal of the American Medical Association*, **295**, 891–894.

Buchdahl, R.M., Taylor, P. and Warner, J.D. (1985) Nebulised ribavirin for adenovirus pneumonia. *Lancet*, **2**, 1070–1071.

Bui, M., Whittaker, G. and Helenius, A. (1996) Effect of M1 protein and low pH on nuclear transport of influenza virus ribonucleoproteins. *Journal of Virology*, **70**, 8391–8401.

Capparelli, E.V., Stevens, R.C., Chow, M.S., Izard, M. and Wills, R.J. (1988) Rimantadine pharmacokinetics in healthy subjects and patients with end-stage renal failure. *Clinical Pharmacology & Therapeutics*, **43**, 536–541.

Carter, B.A., Karpen, S.J., Quiros-Tejeira, R.E., Chang, I.F., Clark, B.S., Demmler, G.J., Heslop, H.E., Scott, J.D., Seu, P. and Goss, J.A. (2002) Intravenous Cidofovir therapy for disseminated adenovirus in a pediatric liver transplant recipient. *Transplantation*, **74**, 1050–1052.

Cass, L.M., Brown, J., Pickford, M., Fayinka, S., Newman, S.P., Johansson, C.J. and Bye, A. (1999a) Pharmacoscintigraphic evaluation of lung deposition of inhaled zanamivir in healthy volunteers. *Clinical Pharmacokinetics*, **36**, 21–31.

Cass, L.M., Efthymiopoulos, C. and Bye, A. (1999b) Pharmacokinetics of zanamivir after intravenous, oral, inhaled or intranasal administration to healthy volunteers. *Clinical Pharmacokinetics*, **36**, 1–11.

Cassano, W.F. (1991) Intravenous ribavirin therapy for adenovirus cystitis after allogeneic bone marrow transplantation. *Bone Marrow Transplantation*, **7**, 247–248.

Cavdar, C., Sayan, M., Sifil, A., Artuk, C., Yilmaz, N., Bahar, H. and Camsari, T. (2003) The comparison of antibody response to influenza vaccination in continuous ambulatory peritoneal dialysis, hemodialysis and renal transplantation patients. *Scandinavian Journal of Urology and Nephrology*, **37**, 71–76.

Chakrabarti, S., Collingham, K.E., Fegan, C.D. and Milligan, D.W. (1999) Fulminant adenovirus hepatitis following unrelated bone marrow transplantation: failure of intravenous ribavirin therapy. *Bone Marrow Transplantation*, **23**, 1209–1211.

Chakrabarti, S., Collingham, K.E., Holder, K., Fegan, C.D., Osman, H. and Milligan, D.W. (2001) Pre-emptive oral ribavirin therapy of paramyxovirus infections after haematopoietic stem cell transplantation: a pilot study. *Bone Marrow Transplantation*, **28**, 759–763.

Chapman, J., Abbott, E., Alber, D.G., Baxter, R.C., Bithell, S.K., Henderson, E.A., Carter, M.C., Chambers, P., Chubb, A., Cockerill, G.S., Collins, P.L., Dowdell, V.C.L., Keegan, S.J., Kelsey, R.D., Lockyer, M.J., Luongo, C., Najarro, P., Pickles, R.J., Simmonds, M., Taylor, D., Tyms, S., Wilson, L. J. and Powell, K.L. (2007) RSV604, a Novel Inhibitor of Respiratory Syncytial Virus Replication. *Antimicrobial Agents and Chemotherapy*, **51**, 3346–3353.

Chik, K.W., Li, C.K., Chan, P.K., Shing, M.M., Lee, V., Tam, J.S. and Yuen, P.M. (2004) Oseltamivir prophylaxis during the influenza season in a paediatric cancer centre: prospective observational study. *Hong Kong Medical Journal*, **10**, 103–106.

Chui, A.K., Rao, A.R., Chan, H.L. and Hui, A.Y. (2004) Impact of severe acute respiratory syndrome on liver transplantation service. *Transplantation Proceedings*, **36**, 2302–2303.

Colman, P.M. (1994) Influenza virus neuraminidase: structure, antibodies, and inhibitors. *Protein Science*, **3**, 1687–1696.

Committee on Infectious (2007) Antiviral therapy and prophylaxis for influenza in children. *Pediatrics*, **119**, 852–860.

Connor, E., Morrison, S., Lane, J. and Al, E. (1993) Safety, tolerance, and pharmacokinetics of systemic ribavirin in children with human immunodeficiency virus infection. *Antimicrobial Agents & Chemotherapy*, **37**, 532–539.

Connor, J.D., Hintz, M. and Vandyke, R. (1984) Ribavirin pharmacokinetics in children and adults during therapeutic trials, in *Clinical Applications of Ribavirin* (eds R.A. Smith, V. Knight and J. Smith), Academic Press, Orlando, FL.

Cooper, N.J., Sutton, A.J., Abrams, K.R., Wailoo, A., Turner, D. and Nicholson, K.G. (2003) Effectiveness of neuraminidase inhibitors in treatment and prevention of influenza A and B: systematic review and meta-analyses of randomised controlled trials. *BMJ*, **326**, 1235.

Cortez, K., Murphy, B.R., Almeida, K.N., Beeler, J., Levandowski, R.A., Gill, V.J., Childs, R.W., Barrett, A.J., Smolskis, M. and Bennett, J.E. (2002) Immune-globulin prophylaxis of respiratory syncytial virus infection in patients undergoing stem-cell transplantation. *Journal of Infectious Diseases*, **186**, 834–838.

de Oliveira, C.B., Stevenson, D., Labree, L., Mcdonnell, P.J. and Trousdale, M.D. (1996) Evaluation of Cidofovir (HPMPC, GS-504) against adenovirus type 5 infection in vitro and in a New Zealand rabbit ocular model. *Antiviral Research*, **31**, 165–172.

De Vincenzo, J.P., Leombruno, D., Soiffer, R.J. and Siber, G.R. (1996) Immunotherapy of respiratory syncytial virus pneumonia following bone marrow transplantation. *Bone Marrow Transplantation*, **17**, 1051–1056.

Dengler, T.J., Strnad, N., Buhring, I., Zimmermann, R., Girgsdies, O., Kubler, W.E. and Zielen, S. (1998) Differential immune response to influenza and pneumococcal vaccination in immuno-suppressed patients after heart transplantation. *Transplantation*, **66**, 1340–1347.

Diggory, P., Fernandez, C., Humphrey, A., Jones, V. and Murphy, M. (2001) Comparison of elderly people's technique in using two dry powder inhalers to deliver zanamivir: randomised controlled trial. *BMJ*, **322**, 577–579.

REFERENCES 421

Dolin, R., Reichman, R.C., Madore, H.P., Maynard, R., Linton, P.N. and Webber-Jones, J. (1982) A controlled trial of amantadine and rimantadine in the prophylaxis of influenza A infection. *The New England Journal of Medicine*, **307**, 580–584.

Duchini, A., Hendry, R.M., Nyberg, L.M., Viernes, M.E. and Pockros, P.J. (2001) Immune response to influenza vaccine in adult liver transplant recipients. *Liver Transplantation*, **7**, 311–313.

Dunn, C.J. and Goa, K.L. (1999) Zanamivir: a review of its use in influenza. *Drugs*, **58**, 761–784.

Dykewicz, C.A. (2001) Guidelines for preventing opportunistic infections among hematopoietic stem cell transplant recipients: focus on community respiratory virus infections. *Biology of Blood and Marrow Transplantation*, **7** (Suppl), 19S–22S.

Emovon, O.E., Lin, A., Howell, D.N., Afzal, F., Baillie, M., Rogers, J., Baliga, P.K., Chavin, K., Nickeleit, V., Rajagapalan, P.R. and Self, S. (2003) Refractory adenovirus infection after simultaneous kidney-pancreas transplantation: successful treatment with intravenous ribavirin and pooled human intravenous immunoglobulin. *Nephrology, Dialysis, Transplantation*, **18**, 2436–2438.

Engelhard, D., Nagler, A., Hardan, I., Morag, A., Aker, M., Baciu, H., Strauss, N., Parag, G., Naparstek, E., Ravid, Z. *et al.* (1993) Antibody response to a two-dose regimen of influenza vaccine in allogeneic T cell-depleted and autologous BMT recipients. *Bone Marrow Transplantation*, **11**, 1–5.

Englund, J.A., Champlin, R.E., Wyde, P.R., Kantarjian, H., Atmar, R.L., Tarrand, J., Yousuf, H., Regnery, H., Klimov, A.I., Cox, N.J. and Whimbey, E. (1998) Common emergence of amantadine- and rimantadine-resistant influenza A viruses in symptomatic immunocompromised adults. *Clinical Infectious Diseases*, **26**, 1418–1424.

Englund, J.A., Piedra, P.A., Ahn, Y.M., Gilbert, B.E. and Hiatt, P. (1994) High-dose, short-duration ribavirin aerosol therapy compared with standard ribavirin therapy in children with suspected respiratory syncytial virus infection. *The Journal of Pediatrics*, **125**, 635–641.

Fanourgiakis, P., Georgala, A., Vekemans, M., Triffet, A., De Bruyn, J.M., Duchateau, V., Martiat, P., De Clercq, E., Snoeck, R., Wollants, E., Rector, A., van Ranst, M. and Aoun, M. (2005) Intravesical instillation of cidofovir in the treatment of hemorrhagic cystitis caused by adenovirus type 11 in a bone marrow transplant recipient. *Clinical Infectious Diseases*, **40**, 199–201.

Garcia, R., Raad, I., Abi-Said, D., Bodey, G., Champlin, R., Tarrand, J., Hill, L.A., Umphrey, J., Neumann, J., Englund, J. and Whimbey, E. (1997) Nosocomial respiratory syncytial virus infections: prevention and control in bone marrow transplant patients. *Infection Control and Hospital Epidemiology*, **18**, 412–416.

Gavin, P.J. and Katz, B.Z. (2002) Intravenous ribavirin treatment for severe adenovirus disease in immunocompromised children. *Pediatrics*, **110**, e9.

Ghosh, S., Champlin, R.E., Englund, J., Giralt, S.A., Rolston, K., Raad, I., Jacobson, K., Neumann, J., Ippoliti, C., Mallik, S. and Whimbey, E. (2000) Respiratory syncytial virus upper respiratory tract illnesses in adult blood and marrow transplant recipients: combination therapy with aerosolized ribavirin and intravenous immunoglobulin. *Bone Marrow Transplantation*, **25**, 751–755.

Ghosh, S., Champlin, R.E., Ueno, N.T., Anderlini, P., Rolston, K., Raad, I., Kontoyiannis, D., Jacobson, K., Luna, M., Tarrand, J. and Whimbey, E. (2001) Respiratory syncytial virus infections in autologous blood and marrow transplant recipients with breast cancer: combination therapy with aerosolized ribavirin and parenteral immunoglobulins. *Bone Marrow Transplantation*, **28**, 271–275.

Glanville, A.R., Aboyoun, C.L., Plit, M.L. and Malouf, M.A. (2005) Intravenous ribavirin is a safe and cost-effective treatment for Respiratory Syncytial Virus infection after lung transplant. *The Journal of Heart and Lung Transplantation: The Official, Publication of the International Society for Heart Transplantation*, **24**, S77–S78.

Gubareva, L.V. (2004) Molecular mechanisms of influenza virus resistance to neuraminidase inhibitors. *Virus Research*, **103**, 199–203.

Guzman-Cottrill, J.A., Anderson, E.J., Kletzel, M., Zheng, X. and Katz, B.Z. (2005) Adenoviral disease and cidofovir in pediatric allogeneic stem cell transplant recipients. 43rd Annual Meeting of the Infectious Diseases Society of America, San Francisco.

Hartline, C.B., Gustin, K.M., Wan, W.B., Ciesla, S.L., Beadle, J.R., Hostetler, K.Y. and Kern, E.R. (2005) Ether lipid-ester prodrugs of acyclic nucleoside phosphonates: activity against adenovirus replication *in vitro*. *The Journal of Infectious Diseases*, **191**, 396–399.

Hatakeyama, N., Suzuki, N., Kudoh, T., Hori, T., Mizue, N. and Tsutsumi, H. (2003) Successful cidofovir treatment of adenovirus-associated hemorrhagic cystitis and renal dysfunction after allogenic bone marrow transplant. *The Pediatric Infectious Disease Journal*, **22**, 928–929.

Hayden, F.G. (1996a) *Antiviral Drug Resistance* (ed. D.D. Richman), J Wiley and Sons, New York.

Hayden, F.G. (1996b) Combination antiviral therapy for respiratory virus infections. *Antiviral Research*, **29**, 45–48.

Hayden, F.G. (2000) *Mandell, Douglas, and Bennett's Principles and Practice of Infectious Diseases* (eds G.L. Mandell, J.E. Bennett and R. Dolin), Churchill Livingstone, Philadelphia, PA.

Hayden, F.G. (2006) Antiviral resistance in influenza viruses – implications for management and pandemic response. *The New England Journal of Medicine*, **354**, 785–788.

Hayden, F.G. and Aoki, F.Y. (1999) *Antimicrobial Therapy and Vaccines*, 1st edn (eds V.L. Yu, T.C.J. Merigan and S.L. Barriere), Williams & Wilkins, Baltimore.

Hayden, F.G., Atmar, R.L., Schilling, M., Johnson, C., Poretz, D., Paar, D., Huson, L., Ward, P. and Mills, R.G. (1999) Use of the selective oral neuraminidase inhibitor oseltamivir to prevent influenza. *The New England Journal of Medicine*, **341**, 1336–1343.

Hayden, F.G., Belshe, R., Villanueva, C., Lanno, R., Hughes, C., Small, I., Dutkowski, R., Ward, P. and Carr, J. (2004) Management of influenza in households: a prospective, randomized comparison of oseltamivir treatment with or without postexposure prophylaxis. [see comment]. *Journal of Infectious Diseases*, **189**, 440–449.

Hayden, F.G., Herrington, D.T., Coats, T.L., Kim, K., Cooper, E.C., Villano, S.A., Liu, S., Hudson, S., Pevear, D.C., Collett, M. and Mckinlay, M. (2003) Efficacy and safety of oral pleconaril for treatment of colds due to picornaviruses in adults: results of 2 double-blind, randomized, placebo-controlled trials. *Clinical Infectious Diseases*, **36**, 1523–1532.

Hayden, F.G., Minocha, A., Spyker, D.A. and Hoffman, H.E. (1985) Comparative single-dose pharmacokinetics of amantadine hydrochloride and rimantadine hydrochloride in young and elderly adults [published erratum appears in Antimicrobial Agents and Chemotherapy 1986 Sep;30(3):579]. *Antimicrobial Agents & Chemotherapy*, **28**, 216–221.

Hayney, M.S., Welter, D.L., Francois, M., Reynolds, A.M. and Love, R.B. (2004) Influenza vaccine antibody responses in lung transplant recipients. *Progress in Transplantation*, **14**, 346–351.

He, G., Massarella, J. and Ward, P. (1999) Clinical pharmacokinetics of the prodrug oseltamivir and its active metabolite Ro 64-0802. *Clinical Pharmacokinetics*, **37**, 471–484.

Hedrick, J.A., Barzilai, A., Behre, U., Henderson, F.W., Hammond, J., Reilly, L. and Keene, O. (2000) Zanamivir for treatment of symptomatic influenza A and B infection in children five to twelve years of age: a randomized controlled trial. *Pediatric Infectious Disease Journal*, **19**, 410–417.

Hoffman, J.A., Shah, A.J., Ross, L.A. and Kapoor, N. (2001) Adenoviral infections and a prospective trial of cidofovir in pediatric hematopoietic stem cell transplantation. *Biology of Blood and Marrow Transplantation*, **7**, 388–394.

Howard, D.S., Phillips, I.G., Reece, D.E., Munn, R.K., Henslee-Downey, J., Pittard, M., Barker, M. and Pomeroy, C. (1999) Adenovirus infections in hematopoietic stem cell transplant recipients. *Clinical Infectious Diseases*, **29**, 1494–1501.

Hromas, R., Clark, C., Blanke, C., Tricot, G., Cornetta, K., Hedderman, A. and Broun, E.R. (1994) Failure of ribavirin to clear adenovirus infections in T cell-depleted allogeneic bone marrow transplantation. *Bone Marrow Transplantation*, **14**, 663–664.

Ison, M.G. (2005) Respiratory viral infections in transplant recipients. *Current Opinion in Organ Transplantation*, **10**, 312–319.

Ison, M.G. (2006) Adenovirus infections in transplant recipients. *Clinical Infectious Diseases*, **43**, 331–339.

Ison, M.G., Gnann, J.W., Jr, Nagy-Agren, S., Treannor, J., Paya, C., Steigbigel, R., Elliott, M., Weiss, H.L. and Hayden, F.G. (2003) Safety and efficacy of nebulized zanamivir in hospitalized patients with serious influenza. *Antiviral Therapy*, **8**, 183–190.

Ison, M.G., Gubareva, L.V., Atmar, R.L., Treanor, J. and Hayden, F.G. (2006) Recovery of drug-resistant influenza virus from immunocompromised patients: a case series. *The Journal of Infectious Diseases*, **193**, 760–764.

Ison, M.G. and Hayden, F.G. (2002) Viral infections in immunocompromised patients: what's new with respiratory viruses? *Current Opinion in Infectious Diseases*, **15**, 355–367.

Jefferson, T.O., Demicheli, V., Di Pietrantonj, C. and Rivetti, D. (2006) Amantadine and rimantadine for preventing and treating influenza A in adults. *Cochrane Database of Systematic Reviews*, CD001169.

Johny, A.A., Clark, A., Price, N., Carrington, D., Oakhill, A. and Marks, D.I. (2002) The use of zanamivir to treat influenza A and B infection after allogeneic stem cell transplantation. *Bone Marrow Transplantation*, **29**, 113–115.

Jones, B.L., Clark, S., Curran, E.T., McNamee, S., Horne, G., Thakker, B. and Hood, J. (2000) Control of an outbreak of respiratory syncytial virus infection in immunocompromised adults. *The Journal of Hospital Infection*, **44**, 53–57.

Jurado Chacon, M., Hernandez Mohedo, F., Navarro Mari, J.M., Ferrer Chaves, C., Escobar Vedia, J.L. and De Pablos Gallego, J.M. (1998) Adenovirus pneumonitis successfully treated with intravenous ribavirin. *Haematologica*, **83**, 1128–1129.

Jurado, M., Navarro, J.M., Hernandez, J., Molina, M.A. and Depablos, J.M. (1995) Adenovirus-associated haemorrhagic cystitis after bone marrow transplantation successfully treated with intravenous ribavirin. *Bone Marrow Transplantation*, **15**, 651–652.

Kaiser, L. and Hayden, F.G. (1999) *Current Clinical Topics in Infectious Diseases* (eds J.S. Remington and M.N. Swartz), Blackwell Science, Malden.

Kaiser, L., Wat, C., Mills, T., Mahoney, P., Ward, P. and Hayden, F. (2003) Impact of oseltamivir treatment on influenza-related lower respiratory tract complications and hospitalizations. *Archives of Internal Medicine*, **163**, 1667–1672.

Kapelushnik, J., Or, R., Delukina, M., Nagler, A., Livni, N. and Engelhard, D. (1995) Intravenous ribavirin therapy for adenovirus gastroenteritis after bone marrow transplantation. *Journal of Pediatric Gastroenterology and Nutrition*, **21**, 110–112.

Kent, R.S. (2000) Important revisions to safety labeling for Relenza (zanamivir for inhalation). *Letter to Physicians, July 2000*, GlaxoWellcome, Ince. Research Triangle Park, NC, 27709. http://www.fda.gov/medwatch/safety/2000/relenz.htm.

Keyser, L.A., Karl, M., Nafziger, A.N. and Bertino, J.S. Jr (2000) Comparison of central nervous system adverse effects of amantadine and rimantadine used as sequential prophylaxis of influenza A in elderly nursing home patients. *Archives of Internal Medicine*, **160**, 1485–1488.

Kumar, S.S., Ventura, A.K. and Vanderwerf, B. (1978) Influenza vaccination in renal transplant recipients. *The Journal of the American Medical Association*, **239**, 840–842.

La Rosa, A.M., Champlin, R.E., Mirza, N., Gajewski, J., Giralt, S., Rolston, K.V., Raad, I., Jacobson, K., Kontoyiannis, D., Elting, L. and Whimbey, E. (2001a) Adenovirus infections in adult recipients of blood and marrow transplants. *Clinical Infectious Diseases*, **32**, 871–876.

La Rosa, A.M., Malik, S., Englund, J.A., Couch, R., Raad, I.I., Rolston, K.V., Jacobson, K.L., Kontoyiannis, D.P. and Whimbey, E. (2001b) Influenza A in hospitalized adults with leukemia and hematopoietic stem cell transplant (HSCT) recipients: risk factors for progression to pneumonia. 39th Infectious Diseases Society of America, San Francisco, CA.

Lalezari, J., Campion, K., Keene, O. and Silagy, C. (2001) Zanamivir for the treatment of influenza A and B infection in high-risk patients: a pooled analysis of randomized controlled trials. *Archives of Internal Medicine*, **161**, 212–217.

Lankester, A.C., Heemskerk, B., Claas, E.C., Schilham, M.W., Beersma, M.F., Bredius, R.G., van Tol, M.J. and Kroes, A.C. (2004) Effect of ribavirin on the plasma viral DNA load in patients with disseminating adenovirus infection. *Clinical Infectious Diseases*, **38**, 1521–1525.

Laskin, O., Longstreth, J., Hart, C. and Al, E. (1987) Ribavirin disposition in high-risk patients for acquired immunodeficiency syndrome. *Clinical Pharmacology & Therapeutics*, **41**, 546–555.

Lawal, A., Basler, C., Branch, A., Gutierrez, J., Schwartz, M. and Schiano, T.D. (2004) Influenza vaccination in orthotopic liver transplant recipients: absence of post administration ALT elevation. *American Journal of Transplantation*, **4**, 1805–1809.

Legrand, F., Berrebi, D., Houhou, N., Freymuth, F., Faye, A., Duval, M., Mougenot, J.F., Peuchmaur, M. and Vilmer, E. (2001) Early diagnosis of adenovirus infection and treatment with cidofovir after bone marrow transplantation in children. *Bone Marrow Transplantation*, **27**, 621–626.

Leruez-Ville, M., Minard, V., Lacaille, F., Buzyn, A., Abachin, E., Blanche, S., Freymuth, F. and Rouzioux, C. (2004) Real-time blood plasma polymerase chain reaction for management of disseminated adenovirus infection. *Clinical Infectious Diseases*, **38**, 45–52.

Liles, W.C., Cushing, H., Holt, S., Bryan, C. and Hackman, R.C. (1993) Severe adenoviral nephritis following bone marrow transplantation: successful treatment with intravenous ribavirin. *Bone Marrow Transplantation*, **12**, 409–412.

Ljungman, P., Ribaud, P., Eyrich, M., Matthes-Martin, S., Einsele, H., Bleakley, M., Machaczka, M., Bierings, M., Bosi, A., Gratecos, N. and Cordonnier, C. (2003) Cidofovir for adenovirus infections after allogeneic hematopoietic stem cell transplantation: a survey by the Infectious Diseases Working Party of the European Group for Blood and Marrow Transplantation. *Bone Marrow Transplantation*, **31**, 481–486.

Machado, C.M., Boas, L.S., Mendes, A.V.A., da Rocha, I.F., Stuarto, D., Dulley, F.L. and Pannuti, C.S. (2004) Use of oseltamivir to control influenza complications after bone marrow transplantation. *Bone Marrow Transplantion*, **34**, 111–114.

Machado, C.M., Cardoso, M.R., Da Rocha, I.F., Boas, L.S., Dulley, F.L. and Pannuti, C.S. (2005) The benefit of influenza vaccination after bone marrow transplantation. *Bone Marrow Transplantation*, **36**, 897–900.

Mack, D.R., Chartrand, S.A., Ruby, E.I., Antonson, D.L., Shaw, B.W. Jr. and Heffron, T.G. (1996) Influenza vaccination following liver transplantation in children. *Liver Transplantation and Surgery*, **2**, 431–437.

Magnani, G., Falchetti, E., Pollini, G., Reggiani, L.B., Grigioni, F., Coccolo, F., Potena, L., Magelli, C., Sambri, V. and Branzi, A. (2005) Safety and efficacy of two types of influenza vaccination in heart transplant recipients: a prospective randomised controlled study. *The Journal of Heart and Lung Transplantation*, **24**, 588–592.

Malakhov, M.P., Aschenbrenner, L.M., Smee, D.F., Wandersee, M.K., Sidwell, R.W., Gubareva, L.V., Mishin, V.P., Hayden, F.G., Kim, D.H., Ing, A., Campbell, E.R., Yu, M. and Fang, F. (2006) Sialidase fusion protein as a novel broad-spectrum inhibitor of influenza virus infection. *Antimicrobial Agents and Chemotherapy*, **50**, 1470–1479.

Malavaud, S., Malavaud, B., Sandres, K., Durand, D., Marty, N., Icart, J. and Rostaing, L. (2001) Nosocomial outbreak of influenza virus A (H3N2) infection in a solid organ transplant department. *Transplantation*, **72**, 535–537.

Mann, D., Moreb, J., Smith, S. and Gian, V. (1998) Failure of intravenous ribavirin in the treatment of invasive adenovirus infection following allogeneic bone marrow transplantation: a case report. *The Journal of Infection*, **36**, 227–228.

Marty, F., Chemaly, R.F., Liaopoulou, E., Dent, J.C. and Powell, K. (2007) A double-blind, randomised, placebo-controlled study to evaluate the safety and efficacy of RSV604 in adults with respiratory syncytial virus (RSV) infection following stem cell transplantation. IX International Syposium on Respiratory Viral Infections, Hong Kong.

Mazzone, P.J., Mossad, S.B., Mawhorter, S.D., Mehta, A.C. and Mauer, J.R. (2004) Cell-mediated immune response to influenza vaccination in lung transplant recipients. *The Journal of Heart and Lung Transplantation*, **23**, 1175–1181.

McCarthy, A.J., Bergin, M., De Silva, L.M. and Stevens, M. (1995) Intravenous ribavirin therapy for disseminated adenovirus infection. *The Pediatric Infectious Disease Journal*, **14**, 1003–1004.

McClellan, K. and Perry, C.M. (2001) Oseltamivir: a review of its use in influenza. *Drugs*, **61**, 263–283.

McCurdy, L.H., Milstone, A. and Dummer, S. (2003) Clinical features and outcomes of paramyxoviral infection in lung transplant recipients treated with ribavirin. *The Journal of Heart and Lung Transplantation*, **22**, 745–753.

McKimm-Breschkin, J.L. (2000) Resistance of influenza viruses to neuraminidase inhibitors–a review. *Antiviral Research*, **47**, 1–17.

Miyamura, K., Hamaguchi, M., Taji, H., Kanie, T., Kohno, A., Tanimoto, M., Saito, H., Kojima, S., Matsuyama, T., Kitaori, K., Nagafuji, K., Sato, T. and Kodera, Y. (2000) Successful ribavirin therapy for severe adenovirus hemorrhagic cystitis after allogeneic marrow transplant from close HLA donors rather than distant donors. *Bone Marrow Transplantation*, **25**, 545–548.

Monto, A.S., Robinson, D.P., Herlocher, M.L., Hinson, J.M., Jr, Elliott, M.J. and Crisp, A. (1999) Zanamivir in the prevention of influenza among healthy adults: a randomized controlled trial. *The Journal of the American Medical Association*, **282**, 31–35.

Morfin, F., Dupuis-Girod, S., Mundweiler, S., Falcon, D., Carrington, D., Sedlacek, P., Bierings, M., Cetkovsky, P., Kroes, A.C., van Tol, M.J. and Thouvenot, D. (2005) In vitro susceptibility of adenovirus to antiviral drugs is species-dependent. *Antiviral Therapy*, **10**, 225–229.

Moscona, A. (2005) Neuraminidase inhibitors for influenza. *The New England Journal of Medicine*, **353**, 1363–1373.

Muller, W.J., Levin, M.J., Shin, Y.K., Robinson, C., Quinones, R., Malcolm, J., Hild, E., Gao, D. and Giller, R. (2005) Clinical and in vitro evaluation of cidofovir for treatment of adenovirus infection in pediatric hematopoietic stem cell transplant recipients. *Clinical Infectious Diseases*, **41**, 1812–1816.

Murphy, G.F., Wood, D.P., Jr, Mcroberts, J.W. and Henslee-Downey, P.J. (1993) Adenovirus-associated hemorrhagic cystitis treated with intravenous ribavirin. *The Journal of Urology*, **149**, 565–566.

Murphy, K.R., Eivindson, A., Pauksen, K., Stein, W.J., Tellier, G., Watts, R., Léophonte, P., Sharp, S.J. and Loeschel, E. (2000) Efficacy and safety of inhaled zanamivir for the treatment of influenza in patients with asthma or chronic obstructive pulmonary disease: a double-blind, randomized, placebo-controlled multicentre study. *Clinical Drug Investigation*, **20**, 337–349.

Naesens, L., Lenaerts, L., Andrei, G., Snoeck, R., van Beers, D., Holy, A., Balzarini, J. and de Clercq, E. (2005) Antiadenovirus activities of several classes of nucleoside and nucleotide analogues. *Antimicrobial Agents and Chemotherapy*, **49**, 1010–1016.

Nagafuji, K., Aoki, K., Henzan, H., Kato, K., Miyamoto, T., Eto, T., Nagatoshi, Y., Ohba, T., Obama, K., Gondo, H. and Harada, M. (2004) Cidofovir for treating adenoviral hemorrhagic cystitis in hematopoietic stem cell transplant recipients. *Bone Marrow Transplantation*, **34**, 909–914.

Nahata, M.C. and Brady, M.T. (1986) Serum concentrations and safety of rimantadine in paediatric patients. *European Journal of Clinical Pharmacology*, **30**, 719–722.

Neofytos, D., Ojha, A., Mookerjee, B., Wagner, J., Filicko, J., Ferber, A., Dessain, S., Grosso, D., Brunner, J., Flomenberg, N. and Flomenberg, P. (2007) Treatment of adenovirus disease in stem cell transplant recipients with cidofovir. *Biology of Blood and Marrow Transplantation*, **13**, 74–81.

Nichols, W.G., Erdman, D.D., Han, A., Zukerman, C., Corey, L. and Boeckh, M. (2004a) Prolonged outbreak of human parainfluenza virus 3 infection in a stem cell transplant outpatient department: insights from molecular epidemiologic analysis. *Biology of Blood and Marrow Transplantation*, **10**, 58–64.

Nichols, W.G., Gooley, T. and Boeckh, M. (2001) Community-acquired respiratory syncytial virus and parainfluenza virus infections after hematopoietic stem cell transplantation: the Fred Hutchinson Cancer Research Center experience. *Biology of Blood and Marrow Transplantation*, **7** (Suppl), 11S–15S.

Nichols, W.G., Guthrie, K.A., Corey, L. and Boeckh, M. (2004b) Influenza infections after hemato-poietic stem cell transplantation: risk factors, mortality, and the effect of antiviral therapy. *Clinical Infectious Diseases*, **39**, 1300–1306.

Nicholson, K.G., Aoki, F.Y., Osterhaus, A.D., Trottier, S., Carewicz, O., Mercier, C.H., Rode, A., Kinnersley, N. and Ward, P. (2000) Efficacy and safety of oseltamivir in treatment of acute influenza: a randomised controlled trial. Neuraminidase Inhibitor Flu Treatment Investigator Group. *Lancet*, **355**, 1845–1850.

Ong, A.K. and Hayden, F.G. (2007) John F. Enders Lecture 2006: Antivirals for Influenza. *Journal of Infectious Diseases*, **196**, 181–190.

Oo, C., Barrett, J., Hill, G., Mann, J., Dorr, A., Dutkowski, R. and Ward, P. (2001) Pharmacokinetics and dosage recommendations for an oseltamivir oral suspension for the treatment of influenza in children. *Paediatric Drugs*, **3**, 229–236.

Paroni, R., Del, P., Borghi, C., Sirtori, C. and Al, E. (1989) Pharmacokinetics of ribavirin and urinary excretion of the major metabolite 1,2,4-triazole-3-carboxamide in normal volunteers. *International Journal of Clinical Pharmacology, Therapy, and Toxicology*, **27**, 302–307.

Patick, A.K. (2006) Rhinovirus chemotherapy. *Antiviral Research*, **71**, 391–396.

Pediatrics, A.A.O. (2006) Red Book: 2006 *Report of the Committee on Infectious Diseases* (ed. L.K. Pickering), American Academy of Pediatrics Elk Grove Village, IL.

Peters, P.H., Jr, Gravenstein, S., Norwood, P., De Bock, V., van Couter, A., Gibbens, M., von Planta, T. A. and Ward, P. (2001) Long-term use of oseltamivir for the prophylaxis of influenza in a vaccinated frail older population. *Journal of the American Geriatrics Society*, **49**, 1025–1031.

Potter, C.W., Phair, J.P., Vodinelich, L., Fenton, R. and Jennings, R. (1976) Antiviral, immuno-suppressive and antitumour effects of ribavirin. *Nature*, **259**, 496–497.

(2007) Tamiflu Package Insert, Roche, Nutley.

Sabroe, I., Mchale, J., Tait, D.R., Lynn, W.A., Ward, K.N. and Shaunak, S. (1995) Treatment of adenoviral pneumonitis with intravenous ribavirin and immunoglobulin. *Thorax*, **50**, 1219–1220.

Sanchez-Fructuoso, A.I., Prats, D., Naranjo, P., Fernandez-Perez, C., Gonzalez, M.J., Mariano, A., Gonzalez, J., Figueredo, M.A., Martin, J.M., Paniagua, V., Fereres, J., Gomez de la Concha, E. and Barrientos, A. (2000) Influenza virus immunization effectivity in kidney transplant patients subjected to two different triple-drug therapy immunosuppression protocols: mycophenolate versus azathioprine. *Transplantation*, **69**, 436–439.

Schleuning, M., Buxbaum-Conradi, H., Jager, G. and Kolb, H.J. (2004) Intravenous ribavirin for eradication of respiratory syncytial virus (RSV) and adenovirus isolates from the respiratory and/or gastrointestinal tract in recipients of allogeneic hematopoietic stem cell transplants. *The Hematol-ogy Journal*, **5**, 135–144.

Shetty, A.K., Gans, H.A., So, S., Millan, M.T., Arvin, A.M. and Gutierrez, K.M. (2000) Intravenous ribavirin therapy for adenovirus pneumonia. *Pediatric Pulmonology*, **29**, 69–73.

Sidwell, R.W., Barnard, D.L., Day, C.W., Smee, D.F., Bailey, K.W., Wong, M.-H., Morrey, J.D. and Furuta, Y. (2007) Efficacy of orally administered T-705 on lethal avian influenza A (H5N1) virus infections in mice. *Antimicrobial Agents and Chemotherapy*, **51**, 845–851.

Smith, N.M., Bresee, J.S., Shay, D.K., Uyeki, T.M., Cox, N.J. and Strikas, R.A. (2006) Prevention and control of influenza: recommendations of the Advisory Committee on Immunization Practices (ACIP). *MMWR Recommendations Reports*, **55**, 1–42.

Soesman, N.M., Rimmelzwaan, G.F., Nieuwkoop, N.J., Beyer, W.E., Tilanus, H.W., Kemmeren, M. H., Metselaar, H.J., De Man, R.A. and Osterhaus, A.D. (2000) Efficacy of influenza vaccination in adult liver transplant recipients. *Journal of Medical Virology*, **61**, 85–93.

Stein, D.S., Creticos, C.M., Jackson, G.G., Bernstein, J.M., Hayden, F.G., Schiff, G.M. and Bernstein, D.I. (1987) Oral ribavirin treatment of influenza A and B. *Antimicrobial Agents and Chemotherapy*, **31**, 1285–1287.

Taylor, G.S., Vipond, I.B. and Caul, E.O. (2001) Molecular epidemiology of outbreak of respiratory syncytial virus within bone marrow transplantation unit. *Journal of Clinical Microbiology*, **39**, 801–803.

Thompson, J., Fleet, W., Lawrence, E., Pierce, E., Morris, L. and Wright, P. (1987) A comparison of acetaminophen and rimantadine in the treatment of influenza A infection in children. *Journal of Medical Virology*, **21**, 249–255.

Treanor, J.J., Hayden, F.G., Vrooman, P.S., Barbarash, R., Bettis, R., Riff, D., Singh, S., Kinnersley, N., Ward, P. and Mills, R.G. (2000) Efficacy and safety of the oral neuraminidase inhibitor oseltamivir in treating acute influenza: a randomized controlled trial. US Oral Neuraminidase Study Group [see comments]. *The Journal of the American Medical Association*, **283**, 1016–1024.

Ventre, K. and Randolph, A.G. (2007) Ribavirin for respiratory syncytial virus infection of the lower respiratory tract in infants and young children. *Cochrane Database of Systematic Reviews*, **1**, CD000181.

Vu, D., Peck, A.J., Nichols, W.G., Varley, C., Englund, J.A., Corey, L. and Boeckh, M. (2007) Safety and tolerability of oseltamivir prophylaxis in hematopoietic stem cell transplant recipients: a retrospective case-control study. *Clinical Infectious Diseases*, **45**, 187–193.

Weinstock, D.M., Eagan, J., Malak, S.A., Rogers, M., Wallace, H., Kiehn, T.E. and Sepkowitz, K.A. (2000) Control of influenza A on a bone marrow transplant unit. *Infection Control and Hospital Epidemiology*, **21**, 730–732.

Welliver, R., Monto, A.S., Carewicz, O., Schatteman, E., Hassman, M., Hedrick, J., Jackson, H.C., Huson, L., Ward, P. and Oxford, J.S. (2001) Oseltamivir Post Exposure Prophylaxis Investigator, G Effectiveness of oseltamivir in preventing influenza in household contacts: a randomized controlled trial. *The Journal of the American Medical Association*, **285**, 748–754.

Wendt, C.H., Fox, J.M. and Hertz, M.I. (1995) Paramyxovirus infection in lung transplant recipients. *The Journal of Heart and Lung Transplantation*, **14**, 479–485.

Whimbey, E., Englund, J.A. and Couch, R.B. (1997) Community respiratory virus infections in immunocompromised patients with cancer. *The American Journal of Medicine*, **102**, 10–18; discussion 25–6.

White-Williams, C., Brown, R., Kirklin, J., St Clair, K., Keck, S., O'Donnell, J., Pitts, D. and van Bakel, A. (2006) Improving clinical practice: should we give influenza vaccinations to heart transplant patients? *The Journal of Heart and Lung Transplantation*, **25**, 320–323.

Whitley, R.J., Hayden, F.G., Reisinger, K.S., Young, N., Dutkowski, R., Ipe, D., Mills, R.G. and Ward, P. (2001) Oral oseltamivir treatment of influenza in children. *Pediatric Infectious Disease Journal*, **20**, 127–133.

Wills, R.J., Belshe, R., Tomlinsin, D., De Grazia, F., Lin, A., Wells, S., Milazzo, J. and Berry, C. (1987a) Pharmacokinetics of rimantadine hydrochloride in patients with chronic liver disease. *Clinical Pharmacology & Therapeutics*, **42**, 449–454.

Wills, R.J., Farolino, D.A., Choma, N. and Keigher, N. (1987b) Rimantadine pharmacokinetics after single and multiple doses. *Antimicrobial Agents & Chemotherapy*, **31**, 826–828.

Wray, S.K., Gilbert, B.E. and Knight, V. (1985a) Effect of ribavirin triphosphate on primer generation and elongation during influenza virus transcription *in vitro*. *Antiviral Research*, **5**, 39–48.

Wray, S.K., Gilbert, B.E., Noall, M.W. and Knight, V. (1985b) Mode of action of ribavirin: effect of nucleotide pool alterations on influenza virus ribonucleoprotein synthesis. *Antiviral Research*, **5**, 29–37.

Young, J. (2007) Numax Update. IX International Symposium on Respiratory Viral Infections, Hong Kong.

Zambon, M. and Hayden, F.G., Global Neuraminidase Inhibitor Susceptibility, N. (2001) Position statement: global neuraminidase inhibitor susceptibility network. *Antiviral Research*, **49**, 147–156.

Index

Pulmonary Infection in the Immunocompromised Patient, Edited by Carlos Agustí and Antoni Torres
© 2009 John Wiley & Sons, Ltd.

Index compiled by Alison Waggitt

3   WF 140
agu